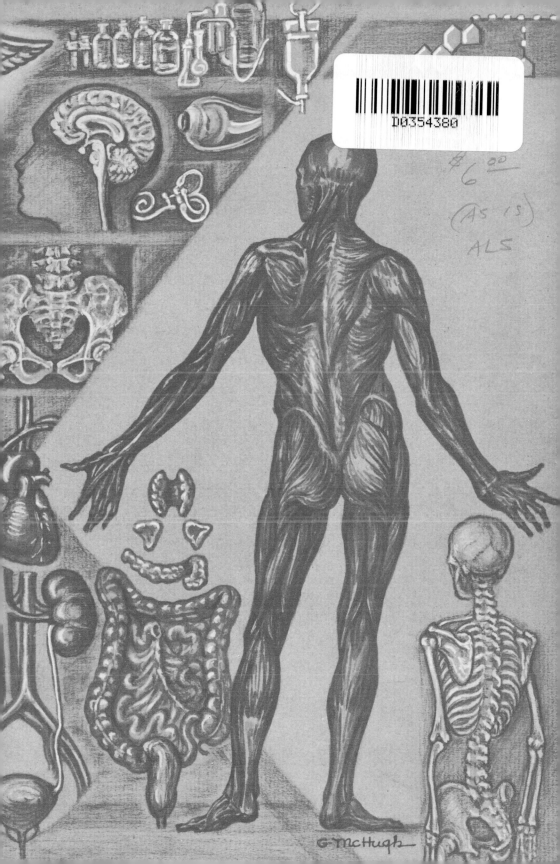

$6⁰⁰

(AS IS)

ALS

G. McHugh

A MODERN MEDICAL AND HEALTH LIBRARY
FOR THE FAMILY . . . INCLUDES ALL THE
CONTENTS OF "THE MODERN HOME
MEDICAL ADVISOR" AND "THE POP-
ULAR MEDICAL ENCYCLOPEDIA"
PLUS ADDITIONAL ARTICLES,
PHOTOGRAPHS AND CHARTS.

ILLUSTRATED

MEDICAL

AND

HEALTH

ENCYCLOPEDIA

VOLUME 5
HAIR (continued) — LOP EARS

ILLUSTRATED

MEDICAL

AND

HEALTH

ENCYCLOPEDIA

EDITED BY

MORRIS FISHBEIN, M.D.

EDITOR, MEDICAL PROGRESS; EDITOR, MODERN HOME MEDICAL
ADVISER; MEDICAL EDITOR, BRITANNICA BOOK OF THE YEAR;
CONTRIBUTING-EDITOR, POST GRADUATE MEDICINE; AND
FOR 25 YEARS EDITOR OF THE JOURNAL OF
THE AMERICAN MEDICAL ASSOCIATION

WITH THE COLLABORATION OF LEADING
SPECIALISTS IN MEDICINE AND SURGERY

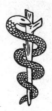

H. S. STUTTMAN CO., *Publishers*
NEW YORK, N. Y.

ILLUSTRATED MEDICAL AND HEALTH ENCYCLOPEDIA
contains new entries and illustrations plus material from
THE MODERN HOME MEDICAL ADVISOR. (Copyright © 1935, 1939, 1940,
1941, 1942, 1948, 1951, 1953, 1956, by Doubleday and Company, Inc.)
and THE POPULAR MEDICAL ENCYCLOPEDIA, revised and
enlarged edition, (Copyright © 1946, 1950, 1953, 1956)
Doubleday and Company, Inc.

PRINTED IN THE UNITED STATES OF AMERICA
BY ROTARY GRAPHIC PRESS INC., NEW YORK 16, N. Y.

INFECTIONS OF THE SCALP

The same bacterial infections that involve the skin may also appear on the scalp. Impetigo, boils, and carbuncles occasionally occur in the scalp and are similar in appearance to the condition when it involves the skin. In impetigo the scalp shows typical honey-colored crusts scattered throughout the hair, often in children having head lice. Boils start as an infection in the hair follicle, with swelling and discharge of pus. In neglected cases they may spread throughout the entire scalp. This is especially true when the boil starts in the back of the neck, and rubbing and friction from the collar cause it to spread. These conditions all respond promptly to local measures with wet dressings, antiseptics, and antibiotics, such as penicillin, terramycin, aureomycin, and chloromycetin. It is of the utmost importance to exercise proper local hygiene if a recurrence is to be prevented. Such measures include frequent washing and shampooing of the scalp and adjoining skin, the wearing of clean, soft collars, and a proper diet, including the avoidance of excessive sweets, starches, fatty and greasy foods.

Ringworm of the scalp is a far more serious condition and is due to the attack of the hair and scalp by a fungus. This organism primarily occurs in children before the age of puberty. It is characterized by the appearance of scaly, bald patches, sometimes covered with brittle and broken hair stubs, and in certain cases with small pustules. Any bald patch in a child's scalp should be considered as a possible ringworm infection until the doctor rubs it out. The disease is highly communicable and may be spread from animals to humans, or, depending upon the type of ringworm, from children to other children. In the epidemic that occurred during the last war it was found that the backs of theater seats and barber shops were often a source of contagion. Insist that your barber clean his instruments before cutting your child's hair, and you may save yourself a serious problem. Also, if your youngster loves to go to the movies and rest his head on the back of the seat, tell him to put his handkerchief on the seat or bring along a little paper towel that he can put on the seat before sitting back and relaxing.

The most common type of ringworm of the scalp is a so-called "gray patch" or human type. In this variety the diseased area is usually round and bald except for a few hairs which have been broken off above the surface of the scalp. It may be impossible to see any bald areas in the scalp, the only sign of infection being the presence of a few scaly or crusted scabs in the scalp. In these instances a doctor should be consulted so that the child can be examined under a special light known as a Wood's filter. Under this very helpful light, the infected areas show up as bright green fluorescent hairs which are immediately both typical and diagnostic. This little gadget has been of great help in screening the scalps of hundreds of school children and in preventing the spread of epidemics of the disease. It is also of value in diagnosing other forms of ringworm, although certain unusual types of the disease do not cause the hair to fluoresce under the light.

The second type of ringworm most commonly encountered is that which is transmitted not only from child to child, but by domestic animals such as dogs or cats. It differs from the simple gray patch type of ringworm because there is a certain amount of inflammation and pus formation present. These are the two most common types of ringworm, although there are many other less common forms observed in different parts of the world. The doctor has a rule that any child showing scaly or bald patches on the scalp must be considered as having a ringworm infection until the Wood's filter and the examination of the hair shows it to be otherwise. In addition to the Wood's light as a means of diagnosis, it is also of importance to the doctor to examine the hairs directly under the microscope and, in suspicious cases, to attempt to grow the organism from the hair by planting the hair in some type of culture medium.

The treatment of ringworm of the scalp depends upon the type of fungus producing the disease. When the organism is of the so-called animal type, which results in infection of the scalp, the use of local remedies such as sulfur, ammoniated mercury, and some of the newer chemicals, combined with frequent shampooing, is usually effective. The reason for this is that the infection around the hair loosens the hair and causes it to be shed from the surface of the scalp. Unfortunately, in the other types of ringworm, where no infection is present, the infected hair is held tightly in the scalp and any attempts to pull it out only result in breaking the hair and the continuance of the infection in the hair under the surface of the scalp. Where this type of infection fails to respond to local measures after a suitable period of time, it is often necessary to treat it by means of X-ray therapy. The X-rays are usually administered at a single session and in a dose sufficient to cause complete falling out of the hair within a few weeks. This procedure requires great training and technical skill on the part of the doctor, and should only be administered by an expert. After the hair has fallen out, regrowth begins after several weeks and the new hairs show no signs of the infection where the X-ray treatment has been properly performed.

HEAD LICE

The head is frequently infected in young children by the head louse referred to medically as pediculosis capitis. The head louse is a small animal approximately 2 mm. long, of a gray color and with black spots around the margins of its body. It inhabits the scalp, especially in children of both sexes and of questionable cleanliness. These lice set up severe itching of the scalp, due to the fact that they feed on and bite the scalp surface. As a result of itching, the child scratches the scalp and often produces a secondary infection. This infection may be so severe that the occasional child develops large glands of the neck due to drainage from the infected areas. Where the social environment is one of absolute neglect, an occasional child may be found to have the head covered with a hairy mess teeming with lice and covered with hundreds of eggs (nits). This combination, plus secondary infection and crusts, leads to a nauseating odor and the accumulation of pus and infected debris on the scalp. Fortunately, these conditions are rare at the present time, although an occasional refugee or neglected child may be seen with such an extreme degree of lousiness. The eggs look like tiny white or grayish grains stuck to the hairs, near the surface of the scalp. In many instances the duration of the infection can be determined by the distance from the egg to the hair shaft, inasmuch as the egg is deposited at the scalp margin and grows out with the hair shaft. In other words, if the egg is approximately one inch from the scalp, the infection would be approximately one month old, inasmuch as hair grows at the rate of approximately one-half inch every two weeks.

There are many local remedies which bring about a speedy and rapid cure of pediculosis capitis. First, it is necessary to remove all sources of the infection and to observe the normal rules of cleanliness if a recurrence is to be prevented. This means that hats, combs, and brushes which have been recently in contact with the scalp should be cleaned very thoroughly or thrown out. The present methods of treatment include the use of DDT in various powders or ointment forms, as well as other newer killers of animal parasites, including benzyl benzoate, Eurax, and Gamergent.

It is also of importance to loosen the eggs with scalp rinses of vinegar or similar substances, and then slide the eggs off the hair shaft with tweezers.

ALOPECIA AREATA

Alopecia areata is a fairly common disease of the hair, occurring more often in children than in adults but not uncommonly in the latter. Often without warning, a bunch of hair may be found upon the pillow in the morning, or a small completely bald patch suddenly noticed in the scalp. There may be only one small spot, but frequently others appear and join to form large, queerly shaped areas. In rare cases this hair loss progresses until all the hair upon the body has disappeared. Such cases are difficult to cure, but to the ordinary case with a limited amount of baldness of the scalp a much more cheerful outlook can be given, for they usually clear up after some months of treatment. In the bald patches the hair may grow in blond at first, even in dark-haired persons; but this usually changes to the normal color later. In those of middle age the hair may come in white and remain so. The afflicted one need not be frightened if the first growth of hair falls out, for continuation of treatment is usually successful in causing a permanent growth. The cause of the disease is not known, but bears a definite relationship to various psychosomatic factors. Within the past year resistant cases of this disease have been successfully treated with cortisone, but this treatment is still in an experimental stage and must be carefully supervised. It is most effective in recent rather than in old cases of alopecia areata. A more permanent cure depends upon a thorough understanding of the physical and mental causes cf the disease.

SUPERFLUOUS HAIR

Undesired hair on a lady's face is a greater trial even than the lack of it upon the head of her husband. This common form of irregular hair distribution often begins in early adult life and causes great mental distress. The mild form appears as lengthening and darkening of the ends of the mustache or groups of long hairs on the sides of the chin; but in severe cases the beard is complete and fairly thick. Efforts to relieve this condition have been made since time immemorial, and the old methods are still in use: the razor, the depilatory, and the resin-wax method. Shaving and the use of an epilating paste are alike in removing only that portion of the hair which projects from the follicle. After their use the hair grows out stiff. The resin-wax method pulls out the whole hair, and it grows again only after a considerable time and then as a young hair, pointed at the end.

When X-rays were first studied, it was thought that they might be the long-desired means of wholesale removal of hair; but it was soon found that it could not be done by this method without great danger of injury to the skin. That such injury might not make itself known for months or years after the treatment did not make it any less serious. All reputable dermatologists have agreed that this method is unsafe. Only the electric needle is left to give lasting relief to the sufferers from this deformity. It is slow and tedious; but safe, certain, and not very painful.

If fine hairs become dark-colored, they can be made less conspicuous by bleaching with peroxide solution, to four parts of which one part of ammonia water is added just before applying it on a cotton pledget. This should not be used often enough to irritate the skin.

THE NAILS

The nails are horny plates designed for protection of the ends of the fingers and toes and also for weapons of defense and offense. These latter uses have to some extent gone out of style, although some women are unaware of that fact. These plates are produced by the epidermal cells much as are the hairs. Normally they are smooth, curved from side to side, and very slightly curved in the long axis. At the base is a light-colored oval area where the active growth of the nail is going on, and over it, next the fold of skin under which the nail grows, is a special membrane, popularly referred to as the "cuticle." As the nail grows, the free end wears off in those doing rough work, or in those who have itching skin disease and keep their nails worn short and highly polished from constant scratching. Nervous individuals often keep their nails short by biting. When protected from friction and injury, the nail may grow several inches long, a good sign of inactivity and the so-called "leisure class."

HYGIENE OF THE NAILS

They should be kept cut fairly short. Fashion decrees at times that they should be trimmed so that they are pointed. This does them no harm. Neither does the polishing, if it is done in a way to avoid infection, nor the various colored nail polishes in popular vogue. Careful pushing back of the cuticle is also harmless if gently done with a smooth, clean instrument, preferably of wood. The manicurist should have some knowledge of cleanliness and should sterilize her instruments by boiling after each use. The polishing pad has gone out of style, and the present-day use of a liquid polish is much more sanitary. After trimming off hangnails, the little tags of skin that become loosened along the sides of the nails, the spot should be touched with an antiseptic. Do not bite or pick hangnails, for these methods favor infection, especially an infected swelling called paronychia or "run-around." Cleansing of the nails should be done after thorough washing, that the dirt under the free edge may be well loosened. A sharp instrument should not be used for this, because it will roughen the inner side of the free portion, dirt will adhere more tightly, and more scraping will be necessary to dislodge it. If the skin of the hands is dry, the nail folds should receive special attention in applying cold cream, for deformities of the nail may result from lack of oil. Dry and brittle nails are common complaints. The causes of nails of this type are not completely known, although in specific instances the reasons are definite. For example, a certain type of nail polish was only applied to the nails after a so-called "base-coat" had been applied first. Many women were allergic to this particular base-coat and their nails became dry, brittle, and deformed. In some cases the reaction was so severe that they lost their nails. Fortunately, the cause was detected and the base-coat taken off the market. In other instances dry and brittle nails may be due to a vitamin deficiency (especially vitamin A), a mineral deficiency (especially calcium), a protein deficiency (especially cystine), or a glandular deficiency (especially thyroid). Don't attempt to be your own doctor, but get professional advice if you are worried about your nail condition. It may be as simple as stopping your nail polish or avoiding soap and water to the best of your ability!

Transverse grooves appear in the nails commonly after illness, sometimes after so trivial a disorder as seasickness, and gradually disappear by growing out to the free end. Any disturbance to the nutrition of the nail may cause this deformity. Even overenthusiastic care of the nails—such as pushing down the cuticle too roughly, cutting it, or injuries received in other ways—may lead to nail deformities. The same is true of other deformities of the nails—longitudinal ridges, pitting, splitting—and often it is impossible to find the cause of these irregularities of growth because they are so slight that the nail changes are the only evidence. Loosening of the nails at the sides may occur in the absence of any other sign of disease; but is usually only temporary. Spoon-shaped nails and other abnormal changes may be hereditary, with accompanying hair and tooth deficiencies, or may result from malnutrition or anemia.

White spots on the nails, "gift spots," may be caused by general disease or local injury. They are the result of imperfect formation of the horny plate as the nail grows and usually disappear in time.

Thickening of the nails may be caused by nutritional disorder, skin disease, or more frequently by ringworm infection of the nail. It occurs most often on the nail of the big toe, and if not due to infection may be kept in check by paring and scraping. Ringworm of the nails is important because, owing to the fact that it is unobtrusive in its manifestations, it is often not noticed, and if treated is very difficult to cure. Therefore, it is likely to remain as a focus of the disease from which infection is spread to other parts. The most successful treatment entails weekly removal of the nail surface by means of an electric drill and the subsequent painting with a fungus-killing chemical such as ammoniacal silver nitrate. These severe nail changes are not hopeless, but take time and skill if a cure is to be obtained.

Ingrowing toenails are caused by improper nail cutting, tight shoes, or local injury. They can be cured, before they become severely inflamed, by carefully cutting out the ingrowing part at the sides of the free border of the nail and preventing regrowth in this direction by padding with wool. This procedure should be performed with the utmost attention to cleanliness in order to minimize infection. Once infection has occurred, wet dressings and some of the newer antiseptics result in rapid cure under medical supervision.

HALITOSIS Most doctors are convinced that a bad odor of the breath arises principally from the mouth, teeth, and throat and is usually due to either decay of the teeth or infection of the tissues.

The word "halitosis," a scientific term for bad breath, was popularized through the promotion of a mouth wash. No mouth wash known has the power to prevent a bad odor arising from a decayed tooth or from an infection. All that it can do is temporarily wash away the infectious material. Only scientific treatment with removal of the source of the infection or decay can prevent the odor permanently.

Decay of the teeth can be determined only by regular dental inspection. Cleanliness of the teeth is controlled only by proper use of the toothbrush and associated therewith such a toothpaste, tooth powder, or solution, as preferred by the individual.

Occasionally an odor comes from an infection in the tonsils. The little crypts or pockets in the tonsils become filled with infectious material, even with decaying particles of food. This material will give off a bad odor with each breath. The physician may squeeze out these crypts and cleanse the surfaces that are left with antiseptic solutions. Gargles occasionally will wash off the surfaces, but few people can get a gargle down to the points that are involved. If the tonsils are seriously infected and if there is an unpleasant odor from an infected throat, surgical removal of the tonsils is necessary to produce a cure.

Infections in the nose with crusting may be associated with a foul breath. The diagnosis and treatment of such a condition is a problem for the specialist. Washing the nose and the cavity behind the nose is a procedure for which special training is required.

Occasionally the lungs or the stomach develop materials which give a bad odor to the breath. Garlic can be eliminated from the blood through the lungs and thus contaminate the breath. In one experiment people swallowed raw chopped garlic in double gelatin capsules, so that none of the garlic could possibly come in contact with the mouth or the teeth. The odor of garlic appeared on the breath just as soon as it was released in the stomach and continued even when the garlic had passed from the stomach into the intestines.

The only way to overcome such an odor is to use flavored oils, which will cover it up with a nice odor. Some mouth washes accomplish this result by substituting for the odor that is to be removed the odor of the mouth wash. Masking of an odor is not in any sense a cure for halitosis.

Recently, preparations of chlorophyll have been urged as efficient in halitosis. The evidence is not good and there is proof that chlorophyll will not prevent mouth odors.

HALITOSIS—See TEETH, article THE CARE OF THE TEETH.

HARDENING OF THE ARTERIES
(See also discussion under *Arteriosclerosis, Blood Pressure, High, Senescence*)

Extensive research has indicated a definite relationship between hardening of the arteries and diets high in fat and high in cholesterol. Apparently cholesterol plays a part in the development of this condition. The cholesterol found in blood is obtained by the body from the diet or it forms from a body chemical called acetate that is a precursor of cholesterol. In the Sloan-Kettering Institute, cholesterol and acetate were tagged with radioactive isotopes and their courses through the body were followed. Apparently, the body has a balancing mechanism for keeping the supply of cholesterol at a normal level. If the diet does not furnish the amount of cholesterol that the body requires, the body manufacturers from acetate enough cholesterol to take care of the deficit. When the cholesterol in the diet exceeds the normal need the body manufactures less cholesterol. Investigations have shown also a relationship between the activity of the sex glands with their hormones and the amount of cholesterol. Derangements in the manufacture of sex hormones by the body may create a cholesterol imbalance that the body does not control and the ultimate effect of this may be hardening of the arteries.

In the biological laboratories of the University of Chicago, investigators determined that feeding of an extract of ground up cattle brain to chickens caused a reduction of cholesterol in their blood. They conceived that this might be a preventive of hardening of the arteries. Even when chickens were fed diets rich in cholesterol the brain extract was able to prevent a rise in the amount of cholesterol in the blood. This effect could be sustained for five weeks. Tests are being made with extracts from sheep and lamb brain. Tests made on humans have heretofore been inconclusive. Conceivably, however, some substance derived from the brain may eventually become the basis of a new drug to be given to persons with hardening of the arteries.

HARELIP   See *Cleft Palate* and *Lips*.

HAY FEVER Hay fever, caused by the giant ragweed, is also called ragweed fever and autumnal catarrh. Seldom is scientific advice needed nowadays to make the diagnosis; the sneezing, watering of the eyes, running of the nose, itching of the nose, throat, and palate that come on coincident with the development of the ragweed pollen have been widely recognized. Oc-

casionally, however, there are still people who feel that the early symptoms of hay fever represent a common cold. Anyone who has these attacks regularly will do well to be tested for sensitivity to make certain that the condition is really hay fever and not some other chronic disturbance.

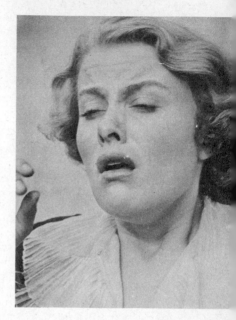

Hay fever victim experiencing a spasm of sneezing. During a hay fever attack the nose burns, is itchy and congested. When the mucous membrane of the nose becomes swollen the passages are obstructed and the person is forced to breathe through the mouth. This aggravates the condition further because greater amounts of pollen are taken in which come in direct contact with the pharynx.

Hygeia

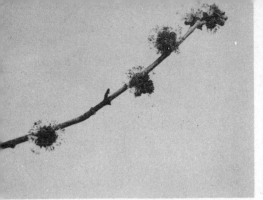

MAPLE

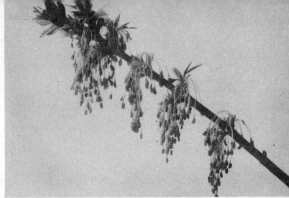

BOX ELDER

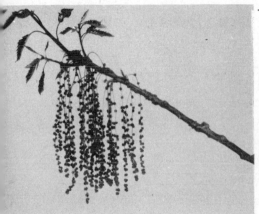

OAK

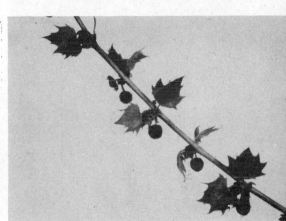

SYCAMORE

Varieties of weeds and trees which cause hay fever. Weeds produce pollen from late August to October. Tree pollen which causes hay fever is prevalent during April and May. There is more pollen in the air in the early part of the day and allergic persons tend to suffer more at that time. American Medical Association

COTTONWOOD

PIGWEED

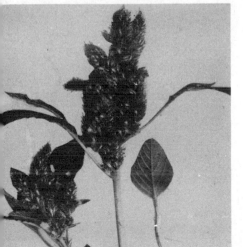

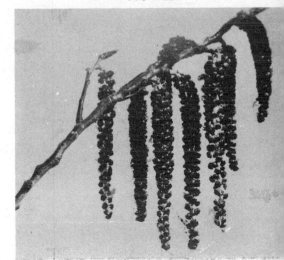

We endeavor now to prevent hay fever rather than to treat it. Some people can go away from home to areas in which the pollens to which they are sensitive are infrequent. For those who stay at home all sorts of protective glasses for the eyes, filters for the nose, and nose masks have been advised. However, the best preventive is a modern air filtration machine which conditions the room in which the patient works or sleeps.

Good general advice for the hay-fever sufferer is to keep out of drafts, avoid automobile trips in the country, stay on the fairway instead of in the rough while golfing, thus avoiding possible contact with the ragweed pollens.

Each section of the United States contains about thirty pollens which are important causes of hay fever. It therefore becomes possible for a physician to test the patient for his sensitivity to these pollens. After having determined the particular pollens to which the patient is sensitive, it is then possible to attempt desensitization. It is unwise for the person with hay fever to wait until the attack begins before he is desensitized. Much better is regular treatment each year with desensitization at regular intervals, so that the patient is protected against the sensitivity up to the time when the pollens begin to fill the air.

There are many methods of treatment by which the person with hay

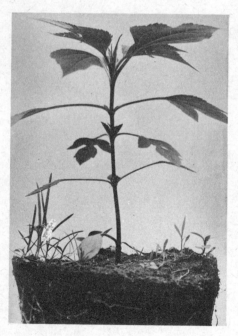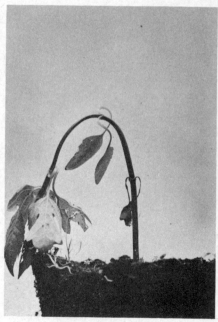

This is ragweed, at left in its healthy, unmolested state, and at right a little while after it has been sprayed with a special poison. The spraying must be done before the plant goes to seed and the pollen starts flying.

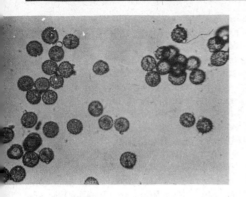

Microscopic appearance of ragweed pollen granules which cause hay fever.

fever may be made more comfortable. Some of the remedies sold in drugstores are of this type. They do not cure hay fever; they merely help to relieve the worst of the symptoms. However, the physician can prescribe or apply remedies which cannot be sold in the form of ready-made drugs and which are known to be much more effective than the type of remedy that is sold without any control.

Such remedies as adrenalin and ephedrine and some of the treatments that are derived from narcotic drugs are immensely important in controlling symptoms but, obviously, cannot be sold or applied without suitable control.

HEADACHE At least one half of all the people who come into the doctor's office complain that they have headaches. The men who have charge of the employees in our large industries say that about one fourth of all of the absences of employees are credited to headaches. Thus this symptom—because headache is not truly a disease—is responsible for much human disability.

Headaches are due to a great variety of causes—indeed a variety so great that the determination of the single cause or multiple causes of any one headache may require the highest art and technic of the doctor. Innumerable classifications have been developed so as to group the causes in various ways and thus to guide the technic of study. One of the simplest methods groups some 203 different causes under three classifications—mechanical, toxic, and functional. Thus the mechanical headaches would be those associated with conditions related to the head itself. For instance, when the sinuses become blocked, changes in pressure will produce headache. When the membranes of the nose swell, this in turn blocks the sinuses and produces headache. When the frontal sinus is involved, the headache is likely to be worse in the morning and to improve during the day as the sinus drains.

The brain lies in a fluid known as the cerebrospinal fluid, which in turn is enclosed in the membranes that cover the brain. These membranes are sensitive to stretching. Anything that causes

the head up and down or against the sides of the crib. In many instances actual bruises result from this action. Some infants will roll the head so hard and so persistently that they will rub the hair away from the back of the head. Sometimes the child will keep up this banging for two or three hours at a time.

Children tend to imitate each other, so that the head rolling and banging will spread through a hospital ward or a dormitory. Seldom does it continue after the fourth year, although a child who has once rolled the head or banged it about may during semisleeping states or in sleep again reproduce this habit.

Parents are likely to become greatly frightened by head rolling or head banging, but they need not be alarmed because rarely indeed is it associated with any organic disease of the brain or any other portion of the body. Some parents are likely to be especially disturbed for fear that it represents a vicious habit or some mental or emotional disturbance. Actually it seems to be a fundamental reaction related to the child's craving for rhythmical activities. Many psychologists are inclined to believe that it is in some way a pleasure-seeking device. One physician felt that it represents a response to some obstruction to breathing, as might be caused by adenoids, and that the rolling of the head is an attempt to obtain relief. When the adenoids are removed, the symptoms clear up, but the rolling and banging of the head, he says, may continue if there is chronic congestion of the nose. Certainly it is worth while to remove enlarged or inflamed adenoids, but there is no certainty that the condition is really related to head rolling or head banging. It has been found that the use of sedatives which cause the child to sleep more deeply will stop the head rolling and head banging.

One observer thought that head rolling was due to the fact that children had been rocked to sleep in an old-fashioned rocking chair or in a crib and that later, when they were put to sleep in a stationary bed, they missed the rocking and therefore rocked themselves. Conceivably the escape from emotional tension brought about by rolling and rocking, that the child may have secured when being artificially rocked, is automatically reproduced when the artificial rocking is discontinued.

Children develop strange habits, many of which are exceedingly difficult to explain by any simple mechanism. Fortunately head rolling and head banging so certainly disappear in the vast majority of cases, as the child gets older, that the matter need not give too great concern to the parent.

HEARING, HARDNESS OF See *Deafness* and *Otosclerosis*.

HEART The heart is essentially a pump that circulates the blood through the body. At birth the heart weighs less than an ounce. In a grown person, if the heart is normal, it weighs about a half pound and is somewhat larger than a fist.

At birth the heart beats about 130 times a minute; at six years it beats 100 times a minute; at ten years about 90, and at fifteen years about 85. Among grownups rates of anywhere from 65 to 80 per minute may well be within the normal. During a lifetime the heart beats 2,500,000,000 times and pumps a total of nearly 15,000,000 gallons.

The heart is a large muscular organ about the size of a fist. You can feel its beat on the left side of your body. The apex, or lower point of the heart is what you feel. The broad side of the heart at the top is where the *coronary arteries* enter the muscle to provide the necessary oxygen for nourishment of the tissue. The arteries are branches of the *aorta,* the largest blood vessel of the body, which leaves the right side of the heart carrying the blood that has been brought back through the veins and passed through the lungs to accumulate more oxygen. The word coronary comes from a Latin word meaning crown. When a coronary blood vessel is blocked by a blood clot, which may originate there, the condition is called *coronary*

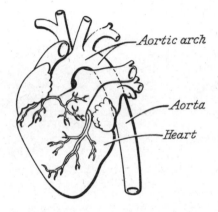

—Aortic arch

—Aorta

—Heart

The aorta is the large blood vessel that carries the arterial blood from the left ventricle of the heart. From the aorta come all the arteries that carry blood to various portions of the body.

thrombosis. A clot of blood or any other foreign material floating in the blood stream is called an *"embolus."* When one of these blocks a coronary blood vessel the condition is called *"embolism."* When a portion of the heart muscle fails to receive blood or oxygen it cannot contract. Then it degenerates. The area is called an *infarct.* A coronary artery can become hardened—*arteriosclerosis*—and such a hardened area blocks more easily. Since the blood vessel walls have

contractile tissue they may narrow or contract with spasm and this lessens blood flow. The result is pain. Any or all of this is called *coronary disease.* A pain in the heart is *angina; angina pectoris* is a pain in the chest, usually resulting from the heart. People with hardened coronary arteries, not functioning normally, do not get enough blood into the muscle of the heart. When they make an effort or put increased strain on the heart it responds with pain. If they stop and rest the pain is likely to go away.

The word for heart is *cardia.* Inflammation of the heart is *carditis.* Inflammation of the inner lining is *endocarditis;* inflammation of the muscle is *myocarditis;* inflammation of the membrane or sac around the heart is *pericarditis.* Such inflammation may result from infection with germs or viruses. If infection is by germ, most often the streptococci a disease results called *subacute bacterial endocarditis* which used to be almost 100% fatal but now yields in many instances to antibiotics like penicillin.

The heart has valves which lie between its various chambers such as the auricles on the left side and the ventricles on the right side. These valves may be damaged by infections or by changes in the muscles of the heart. They may be narrowed, called *"stenosis"* or *"dilated."* If a valve is narrowed not enough blood gets through during heart action. If it is dilated the blood going through may leak back. This is called *"regurgitation."* The valves are *mitral, aortic, tricuspid* and *pulmonic.* Thus there may be mitral stenosis or mitral regurgitation, or similarly for the other valves. When this occurs the sounds that the doctor hears with a stethoscope change; these sounds are called *murmurs.* From the sounds the doctor can tell whether these valves are opening and closing as they should. If the heart

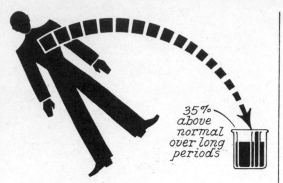

35% above normal over long periods

HEART FAILURE

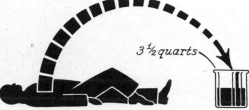

3½ quarts of blood each minute through the arteries

3½ quarts

EMOTIONALLY CALM MAN

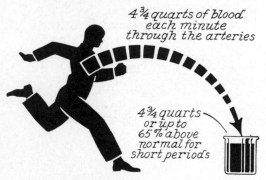

4¾ quarts of blood each minute through the arteries

4¾ quarts or up to 65% above normal for short periods

AFTER EXERCISE, SUCH AS RUNNING

Indication of manner in which extra work is thrown on the heart by exercise, forcing unusual amount of blood through the heart and giving the heart increased work.

muscle enlarges because of increased work the resulting condition is called *hypertrophy.*

One type of inflammation of the heart associated with infection is *rheumatic fever.* Just why infections of the throat of some children result in damage to the heart by the inflammation and degeneration that occurs is not known. Many believe these children are by nature especially susceptible.

When a heart cannot do its work or fails the condition is called *heart failure.* In such cases the blood does not go around the body as it should and fluid collects in the tissues particularly of the limbs. This is called *edema.* Fluid collecting in the abdomen is *ascites,* also called *dropsy.* If the heart recovers sufficiently to do its work the condition is said to be *compensated.*

A *heart attack* is a term used by people generally to mean some condition that affects the heart that causes the person concerned to suffer pain and often to faint or collapse.

Sometimes nervous people think the heart is fluttering or beating irregularly. The sensation is called *palpitation.* Sometimes murmurs are heard by the doctor which do not really mean anything is wrong. These are called *functional murmurs.* Occasionally the automatic nervous mechanism which controls the action of the heart is disordered. Then the muscle may not work rhythmically and efficiently but twitch irregularly. This is *fibrillation,* either auricularl or ventricular.

The impulse which causes the heart to contract develops in some nerve tissue which is called the pacemaker of the heart. An attempt to measure this impulse indicates that its energy is the equivalent of one thousandth of a volt.

The blood comes into the heart after having been collected from the veins of the body and passed through the lungs, where new oxygen is taken up.

When the heart muscle contracts, the blood is forced out of the heart and then goes by way of the large arteries and blood vessels to the farthest extremes of the body.

The heart moves a total of 500 gallons of blood a day. Since there are about 6 quarts of blood in the whole body, the heart moves the same fluid, slightly modified chemically as it travels about, over and over again.

The heart never gets a complete rest until we die; then of course the rest is too late. It begins working before the child is born and is never quiet until death. The only rest it gets is when its beat is slowed a little or decreased somewhat in its force.

The heart is one of the involuntary muscles of the body. A few instances are recorded in medicine in which people have been able voluntarily to control their heartbeat. Most people, perhaps fortunately for them, do not have this power. If they did, they might want to try it once too often.

NATURE PROTECTS THE HEART—The vital organ must, therefore, be protected in every way possible against overstrain and damage. By its situation in the body the heart is reasonably well protected against most ordinary dangers. The heart lies just below and to the left of the lower two thirds of the chest bone. Its shape is like that of a large pear with the broad end upward and under the chest bone, and the pointed end downward and to the left. If you put your finger in the space just below the fifth rib and slightly to the left of the breastbone, you can feel the impulse of the heartbeats.

The heart lies inside a sac which is called the pericardium. This serves to separate the heart from the other organs in the chest and to hold it in position. Sometimes the strain and pressure on the heart may be so great that it would swell like a balloon if it did not have this sac around it to keep it from stretching too far. The outside of the heart, too, is enclosed in a membranous sac. A thin layer of fluid keeps these two layers of tissue from being rubbed together when the heart beats.

The heart is a muscle. This muscle is called the myocardium. The interior of the heart is lined with another membrane which is called the endocardium.

CORONARY ARTERIES—The heart gets its own nourishment from small blood vessels which pass into the muscle tissue from the large blood vessels that carry the blood away from the heart. These small blood vessels which nourish the heart itself are known as the coronary arteries. Remember this name. Today trouble with these coronary arteries is responsible for a good many cases of sudden death in people past middle age.

All of the openings leading into the heart and passing out of it are controlled by valves which open and shut as the blood comes in and passes out. There are similar valves governing the passing of the blood from one portion of the heart into another.

HEART FAILURE—Heart disease and failure of the heart to carry on its work are among the commonest and most serious conditions that affect human beings. This is particularly the case since man has increased his life expectancy. When human beings died young of infectious diseases, the number of cases of breakdown and degeneration of important organs was not nearly so great as now.

The human body is built ordinarily to run about seventy years. If it is used to excess or if it is attacked by infections or in other ways damaged, it sometimes fails to last that long. Even when the human being lives much longer, however, the tissues begin to break down somewhat past middle life and, having broken down, fail in their capacity to carry on their functions.

The failure of the heart to do its work is especially serious because the whole body depends on the blood as a means of sustaining its life. When the heart fails to get blood out to the cells, they cannot function satisfactorily. Failure of the heart to do its work may be due to inability of the muscle to pump, failure of the pump to force out a sufficient amount of blood at each beat, or failure of the pump to force the blood all the way around and back again, since the blood must circulate continuously. When the heart is insufficient to force the circulation completely around, there is a tendency for blood to remain in various portions of the body, particularly in the feet; fluid collects in the abdomen, and there occurs finally what is known as congestive heart failure. Sometimes when the heart has become weakened, rest of the patient and aid given to the body by other means of modern medicine will permit the heart to carry on its work satisfactorily. With time, the muscle of the heart may increase in amount, so that the heart, though enlarged, is able to do its work. This is known as compensation.

Some of the ordinary signs of failure of the heart to do its work are shortness of breath, collection of fluid in various portions of the body, and swelling of the tissues. Shortness of breath is particularly a sign of the failure of the heart to push the blood into the large blood vessels. The tendency is, therefore, for the blood to back up, and the first signs of congestion are seen in the lungs, from which the blood comes to the heart. The result is a distressful, rapid, shallow breathing which demands again the most careful consideration by the doctor in order to overcome the disturbance before permanent changes in the structure of the tissues occur. Sometimes

these patients have trouble when they lie down because of the increased amount of fluid that moves promptly into the circulation.

All of the difficulties that have been described are so serious and so definitely progressive unless properly cared for that physicians have never hesitated to advise again and again a regular examination of the human body at least once each year, or, better perhaps, once every six months, after middle age. With such an examination serious breakdowns are detected early, and proper treatment can stop progress in the early stages.

THE PROBLEMS OF HEART DISEASE—Today heart disease is the outstanding cause of death. The attack on heart disease is directed primarily against those forms of infection and overstrain of the human body which primarily affect the heart.

Rheumatic fever is one of the foremost foes of health in children.

The second great problem in heart disease is the deaths of people of advanced years from breakdown of this vital organ. This is associated with the fact that more people are living longer than people used to live. The diseases involving breakdown of the heart, and especially blocking of the coronary arteries, affect men far more than they do women. Certainly this should indicate that many of these deaths may be prevented by taking from the male workers, and particularly people occupying positions of stress and strain, much of the demand that is now placed on them.

The third group of heart conditions to which attention should be given is the group of old people who have gotten so old that their hearts are in constant danger of breakdown. Here the necessity is for additional facilities for examination and diagnosis of such cases, facilities for home care, including

WHAT YOUR HEART DOES

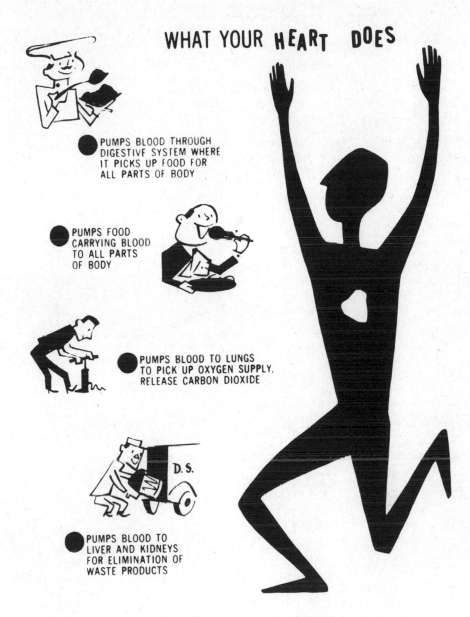

PUMPS BLOOD THROUGH DIGESTIVE SYSTEM WHERE IT PICKS UP FOOD FOR ALL PARTS OF BODY

PUMPS FOOD CARRYING BLOOD TO ALL PARTS OF BODY

PUMPS BLOOD TO LUNGS TO PICK UP OXYGEN SUPPLY. RELEASE CARBON DIOXIDE

D. S.

PUMPS BLOOD TO LIVER AND KIDNEYS FOR ELIMINATION OF WASTE PRODUCTS

- BEATS 100,000 TIMES DAILY
- PRODUCES ENOUGH DAILY ENERGY TO LIFT AN AVERAGE PERSON TO TOP OF EMPIRE STATE BUILDING

Graphics Institute for Eye Magazine

adequate nursing, and, finally, institutions where such people may be given hospital attention.

Primary in the treatment of all types of conditions affecting the heart is the provision of adequate rest. This means not only relaxation, but in many instances long-continued actual rest in bed. The number of beds available in hospitals and institutions in the United States for patients with heart disease is far below the number actually required. This applies to beds in hospitals for all types of convalescents from disease and for all types of chronic disease.

RHEUMATIC FEVER (See also *Rheumatic Fever*)—Today rheumatic fever is among the foremost health problems of youth. Most of the cases occur in the months from March to June, with the smallest number of cases in the months from August up to December.

In most instances the condition appears following infections of the nose and throat. It may also, however, be associated with an infection of the ear, with scarlet fever, St. Vitus' dance, or other similar conditions. In at least one fifth of all the cases of rheumatic fever the most serious associated condition is the attack on the heart.

The child who is likely to have rheumatic fever is one who has frequent illnesses, especially sore throat, tonsillitis, and infections of the nose and throat. Such children seldom gain weight as they should, they become easily tired, and frequently they have deficiencies in the blood. Whenever there are frequent fevers of unknown cause, with fleeting pains in the joints, special attention should be given to the possibility that the child is getting rheumatic fever. The so-called growing pains so commonly talked about in a previous generation are now recognized to be, in the vast majority of cases, early attacks of this disease.

Rheumatic fever is dangerous because it comes on insidiously. Often the family does not suspect that the child is ill until so much damage has already been done to the heart that recovery is impossible. A child acutely ill with rheumatic fever will have a high fever, a rapid heart, difficulty in breathing, drowsiness, weakness, profuse perspiration, and prostration.

Sometimes the joint involvement is serious; other times it is absent. The joints when involved are swollen, red, and tender. Sometimes a child who seems to be recovering from the disease suddenly seems to be reinfected with an acute period as bad as or worse than the initial attack.

Most difficult are the smoldering forms of the disease in which the child never seems to be seriously sick but at the same time is constantly suffering from an infected heart. Such children may appear fretful and indisposed with poor appetite and restless sleep. A careful examination may show, however, that the heart is already subject to murmurs and difficulty in its functions.

Some years ago it was discovered that a sudden and severe abdominal pain might be the only sign of an acutely inflamed heart. Such cases have been mistaken for appendicitis. In the absence of the other positive signs of appendicitis, the doctor nowadays always suspects the possibility of rheumatic fever.

Seven years of age is the time when most children are attacked but many are attacked even as early as five years of age. Since children of school age are the ones chiefly affected, many communities have been trying to develop suitable plans to meet the situation.

In New York City classes for children with heart disease have been developed in the public schools. Such children have to be continuously under medical supervision. Moreover, their instruction

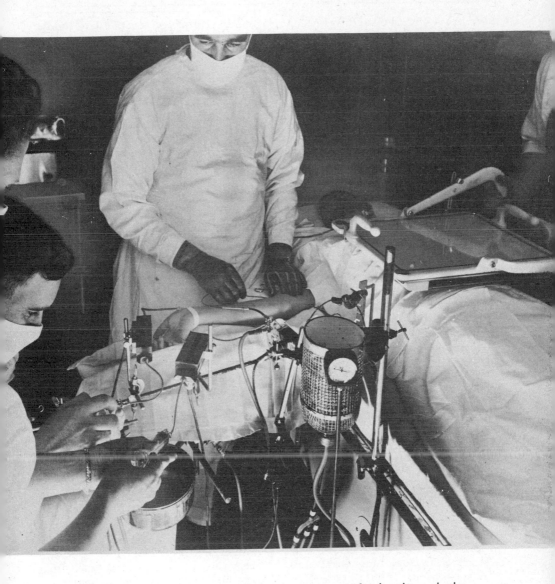

The physician is inserting a slender, wet-proof tube through the patient's arm vein. The catheter will travel up the arm vein and be directed into the right side of the heart. With the catheter, blood samples can be drawn, and pressures recorded at various sites in the chambers. This procedure is called cardiac catheterization and is used in the diagnosis of congenital heart defects and in research on the heart's action. American Heart Association must be conducted by teachers who have had special interest in heart disease and who know how to watch developments in such patients. In most instances special transportation has to be provided to get the children to schools. There must also be definite rest periods for them in order to relieve them of the possibility of strain.

Prevention of Rheumatic Fever—In the prevention of rheumatic fever, attention must be given to many details which are important for improving general health. The whole life should be quiet and restful. There must be particularly plenty of periods of rest and recreation. If a child becomes fatigued and exhausted, his digestion is interfered with and he becomes easily subject to infection. For children who are exceedingly nervous and who tire easily, a rest period of a half hour before and after meals is useful.

Damp, wet clothing should always be removed from the child when he comes indoors. Research has proved that attacks of rheumatic fever can be prevented by giving sulfadiazine or penicillin at the first indication that a child has a sore throat. This controls the streptococcus.

A new form of penicillin has been found called depot penicillin which when injected will keep up the level of penicillin in the body for a month.

Wholesome Diet—The child requires a diet with plenty of milk, butter, eggs, leafy green vegetables, fruits, cod-liver oil, and other foods. These give adequate amounts of protein, carbohydrate, fat, mineral salts, and vitamins for satisfactory nutrition. If there is a tendency to persistent underweight, if the child eats without appetite, and if his digestion is constantly disturbed, he will become more easily a victim to heart disease.

Particularly important is prompt attention to every cold and sore throat and avoidance of cold and sore throats as far as possible. Children who suffer constantly from sore throats or infections of the nose and sinuses should be carefully watched by a physician and should be given, if possible, the benefit of a warm climate in order to permit opportunity for complete recovery.

There is no certain cure for rheumatic fever, no drug or serum that has specific effect on which dependence may be placed. The child, as has already been said, must be put to bed promptly if this condition occurs. He must be constantly under the care of a doctor who understands heart disease. He should be allowed out of bed only gradually, remaining in bed for at least two weeks or even longer after the fever has completely disappeared.

Many cities now have hospitals and sanitariums specifically designated for care of patients with rheumatic fever. Clinics are being established to provide sulfadiazine or antibiotics to children with possible rheumatic fever and to control relapses.

Convalescence (See also discussion under *Rheumatic Fever*)—The doctor can determine, after the child has recovered, how much damage has been done to the heart. He will have to regulate the amount of exercise and the amount of work that the child may do day by day, in order to see that strain and overwork are not put upon this vital organ. If a heart has been damaged by rheumatic fever, it will not do its duty adequately as a pump. This will be shown by discomfort after exertion, shortness of breath, swelling of the feet, blueness of the complexion, and other symptoms which indicate that the tissues of the body are not receiving adequate amounts of oxygenized blood. Such cases demand constant, careful watching.

ENDOCARDITIS—Among the most fatal of all diseases affecting the heart is bacterial endocarditis. In this condition the germs which have infected the heart will frequently be found circulating in the blood. This form of heart disease is most often seen after the patient has had rheumatic fever or some other form of heart disturbance. If the valves of the heart have been damaged by any previous disease, the bacteria which get into the blood may adhere to the valves of the heart, survive, and grow.

As a result of this infection, blood clots accumulate and form a material in which the germs may grow and multiply with facility. Sometimes this form of infection of the valves of the heart may occur without the germs being found in the blood. But it must be remembered that the streptococcus, which is the germ most frequently responsible, is found in almost all noses and throats throughout life.

The condition has been produced experimentally in animals by injecting the germ into the blood of the animal. The germs settle on the heart valves and begin to destroy the tissue. One of the great difficulties in attacking this disease is the fact that the germs penetrate into the tissues of the heart and into the accumulation of fibrous tissues on the valves of the heart, so that it is difficult for remedies to reach the germs. Several suggestions have been made for the prevention of the formation of these fibrous deposits. One of them was the use of a new substance called heparin, which prevents the formation of clots, with the idea that this substance would loosen the clots. Another substance with similar effects is known as dicumarol. Sulfanilamide, or one of the new derivatives, or penicillin may be given to attack the germs.

The patient who recovers from infection of the heart valves may die subsequently as the result of damage which has been done by this condition to the kidneys, the blood, or the brain. Unfortunately, when clots or fibrous formations occur on the heart valves, they sometimes break off and circulate in the blood, coming eventually to an artery through which they cannot pass, thus blocking that artery. This condition is called an embolism with thrombosis. Should the artery that is blocked be an artery in the brain or one associated with any other vital organ, that in itself may cause death.

CORONARY THROMBOSIS (See also *Angina Pectoris*)—Thrombosis means blocking by a clot of blood. The coronary arteries are the blood vessels which furnish blood to the heart. The term "coronary thrombosis" therefore means blocking of the blood vessels to the heart by a clot of blood.

If the person has been well previously, or if the person has had previous attacks of pain referred to the heart, the diagnosis is usually justified. If the blocking occurs gradually, the symptoms may have developed over a period of weeks.

Far too often the symptoms suggest a disturbance of digestion. There is a sense of fullness in the abdomen relieved by the belching of gas.

There may be nausea and vomiting; discomfort associated with the stomach often follows a meal, and there may be other symptoms of indigestion, so that far too often the condition is passed over with a diagnosis of acute indigestion.

Most people with this disease are past fifty years of age, but occasionally there are cases between forty and fifty.

If the attack takes place gradually, the other blood vessels which supply blood to the heart may take over the function of the one which is blocked. There may be slight changes in the heart with symptoms during this process, but under such circumstances the condition is not necessarily fatal.

In an acute attack of coronary thrombosis there is pain—sudden, severe, and persisting. There is also a feeling of impending death, so that the person becomes pale and is in a cold sweat.

Most often the pain, which is described as deep-seated, cutting, or tearing, is referred to the heart. It may persist for minutes or even hours. As the pain lessens into a dull ache, there is still a feeling of apprehension.

A physician is able to make examinations which will verify the diagnosis. This he does by studying the pulse, the blood pressure, the breathing, and sometimes by using an electrocardiographic device, which gives him an indication of the action of the heart.

There are, however, some cases in which even such methods fail to show definitely the nature of the change. An experienced physician, particularly someone who has studied heart disease, is able to make the diagnosis by the use of observation, by listening to the heart, and by the type of study called physical as contrasted with laboratory diagnosis.

No doubt many patients die almost with the onset of the attack. However, an equal number of patients recover and remain free from attacks for several years or even longer.

Dr. Paul D. White records several instances in which patients have survived seven or eight years or more. Dr. Arthur D. Master found 50 per cent of his patients surviving more than ten years.

One man had his first attack at the age of sixty-three, passed a life-insurance examination two years later, and at the age of seventy-two climbed mountains without symptoms. He died at the age of eighty of brain hemorrhage, without any sign of heart disease except the healed scar in the heart.

The post-mortem examination showed definitely the scar associated with the attack of coronary thrombosis seventeen years previously.

This case serves to illustrate the wonderful recuperative power of the seriously injured heart muscle, and indicates that the occurrence of one attack may not necessarily mean permanent crippling.

The moment an attack of coronary thrombosis occurs, the person affected should be put immediately at complete rest in bed. Then a competent physician will be able to prescribe drugs according to the symptoms, relieving the pain, making sure that the patient stays quiet until the condition of the heart warrants slight exertion, then controlling bodily exertions so that activity is gradually resumed.

Some patients die immediately, regardless of what the physician can do, because the heart is mortally wounded with the first blocking that occurs. Others have such a small area of heart tissue involved that they incline to recover. There is a large group in whom control of the condition and treatment mean the difference between life and death.

Most important of all, however, is the advice to persons past forty-five years of age that what seems to be an attack of acute indigestion should never be disregarded, particularly when the pain is referred largely to the heart.

Most patients who feel the first symptoms of this disease do not feel them-

A mechanical heart being used in substitution of a human heart during surgery. The machine takes over the heart's blood-pumping function so that the surgeon can repair heart defects without the interference of blood in the operative field.

General Motors

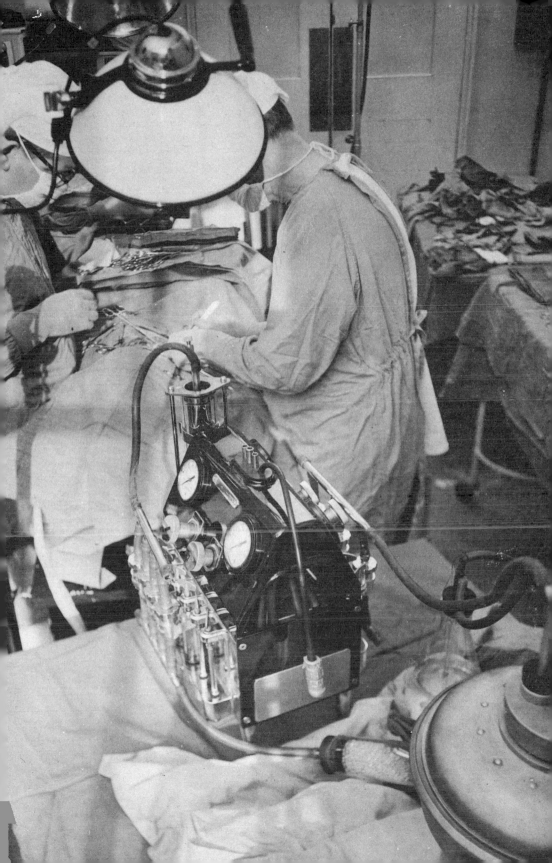

selves sick enough to call a doctor. If they do not recover by good luck, they make their first medical contact with the coroner.

Every means of publicity available ought to be used, even at the risk of creating some unnecessary fears, to teach middle-aged and older people that diagnoses of ptomaine poisoning and acute indigestion are usually serious cases of mistaken identity, and that every case of pleuritic pain and neuritis of the chest, neck, jaw, or arms demands the most prompt and painstaking diagnostic scrutiny possible.

The only advice that can be given for prevention is that best advice of medical science—moderation in all things. The avoidance of overeating and of over-strenuous life are the two main points to be considered.

Here are ten heart commandments which you should keep to prolong your life:

1. Do not subject your heart to sudden, strenuous, or prolonged physical exertion.

2. Eat regularly, slowly, and temperately.

3. If you are excessively overweight, seek sound counsel as to how best to dispense with this form of heart handicap.

4. Try to avoid physical activity for at least thirty minutes after eating, particularly after the heaviest meal of the day.

5. Avoid emotional stress and strain. Worry is an important factor in its relation to heart strain.

6. By appropriate measures, keep your body as free as possible from so-called foci of infection.

7. Regular intestinal elimination is highly important.

8. Average not less than eight hours of sleep in a room abundantly supplied with fresh air.

9. Perennial health demands a proper balance between work, play, and rest.

10. A periodic examination may often reveal defects of which you are totally unaware. A stitch in time saves nine!

CARDITIS—See HEART, article DISEASES OF THE HEART AND CIRCULATION.

CORONARY THROMBOSIS—diabetes: See article DIABETES.

CORONARY THROMBOSIS—hypotension following: See article BLOOD PRESSURE.

CORONARY THROMBOSIS—resulting from hardening of coronary arteries: See article BLOOD PRESSURE.

HEART—anatomy: See HEART, article DISEASES OF THE HEART AND CIRCULATION.

HEART—angina pectoris: See HEART, article DISEASES OF THE HEART AND CIRCULATION. See also entry ANGINA PECTORIS.

HEART—associations: See HEART, article DISEASES OF THE HEART AND CIRCULATION.

HEART—asthenia, neurocirculatory: See HEART, article DISEASES OF THE HEART AND CIRCULATION.

HEART—attack: See references CORONARY THROMBOSIS above.

HEART—attack mistaken for acute indigestion: See article DIGESTION AND DIGESTIVE DISEASES.

HEART—auricle: See HEART, article DISEASES OF THE HEART AND CIRCULATION.

HEART—bacterial endocarditis: See HEART, article DISEASES OF THE HEART AND CIRCULATION.

HEART—beats: See HEART, article DISEASES OF THE HEART AND CIRCULATION.

HEART—carbon dioxide given up by blood in right ventricle: See HEART, article DISEASES OF THE HEART AND CIRCULATION.

HEART—cardiac insufficiency: See HEART, article DISEASES OF THE HEART AND CIRCULATION.

HEART—changes: See HEART, article DISEASES OF THE HEART AND CIRCULATION.

HEART—changes during stress: See article STRESS AND DISEASE.

HEART—chorea: See HEART, article DISEASES OF THE HEART AND CIRCULATION.

HEART—circulation (figs.): See HEART, article DISEASES OF THE HEART AND CIRCULATION.

HEART—congenitally defective: See HEART, article DISEASES OF THE HEART AND CIRCULATION.

HEART—contusion: See HEART, article DISEASES OF THE HEART AND CIRCULATION.

HEART—coronary insufficiency: See HEART, article DISEASES OF THE HEART AND CIRCULATION.

HEART—coronary occlusion: See HEART, article DISEASES OF THE HEART AND CIRCULATION.

HEART—coronary system: See HEART, article DISEASES OF THE HEART AND CIRCULATION.

HEART—defective because of disease: See HEART, article DISEASES OF THE HEART AND CIRCULATION.

HEART—diastole: See HEART, article DISEASES OF THE HEART AND CIRCULATION.

HEART—diphtheria: See CHILDHOOD DISEASES, article INFECTIOUS DISEASES OF CHILDHOOD.

HEART—diseases: See HEART, article DISEASES OF THE HEART AND CIRCULATION; article DIABETES.

HEART—disordered action: See HEART, article DISEASES OF THE HEART AND CIRCULATION.

HEART—"effort syndrome": See HEART, article DISEASES OF THE HEART AND CIRCULATION.

HEART—endocarditis: See HEART, article DISEASES OF THE HEART AND CIRCULATION.

HEART—endocardium: See HEART, article DISEASES OF THE HEART AND CIRCULATION.

HEART—energy: See HEART, article DISEASES OF THE HEART AND CIRCULATION.

HEART—enlarged: See HEART, article DISEASES OF THE HEART AND CIRCULATION; article BLOOD PRESSURE.

HEART—fibrillation: See HEART, article DISEASES OF THE HEART AND CIRCULATION.

HEART—function: See HEART, article DISEASES OF THE HEART AND CIRCULATION.

HEART—inflammation, rheumatic: See reference CARDITIS above.

HEART—involuntary muscle: See HEART, article DISEASES OF THE HEART AND CIRCULATION.

HEART—mechanism of beating: See article BLOOD PRESSURE.

HEART—murmur: See HEART, article DISEASES OF THE HEART AND CIRCULATION.

HEART—muscles: See HEART, article DISEASES OF THE HEART AND CIRCULATION.

HEART—myocardium: See HEART, article DISEASES OF THE HEART AND CIRCULATION.

HEART—overweight a handicap: See article DIABETES.

HEART—oxygen taken on by blood in right ventricle: See HEART, article DISEASES OF THE HEART AND CIRCULATION.

HEART—pain: See entry ANGINA PECTORIS.

HEART—pericardium: See HEART, article DISEASES OF THE HEART AND CIRCULATION.

HEART—position in chest cavity (fig.): See HEART, article DISEASES OF THE HEART AND CIRCULATION.

HEART—pulse irregularities: See HEART, article DISEASES OF THE HEART AND CIRCULATION.

HEART—rheumatic fever: See HEART, article DISEASES OF THE HEART AND CIRCULATION.

HEART—scarlet fever: See CHILDHOOD DISEASES, article INFECTIOUS DISEASES OF CHILDHOOD.

HEART—shape and size: See HEART, article DISEASES OF THE HEART AND CIRCULATION.

HEART—subacute bacterial endocarditis: See HEART, article DISEASES OF THE HEART AND CIRCULATION.

HEART—symbol of human spirit: See article STRESS AND DISEASE.

HEART—syphilis: See HEART, article DISEASES OF THE HEART AND CIRCULATION.

HEART—thyroid, toxic: See HEART, article DISEASES OF THE HEART AND CIRCULATION.

HEART—traumatic injury: See HEART, article DISEASES OF THE HEART AND CIRCULATION.

HEART—vena cava: See HEART, article DISEASES OF THE HEART AND CIRCULATION.

HEART—ventricle: See HEART, article DISEASES OF THE HEART AND CIRCULATION.

HEART—weight: See HEART, article DISEASES OF THE HEART AND CIRCULATION.

HEART—whooping cough: See CHILDHOOD DISEASES, article INFECTIOUS DISEASES OF CHILDHOOD.

Diseases of the Heart and Circulation

BY

NEWELL C. GILBERT, M.D.

Chairman, Department of Medicine, Northwestern University Medical School, Chicago.

INTRODUCTION

THE HEART OF A CHILD *at birth weighs less than an ounce; that of an adult, a half pound. The energy which causes the heart to contract develops in some nervous tissue called the pace-maker of the heart. Apparently its energy is the equivalent of a thousandth of a volt. The heart beats one hundred times a minute in a small child, and on an average of seventy-two times a minute in an adult.*

This pump, because the heart is a pump which circulates the blood throughout the body, moves five hundred gallons of blood a day. During a lifetime the heart beats two and a half billion times and pumps a total of nearly thirty-five million gallons. The heart begins working before a child is born and is never quiet until death. The only rest it gets is when its beat is slowed a little or decreased somewhat in its force. The heart never gets a complete rest. This vital organ must therefore be protected in every possible way against damage.

The one disease of the heart which has baffled medical science is known as rheumatic fever. This disease is responsible for a vast amount of crippling and handicapping of young children. Because of its great importance, it is given more than usual consideration in the pages that follow.

About two hundred and twenty-five thousand people die in the United States each year from heart disease. The condition is more expensive in cost of human lives than cancer, but somewhat less expensive than tuberculosis. On those who live, however, the burden of heart disease falls heavily.

Because of the greater realization of the importance of heart disease in relation to the cause of death, and since today it leads all other causes, and since it is estimated that there are at any time at least two million people in the United States suffering from heart disease, this section of any modern home medical book is important.

From the earliest times the heart has aroused the curiosity and interest of man to an extent not equaled by any other organ in the human body except the brain. Most people who get sick are inclined to refer unusual symptoms to the heart. This organ has often been associated with the idea of courage, as in the phrase "faint heart," and the average man is likely to speak of the other person as either "weak-hearted" or "strong-hearted." It was once believed that the heart was the seat of the soul. It is still referred to as the seat of one of life's most interesting emotions.

The heart is one of the involuntary muscles of the body. There are but few instances recorded in medicine in which people were able voluntarily to control the heartbeats. Nevertheless, there is plenty of evidence to indicate that the speed of modern life and the stress of modern emotions modify greatly the work of the heart. There is also evidence that a suitable hygiene in relationship to this organ will lead to longer life.

The circulatory system is in reality the transportation system for the body. It carries to the cells, of which every organ and tissue of the body is built, essential materials for construction, reconstruction, and replacement of the tissues broken down by wear and tear. The blood carries fuel, and oxygen to burn the fuel, so that the necessary energy for repair and rebuilding may be obtained; each cell is thus enabled to perform its special function. Many other products, for instance, the secretions of certain glands, must be carried to the cells. The waste products from the cells must be carried away and taken to organs whose duty it is to excrete the waste or the waste may be utilized elsewhere, and made over for certain needs of the body. This circulation system acts perfectly under normal conditions and takes care of the changing needs of each part of the body. When an organ or tissue is doing active work, that part receives an increased flow of blood, while parts at rest receive a reduced amount.

The Anatomy of the Heart

The heart is the great central pump which moves the fluid carrying the necessary supplies through the blood vessels to every part of the body. It is a hollow organ with strong muscular walls. Its size is about that of the clenched right fist of its owner. The heart lies just below and to the left of the lower two thirds of the breastbone. Its shape is similar to that of a large pear with the broadened end upward and under the breast bone, and the pointed end downward and to the left, where one may feel the impulse as the heart beats.

THE PERICARDIUM

The heart lies inside a fibrous sac, called the *pericardium,* which is a resistant membrane and which forms a chamber, separating the heart from the other organs of the chest and holding it in position. In case of necessity this sac prevents the heart from dilating or stretching beyond a certain point. The surface of the heart itself is enclosed in a second fold of the same membrane. The two surfaces of the pericardium which lie against each other are covered by a smooth glistening layer of tissue, kept moist by a thin layer of fluid. This fluid prevents any friction between the layers as the heart beats.

CONSTRUCTION OF THE HEART

When the heart is opened it is seen to be separated into two halves with no communication between them. The halves are right and left in position and similar in arrangement. They act in unison. Each of the halves is also divided into two chambers. Above, on either side, is a thin-walled chamber which acts as a receiving reservoir for the blood returned to the heart. This chamber is called the *auricle.* Below the auricle is a chamber with thick, strong muscular walls, called the *ventricle.* This connects with the upper chamber by means of an opening provided with *valves,* which admit the blood freely into the ventricle when it relaxes, but close tight when the ventricle contracts, and thus prevent the return flow of blood back into the auricle during the contraction of the ventricle. The only essential difference between the right and left sides of the heart is that the muscle walls on the left side are thicker; for the left side must propel the blood through the entire body, while the right side needs to pump the blood only through the lungs. Leading from each ventricle is a large artery or blood vessel which carries away the blood forced out of the ventricle when it contracts. At the point where the blood leaves the ventricle and enters the artery there are other valves to prevent the reflow of blood into the ventricle, when its muscular walls relax again after contraction.

THE HEART MUSCLE: THE MYOCARDIUM

The muscle wall of the heart is referred to as the *myocardium*. The entire hollow interior of the heart is lined with a thin smooth membrane called the *endocardium*. This is continuous with a similar membrane lining the arteries. From these terms come the names of diseases in which these tissues are inflamed, such as myocarditis and endocarditis.

The heart muscle itself is supplied with a system of arteries and veins for its own fuel and repair requirements. This is called the *coronary system*. The coronary arteries open from the interior of the *aorta* (the large artery leading off from the left side of the heart). They begin just below the valves which separate the aorta from the ventricle. The flow through these arteries, then, will be greater or less as the blood pressure in the aorta is greater or less.

The Function of the Heart

The blood returning from every part of the body is brought back to the right auricle by two large veins, one coming from the upper, the other from the lower, part of the body, called respectively the superior and inferior *vena cava*. From the right auricle, the blood enters the right ventricle, which forces the blood through the lungs. There it gives up its carbon-dioxide, carried from all parts of the body, and takes on a fresh supply of oxygen. The blood returning from the circuit through the lungs is returned to the left auricle by the pulmonary vein. The auricles act as receiving reservoirs for the blood. Between the beats of the heart, their muscle walls relax and the chambers become distended with the returned blood. The period between each contraction or beat is referred to as the *diastole,* and is a period of rest and recuperation for the heart.

When the walls of the ventricles relax in their turn, after each contraction, the blood from the distended auricles flows into the ventricles during the relaxation or diastole of the ventricle. Just before the end of the ventricular diastole or period of relaxation of the walls of the ventricle, the muscle walls of the auricle contract, further emptying the auricle and more completely filling the ventricle. A fraction of a second later, the ventricle begins to contract. As the walls of the chamber contract and draw together, the pressure of the contained blood increases; the valves leading back into the auricle are closed and held firmly shut by the blood in the ventricle pushing against them.

When the pressure in the contracting ventricle becomes greater than the pressure in the artery, the valves leading into the artery are opened and the contents of the ventricle forced into the artery. At the end of the ventricular contraction or *systole,* the ventricle in its turn relaxes. As it does so the valves leading back into the ventricle from the aorta are closed by the pressure of the blood, thus preventing a reflow of blood back into the ventricle. During the period of ventricular systole the relaxed auricle has again been filling with blood, whereupon the now relaxed ventricle is again filled. This cycle is repeated, many times a minute, hour after hour, and year after year during life. The heart works constantly, but the amount and speed of its work may be varied.

The heart and the blood and lymph vessels which make up the circulatory system of the body constitute a mechanism equipped to meet every need of the body under normal conditions. This mechanism automatically adjusts itself to changing and varying needs in every part of the body. Provision has been made for almost every contingency that may arise. In addition, nature has given this mechanism a wide margin of safety so that it may still continue to do its work, even after a considerable amount of damage to the heart has been sustained.

Nothing that is said in this chapter should ever lead the reader to form his own opinion without the consultation of a well-trained physician. The purpose of the chapter is only to help the reader to understand the mechanism of the heart, and to understand the disorders to which it may be subject, so as to better understand the physician and his counsel and his advice.

Except in the rare instances in which the structure of the heart is defective from birth, it continues to do its work day after day and year after year without its possessor being conscious of its activity.

Frequently our attention is called to the heart by symptoms which we interpret as symptoms of heart disease, but which are not due to any disease of the heart or to disease of any organ. Sometimes such symptoms may be troublesome. Usually they are due to an instability of the nervous mechanism which regulates the rate at which the heart beats, or to disturbances of the digestive tract, or other organs. Such simple conditions as over-fatigue, worry, or emotional excitement tend to produce such effects. Rest and care usually provide a cure, or at least substantial improvement. Whether the heart is really damaged or not is a question for your physician to decide. He will be guided by an evaluation of the symptoms, by a physical examination and by laboratory methods. If a murmur is present, it does not necessarily have any significance. Murmurs may come and go in a heart that is quite normal. A heart that is normal in size and contour may almost always be assumed to be a normal heart.

Changes in the Heart

Structural changes in the heart are largely permanent. They may be compensated for in many ways by the body, and there is such a wide margin of safety that the heart may continue to do its work for a normal lifetime in the presence of extensive damage. But such changes are never to be ignored. They are usually due to one of two causes: Infection or disease or the degenerative changes which follow the disease, and which may appear in any of us as we grow older. But a third less frequent cause must be considered, and that is a contusion of the heart due usually to a sudden, sharp blow. The most frequent of such contusions are "steering-wheel accidents," or other incidents in which the chest has received a severe blow. A heart muscle which is forced to work with a blood supply which does not bring it sufficient material for repairs, or sufficient fuel, or sufficient oxygen to burn the fuel, is bound to suffer some damage. Changes in the blood flow to the heart muscle are due in large part to structural changes in the vessel walls, which narrow the vessels. Such changes may result from infection, especially rheumatic fever, or they may occur with advancing years because of reasons which we do not fully understand. There are a very few people who are born with deficiencies in the arterial blood supply to the heart muscle. In many cases the blood supply to the heart muscle is inadequate, not so much because of changes in the arteries, but because the territory which the arteries supply has been greatly increased by an overgrowth of the muscle. This overgrowth has been made necessary by demands for increased work. This increased work may be the result of damage to the valves. It may also be the result of the necessity of pumping blood through narrowed vessels over the entire body, as is the case in high blood pressure.

Temporary, and often only momentary narrowing of the vessels may result from nerve impulses. They may be due to reflex nerve impulses from other organs, as the stomach, gall bladder, or other sources. They may be due to working under extreme nervous tension with insufficient rest and relaxation. Emotional stress may be a factor. Such temporary narrowing of the vessels, oft repeated, may bring on permanent changes.

Overexertion does not injure a normal heart. Uncomfortable symptoms, or if these are not heeded, unconsciousness, stop the overexertion long before the heart is damaged. But overexertion can cause great and perhaps irreparable damage in a heart in which an active infection is present or in a heart previously damaged by infection.

Except, then, for the small group of hearts which are defective at birth, permanent changes in the structure of the heart which interfere with its function as a pump, and which are crippling, are due for the most part to infection, or to the inevitable changes which appear with age, or, very much more rarely, to trauma. If a heart is not able to perform its functions, either structural defects present at birth or structural changes acquired as the result of disease or as a result of a blood supply to the heart muscle insufficient for its needs may be responsible.

Congenitally Defective Hearts

A small number of children are born with hearts which are structurally defective. This defect may occur as a narrowing of the two large vessels which leave the heart, or as defects in the valves of these vessels. There may be defects in the structure of the heart itself which interferes with its work. A rather frequent cause is the persistence after birth of an arterial connection which diverted the blood from the lungs before birth. Such congenital defects may be so serious that the child dies at birth or soon after. In other cases, where the defect is less serious or where its presence is compensated for by some other abnormal condition, the child may survive for varying periods, with some disability, or may even lead a normal life, with the heart doing its work in spite of its handicap.

In some of the children in whom the only evidence of a congenital defect is perhaps only a loud murmur over the heart area and who are normal in growth and development, it is probably safe to disregard the condition if there are no symptoms on exertion. These children should be allowed to live the life of normal children with the usual attention to health and hygeia, but under careful observation. They do not require any medicine for the heart.

However, it is quite a different thing if the child does have symptoms. Such symptoms are shortness of breath on exertion, or occasional fainting spells, or a lack of growth and development for the age. The skin may have a bluish cast, and the fingers may be "clubbed," that is, the ends may be broader and flatter than normal. Formerly such children did not survive, or were invalids or semi-invalids. Now surgical procedures can do a very great deal to restore such children to normal. The risk of doing such an operation is small compared with the risk to future health and life if it is not done. The decision is a matter for the careful judgment of your physician, as is also the choice of a surgeon with special training who is skilled in such work. One point of especial importance should always be kept in mind, that is, the increased likelihood of infection. Particularly to be guarded against is the predisposition to tuberculosis and to those infections which cause additional heart damage, as infective endocarditis. The child must be carefully guarded against exposure to infection, or to conditions which predispose to infection; and the general health must be kept at the highest possible level. Such children should receive the same care as those whose hearts have been previously damaged by rheumatic fever, and the same precautions should be taken. They should be examined at frequent and regular intervals, and any possible question of doubt should be referred at once to the physician for advice.

HEARTS DEFECTIVE BECAUSE OF DISEASE

The illness responsible for more heart disease than any other, and for almost all the heart disease of childhood and early life, is known variously as rheumatic fever, acute rheumatic fever, or inflammatory rheumatism. Chorea, or St. Vitus's dance, is only a manifestation of rheumatic fever.

The name "rheumatic fever" is not apt! The name "rheumatism" calls to mind symptoms of disease of the bones and joints, and rheumatic fever may exist and cause severe damage to the heart without any such symptoms or with symptoms so slight that they do not attract attention.

Fever, while it is doubtless present in some degrees at times during the disease, may be a minor symptom or may remain undiscovered. However, the name "rheumatic fever" has been in general use for so long that it would be confusing to attempt to change it.

MANIFESTATIONS OF RHEUMATIC FEVER IN CHILDHOOD

While we think of rheumatic fever as a disease of the joints and of the heart, it is really a very generalized disease. Its effects are not evenly distributed and it may affect some organs greatly, such as the joints and the heart, while other organs may be only slightly affected, or not at all. The joints may escape damage and the heart may be involved, without any joint symptoms. But the characteristic changes in the smaller arteries may appear anywhere, from the brain down. It is essentially a chronic disease and its course in one form or another may cover a period of months or even years. One does not acquire an immunity as the result of one attack, but the whole process may recur following some slight "cold" or other infection. The disease should never be regarded as cured no matter how complete the apparent recovery after an acute attack, nor how long the apparent recovery may have lasted.

There may never be any acute symptoms. It is, however, usually characterized by intervals of varying duration which come on more or less suddenly and sharply, and by much longer intervals of apparent quiescence, when but slight symptoms or none at all are apparent.

Most of the damage done to the heart occurs during the acute stages, but damage may also be going on slowly, though none the less certainly, during the periods when the disease is apparently inactive.

Rheumatic fever may exist and cause structural damage to the heart without any recognizable symptoms. Frequently unquestionable evidence of heart damage due to rheumatic disease is found in patients whose record, after the closest questioning, furnishes no clue to the time when the damage might have occurred.

The earlier and milder manifestations of rheumatic fever, unless accompanied by some more definite sign, such as rheumatic nodules, or the so-called growing pains, are difficult to differentiate from symptoms occurring in other conditions.

The child may only appear to be below what would be considered the normal health level. Colds and sore throats may appear with more than usual frequency. The weight may be below the normal average, or a loss of weight may occur rather conspicuously and suddenly. Fatigue is present out of all proportion to the play or exertion which brought it on. There may be loss of appetite, symptoms of stomach or intestinal disturbance, headache, nervous instability, or many other symptoms which are not characteristic of rheumatic fever particularly, but which are indicative of mild illness. There may be pallor, and a blood examination may reveal mild anemia, although sometimes the pallor is out of proportion to the anemia actually present. Blood examination may also show an increase in the number of white cells, indicating the presence of an infection, even during these mild and doubtful stages. The pulse may be more rapid than normal. Careful and repeated trials may indicate the presence of fever. A reliable temperature record, especially when only a slight rise is present, requires that even the best thermometer be held under the tongue for fully five minutes. Rectal temperatures are more reliable in children.

In some of these doubtful cases, repeated examination of the urine may show evidence of a mild inflammation of the kidney. This may be related to a silent rheumatic fever, or to one of several mild and more or less silent infections. It should never be neglected, and should be cared for especially by rest and by medication in addition, if the physician thinks it advisable. If such mild cases are cared for thoroughly the occurrence of chronic kidney disease would be reduced to a point where it is very rare indeed, if not ruled out altogether.

There is nothing characteristic of any one disease in the symptoms described. These cases do, however, demand careful examination and reëxamination by the family doctor. It is significant that there is a period of a few months up to three to five years of such indefinite symptoms, which have been called "toxic debility," in the majority of cases, before there is definite evidence of rheumatic fever. It is also significant that in many of these cases of "toxic debility" some evidence of rheumatic fever may occasionally be found on examination. It is during these silent and doubtful stages that some of the unexplained permanent changes may occur. Also, mild infections precede and predispose to rheumatic fever.

"Growing pains" are usually an important symptom and may occur during the doubtful stages. Many such indefinite pains are not significant, but there should always be careful questioning to determine their true nature. If there is any doubt, careful and repeated physical examination by the physician is of the greatest importance. About three fourths of all cases of rheumatic fever have had such pains. They are rather indefinite nagging muscle or joint pains, occurring anywhere, but most often in the legs, in front of the thighs, or behind the knees, or in the so-called "hamstring muscles." Sometimes the child complains of neck pains. Similar pains may occur from many natural causes. But no matter how mild they may be, they constitute an early danger signal. The watchful mother should listen to the child's story in order that the true nature of the pains may be determined.

Another minor manifestation which occurs with variable frequency is the "rheumatic nodule." It is a small round nodule, visible under the skin and movable. It is not tender. The size varies with the location, but on the average is about the size of a small pea. These nodules are most easily found where the tendons join the muscles with the bones, as close to the elbows or wrists, the knees, or the nape of the neck, or over the shoulder or hips, and less frequently over the shoulder blade or the collar bone. The presence of these nodules may be presumed to indicate rheumatic fever, although they have been observed in apparently healthy children, in cases in which rheumatic fever could not be definitely proved.

More frequently the actual onset of rheumatic fever occurs abruptly. It begins with the immediate appearance of joint symptoms or sometimes heart symptoms. There may be a short premonitory stage of fever. Some infection of the upper respiratory passages, such as a cold or sore throat, usually precedes the attack, and there may have been exposure to cold or dampness. In more than half the cases, the attacks begin with an inflammation of one or more joints. There is pain in the joint, which is swollen, tender, reddened, and feels hot to the touch. The symptoms may be severe or mild. The joints may be tender with little or no swelling, or slightly swollen with little or no tenderness. Characteristically the symptoms migrate from joint to joint, with a duration of one to eight days or more for each joint. At a given time, one or several joints may be involved. Fever is present from the start during these stages, and its height varies with each case. Its severity or lack of severity must never be taken as an index of the involvement of the heart.

Pleurisy or inflammation of the membrane lining the chest cavity may be the first symptom of the onset of rheumatic fever. Severe pain on breathing may occur suddenly, without any previous warning, or may follow after a few days of what is apparently only a "cold." The symptom of pain may disappear, and the pleura, or lining membrane of the chest, escape further trouble. Sometimes the pain may be followed by a collection of fluid in the chest cavity. Occasionally the fluid may appear silently without any preceding pain. A form of pneumonia, peculiar to rheumatic fever, may appear at the onset, but is more likely to occur later in the disease.

CHOREA

Chorea, or St. Vitus's dance, is another manifestation of rheumatic fever, occurring rather more frequently in girls, and is limited usually to the early school age. Most cases occur between the ages of five and ten, and most frequently independently of the joint symptoms. The child who has had choreic twitchings will probably have chorea when rheumatic fever recurs, just as the one with symptoms affecting the joints most frequently has joint symptoms when there is a recurrence. In a part of the cases chorea and joint symptoms are present at the same time, or the child may show chorea at one time and joint symptoms at another.

Heart disease ensues in the children with choreic manifestations as frequently as it follows with other signs and symptoms. It does not always follow so promptly, however. Children with the joint symptoms usually develop the heart disease while they are still under observation because of the acute attack, or shortly after, although the appearance of heart disease is often delayed in them also. In chorea the heart disease frequently appears later, after the symptoms of chorea have subsided, or even after a period of years. Chorea is less disabling and is often mild, and does not always attract the attention it should. Occasionally it occurs without being noticed. Sometimes there are only minor symptoms, such as fidgeting, restlessness, or lack of attention and concentration. The lack of concentration may be noticed only at school, or the nervousness may show in the handwriting. There may be loss of appetite, headache, and general nervous instability. The child may be forgetful, irritable, emotional, and may have crying spells. In the less mild cases the nervousness is more evident. There are spasmodic involuntary movements of the face and hands. The child may drop things that he is carrying and be unable to sit still. The more severe cases cannot escape attention. The spasmodic movements are more extreme and pronounced; the face is distorted, and there are uncontrollable grimaces. The tongue may be involuntarily thrust out; the speech may be interfered with.

Choreic manifestations are always worse during excitement or when attention is attracted to them. The choreic movements disappear during sleep. A child with chorea requires rest and quiet surroundings and should never be sent to school. Chorea should be considered as active rheumatic fever and treated as such.

RHEUMATIC INFLAMMATION OF THE HEART (CARDITIS)

Inflammation of the heart and its consequences are as much a manifestation of rheumatic fever as are the joint symptoms or the nodules. It is not to be regarded as a complication or as an aftermath of rheumatic fever, but as an essential part. Rheumatic fever is a generalized chronic infection, doing similar damage to similar tissue in many parts of the body. The damage may be much greater in one part of the body than in another, or it may be more evident, because it may interfere with functions, as in the heart, or cause pain, as in the joints; or it may occur where it produces no symptoms and be silent. The heart may escape, or apparently escape, or the joints may escape, or both may escape and the infection manifest itself in some other way.

The infection may seem to expend all of its energy on the heart, and the effects of rheumatic fever on the heart may appear without evidence of rheumatic fever elsewhere. Occasionally when a child is examined because of an acute attack of rheumatic fever with joint symptoms, or other manifestations, the heart is found to have been already involved at some previous time. In such cases there is always the probability that minor manifestations of rheumatic fever had occurred and were unobserved.

Such cases are not the common rule; more frequently involvement of the heart is associated with or follows one or more of the other manifestations of rheumatic fever. Unless there are symptoms of pericarditis or inflammation of the heart sac, the inflammation of the heart may not be noticed at the onset and for a long period give no indication of its presence.

Pericarditis is an inflammation of the walls of the sac in which the heart in enclosed. As these inflamed walls rub past each other with each beat of the heart, they may cause intense pain. In some cases the pain is absent. Frequently fluid appears between the two walls of the pericardium, separating them, and sometimes causing great distention of the pericardial sac, even to the point of interfering with the work of the heart. This is referred to as *pericarditis with effusion.*

Pericarditis may be the first manifestation of rheumatic fever and may come on suddenly. It more frequently occurs in the course of the disease and in the presence of other manifestations. It always means that an inflammation of the heart is present. Rheumatic inflammation of the heart is to be considered as an inflammation involving all of the tissues of the heart. While one tissue, as the pericardium or the endocardium, may give more evidence of involvement than the other tissues, or may be more extensively involved than the other tissues, the other tissues do not escape.

Except when pericarditis makes an inflammation of the heart evident, signs of heart involvement, or changes in the heart which interfere with its function, may not appear for a long period after the onset of rheumatic fever or even after actual involvement of the heart. Indeed, such changes may not appear until long after all the other symptoms of rheumatic fever have subsided and the patient is apparently well.

Usually in such cases there is evidence that an inflammatory process is still active somewhere. A slight fever is found on careful examination, the pulse is more rapid than normal, and an increase in the number of white cells in the blood may be found on examination. Such a child should be kept in bed under the supervision of a doctor until all possible chance of an active infection of the heart has been ruled out.

The absence of signs of damage to the heart does not mean that an active inflammation of the heart is not present. Such signs of damage are the results of the inflammation, and not signs of the inflammation itself. No child in whom rheumatic fever is even suspected should be allowed out of bed while there remains any elevation of temperature or until after the temperature has been normal for at least two weeks or more and until the sedimentation rate is normal.

Heart damage may be found three or four years or more after an attack of rheumatic fever, without any of the manifestations of the disease having been observed during this period. The patient may appear in good health during the intervening period. In many of these cases, a mild infection may have occurred which escaped observation. In some of these patients, the late appearance of the heart symptoms may be that the vessels which nourish the heart muscle have been narrowed by the previous rheumatic infection. Because of this slow, but progressive damage has been done to the heart muscle. This would be especially true if the earlier attacks had caused changes which resulted in an overgrowth of the heart muscle. New vessels do not come with the overgrowth of heart muscle, and the heart must do its work with the same vessels it started out with at birth.

Because of this possibility of progressive damage occurring after an attack of rheumatic fever, the child should be carefully watched by the parents, and frequently re-examined by the physician.

Rheumatic fever causes what is essentially an inflammation of the whole heart, the enveloping membrane or the pericardium, the heart muscle or the myocardium, and its lining membrane or the endocardium. Because of the inflammation of the endocardium, deformities of the valves develop so that they cannot close properly. This may affect any of the valves, but most frequently the mitral valve between the left auricle and ventricle, and the aortic valve are involved. Less frequently the tricuspid valve, between the right auricle and ventricle, and rarely the pulmonic valve are concerned. The mitral valves may have a deformity which is specially characteristic of rheumatic fever, a narrowing of the valve due to scar contraction following the inflammation, referred to as *mitral stenosis*. Such a deformity also prevents the valve from closing properly when the ventricle contracts. This makes an *"insufficiency"* of the valve (*valvular insufficiency*), so that the blood flows back into the auricle during contraction of the ventricle. This insufficiency of the mitral valve also occurs without the narrowing. It is what people refer to when they say they have a "leaky valve" or a "heart leak."

The heart muscle is invariably involved in the inflammation to some degree, perhaps slightly, or perhaps to a degree which interferes with its efficiency.

Permanent changes may also persist in the pericardium, increasing the work of the heart. The two layers, the one covering the heart and the one forming the sac in which the heart is suspended, may adhere together, so that at each beat the heart not only has to pull against the normal attachments of the pericardium, but frequently against new and abnormal attachments due to inflammation of the outer sac and its attachment to surrounding tissue.

In order to compensate for damage done to the heart, nature causes the heart to enlarge and the muscular walls to become stronger and thicker. In this way it can pump more blood at each stroke and make up for reflow of blood through the damaged valves, or it can pull against the adhesions of the pericardium to adjacent structures. A heart that has been damaged is almost always enlarged and in rheumatic fever may become greatly enlarged. When the heart enlarges in order to compensate for the additional work which it must do, the muscle fibres become longer or thicker, or both. The bulk of the muscle is increased. But as the heart muscle increases in size, it cannot grow any new blood vessels, so that the enlarged muscle must be nourished by the same number of blood vessels that supplied it before it became enlarged. The blood vessels per unit of size are fewer in number, in spite of the increased needs. The body may compensate for this in part by increasing the blood flow through the vessels which are present. But a decreased blood flow, with increased blood needs, may eventually cause serious changes in the heart muscle and the person with an enlarged heart should not leave the entire burden of care to nature, however kindly nature may be, but he should help by not throwing any greater burden upon an already burdened heart muscle. A heart muscle forced to work without sufficient material for repair and without sufficient fuel and oxygen to burn the fuel may suffer further permanent damage.

THE ATTACK ON RHEUMATIC FEVER

Most acute infections are produced by a specific variety of germ, which always causes the disease characteristic of that germ when it enters the body under conditions favorable for its growth. In such cases the actual causative organism can be demonstrated in the infected part or in the blood.

In rheumatic fever we have very good reason for thinking that the disease is caused by the hemolytic streptococcus, and usually, if not always, by a group known as Type A, but we can not show the responsible organism in the blood or in the tissues affected. There is a lag between the onset of infection and the symptoms of rheumatic fever. Also, this infection does not cause an immunity, as it usually does in other streptococcus infections. This has led many to assume that rheumatic fever is an allergic response to the infecting organism. Similar responses of sensitization to bacteria or to foreign blood proteins, or even to chemical agents, are seen in other of the so-called "collagen diseases," of which rheumatic fever is one. Perhaps in some cases different streptococci may cause a similar response.

We have reason to think also that very often some mild or not so mild upper respiratory infection, or "cold," may prepare the ground for the advent of the streptococcus infection with its resulting symptoms of sensitization. Usually we do see such a preceding infection.

Rheumatic fever is probably the resultant of many factors in addition to the invading organism. The effects of many different environments on the growth of the germ and of different responses by different bodies to the growth of the organism must be considered. Some of these differences in environment or response may be determined by hereditary predisposition, by the effect of fatigue or exercise, by the effect of previous infections or ill health, or by many factors not accurately known.

There are several general conditions which seem to influence the incidence of rheumatic fever. In the first place it is much more frequent in the Caucasian or white race, although it does occur among all races. While it occurs all over the world, it is much more frequent in the temperate zones. When it does occur in the tropics, it is likely to run a milder course.

Damp climates have been considered an important factor; but apparently a damp climate does not necessarily predispose to rheumatic fever, nor does a dry or warm high climate prevent its occurrence. Rheumatic fever is not especially common in Holland, and is much less frequent there than in England or the northern United States. It is more common on the Mexican plateau than on the Mexican seaboard. In the West Indies it is infrequent. In Puerto Rico, in spite of poor living conditions, it is uncommon among the native population. It does occur in Egypt, but is unknown in the Malay peninsula. Much remains to be learned in regard to the influence of climate as a single factor in the incidence of rheumatic fever. This much can be said, however: that it is less frequent in warm climates and less common where there are no abrupt or sudden changes in temperature. It has been supposed to be less common where there were no abrupt or sudden changes in climate. But in the Malay peninsula it is just as uncommon in the highlands, where such changes occur, as on the coast, where the changes are minimal. The decreased occurrence in warm climates is probably due in large part to a life lived more out of doors.

Bad housing, cold, damp surroundings, or proximity to water courses have been considered important causative factors. There is much to indicate that such conditions may be a determining influence in the occurrence of rheumatic fever, but again there is the low incidence in Holland, and there was a low incidence in the late war among the troops in the trenches.

Rheumatic fever is less common among the well-to-do. While it is probable that social status is a factor, it is probably not as important a factor as would appear at first glance. Perhaps among the well-to-do predisposing ill health and minor infections are better cared for than among the poor. When rheumatic fever does occur it is recognized earlier and managed more adequately, so that there is less probability of serious consequence. Among the well-to-do classes there is less crowding and less frequenting of crowded places of amusement and crowded conveyances. There is much greater chance of transmitting minor infections of the nose and throat from one to another in crowded surroundings.

Probably there is a family predisposition to rheumatic fever. It is also difficult to be sure just how to evaluate the importance of contagion. Rheumatic fever is not contagious in the sense that it is transmissible from one developed case to another. Local epidemics have been reported and ward epidemics have occurred in hospitals. Epidemics of recurrences have been reported in convalescent homes for rheumatic fever patients. These may be explained as epidemics of "colds," or of sore throats, referred to as "upper respiratory infections," which have paved the way for the ever ready streptococcus, and which have resulted in rheumatic fever. It must be remembered that those who have already had rheumatic fever are not immune, but are very prone to have a recurrence with any infection.

Rheumatic fever, as such, is not contagious, but the causative streptococcus infection is contagious.

Rheumatic fever does show annual variation, in which there are years of increased incidence and years of lower incidence. This would suggest some epidemic influence, although it may be that these variations are due to climatic or other causes.

There are seasonal changes also. In the United States rheumatic fever is more frequent in late winter and early spring. In England it is more frequent in the fall months.

Rheumatic fever is much more common in childhood; indeed, it is largely a disease of childhood. There are a few cases from three to five years of age, but after five the frequency steadily increases until the twelfth year. After twelve the frequency of the initial attacks decreases, and they are much less frequent after twenty, but do occur with constantly diminishing frequency through old age.

Rheumatic fever, generally considered, is somewhat more frequent in girls, and the choreic manifestations are much more frequent in girls.

The weak and undernourished child seems to have the pre-rheumatic state. This may be a definite constitutional state, due to inherited tendencies, or to repeated minor infections, or deficiencies in diet and general care; or perhaps it is actually a stage of the disease itself. The truth probably includes both views: that it is a definite predisposing constitutional state, and that among the group are many who already show the minor manifestations of rheumatic fever. Such conditions either predispose to rheumatic fever or actually may be a part of it.

Some children are under the standard of weight for their age, are prone to listlessness, and tire more easily than a normal child. Such children have poor appetites, constipation, and other minor and indefinite symptoms. These children are especially liable to recurrent upper respiratory infections, or colds. By the upper respiratory tract is meant the upper air passages, the membrane of the nose and pharynx and the lymphoid tissue of the tonsils, adenoids, and walls of the pharynx. It is a question as to whether these recurring infections are a cause or a result of the subnormal condition of the health. The same question applies to the gastro-intestinal symptoms.

However indefinite may be the effect of these factors on the incidence of rheumatic fever, there can be no doubt of the importance of infections of the upper respiratory tract as a whole. Such infections are almost always associated with the occurrence and recurrence of the different manifestations of rheumatic fever, with the single exception that there is a less close relationship with the occurrence of chorea.

This of course brings up the question of the relation of the tonsils to rheumatic fever. The tonsils are frequently the portion of the upper respiratory tract most obviously infected, although similar infection may be and usually is present in other portions. The tonsils are only a part of the tissue which may be involved in such infections. Their normal function is to act as a barrier to infection.

The fact that the tonsils are only a part of the tissues which may serve as a point of entrance for the infection must be borne in mind in considering the prevention of rheumatic fever. Normal tonsils serve as a barrier to infection and should not be removed under any circumstances, even if they are larger than normal. The same applies to tonsils which have recurring attacks of infection but are normal between the attacks. The inflammation at such times is due to the fact that the tonsils are acting as a barrier to infection and are bearing the brunt of the attack. Not infrequently, when tonsils of this type are removed, the attacks still recur, in the tissues similar to the tonsils which are part of the throat membrane and which also serve as a barrier.

If the tonsils, however, have constant, chronic infection, they should be removed. Such chronically infected tonsils need not be large. Small tonsils which show signs of chronic infection, associated with enlargement of the glands of the neck and large, ragged chronically infected tonsils, should be removed. Adenoids which are infected or are an obstruction to breathing should of course always be removed. Such a procedure will at least aid in conserving the health of the child and will tend to make attacks or recurrences less likely.

PREVENTION

The prevention of rheumatic fever is largely a matter of attention to the many details which go to insure the best possible general health. Absolute rules for this care cannot be set forth in detail, for just what are the best conditions vary with the individual child. In general they may be summarized in the words "good maternal care." This will mean first of all a quiet, restful home life, free from the disturbing influences which make a "nervous child," with the attendant disturbance of digestion and sleep. It will mean well-ordered and adequate rest periods and supervised recreation. Overfatigue interferes with digestion and rest and predisposes to infection. A rest period of a half hour before and after meals will aid in digestion and nutrition.

The clothing should be warm and adequate. Damp, wet clothing should be changed at once. Fresh air in the home and sleeping quarters is essential. Fresh air need not be damp, irritating air and warm air can be fresh air. Certainly infections of the nose and throat have been made worse by overenthusiasm in the matter of fresh air. Here again individual judgment must be applied to each child.

The diet should be a sensible, easily digested, nutritious diet. Vitamins are sometimes deficient, even in good American homes. That is a matter for your physician to advise you upon.

It is always to be borne in mind that in rheumatic fever in actual practice and in experimental animals, "colds" and upper respiratory infections and the so-called virus infections are found to predispose to streptococcus A infection.

It is also important to remember that rheumatic fever is usually preceded by some minor "cold" or so-called virus infection.

Colds and sore throats are more apt to be contracted from the "droplet infection" of crowds, or crowded places of amusement or public conveyances. Minor colds and sore throats should be watched and treated carefully, and the child should be kept in the house for a period after all temperature has subsided.

Children with chronic throat, nose, and sinus infections should receive especially watchful care at home and be under the observation of a physician. When possible they should be given the benefit of a warm, equable climate, if only for a time, where such infections are at least less frequent.

Antibiotics, and especially penicillin, have been shown to be of value in the prevention of rheumatic fever in two ways. One method is their prompt use in any hemolytic streptococcic infection, in adequate dosage, combined with bed rest and an adequate period for convalescence. This applies to any "cold" of any origin, any one of which may precede an attack of rheumatic fever.

Another method of prevention is the daily use of the antibiotics over a long period of time in cases where there are recurring attacks of "colds" and a history of previous rheumatic fever.

The possibility of sensitization to the drug must of course always be considered. Such sensitization may cause joint pains or hives. There is a possibility, too, that a race of organisms may develop which will not yield to penicillin, or whatever antibiotic is used. Neither of these deterrents is very important, as the drug can be taken by mouth.

On the other hand, sulfa drugs used to prevent rheumatic fever may result in a sensitization which has very serious possibilities. Such a sensitization is rare, but it is too serious to chance. Other drugs are much safer and just as effective, or more so. The treatment of rheumatic fever when it has once occurred is a matter for the best judgment of a good physician. Pressure should not be exercised upon the physician to use some new drug just because it has received a great deal of newspaper or magazine publicity.

ACTH AND CORTISONE IN RHEUMATIC FEVER

One of the most remarkable discoveries of modern times is the value of Cortisone and ACTH in many conditions. They are two of the most active agents which we possess in medicine, but like all extremely active agents, they have great powers for harm as well as for good, and they are to be used only in specific circumstances, according to the judgment of your physician.

Rest and quiet and time, and some of the old, long-tried remedies are often just as effective in the long run, and do not possess dangerous side effects.

ENDOCARDITIS

While rheumatic fever is the one largest single factor in the production of heart disease, other illnesses arise later in life which are also causatives. Just at the time when rheumatic fever is becoming less frequent, endocarditis, or inflammation of the interior of the heart, begins to appear. It may occur in childhood but is uncommon until after puberty, when its frequency increases until some time in the early twenties, at which time it gradually decreases, although it may persist through all ages.

Endocarditis occurs much more frequently in those who have previously had rheumatic fever, and this is especially true of the less acute forms.

There is an acute, sudden, sharp form which may occur at any age, and usually occurs in the course of some severe illness such as pneumonia, childbirth fever, multiple abscesses with pyemia, severe gonorrheal infection, influenza, severe tonsillitis, or recurrences of rheumatic fever. The causative germ is in each case the causative germ of the original infection. This acute severe endocarditis does not bear the same intimate relation to previous heart involvement as does the more mild and more frequent form to be described later and which is known as subacute bacterial endocarditis.

The symptoms of the acute endocarditis are those of a severe acute infection with high fever, chills, and prostration. It is important only as a complication of a very severe infection of some sort quite apart from the heart, but a complication which involves the heart. Recovery is very rare indeed.

The milder, subacute form is of more concern because some cases of this form do actually recover, and others might recover if recognized more promptly. This form is much more closely related to rheumatic fever, and at least 80 to 90 per cent of cases follow rheumatic fever infection. The connection is so close that in many cases there is some doubt as to the separate identity. In the acute form only a little over half are due to the streptococcus, while in the subacute form about 95 per cent are due not only to the streptococcus, but to one type of streptococcus, the *S. viridans,* and the remaining 5 per cent are divided between other forms of streptococci, the influenza bacillus, the gonococcus, and other organisms.

As in the acute form, the infection is practically confined to the endocardium, especially to the valves, where it results in a productive inflammation, causing vegetation upon the valves, with underlying ulceration of the tissue.

The symptoms may be mild indeed at the onset, so mild as to attract little or no attention for a long time. The condition is frequently similar to mild, incipient tuberculosis. There may be only fatigue on slight effort, weakness, feeling of malaise, or slight digestive disturbance, or loss of weight and strength. There may be some pallor, and an actual anemia is often present.

Fever is invariably present, although there may be periods of days when it is absent. It varies from a rise of only a fraction of a degree in the milder cases to higher temperatures in the more sharp types. In the cases associated with the higher temperatures, chills may occur. The pulse rate is usually faster than normal.

The fingers may show clubbing, the spleen is usually enlarged, and the symptoms of the preëxisting heart disease may be accentuated. At some time during the disease what are known as petechiæ, or spots, always occur. They should be watched for constantly, as they occur in crops with sometimes long intervals between them, and last only for a day or two or longer. They are small round red dots, not appreciably raised, and differing in size, rarely larger than a pinhead in diameter, and do not disappear on pressure. They occur most frequently above and below the collar bone and over the chest, but may extend over the abdomen, down the arms, or to the back. They are frequently seen in the white of the eye, where they cannot be confused with minor blemishes of the skin.

Still another sign of the disease is the occurrence of emboli in various parts of the body. These are small fragments which have become detached from the growths on the valves of the heart, and are carried by the blood stream through the arteries to lodge in some distant part. The symptoms and signs will vary with the site of the artery which is occluded by the embolus. Occasionally the lodgment of such an embolus in the brain, with consequent paralysis, or in the spleen, with intense pain, or in the kidney with pain and the appearance of blood in the urine, or in one of the arteries of the extremity, is the first symptom which brings the disease to the attention of the patient and his physician.

Subacute bacterial endocarditis may start with a mild, almost unnoticeable infection, very much like a beginning tuberculosis, or it may start with severe and definite symptoms and a fever which is high from the first. It seems to have lost much of its former significance. We can not be too sure of this, however, as waves of this infection have come and gone. Just at present it does not seem to appear as frequently as it did, due to better general care of rheumatic fever, and better care of other acute infections. The sooner this infection is recognized, the better. The outlook, with penicillin and the other antibiotics, is immeasurably brighter than formerly. In these days most cases recover, instead of just a few, but it is still an extremely serious disease.

SYPHILIS OF THE HEART

Syphilis of the heart and aorta may occur in the twenties but is more common in middle and in later middle life; it is the causative factor in much heart disease first appearing at this time, and especially among certain elements of the population.

Syphilis of the heart may exist silently until extensive or irreparable damage has been done. For this reason repeated blood examinations, like Wassermann or Kahn tests, should be made on those in whom there is any reason to suspect the disease to have occurred, no matter how well it has been treated. Too much confidence should never be placed upon any supposed cure by any method. The heart should be carefully watched, and the observations checked by X-ray examination, for the infection does not always show in the blood examination.

When syphilitic disease of the heart is known to be present, treatment should be directed primarily at the heart condition, and the underlying syphilis may be treated secondarily and with great caution.

HEART CHANGES IN TOXIC THYROID

In the cases known as toxic thyroid, or exophthalmic goiter, or more popularly known by the misleading name "inward goiter," there is an oversecretion of thyroid material or a secretion which is in some way abnormal.

In these cases there is almost invariably one symptom referable to the heart: the rapid pulse rate. Occasionally there may be an abnormal rhythm, or some shortness of breath, or even pain. The presence of a definite increase in the metabolic rate will confirm the diagnosis.

Such symptoms subside when the abnormal condition of the gland is remedied, by operation or use of new drugs like propylthiouracil or similar agents which control excessive action of the thyroid. Iodine is useful now, as it has always been. In some cases there is some degree of permanent damage, but this is rarely serious and can usually be readily cared for. An abnormal rhythm, such as auricular fibrillation, may be present in cases which have remained untreated for some time. If the rate is too rapid, it can be readily controlled by digitalis, under the advice and direction of a physician.

ANGINA PECTORIS AND CORONARY OCCLUSION

The heart muscle is supplied with the blood necessary for its activity by means of blood vessels which run through the heart itself, dividing and subdividing finally in small capillaries in close contact with each muscle fibre. They bring to the heart muscle material for repair, fuel to furnish energy and oxygen to burn the fuel. They carry away the waste and the results of combustion. They are essential for the life and the activity of the heart muscle.

These arteries have their origin in the aorta, the large vessel leading from the heart, at its beginning, just as it leaves the left ventricle or left chamber of the heart, and just above the valves which separate the aorta from the ventricle. Hence the flow into these arteries will depend upon the pressure in the aorta, at their origin.

The coronary flow is a very perfect mechanism, and an excellent example of the "wisdom of the body." It works constantly all through our lives, supplying the heart muscle according to its needs, with more blood or less, as the occasion demands. Any condition which interferes with the coronary flow, or tends to make it inadequate, may shorten life or result in incapacity.

Some people, very few indeed, are born with a coronary blood supply which is insufficient. They may do very well until the artery walls in middle life change and become narrowed. When this does happen, these patients may have symptoms of coronary insufficiency. On the other hand, these patients may lead a perfectly normal life and die of old age.

In some patients the coronary vessel walls are constricted by the inflammation of the wall which accompanies rheumatic fever, and symptoms of deficient circulation to the heart muscle appear in later life. Other more rare diseases may have a similar effect.

In all of us changes in the coronary vessels occur as we grow older. These may be of very minor importance, or of very great importance. It is interesting, in this connection, to observe how many people live to a ripe old age, with no symptoms at all, even though they may have very hard arteries indeed. Probably "hardened arteries" receive more attention than they deserve. So called "hardening of the arteries" begins early in life in everyone, and should never alarm us too much.

Nature, too, has provided a safeguard by increasing the connections between the different arteries as we grow older, so that if the flow in one artery in one locality is insufficient, blood may be detoured to it through other highways.

A deficient blood supply to the heart muscle results in definite symptoms, the severity and duration of which depend upon just how seriously the blood supply is interfered with and upon what is interfering with it. When a muscle anywhere in the body is obliged to contract when it does not have a blood supply sufficient for its needs, pain results. The same thing occurs in the heart muscle when it is forced to work with an insufficient blood supply. In addition, it may not be able to do its work adequately, and shortness of breath may result, or even what we refer to as heart failure.

ANGINA PECTORIS

One of the most frequent and best known episodes resulting from an inadequate blood supply is referred to as angina pectoris. In angina pectoris symptoms are of short duration, because the blood supply is only temporarily diminished, or because it is insufficient for the work of the heart just at that time, as when some extra demand is made on the heart. Such a decrease in the blood supply of the heart might be due to a temporary and transient narrowing of the vessels supplying the heart with blood, due to nervous impulses having their origin elsewhere. Since the flow through these arteries rises and falls with the blood pressure in the aorta, a fall in blood pressure, as occurs during sleep, or as occurs during the day from many causes, might decrease the flow to a point at which it would cause pain. This is particularly the case in a heart whose arteries show the hardening which comes with age, but would probably not cause any symptoms in a more normal heart. Whatever may cause the temporary decrease in the flow of blood in the vessels of the heart itself, it is this decrease and the consequent transient inadequacy of the blood supply to the heart which causes the symptoms.

Pain is the one most important symptom in angina pectoris. The pain is usually under the breast bone, and more frequently under the upper portion of the breast bone, or just to the left of the upper portion. It may remain in that region, or it may radiate to the shoulder, or down the left arm, perhaps only as far as the elbow, or the wrist, or it may extend to the tips of the fingers. Occasionally it may radiate to the right shoulder and down the right arm, or it may radiate to both shoulders, and down both arms. In other persons it may radiate to the left side of the neck or be referred to the lower back teeth. In others it may radiate to the pit of the stomach and be considered as having its origin in the stomach, or it may be felt just below the ribs on the right side. Frequently the pain may never be felt in the chest at all, and be felt only at the points to which it may radiate, as the left shoulder, the elbow, or the little and the ring finger, or the left lower jaw, or the pit of the stomach. The pain is often severe and agonizing, but it is not necessarily so, and may be mild.

Except for these symptoms, associated or appearing singly, there is nothing which characterizes an attack, except that it is of short duration, a matter of seconds or minutes. Attacks lasting hours, or with other symptoms, are not merely angina pectoris.

There are no certain signs which enable the physician to recognize the presence of an attack or to judge of the probability of the future occurrence of such an attack. Nothing characteristic can be found by examination of the heart, or the pulse or blood pressure, or by laboratory methods. The physician must be guided altogether by the story of the attack and such characteristics as the patient tells him.

Attacks are most frequently brought on by exertion. In some persons they are brought on by moderate exertion at any time; in others by moderate exertion only under certain conditions; and in others the attacks may accompany only unusual exertion. Attacks are especially apt to accompany exertion soon after a meal. With an empty stomach a man may be able to walk briskly for a long distance without distress and find himself unable to walk a hundred feet after a meal without symptoms of pain. In some the attacks may follow exertion after any meal, or may follow especially some one meal, as in the evening or in the morning. Attacks are likely to follow a meal which is too hastily eaten, or one which is indigestible, or too full a meal, or one eaten when too tired.

For these reasons, it is best not to eat when tired, nor to eat heavily at any time. It is well to take a rest period before and after each meal and to eat leisurely. The diet should be chosen so as to avoid those foods which are indigestible or which in the patient's experience cause gas.

Anginal pain may occur almost equally easily on an empty stomach. In addition to oxygen the heart muscle also needs sugar to burn with the oxygen. Too low a blood sugar, or exertion with too low a blood sugar, may cause typical anginal pain. This condition may occur with a poorly proportioned diet, or too much insulin, etc. It is a matter of careful consideration by your physician.

A reflex narrowing of the coronary vessels due to impulses arising from various sources may occur. One very frequent such reflex is that resulting from breathing cold air through the nose or walking against a cold wind. This can readily be obviated by holding a muffler over the nose and breathing warm air through the mouth.

Other sources of such reflex effects are gall stones or stomach disorders, duodenal ulcers, diverticula of the duodenum or of the esophagus. A fairly frequent cause is a hiatus hernia, where the stomach pushes up through the opening through which the esophagus descends to the stomach. Just too full a stomach, or an indigestible meal, may be a cause, or an abdomen distended with gas.

Exertion does not necessarily bring on an attack. An attack may come when sitting quietly, especially after a meal. An attack may occur in the early morning hours in the midst of a normal sleep.

Attacks are more frequent in the emotionally and nervously unstable. Any emotion may bring on an attack, but especially anger, grief, or worry. Attacks are more frequent also in the presence of fatigue, and especially of nervous or mental fatigue. While angina pectoris may occur in people in any walk of life,

---

it is much more common in those whose work demands an undue proportion of strain and energy and worry, and who are obliged to do their work under tension, or, what is especially true, those who are so constituted that they do any work under tension, and with an undue amount of nervous energy. This is probably one reason why angina pectoris is more frequent in cities and why it is much less frequent in the more leisurely tropics.

Angina pectoris is by no means the hopeless disease which is often pictured. It may be serious, but it is possible in many cases for patients to go on for years with recurring attacks, or the attacks may cease to occur and the patient lead a normal life with only moderate restrictions, living within his physicial means. Sources of reflex irritation should be overcome. Patients with angina pectoris usually know about how far they can go without bringing on an attack, and they should conduct their lives accordingly. They should keep in touch with their physician and report at regular intervals. It is possible, also, that the physician may wish occasional electrocardiographic tracings made to confirm his observations. If an attack occurs which is different from those usually experienced, which is more painful, or lasts longer, the patient should get to his home with just as little effort as possible and as soon as possible, and have his family physician called immediately.

CORONARY OCCLUSION

In occlusion of one of the branches of the coronary artery, as well as what is referred to as acute coronary insufficiency, the pain is identical with that of angina pectoris and occurs for the same reason. In angina pectoris there is only a temporary disproportion between the blood supply to the heart muscle and its needs for blood. The pain usually quickly passes away, and no damage to the heart muscle results from the isolated attack. Oft-repeated attacks may eventually cause permanent damage. In coronary occlusion one of the branches of the coronary artery is occluded, just as the term suggests. Whatever the occlusion is due to, the area of muscle supplied by that particular branch is deprived of blood for a length of time sufficient to do serious damage to the muscular wall of the heart, and weeks of time and rest are necessary for the body to make sufficient repairs.

In what is referred to as acute coronary insufficiency an area of the heart muscle is again deprived of its blood supply for a length of time sufficient to do serious damage, although here an actual obstruction of one particular vessel is not seen. The results may not be as serious as when one branch is actually occluded. The differentiation between the two incidents is not defined clearly enough, however, to warrant drawing a conclusion in any one case as regards future outlook or treatment. They should be treated alike.

1146

A patient with coronary occlusion or coronary insufficiency is best cared for in a hospital, where laboratory methods are available to confirm the diagnosis and to check on progress toward recovery. Electrocardiographic tracings are almost always diagnostic, but their absence or lack of characteristic findings should not outweigh the clinical evidence. Oxygen and other emergency agents are always at hand in the hospital, as well as trained observers.

DISORDERED ACTION OF THE HEART

In a large group of cases, especially in early life, there are symptoms regarded often as due to the heart and variously referred to as disordered action of the heart, neurocirculatory asthenia, and, most apt of all, "effort syndrome." In these cases the heart and the circulatory system are perfectly normal structurally. What is abnormal is the automatic nervous mechanism controlling the heart and controlling all of the activities of the body. This automatic nervous system temporarily responds to smaller stimuli than normal, and when it does respond, overresponds. An exertion which would make the pulse of a normal individual beat only a little more rapidly than normal causes the pulse of such a person to beat exceedingly rapidly. An exertion which would hardly affect the rate of breathing in a normal person would cause rapid breathing in such a person.

During sleep, or when resting quietly or unobserved, the pulse and the respiration are normal. On exertion, and in some cases on slight exertion, the pulse becomes rapid, and there is severe shortness of breath. The hands and feet may appear blue. The hands are cold and wet, even in a warm room. Such patients often complain of what they refer to as dizziness; this is not a real dizziness, when there is a sense of rapid rotation, but is rather a giddiness, a sense of unsteadiness; surrounding objects may appear to sway or turn slowly. Fainting attacks are frequent among such patients and rare in actual cases of heart disease. Some of these patients complain of pain in the heart region.

When they are examined, the heart is always normal in size and normal in every determinable way. If it is not normal, the case does not belong to this group. To add to the difficulties, what is called a heart murmur is often heard. It is the kind of murmur which, although it is heard in heart disease, is also heard in normal hearts, and is not of significance in a heart of normal size. In those belonging to this group, the murmur is rarely constant. It may be heard at one time and a few moments later may have completely disappeared.

Such patients often complain of various other symptoms, which are on a nervous basis. They will in addition show a lack of initiative, an unwillingness to go about their normal duties, and be subject to worry, and fear, and apprehension. Others may lead a normal life, be energetic in their work, but still show the symptoms referable to the heart.

There is always a certain proportion of such people in any population. They are frequently classified as having real heart disease or as having thyroid disease, or early tuberculosis, or as being simply neurotic. Such hearts have been a source of disability in every war, for many decades past.

In the army a period of rest and recreation usually restored the soldier to normal. Of the large number who showed the symptoms on entrance into the army from civil life, or who developed the symptoms in the army, more than half were restored to normal in camps where they were given special care and put on gradually increased exercise.

Care should be taken that there is no underlying minor infection in such cases. An adequate period for convalescence should always be allowed after illness or even a minor operation. When these symptoms are present, rest, recreation, exercise increased gradually and carefully, and attention to the general health should restore the patient to normal.

IRREGULARITIES OF THE PULSE

Some irregularities of the pulse beat are quite normal; others may be significant of conditions which demand the physician's advice. In youth, and again in later life, there is a slowing of the pulse in breathing out, and a quickening in breathing in, which is normal. Sometimes the alternating change in rate may be noticeable. It is never of any significance.

In many people over forty years of age, an irregularity which may frequently attract attention is really an extra beat of the heart coming before the anticipated time, but the long pause following the beat makes it appear as though a beat had been dropped. It is usually described by the patient as a feeling of the "heart flopping over." It is more noticeable with fatigue, or with indigestion, or after too hearty a meal. It often appears with worry or apprehension. The irregularity tends to disappear on exertion and then is more noticeable during the rest which follows exertion. This irregularity is usually of no significance in itself, but is a matter for the physician to decide.

Attacks of rapid heart action coming on instantly, and stopping just as suddenly, occur in some people. They rarely last more than a few seconds or minutes, but they may persist for longer periods. They usually begin in early life. They are inconvenient and troublesome, but not serious. Such paroxysmal attacks occurring later in life may be of real significance, and a physician should be consulted at once.

Another form of irregularity occurs, especially in those who have had a rheumatic infection of the heart, but may accompany other conditions, such as toxic thyroid. In this, the pulse is absolutely irregular in both rate and volume and is more irregular on exertion and more quiet at rest. Because of the usually rapid rate, the ventricle of the heart does not have sufficient time in which to fill at each beat; hence the volume of blood pumped by the heart is less, and is insufficient for the needs of the body. The patient may be short of breath and the limbs may swell.

This condition and the rapid heart rate can always be controlled by digitalis or similar drugs, and may be adequately controlled for an indefinite period of time. This should always be under the guidance of a physician, but the physician should also teach the patient just how to adjust the dosage to meet changing needs. If too little is used, the heart will beat too rapidly, and the volume pumped will be insufficient. If too much is used, there may not be enough beats per minute, and the volume of each beat may be too small, because the drug also tends to make the chamber of the ventricle smaller. The patient cannot have the doctor at his elbow every minute, and the doctor must teach the patient just how to use the drug. Paroxysmal attacks of fibrillation coming on early in life may be of short duration and will go away of themselves, without medication.

Accidental injuries to the heart are often overlooked, because there may be little in the way of symptoms and signs at first, and because the possibility of injury is not considered as often as it should be. Traumatic injury to the heart may result from a variety of chest injuries. By far the most frequent cases occur as the result of motor accidents, and especially steering wheel accidents where the chest is thrown violently against the steering wheel. When ribs are broken or there are bruises and obvious signs of injury, it is not so apt to be overlooked, although even then it may be. However it is possible for the breastbone to be pushed clear back against the spinal column without any fracture of the ribs or breastbone or any bruising of the skin. While this is most apt to occur in youth, it may occur in adult or middle life or later. In such cases the heart can not very well escape damage.

There may be bleeding into the pericardial sac or actual bruising of the heart muscle. There may be hemorrhages beneath the lining membrane or interior of the heart. There may be no evidence of these hemorrhages at first, but they initiate a necrosis of the heart muscle and a rupture of the heart wall days or weeks later.

After such injuries there may be immediate shock with obvious signs of heart damage. In some cases the symptoms may be very slight or none and the injured person protests that he is quite unhurt. Between these two extremes, there is every possible gradation. The symptoms may remain slight, or they may progress to severe symptoms and death. No matter how mild the immediate symptoms may be the heart should be considered one of potential damage, and watched and investigated. In an English hospital seventy-five cases of chest injury had electrocardiographic tracings made, and twenty showed heart damage. Of the twenty, two died, and one suffered some permanent heart damage.

CARDIAC INSUFFICIENCY

When the heart is unable to fulfill its function adequately as a pump, supply sufficient circulation to all of the tissues of the body, such symptoms as shortness of breath, or swelling of the limbs, or swelling of the abdomen may result. Such conditions always, in every case, demand the advice and the care of a physician at once.

SURGERY OF THE HEART

Among the greatest advances in modern medicine are the applications of surgical techniques to correcting deficiencies of the heart, either congenital or acquired. Operations are done to re-route the circulation, to widen large blood vessels like the aorta, to transplant blood vessels from blood vessel banks, to stimulate formation of new blood supply to the heart, and to open constricted valves of the heart. Such procedures are carried out only in hospitals by experienced surgeons with all the special equipment and facilities necessary.

HEART BLOCK When the heart is damaged by disease so that the muscular interconnection between the auricles and ventricles (the upper and lower portions of the heart) is interrupted they will beat independently of each other, and the condition is called heart block. As a result the beat of the heart becomes slowed and occurs in paroxysms or spasms.

HEART DISEASE, SURVIVAL AND REHABILITATION AFTER Dr. Master and his associates in the Cardiographic Laboratory of the Mount Sinai Hospital, New York, followed up 500 patients who had survived a coronary occlusion for from 1 to 29 years. Two out of every five patients had made a complete functional recovery. Three-fourths of all the patients were working and more than half of them had already lived more than five years after the attack. One out of every five patients survived the attack for more than 10 years. Death usually occurred as a result of another coronary occlusion or of congestive heart-failure.

Dr. Master emphasizes that the most reliable measure of recovery after coronary occlusion is the absence of symptoms related to the heart. When the physical examination, electrocardiogram, heart size and cardiac pulsuation are normal, according to his observations, the patient has almost always made an excellent recovery. Important is the observation that the site of the infarction does not affect the prognosis after occlusion of a coronary vessel. The prognosis is better in younger patients, but on the whole the patient and the physician may be optimistic about the prognosis in coronary occlusion. Statistical studies have established that the majority of patients survive for many years and lead productive lives and those patients who return to work do at least as well as those who retire.

HEART FAILURE (See also discussion under *Angina Pectoris, Arteriosclerosis, Ballistocardiography, Bee Stings, Blood Pressure, High, Cardiac and Coronary, Cathode-Ray Oscilloscope, Climate, Coronary Thrombosis, Cyanosis, Delirium Tremens, Diamox, Digitalis, Electrocardiograph, Embolism, Fibrillation, Heart, Obesity, Pericarditis, Pulse, Rheumatic Fever, Surgery of the Heart, Uremia*) When the heart fails to carry on its work, the rhythm of the heart changes, the beat may become more rapid, the sounds of the heart as they are heard by the doctor with his stethoscope will change, the pulse becomes irregular and shortness of breath occurs at night and on exertion. With all of this may come swelling of the body due to accumulation of fluid. When the right ventricle or pumping chamber of the heart fails, the veins and neck become swollen, the liver becomes swollen, often painful and tender, and much fluid accumulates. Formerly such conditions were viewed askance by physicians and the future was dubious. Today patients with failure live much longer than they used to and they are kept comfortable by the proper use of the many new methods that have been discovered. The original digitalis has been supplemented by a wide variety of more active and dependable preparations although many physicians still depend on the early preparations. Lately drugs have been developed which depend upon mercury as their chief ingredient which has the power of causing the elimination of fluid. However, the most recent discovery is a drug called "diamox" which acts to inhibit the prevention of flow through the kidney by an enzyme. "Diamox" has proved to be a veritable blessing for patients with this condition because it does not have some of the side effects of the mercurial drugs.

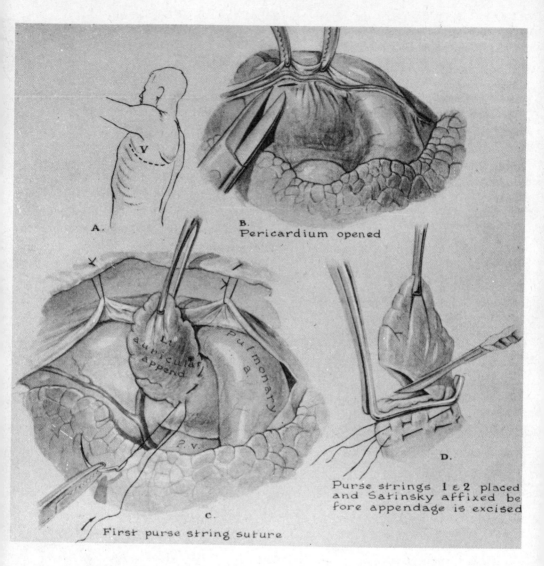

A.

B.
Pericardium opened

C.
First purse string suture

Lt. auricular append.

Pulmonary a.

? v.

D.

Purse strings 1 & 2 placed and Satinsky affixed before appendage is excised

Blood from the lungs goes to the left auricle of the heart and passes to the left ventricle through the mitral valve. This valve prevents the return of blood to the auricle. Growths or disease in the valve reduce the size of the opening and interfere with blood flow from the auricle to ventricle. Surgical technic used to repair this valve is called commissurotomy. The dotted line in drawing A indicates where the incision will be made. Draw-

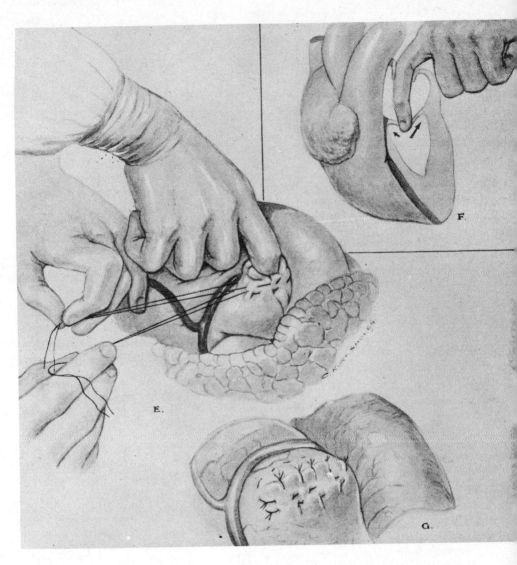

E.

F.

G.

ings B, C and D show cutting into the tissue covering the heart (pericardium) and the auricular appendage. E and F show the finger in the auricular chamber and making contact with the mitral valve. Purse string sutures are pulled around the finger to prevent loss of blood. Arrows in F show the directions of force applied to widen the valve. The operation is complete and wound closed (G).

Postgraduate Medicine

Finally, the accumulation of fluid can be controlled to some extent by restricting the total amount taken in the diet and a wide campaign of education in this regard has brought successful results. In one great city a restaurant was established which specialized in providing low sodium diets for patients who needed them.

The rate of the heart has been controlled in many ways. Sometimes when there are premature beats or double beats or fluttering of the heart, drugs such as quinidine or digitalis act successfully in eliminating the symptoms and in quieting the apprehension.

Mention should also be made of the widespread use of oxygen for persons with varieties of heart disturbances. The serious shortness of breath and the apprehension which ensue in heart attacks are controlled by the administration of oxygen; nowadays this is almost routine.

HEART, SURGERY OF THE (See also *Open Heart Surgery, Surgery in Pulmonic Stenosis, Cathode-Ray Oscilloscope*) Some years have passed since the treatment of blue babies born with congenitally damaged hearts by surgical operations which changed the nature of the circulation were announced and established. Already thousands of such operations have been done with great success in the vast majority. Mention has also been made of the operations for widening constricted valves of the heart in which case the heart itself is opened and the physician either with a finger or with a blade on the end of a finger cuts or breaks the valve and increases the flow of blood through it.

More recently artificial pumps have been invented so that the blood can bypass the heart or even bypass both the heart and the lungs, with the idea of doing intricate operations, the circulation being carried on outside the body by such mechanical devices. Many cases have now been reported in which this has been done successfully.

Several operations have been devised to bring new blood supply to the heart by operations which stimulate the formation of new blood vessels in the heart or which transfer by an attachment to the heart tissues which contain a fresh blood supply. In some operations talcum powder has been sprinkled on the heart to roughen its surface and to cause adhesions which will bring in new blood. One surgeon has operated on 23 cases in which a plastic valvular ball was introduced into the heart for severe insufficiency of the aortic valve. This served to control the blood pressure in the legs and resulted in reduction of the size of the heart in a number of the patients who were subjected to this operation. In some instances, the partition which separates the various chambers of the heart does not close completely which means that the pressure of the circulation is not maintained. In order to correct such deficiencies, operations have been done to mend the septum and in at least one case done by Gibbon of Philadelphia, using an artificial pump to bypass the heart, the operation was a success.

Special mention must be made also of the establishment of blood vessel banks in various large cities from which tissues may be obtained to repair large blood vessels. This has been done particularly in the cases of aneurisms or weak places in the wall of the aorta. The operation is now recognized as desirable and successful because of the excellent progress that has been made particularly through the work of such leading surgeons as Ochsner and DeBakey.

An amazing accomplishment in the field of heart surgery was the repair of congenital anomalies of the heart of various kinds by Lillihei of the University of Minnesota. This was accomplished by isolating the heart of the patient from the general circulation; then a donor supplied blood from his own heart to keep both himself and the patient alive during the operation. In order to carry out this procedure, the blood of the patient and that of the donor are matched carefully so that reactions do not occur from the mixing of the circulation.

HEAT SICKNESS (See also *Sun-* and *Heat Stroke*) Workers at glass and metal furnaces, rolling mills and open pit mines, women in laundries, and bakers may be overcome by heat, owing not only to the summer season but also to fatigue.

A few salt tablets taken during the day help to prevent heat stroke. These tablets replenish the salt lost from the body by excessive sweating. Loss of salt is not, however, the only factor in heat stroke.

In summer, workers need a diet low in fat. They should take plenty of water. If they wish, they may take fresh fruit juices, milk, or carbonated drinks to keep up the water supply. Although beer and ale are permissible in small quantities, drinks high in alcohol content are likely to increase the possibility of heat stroke. Small amounts of fluid taken frequently are better than a large amount taken at one time. Ice-cold drinks should always be consumed slowly.

Among foods not easily digested in hot weather are fried foods, heavily spiced foods, and material that is thick with fiber.

Short periods of recreation between the hours of work are especially important during the hot season. A cool shower or tub bath before going to work and after coming home will do much to minimize effects of a job in an overheated plant.

Most plants provide workers with salt tablets of five grains each, which they may take as needed. Two tablets every two hours are plenty for the purpose.

Here are good rules for health during the hot season:

Wear cool clothes—loose and light-weight.

Eat "light" food—fruits, vegetables, and milk. Do not overeat.

Drink cool water—iced drinks in moderation.

Avoid exposure to the sun in the middle of a hot summer day.

Avoid strenuous exercise on a hot day.

Wear a helmet or hat of a porous material when working in the sun.

HEIGHT The impression is increasingly prevalent that boys and girls are growing taller than they used to be. Nevertheless, the records of the Selective Service indicate that the average height of the American boy over twenty-one years of age was just about the same during the Civil War, World War I, and during World War II.

Children do not grow constantly from birth to maturity at an even rate. Like plants, they grow more during some seasons and less during others. The rate of growth of a child is influenced by the weather, sunlight, exercise, diet, and particularly by the actions of his glands.

There is in the pituitary gland a secretion known as the growth hormone, which definitely controls growth. There are also glandular materials coming from the parathyroid glands which are related to this activity.

For years there has been a belief that the boys in California grow bigger than boys elsewhere in the nation. Coaches of football and track athletics, and particularly of basketball teams, assert that the boys who come from California with the teams are much taller and stronger. However, in 1944 the tallest boys on basketball teams came from Oklahoma. Nevertheless, a study made on children in California revealed the fact that the Los Angeles children are on an average over an inch taller than children from San Francisco and from Oakland. In attempting to account for a superiority in height of children from one section of the country as compared with those from another, the environment is given chief credit. The items in environment especially emphasized are increased sunshine, greater variety in diet, including many fresh vegetables and fruits, and more hours of outside play. Incidentally, however, there has also been for some time consistent drill in posture of children who attend the Los Angeles schools. To some extent the improvement in posture is reflected in the increased height.

When there is overactivity of the pituitary gland, there is a tendency to acromegaly and giantism. When there is underactivity of the anterior lobe of the pituitary gland, dwarfism results. The glandular principles, given sufficiently early in life, can definitely affect height. Unfortunately, once a person has attained adult age, there is nothing that can be done to increase height. Occasionally advertisements appear of strange devices which are supposed to bring about stretching or in other ways extend the length of the human body. There is no scientific evidence to indicate that any of these can accomplish the purpose for which they are sold. About all that can be done is to practice good posture and then to supplement the height by raised heels and similar means.

HEIGHT—height at various ages: See DIET, article ADVICE ON THE DIET.

HELIOTHERAPY The use of the sun's rays to treat disease is called heliotherapy. This may be either by the natural sun or by the use of artificial ultraviolet rays. Treatment with light generally is called phototherapy. One form of this can be the infrared therapy which is the use of the heat rays from the sun or artificial heat rays.

HEMATURIA Abnormally the urine contains blood. In a small percentage of cases the source of this blood cannot be determined, but in the majority the doctor is able, by a careful examination, to find out the source of the bleeding.

For about 2 per cent of all cases bleeding in the urine is said to be of unknown origin. In such cases the blood appears spontaneously and without any pain. Seldom is it sufficient in amount to lead to a state of anemia or to faintness. In many instances such blood appears to have oozed from a varicose vein somewhere along the urinary tract. The condition is usually found in people less than thirty years old.

Other causes of blood in the urine are related to the portion of the urinary tract through which the urine passes. Urine is developed in the kidney and passes down a long tube known as the ureter to the bladder. Here it is collected and at intervals passes out of the body along another tube that is known as the urethra. A severe infection, inflammation, or congestion of the kidneys can cause some red blood cells to escape into the urine. A tumor that breaks through the blood vessels can do this. Certain chemicals like turpentine, cantharides, and carbonic acid can so damage the tissues that blood will appear in the urine. Occasionally the sulfonamide drugs act on the kidneys of some people and cause blood to appear in the urine.

Not infrequently a stone, by its irritation and damage to the walls of the tissues in the urinary tract, can cause the appearance of blood. A rupture or breaking of the kidney, the bladder, or the tubes that have been mentioned, due to any cause, is followed by the appearance of blood in the urine.

Instances are known in which exhausting physical exercise or exposure to cold have been followed by the temporary appearance of a few red blood cells in the urine without any evidence of great damage to the kidney.

There are cases of blood diseases like hemophilia and thrombocytopenia or purpura—easy bruising—in which blood passing from the body by way of the urine is not an infrequent sign.

When the doctor is called on to determine the nature of such disturbances, he is likely to make certain, first, that blood actually is present, and, second, the spot from which the blood is coming. This he can do by a number of observations, including the nature of the coloring material and the state in which it appears. Certainty, however, is brought about by those methods which involve the passing of a tube into the bladder and from the bladder into the ureter so as to determine exactly the point from which the blood emanates.

Incidentally, children occasionally pass urine which is bright red because of eating too many beets containing red pigment.

Whenever blood is found in the urine in any amount, it is desirable that the person get to bed at once and that the physician determine as soon as possible what is wrong. Uncontrolled or continuous bleeding invariably threatens life itself.

HEMOGLOBIN The portion of the red blood corpuscles that carries oxygen is the red pigment. This is called hemoglobin. The amount of hemoglobin is measured in order to determine whether or not the blood is normal as relates to this constituent. Usually nor-

mal is called 100 per cent. Modern scientific measurements determine the hemoglobin by weight in relationship to a definite volume of blood. Various devices have been invented for measuring the hemoglobin. When the red blood coloring matter appears in the urine, the condition is called hemoglobinuria.

HEMOGLOBIN—See BLOOD, article THE BLOOD AND ITS DISEASES.

HEMOPHILIA Among the most dramatic of the diseases that affect mankind is hemophilia. This is the disease that affects the royal families of Spain and of Russia—a condition with a peculiar hereditary basis, limited to the males of the family but transmitted by the females.

In hemophilia the clotting time of the blood is much prolonged; the person with this condition may bleed to death because means have not been found to cause the blood to clot successfully. In these cases the number of red blood cells and white blood cells is usually normal at the beginning of the bleeding. The condition is distinguished from purpura by the fact that the blood platelets are not diminished as they are in purpura. In fact they are sometimes increased over the normal in response to the bleeding that occurs. Hence in hemophilia some other element in the blood-clotting process is missing rather than the platelets.

Innumerable investigations have been made in the attempt to find out what happens in the blood of a person who is hemophilic. The defective coagulation in some cases may be due to difficulty in the formation of the blood-clotting element called thrombin, but the cause for the deficiency in this element has not yet been determined. Another element in the blood called antithrombin may interfere with the clotting, and an excessive amount of this substance may be responsible.

The chief symptom in hemophilia is the bleeding. Bleeding frequently follows an injury which would not cause bleeding in a normal person. Cases are known in which the pulling of a tooth, a scratch with a needle, or a slight nosebleed has progressed to a hemorrhage which resulted in death.

The person with hemophilia will have bruises under the skin, with the formation of large masses of blood, but will not have spots of the type that occur in purpura. Occasionally bleeding from a slight injury will occur into a joint— a severe symptom that will cause much distress.

Because of the severe character of this condition and the inability of medical science to control it, children with hemophilia seldom live to adult age. It is almost impossible for the average person to avoid slight bruises or accidents; the hemophiliac is therefore in constant danger of some accident that will cause death.

The most important measure of treatment in cases of hemophilia is to stop the bleeding when it occurs. Many different procedures have been used for this purpose. It is possible to pack a wound with gauze or cotton or to sew it together tightly. Various substances have been discovered which the doctor may apply to the wound in an effort to aid clotting by supplying the missing elements. It is also possible to supply these elements by the transfusion of blood directly into the veins. New research suggests that the missing principle in the blood, responsible for hemophilia, has now been determined.

Investigators have found the specific substance lacking in the blood of hemophiliacs and such preparations can now be injected and will control the bleeding.

New hope for hemophiliac patients came with the introduction of a plasma which has the effect of stopping hemophilia. The plasma is the fluid portion of the blood. The plasma which is useful is so processed as to prevent loss of that component of the plasma which has the ability to control hemophilia. Its administration provides a temporary reduction of the time required for the plasma to coagulate which is long in patients with hemophilia. The new product is administered intravenously. The substance which is derived from ordinary blood is available as a powder. To this substance fluid is added and the solution is injected as the physician finds it needed. A single dose of this antihemophilic plasma will usually maintain the 'normal clotting time for several hours to as long as two days. The dosage required to maintain the person with normal clotting time depends on the extent to which he responds to the treatment. Obviously the method is repeated as often as is necessary to maintain a normal blood clotting time.

HEMOPHILIA—See BLOOD, article THE BLOOD AND ITS DISEASES.

HEMOPHILIA—arthritis: See article ARTHRITIS, RHEUMATISM, AND GOUT.

HEMOPHILIA—nose-bleed: See EAR, article THE EAR, TONGUE, NOSE, AND THROAT.

HEMORRHAGE Bleeding at any time and under any circumstances is a serious symptom. Some people bleed more easily than others. Some people bleed longer than others because the blood does not clot easily. When bleeding is difficult to stop, the condition menaces life itself.

Many factors are concerned in bleeding. The cutting of a blood vessel will result in bleeding that is not easy to stop, particularly if it is a large blood vessel. For the formation of a blood clot, calcium is necessary and also certain materials from the fluid portion of the blood which, with the calcium and with a substance called fibrinogen, make up the product called fibrin. Fibrin is the material of a blood clot.

The blood of a normal person contains materials necessary for forming a blood clot. In abnormal instances some of these materials are absent. This is particularly the case in a condition called hemophilia, also in another condition called thrombocytopenia. People with thrombocytopenia have an insufficient number of blood platelets. They tend to bleed easily and to bruise easily. They bleed particularly from the gums, from the sockets of extracted teeth, from the nose, and occasionally from the internal organs. Hemorrhage into a vital organ, such as the brain, may cause death.

When a doctor finds that a patient bleeds too often and too easily, he will try first to determine the cause. The normal blood contains as many as 200,000 or more blood platelets for every cubic millimeter. However, a fairly good blood clot can occur with as little as 50,000 platelets in each cubic millimeter of blood. When the number is below 50,000, the formation of a good blood clot is less likely to occur.

Every person who bruises easily, who bleeds a long time without forming a blood clot, or who tends to have an insufficient amount of the red blood cells or of the red coloring matter of the blood should have a careful examination to determine the deficiencies that exist and should have treatment to bring the amounts of the deficient materials up to the normal.

When bleeding occurs, regardless of the cause, it is important to stop the hemorrhage. One of the simplest ways to stop bleeding is to put on a pack of sterile gauze and to cover this with a tight bandage. This will control the flow of blood in the majority of wounds. If a large artery of an arm or a leg is cut, a tourniquet may be necessary to stop the flow of blood. When there is bleeding from the socket of a tooth after a tooth has been pulled, the hemorrhage can easily be controlled by plugging the socket with sterile gauze or applying hot water. If the bleeding continues, a doctor or dentist should be called immediately. He will have available various drugs which he can apply directly to the bleeding spot and thus stop the hemorrhage.

In persistent nosebleed the person should be put flat, preferably with the face down. Ice water or hot water may be applied to the nose or the nose may be temporarily packed with sterile gauze. If nosebleeds occur frequently, proper study of the blood and the tissues generally should be made to determine the cause.

Hemorrhage from the skin or from wounds may be prevented by avoiding the sources of injuries that produce hemorrhage. All broken glass, razor blades, or sharp instruments should be carefully put away so that children particularly cannot get at them. Tools with sharp edges should be used with the greatest of care. All sharp knives and other sharp utensils should be kept in a special drawer with the handles pointing in one direction. Among the most frequent causes of cuts on the hands is carelessness in opening cans. The use of a proper can opener will prevent a jagged edge on the can.

HEMORRHAGE—benzene poisoning: See article OCCUPATION AND HEALTH.

HEMORRHAGE—bowel: See article TRANSMISSIBLE DISEASES.

HEMORRHAGE—cerebral: See article DIABETES.

HEMORRHAGE—first aid: See article FIRST AID.

HEMORRHAGE—meant to protect the

individual: See article STRESS AND DISEASE.

HEMORRHAGE—ulcers: See article DIGESTION AND DIGESTIVE DISEASES.

HEMORRHAGE—vitamin K not absorbed: See article DIGESTION AND DIGESTIVE DISEASES.

HEMORRHAGE—vitamin K to prevent: See article DEFICIENCY DISEASES.

HEMORRHOIDS Hemorrhoids, or piles, are actually varicose veins that occur at the lower end of the bowel. Doctors estimate that at least one third of all grown people have hemorrhoids.

Hemorrhoids can be classified into two kinds—external and internal, de-

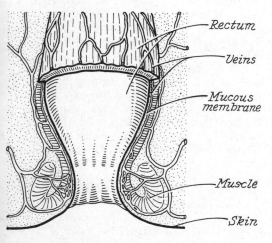

Rectum

Veins

Mucous membrane

Muscle

Skin

Structure of the rectum and anus. The anus is the external opening at the end of the rectum. Strong ring-like muscles surround the anal opening and are able to close it. The rectum is a common site for cancer. Cancer of the rectum may develop in either sex, but the incidence is greater in men.

pending on whether they are inside or outside the muscular ring that closes the lower end of the bowel.

Among the many causes of hemorrhoids are any kind of condition which interferes with the proper flow of blood in these blood vessels. Therefore an extremely sedentary life, the development of overweight, pregnancy, constipation, or the excess use of cathartics may be associated with the appearance of such varicose veins. The most that can be done to prevent the occurrence is the opposite of the things that are associated with the cause. People who are sedentary must get more exercise. Those in whom the circulation is poor should do what can be done to improve the circulation. Overweight is benefited by weight reduction. It is known, however, that many irritant substances, such as vinegar, spices, coffee, and tobacco, help to increase congestion in the blood vessels at the end of the bowel. Also much can be done to prevent the blocking that comes from hardened material in the rectum. The bowel movements may be made regular by practicing good habits, and softness may be encouraged by the use of small amounts of mineral oil.

Hemorrhoids become painful when the blood in a dilated vein becomes clotted. This occurs when the person concerned has been sitting for a long time or when he has been using violent cathartics. There may also be secondary infections in the area where the hemorrhoids are present. Secondary infection with the fungi of the type that cause athlete's foot will produce severe itching. Indeed this itching may become of such torment that people actually scratch and tear their tissues to get relief. The more damage that is done in this way, the more likelihood is there for spread of the infection.

Occasionally hemorrhoids inside the circular muscular ring will be pushed through at the time when the bowels have an action. They are then called protruding hemorrhoids. If these blood vessels are scratched or broken by straining, the dilated veins will bleed until the blood clots. Then the hemorrhoids are called bleeding hemorrhoids. The quacks and the people who sell remedies for treating these conditions have a great deal to say about itching, bleeding, and protruding hemorrhoids. When hemorrhoids get to the point where they are simply intolerable, most people are willing to have them treated by surgical care. There are innumerable ointments, suppositories, and other preparations that can be applied to hemorrhoids to relieve the symptoms that have been mentioned; such relief is, however, frequently only temporary rather than permanent. Surgical control, whether done by the kind of injection that is used for varicose veins elsewhere in the body or by electric coagulation or by removal with the knife, is a matter for special consideration.

HEMORRHOIDS—hypertension may be aggravated by: See article BLOOD PRESSURE.

HEMORRHOIDS—old people: See article OLD AGE.

HEMORRHOIDS—pregnancy: See BIRTH, article CARE OF MOTHERS BEFORE AND AFTER CHILDBIRTH.

PILES—cancer mistaken for: See article DIGESTION AND DIGESTIVE DISEASES.

HEPATITIS, INFECTIONS (See also, *Infections and Immunity*) Infectious hepatitis is an infectious disease caused by a virus. Formerly the condition was simply called jaundice; now we know that catarrhal jaundice is produced by an inflammation of the liver resulting from an attack by the virus which is specific for that disease. Epidemiologists

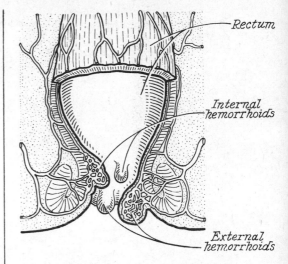

Hemorrhoids, often called "piles," are painful swellings at the anus. Infection or strain weaken and dilate the walls of the veins of the rectum, causing blood clots to form in the vessels or surrounding tissue. The above drawing distinguishes between external and internal hemorrhoids. External hemorrhoids develop in the anal area outside the muscular ring that closes the opening. Internal hemorrhoids form inside the muscular ring, but they may be pushed toward the outside and protrude through the muscle during bowel action.

believe that the virus gets into the human being by two possible routes: 1) by inhaling a droplet from the throat coughed into the air by people who are infected, and 2) by consuming contaminated food or water.

A similar condition called homologous

serum jaundice follows the injection of blood or serum from certain donors who harbor a virus that attacks the liver. This type of jaundice has a longer incubation period than infectious hepatitis—namely, from 50 to 140 days after the tranfusion compared to 25 or 46 days after receiving the virus by the routes previously mentioned.

Since the use of one syringe and a different needle for each person in a series of mass injections has been shown to be involved sometimes in causing homologous serum jaundice, doctors urge the only sure way to prevent this is to provide a heat-sterilized needle and a separate syringe for each person. Usually infectious jaundice causes gastro-intestinal trouble, including nausea and loss of appetite, occasionally with fever, before the jaundice which is characteristic of this condition first appears. Symptoms include some upper abdominal pain on the right side and a loss of appetite associated with nausea. Vomiting and diarrhea occur in about one-fifth of the cases. Occasionally the liver is found to be enlarged and tender.

The jaundice and the symptoms gradually subside in from one to three weeks. When the jaundice has cleared completely and the patient is becoming convalescent, relapses may occur and the jaundice will reappear. Rest in bed is one of the most important treatments. Most of the patients get well and do not have any after-effects; about 90 per cent recover in this way. The number of people who die is exceedingly small, perhaps something like one in every 500 people who are infected with this virus. In one or two per cent of the infected chronic liver damage occurs and these people can be troubled thereafter with hardening and scarring of the liver.

Certain factors seem to predispose people who have infectious hepatitis to having a serious case instead of a mild one. Probably the most important factor is a low state of nutrition. The high mortality observed in outbreaks among native people in such areas as India where famine has been prevalent is not seen in healthy European countries where mortality rates are much less. In undernourished communities, the mortality rate may be fifteen times that among well nourished people. Severe injuries or burns associated with infectious hepatitis make the condition much worse, and pregnancy is reported to increase the risk of serious and permanent damage to the liver. Since malnutrition, injuries, burns and pregnancy all are related to disturbance of the protein metabolism, the massive damage to the liver that occurs when people have diets deficient in protein seem to bear a definite relationship to the severity of infectious hepatitis.

Although various methods of treatment have been tested, no specific chemical substance has been found which is effective against the virus of infectious hepatitis. Rest in bed for as long as the illness persists is one of the most important forms of treatment. When the bile has disappeared from the urine of the patient, he is allowed to leave his bed in order to attend to his toilet. Otherwise he must have complete rest in bed until the enlargement of the liver and the tenderness have disappeared. After infectious hepatitis, return to work must be gradual since the condition leaves the patient seriously exhausted.

Protein is necessary to maintain the integrity and function of the liver. The diet in infectious hepatitis should be rich in protein and carbohydrate but poor in fat. The fats must not, however, be so severely restricted that the food will become unpalatable and the patient will lose his appetite and quit eating. The diets recommended are 150 grams of protein, 350 grams of carbohydrate and 50 grams of fat which provide about 2,500 calories. This is more than ample for a person confined to bed. Since the appetite is weak, the meals are to be small and given at frequent intervals. People who are severely undernourished and who sustain infectious hepatitis may have extra amounts of certain basic amino acids, methionine, cystine or choline which deficiencies seem to enhance the virulence of the virus. British investigators suggest that water-soluble vitamins, particularly ascorbic acid, must be provided in adequate amounts to these patients and also the vitamins of the B complex.

Therefore, in addition to rest and careful supervision of diet, the treatment of infectious hepatitis is applied to control of unpleasant symptoms like constipation, the use of sedatives to insure rest and sleep and other methods of treatment to control nausea and vomiting. If much water is lost by vomiting and diarrhea, the provision of extra fluid is important.

HEPATITIS—See article DIGESTION AND DIGESTIVE DISEASES.

HEPATITIS—diet: See article DIGESTION AND DIGESTIVE DISEASES.

HEREDITARY FACTORS IN OVERWEIGHT (See also, *Glands and their Affect on Weight*) From twin and pedigree studies and from other available information, variations in hereditary factors contribute considerably to variations in weight in man. To what extent they do so and how many pairs of genes are involved are questions which at this stage of the development of the problem cannot be answered in specific terms. The evidence suggests, however, that overweight, at least in some families, is inherited in a relatively simply fashion and that some genes for overweight exist which tend to be dominant over some of those which tend to produce leanness. This means that the children of two lean parents will in most

instances be lean, whereas a majority of the children of two stout parents will tend to grow stout. If only one parent is stout, then about half of the children may be expected to grow stout.

Since hereditary factors quite certainly contribute to overweight in man, how do the involved genes produce their effects? One possible way is for them to produce their effects through the endocrine system, since variations in the secretions of several endocrine glands affect weight. Another possible way is for the responsible genes to produce their effects through variations in the absorption and distribution systems of the body. A further possibility is an effect by way of the nervous system. It would be possible for genes to produce more or less directly a greater appetite in some people than in others or a greater taste for sweet or starchy foods. In this connection the ability to taste different substances is known to have a hereditary basis. One substance called phenyl-thiocarbamide (P.T.C.) tastes bitter to some people, whereas others experience no taste at all. This difference in ability to taste P.T.C. is inherited in a simple fashion. A person who can taste the substance possesses at least one dominant gene called T, whereas a person who cannot taste the substance possesses two recessive genes, tt. Finally, the genes responsible for differences in weight might produce their effect through the nervous system by producing people who differ simply in the delight of eating.

These comments are speculations and not conclusions supported by specific facts. Yet they are suggestions well within the range of ways in which other genes are known to produce an effect.

What can be done to control weight if it does have some hereditary basis? Many persons believe that nothing can be done to modify or control a characteristic which has some hereditary basis.

This is absurd! A characteristic which varies both as a result of variations in heredity and as a result of variations in environment can often be controlled in large measure by controlling the environment. Many cases of overweight in man are the natural consequences of a hereditary predisposition in this direction. However, it is possible to modify or control the development even of such cases.

HEREDITY Our bodies are a reflection of our inheritance from our ancestors. A special branch of science, which deals with the origins of man, the kind of material from which he is constructed, and the effects of his constitution on his life, is known as the science of genetics.

The belief that thoughts held by a prospective mother may induce changes in the body of her child is not borne out by any facts. There is good evidence, however, that the color of the hair and its form—whether curly or straight—the pigmentation of the skin and color of the eyes are characteristics that are inherited to a considerable extent by the child through his father and mother. Tall parents are likely to have tall children, and short parents to have short children. However, each of us is the accumulated result not only of factors coming from the mother and father but also from their mothers and fathers and even further back. Occasionally a child will represent apparently far more of some ancestor two or three generations previous than of the immediate ancestors.

We inherit a type of constitution which seems to make some of us more susceptible than others to certain diseases. People do not inherit tuberculosis. The germ of the disease must be present before it can occur in the human body.

Inheritance in cancer is of the same type. Conditions of marriage among human beings are such, however, that the control of cancer by the control of marriage is hardly feasible. Many an old-time novelist and dramatist created an absorbing plot by presupposing that every family that shamefacedly admitted it included a drunkard had in it a hereditary strain of drunkenness. Modern students of heredity say that there is no proof of the inheritance of a strain of drunkenness. It has been said that fat parents are likely to have fat children because the parents eat too much and the children imitate the parents. Conceivably the tendency to drink alcohol can be begun in much the same manner.

Certain mental characteristics may be inherited, as for example musical memory or memory in general.

What the child inherits is not a series of fixed traits or characteristics but a multitude of substances called genes which interact with each other to produce certain characteristics in the organism. When it is realized that a great variety of such genes enter into combination, it is not at all surprising that several children in one family will differ greatly from one another. The chances in the combinations are tremendous.

Among the constitutional diseases in which heredity seems to play a part, the tendency to allergies or sensitivities to various protein substances should be mentioned. The condition called hemophilia, the tendency to bleed, which was inherited in the royal families of Russia and Spain, is transmitted to the sons of the families by the mothers, who did not themselves suffer from the disease. Some forms of mental defect may be inherited because of the inheritance of the wrong structure of the brain, exactly as high qualities of brain tissue may be inherited. Many a state now has laws which control the propagation of persons who are insane, mentally defective, or possessed of other characteristics which might be passed on to their children.

HEREDITY—diabetes: See article DIA-BETES.

HEREDITY—spherocytosis: See BLOOD, article THE BLOOD AND ITS DISEASES.

HERMAPHRODITISM A hermaphrodite is a person who has or appears to have both male and female characteristics. Modern research shows that these cases vary from cases in which the organs of one side are male and the other female to those in which the sexual organs are predominantly female with some of the characteristics of the male and vice versa. Sometimes the external organs are female and the outer male, and vice versa. Such cases are treated successfully with glandular products, surgery, and psychotherapy combined.

HERNIA The examination of millions for entrance into the United States armed forces has focused attention particularly on rupture as a cause for rejection. A rupture is merely the protrusion of the contents of the abdomen through a weak place in the abdominal wall. There may, however, also be ruptures at other portions of the body, as in the groin or even in the back.

When the tissues underneath the surface force their way through an opening in the body wall a lump appears. Certain portions of the wall of the body are weaker than others. One of the weak spots is in the midline between the large muscles that pass between the breastbone downward toward the groin. Another common spot for a rupture is in the groin itself at the bottom of the abdominal cavity. Still another place for a rupture is in the sex organs.

There are many different causes for ruptures. Sometimes they are present at birth. Frequently the pressure inside the abdominal cavity is increased in an attempt to lift a heavy object. Occasionally an athlete will strain in competition and a rupture will apear. Occasionally ruptures are associated with excessive fat. Sometimes also they occur from failure of the tissues to heal properly after a surgical operation.

Many people who have small ruptures obtain relief by wearing a truss or a support which holds the tissues in place and, if the person concerned is young enough, may give opportunity for healing. However, a hernia or rupture that has been present for a long time is more likely to increase in size, if it is not properly controlled, rather than to heal. As the tissues inside push out more and more, the opening is enlarged, so that eventually the tissues may completely fill the opening. Then the walls of the opening may so constrict or press upon the tissues inside that the blood flow stops. When this occurs, the hernia is said to be strangulated. The stopping of the blood supply to any tissue is exceedingly serious because the tissues will die without a blood supply. Therefore the tissue that is pushed through may become gangrenous or secondarily infected, at which time, of course, the condition threatens life itself.

The treatment of hernia naturally depends on the place where the hernia is located and on the technic decided upon by the doctor. He may wish, although this is rare, merely to push back the material and to apply a support. Such treatment is tried only in very small babies and is seldom recommended in older people. In older people the methods of treatment usually include the permanent wearing of a support, the injection method, or surgery. The decision as to the method to be employed must obviously be made on the basis of the condition that exists in each case.

The injection method aims to produce irritation of the separated tissues so that they will heal together. This method does not have the certainty that is associated with surgical care.

In the surgical method the tissues are observed during operation and the stitching is placed in such a way as to bring about healing. The operative method for the treatment of hernia is exact. The risk is relatively slight, particularly since the operation is often done nowadays without a general anesthetic. If the patient will consent to remain in bed for anywhere from ten to fifteen days so that healing occurs completely, there is little if any chance that the operation will not be completely successful.

Improvement in surgical procedures involves the use of metallic woven material which integrates with the tissues.

An unusual form of hernia is diaphragmatic, with a weak spot in the muscle between the chest and the abdomen.

HERNIA—angina pectoris caused by: See HEART, article DISEASES OF THE HEART AND CIRCULATION.

HERNIA—infants: See INFANCY, article CARE AND FEEDING OF THE CHILD.

HERNIA—intestinal obstruction: See article DIGESTION AND DIGESTIVE DISEASES.

HERNIA—whooping cough: See CHILDHOOD DISEASES, article INFECTIOUS DISEASES OF CHILDHOOD.

RUPTURE—appendicitis: See article DIGESTION AND DIGESTIVE DISEASES.

RUPTURE—spleen: See BLOOD, article THE BLOOD, AND ITS DISEASES.

HERPES SIMPLEX The common name for ordinary herpes is cold sores or fever blisters. Everybody knows what a cold sore looks like. It is usually just an accumulation of blisters, most frequently around the lips. However, any part of the skin may be affected. Fre-

quently cold sores are associated with infectious diseases like pneumonia, malaria, and meningitis. Indeed 40 per cent of all such cases develop fever blisters.

Often a sensation of heat and burning will be followed by the development of a lot of small blisters containing clear serum. Later the small blisters may run together. Then the large blister breaks and a crust forms, followed by healing in a few days.

Another favorite site for fever blisters is the genital area. The possibility of secondary infection in this area is more common and occasionally the blisters may be filled with infected material or blood.

Most experts today believe that cold sores represent a reaction which comes primarily through the nervous system but which may be induced by a variety of causes. Sometimes these causes are physical changes like the rays of the sun, a draft of cold air, or simple rubbing. In other instances an infection may be concerned, as has already been mentioned. The simple cold sores frequently occur in women at the time of menstruation.

Obviously there is little that can be done to prevent cold sores. Fortunately, however, they tend to be self-limited and in most instances should disappear, recurring at intervals. Such danger as they represent is associated with the possibility of secondary infection. There is also, of course, the chance that women particularly will become much too seriously concerned about them and overtreat them, using all sorts of astringent lotions, covering ointments and, even worse, constantly picking off the crusts. The ordinary camphorated ointment or other similar care that the dermatologist prescribes is sufficient in most instances to keep the condition under control until it disappears.

HERPES SIMPLEX—See SKIN, article THE SKIN.

HERPES ZOSTER See *Shingles.*

HICCUPS Way back in the days of Plato, who lived about four hundred years before the Christian Era, a Greek was talking to another Greek who was suffering with hiccups. He said, "Let me advise you to hold your breath, and if this fails, then to gargle with a little water, and if the hiccups still continue, tickle your nose with something and sneeze, and if you sneeze once or twice even the most violent hiccup is sure to go."

Now more than two thousand years have passed and people still treat hiccups first with these measures.

Hiccups are due to a spasm or constriction of the diaphragm, the large muscle that separates the abdominal cavity from the chest cavity. When the diaphragm constricts, the nerve that shuts off the breathing tube from the throat (called the glottis) is closed. Ordinarily the motions of the glottis opening and closing are co-ordinated with the activities of breathing, so that breathing takes place noiselessly. Anything that disturbs the co-ordination can cause a hiccup.

The causes of hiccups include naturally anything that can bring about a failure of co-ordination in the action of the nerves and muscles involved in breathing. A sudden distention of the stomach will disturb the action of the diaphragm and bring on hiccups. An irritation of the center in the brain which is connected by a nerve with the diaphragm can set up a contraction of the diaphragm and hiccups. Trouble along the nerve which controls the diaphragm can also produce hiccups. Finally, hiccups may be associated with nervousness, worry, anxiety, shock, or accidents, since we now recognize the close relationship between the mind and the body and realize the possibility that an emotional cause can be reflected in a physical reaction.

Among the popular treatments for hiccups in addition to coughing, sneezing, swallowing ice, vinegar, or cold water, we include pulling on the tongue, pressing the upper lip with the finger, and breathing into a paper bag so that the breath is reinhaled. The reinhaling of the breath fills the body with carbon dioxide and thus stimulates breathing.

When, however, hiccups persist to the point of exhaustion, more serious remedies must be used. In such cases it may be necessary to try narcotic drugs, to inject potent remedies, to anesthetize the patient, or even to operate.

A new drug called chlorpromazine or Thorazene has been used successfully in treating persistent hiccups.

Since hiccups may have both physical and mental factors study is required to determine just which causes are concerned and to treat the patient accordingly.

Among other technics that occasionally work doctors mention the use of an icebag on the neck, the spraying of ethyl chloride as a refrigerant on the front of the abdomen, slight pressure on the eyeballs, and pressure on the ribs near the place where the diaphragm is fastened.

HICCUPS—first aid: See article FIRST AID.

HIGH BLOOD PRESSURE, SURGERY OF (See also discussion under *Arteriosclerosis, Blood Pressure, High, Goiter, Hypertension, Pituitary*) The surgery of high blood pressure has included particularly the operations on the adrenal glands and the sympathetic nervous system. Formerly operations on the adrenal glands were not even considered but since the discovery of drugs that can supply the adrenal hormones,

the operation is more frequent. Symptoms following removal of the thyroid may sometimes be mitigated by the giving of thyroid extract. The entire role of surgery in the treatment of hypertension is again being re-evaluated because of the discovery of new drugs which are of so much greater value than any medical treatments which were available previously.

HIRSUTISM (See also *Hair, Precocious Hair*) Excessive growth of hair is particularly disturbing to women. The condition is called hirsutism. Investigations have shown that certain glandular disorders may produce this symptom. In some instances women have hair on the upper lip which is annoying when it is dark. Sometimes women have what is the usual masculine distribution of the hair on the body. The commonest places for excessive hair to appear are the upper lip, the cheek, the upper arms, the thighs, the breasts, the skin between the breasts and occasionally over the shoulders. Recent investigation has shown that there is a genetic or familial influence involved in growth of hair and distribution of hair on the body. Attempts have been made to treat excess growth of the hair with various glandular preparations applied either directly to the growth or taken internally and for a while it seemed that this would be the answer. However, many experiments have not been able to establish routine effectiveness with this method. Use of x-rays has not been effective in causing falling of the hair because in the doses that can be given without danger, the results are dubious. Most dermatologists are convinced that electrolysis for the destruction of the hair is the best method but this method is expensive and requires a long time.

HISTAMINE (See also discussion under *Allergy, Antihistamines, Asthma,* *Benadryl, Blood Transfusion, Colds, Hay Fever, Hives, Itching, Psoriasis*) Histamine is a chemical substance that normally is formed in many tissues of the body. In allergic diseases, histamine is released in the body in excessive amounts; for instance, in many eruptions, such as blisters or wheals on the skin, excessive amounts of histamine or substances like histamine are liberated in the skin. In hay fever, excessive histamine is liberated in the membranes of the eyes and nose. The antihistamine drugs of which there are now more than 25 are used in controlling the excessive histamine. These drugs are now available in many combinations with antibiotics and with constrictive preparations and have a tremendous use in the control of allergic conditions.

HIVES The hive is also called a wheal and is a manifestation of a condition that is known technically as urticaria. Abscesses sometimes develop by secondary infection, however. Wheals develop after insect bites, and conditions like hives are associated with poison ivy. A common name for the hives is nettle rash.

Usually hives follow the eating of certain foods to which people are sensitive, like shellfish, pork, nuts, mushrooms, cucumbers, or indeed any one of a variety of foods. Sometimes hives are caused by reactions to light, heat, cold, or scratching, to which a person may be sensitive, the common belief being that these physical conditions bring about changes in the chemistry of the skin so that absorption of certain substances produces the reaction of hives.

Some people have a much more sensitive skin than others. The sensitivity of the skin may be indicated by a phenomenon that the doctors call dermographism, which means simply that it is possible to write on the skin with pressure. Thus the drawing of a pencil point or a fingernail along the skin will be followed by the appearance of an elevated area which, if sufficiently severe, is actually like a hive.

There are many different varieties of urticaria, so that doctors call them acute, chronic, recurrent, or persistent. Sometimes a crop of hives appears and goes away within three or four days, only to be followed by the appearance of new crops. Fortunately most hives tend to disappear in time, but people will scratch them, irritate them, or infect them, so that they may be much more serious than they would be if merely palliated or let alone. If the doctor can find out, with the aid of the person who is affected, the special substance to which the person responds

with hives and then eliminate that from the diet, the hives are kept under control. A new technic is to desensitize the person with gradually increasing doses of the extract of the protein concerned. Particularly useful for hives are the new antihistaminic drugs like pyribenzamine and benadryl. In the treatment of intractable urticaria, Cortisone and ACTH have proved successful.

In very serious cases of hives the symptoms are aided by stopping foods, cleansing the intestinal tract, and using applications directly on the skin of lotions which contain substances that help to control the itching. Most specialists in diseases of the skin prefer lotions to ointments. Some, however, like powders rather than lotions. The

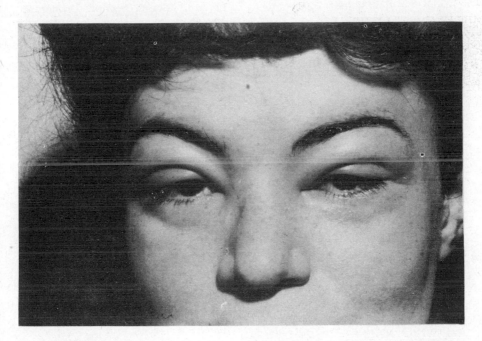

Giant hives of both eyes in a young girl who presents marked dermographism and hives. The wheals seen in a case of hives are caused by an accumulation of fluid in the tissues.

1169

advantage of the powder is the part that it plays in keeping the area dry, while allaying the itching.

Garments that produce much warmth of the skin and perspiration are certainly to be avoided in the presence of hives, since they will tend to increase the amount of the eruption and irritation of the broken blisters.

HIVES—See article ALLERGY; SKIN, article THE SKIN.

HIVES—ACTH: See article ENDOCRINOLOGY.

HIVES—allergy: See SKIN, article THE SKIN.

HIVES—antihistamines: See article ALLERGY.

HIVES—drugs may cause: See SKIN, article THE SKIN.

HIVES—how produced: See article ALLERGY.

HIVES—inhalants may cause: See article ALLERGY.

HIVES—reaction to noxious interpersonal relations: See article STRESS AND DISEASE.

HIVES—skin reaction: See SKIN, article THE SKIN.

HOARSENESS (See also *Laryngitis*) When the human voice suddenly assumes a pitch well below that to which its user has become accustomed, the condition is called hoarseness. Usually such a sign means that the cords in the larynx, or voice box, which vibrate during speaking, have become inflamed. In most instances mere rest and discontinuance of the use of the voice will bring about improvement. However, hoarseness occasionally persists. Continuous hoarseness demands an immediate, direct examination of the vocal cords and of the larynx by a physician who specializes in such conditions. There should, moreover, be a complete physical examination to determine the presence of any constitutional disease.

The vocal cords must come together properly or the voice will not be normal. They must be under proper tension and they must vibrate properly. Therefore any factor that produces swelling and inflammation of the vocal cords may so damage them that they will not work as they should.

Among the dangerous conditions that may interefere with the proper use of the vocal cords are tuberculosis, cancer, and syphilis. However, the most frequent causes are simple infections with the kind of germs that cause sore throat and colds.

Singers who use the voice too freely for long periods of time sometimes develop small nodules on the cords. The result is hoarseness. Means have been found for controlling the development of such singers' nodes. Businessmen frequently complain of hoarseness after long conversations associated with excessive eating, drinking, and smoking. The throats and vocal cords of some people are especially sensitive to various ingredients of tobacco smoking. People with intelligence soon learn to associate attacks of hoarseness with excessive smoking or with other determinable factors. Then if they are really intelligent, they discontinue the exposures.

The voice is also modified by infection in the nose and in the sinuses. Under such circumstances it develops a nasal twang or tone. Frequently treatment of the nose will take care of the condition and at the same time eliminate the continued infection in the vocal cords.

Fortunately the venereal diseases are now being controlled by new remedies like penicillin and terramycin.

Tuberculosis of the throat, if seen early, may be treated not only as tuberculosis elsewhere in the body but also by direct application of ultraviolet rays.

If a cancer of the larynx is seen early, it may be removed early and in many instances may be treated successfully with radium. Already there are many reports of the saving of life when it was threatened by cancer of the larynx. However, the most important single step is early diagnosis so that proper treatment may be administered before the condition can spread too freely.

HOARSENESS—cancer danger signal: See article CANCER.

HOARSENESS—cancer of larynx: See article CANCER.

HOARSENESS—diphtheria: See CHILDHOOD DISEASES, article INFECTIOUS DISEASES OF CHILDHOOD.

HODGKIN'S DISEASE In 1852 an English doctor named Thomas Hodgkin first described a disease in which the lymph glands of the throat, the spleen, and the tonsils become swollen and remain swollen, thus differing from the kind of inflammation that occurs when there is an infection by the ordinary types of germs. Because there are so many other conditions that may cause swelling of the lymph glands, the condition called Hodgkin's disease is sometimes overlooked in its early stages. The cause of Hodgkin's disease is still unknown. The only way that the doctor can be certain that the disease is actually Hodgkin's disease is to take out a piece of the lymph gland and examine it under the microscope. This is not too difficult when the glands are near the surface of the body.

Hodgkin's disease occurs about twice as often in men as in women. Whereas it may develop at any age, the largest number of patients are young adults between the ages of twenty and thirty.

The first symptom of Hodgkin's disease is frequently just a painless enlargement of the gland on one side of the neck. However, this spreads to the other side of the neck and to glands elsewhere in the body. Persistence of the swelling is the vital factor that differentiates Hodgkin's disease from other glandular enlargements.

The average person with Hodgkin's disease lives two or three years after the earliest symptoms are noted, since it is a form of malignant swelling of the lymph glands. In rare cases people have survived for ten to fifteen years. Instances are on record of patients who have lived for seven years and of one patient who lived fifteen years after a positive diagnosis of Hodgkin's disease had been made.

Unfortunately a specific method for treating Hodgkin's disease has not yet been discovered. However, experimentation goes on and new technics are being developed which offer encouragement. At present the methods of treatment most in use include radium and X ray. The irradiation is applied to the enlarged glands, particularly those in the neck. The use of X ray or radium reduces the size of the tumor masses and thus controls much of the discomfort as well as the pain that comes from pressure of the swellings on the nerves. From time to time experiments have been made in the use of vaccines, arsenic, iron, liver extracts, and blood transfusions. Experiments are now being made with the use of what are called radioactive isotopes, and with chemical substances derived from war gases. Aminopterin, which is an anti-folic acid, is also being tried.

HODGKIN'S DISEASE—See BLOOD, article THE BLOOD AND ITS DISEASES; article CANCER.

HODGKIN'S DISEASE—chemotherapy: See article CANCER.

HORMONES Hormones are chemical substances which are produced in some of the organs of the body and then

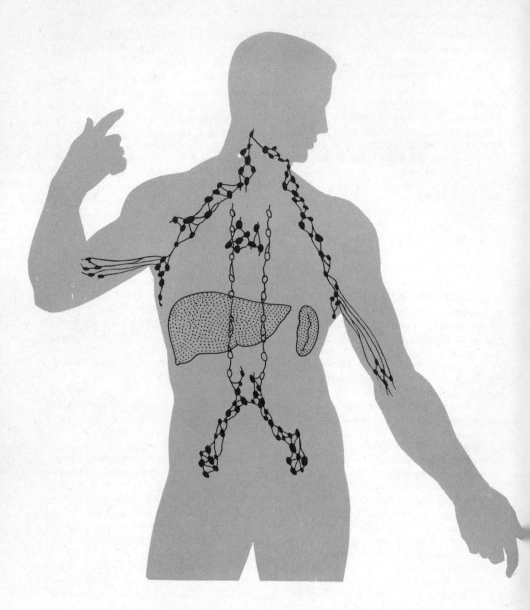

Diagram showing the lymph nodes, liver and spleen which are markedly enlarged in Hodgkin's disease. The enlarged lymph nodes are painless and usually begin in one side of the neck. Enlargement of lymph nodes in the axilla, chest and abdomen follow.

Chas. Pfizer & Co.

transported by the blood to other areas where they produce specific effects. Hormones are secreted by most of the glands of the body.

HORMONES—See article BLOOD PRESSURE. See also entry GLANDS.

HORMONES—acne: See SKIN, article THE SKIN.

HORMONES—adrenal, relation to allergy: See article ALLERGY.

HORMONES—arthritis: See article ARTHRITIS, RHEUMATISM, AND GOUT.

HORMONES—artificially made: See article ENDOCRINOLOGY.

HORMONES—baldness: See HAIR, article THE HAIR.

HORMONES—cancer: See article CANCER.

HORMONES—cold creams: See SKIN, article THE SKIN.

HORMONES—digestive: See article ENDOCRINOLOGY.

HORMONES—endocrine glands produce: See article ENDOCRINOLOGY.

HORMONES—estrogenic: See WOMEN, article HYGIENE OF WOMEN.

HORMONES—gout: See article ARTHRITIS, RHEUMATISM, AND GOUT.

HORMONES—growth: See article ENDOCRINOLOGY.

HORMONES—pituitary gland supplies: See article ENDOCRINOLOGY.

HORMONES—rheumatism: See article ARTHRITIS, RHEUMATISM, AND GOUT.

SEX HORMONES—female: See CHILDHOOD DISEASES, article INFECTIOUS DISEASES OF CHILDHOOD; article CANCER.

SEX HORMONES—male: See WOMEN, article HYGIENE OF WOMEN; SKIN, article THE SKIN.

HYDROCEPHALUS (See *Spina Bifida*) Water on the brain.

HYDROCEPHALUS, SURGERY IN (See also *Spina Bifida*) An amazing surgical procedure has been devised to help children with hydrocephalus (enlarged head caused by accumulation of fluid within the skull). The operation has been performed on 50 infants, mostly between the ages of three and six months. The operation consists of removal of one kidney, usually the left, and placement of one end of a polyethylene tube into the ureter, the duct that carries the urine from the kidney to the bladder. The other end of the tube is placed in the lower portion of the spinal column. Seventeen infants have died, 33 are still living. The investigator reports that satisfactory results have been obtained with 31 of these children. In all, 30 of the children have been followed for more than two years. Only one is mentally retarded to the point of needing institutional care. Five others are slightly behind the normal development schedule, but they are making progress. Twenty-four are said to be in excellent health with normal or nearly normal mental and motor development. Where death occurred, the cause was usually meningitis.

HYGIENE, PERSONAL (See also discussion under *Clothing*) Doctors are often asked to supply a simple set of rules for health. Many years ago at Salerno, Italy, there was a medical school which published a list of rules for health known as the regimen of the school of Salerno. One of the most important lines in that regimen was one which said that three doctors were necessary for health—namely, Dr. Diet, Dr. Merryman, and Dr. Quiet. In other words, proper understanding of food, a good mental attitude, and plenty of rest are the very basis of good hygiene.

One set of rules, developed by Irving Fisher and E. L. Fisk in their book called *How to Live*, gives sixteen important recommendations. They are:

AIR

1. Ventilate every room you occupy.
2. Wear light, loose, and porous clothes.
3. Seek outdoor occupations and recreation.
4. Sleep outdoors if you can.

FOOD

5. Avoid overeating and overweight.
6. Avoid excess of high-protein foods, such as flesh foods, eggs; also excess of salt and highly seasoned foods.
7. Eat some hard, some bulky, some raw foods daily.
8. Eat slowly and taste your food.
9. Use sufficient water internally and externally.

POISONS

10. Secure thorough intestinal elimination more than once daily.
11. Stand, sit, and walk erect.
12. Do not allow poisons and infections to enter the body.
13. Keep the teeth, gums, and tongue clean.

ACTIVITY

14. Work, play, rest, and sleep in moderation.
15. Take deep-breathing exercises several times a day.
16. Keep serene and wholehearted.

Concerning two of these there might be some doubt. Most competent observers of the human body would disagree with No. 10. They would say that the majority of people get along rather well with only one elimination of the bowel daily or perhaps at most two. It was the concept of Fisher and Fisk that repeated eliminations were desirable.

Rule No. 15 suggests that deep-breathing exercises be practiced several times each day. Most experts would consider this a health fad. There is no doubt that thorough ventilation of the lungs is desirable, but ordinary breathing does well for thorough ventilation. Careful studies that have been made on marathon runners have not shown that excessive breathing, in which they must indulge in practice, improves their ability to breathe or improves their "wind" beyond that of people generally.

Dr. Alfred Worcester of the Harvard Medical School emphasized four factors as most important for the health of the aged. These are more warmth, more rest, less strenuous work, and less food.

Finally, the one word on which most emphasis must be placed in personal hygiene is cleanliness. Frequent washing of the hands and a bath at least once daily are now recognized as essential to good health.

Assume that you are in good physical condition and that your doctor has made a complete physical examination and found nothing that needs to be corrected. You probably want to know how to conduct yourself so as to avoid disease in the future. Certain health habits are conducive to the maintenance of good health.

As I have observed people over a good many years, I have found that most of them incline to pick some single point on which to put emphasis in relation to the maintenance of health—exercise, rest, bathing, or diet. From the point of view of good general health with relation to the prevention of infections, most doctors would emphasize cleanliness as the number one point for maintaining health. Cleanliness means more than just bathing. Everyone ought to take a bath, if possible, at least once each day. There are great varieties of baths—hot, cold, warm, steam, carbonated water, and other baths. The moderately warm bath cleanses the body, draws the blood to the surface, increases perspiration, and has a soothing effect. Bathing in very hot water may be dangerous, particularly to persons not in the best of health. A cold bath taken in the morning stimulates the nerve endings in the skin and drives the blood from the surface, to which it returns with a rush when the person emerges from the bath and has a rubdown with a towel. Cold-bath fanatics who submit themselves to exposure unduly with the notion that they will in this manner harden themselves against catching cold are simply indulging in a notion. There is no good evidence that the taking of a cold bath every morning is an effective protection against colds. One way to take a cold bath with a reasonable amount of safety is to fill the tub with water, step in, sit down, immerse the body completely and promptly step out again. A cold bath is preferably taken under a shower.

Baths in which all sorts of materials are placed have little effect, since few materials are absorbed through the skin. The chief value of salt-water bathing is credited to the air, the breeze, the sunlight, and the buffeting of the waves. Sea salt in bags thrown into a tub does not carry with it the sunlight, the buffeting of the waves, the brisk ocean breezes, running and playing on the beach, or the pleasures of conversation with the surrounding company.

Hot vapor baths stimulate excretion of material through the pores of the skin. They are not especially health-inducing for the normal person and should be considered a special bath to be taken only when recommended by the doctor.

All human society may be divided into classes according to bathing habits. The hygienic person bathes daily and sometimes includes a cold bath in the morning and a cleansing warm bath at night. The average person seems to be one who bathes every three days whether he needs it or not. Finally, there are the Saturday-night bathers, who are limited in their conveniences to a galvanized iron tub and the water they can carry in a bucket.

In addition to bathing the body as a whole, good personal hygiene demands some attention to the cleanliness of various special portions of the human body.

Hand-to-mouth infection is one of the most common causes of illness. Many of the early religious bodies incorporated washing of the hands into religious ritual in order to make certain that people would thus protect themselves against the danger of infection. Thorough washing of the hands before eating and after attending to excretion of material from the body is recognized as the most important step in all hygienic practice. Washing of the hands can, of course, be made a fetish, so that people rush to the washroom on the slightest appearance of soiling. More important is the decision, however, to keep the fingers out of the nose, mouth, ears, or other openings into the body. With the minimum amount of washing of the hands, there would be the following: On arising, before and after meals, before and after attending to the excretions of the body, before going to bed and whenever there is exceptional soiling. Finally, the hands should always be washed thoroughly whenever one has been in contact with infection of any kind.

It is customary also to clean the teeth with a brush and a suitable paste, powder, or other material at least twice a day—on arising and before going to bed. Some people, however, find it necessary to give more attention to the teeth than this minimum, particularly those who have artificial dentures or plates. They may find it necessary to practice washing of the teeth and of the artificial dentures on more frequent occasions.

The use of a mouth wash or gargle accomplishes little beyond the actual washing that takes place, so that most physicians are inclined to attach little value to using medicated mouth washes or gargles. Strong solutions should be used on the advice of the physician or dentist only.

The third type of cleanliness to which attention often is called is internal washing of the body such as is brought about through the taking of cathartic substances that cause fluid to be poured into the bowel—the so-called saline cathartics or salts—and the use of enemas for washing out the bowel from below. The routine use of enemas is unnecessary for a person in a healthful state. Such enemas should never be used unless prescribed for a special purpose by the doctor. Neither should saline cathartics be taken except with the advice of the doctor, since the harm that they may do by establishing habits is greater than the good that they may accomplish through sweeping waste material out of the body.

Finally, there is the cleaning of the fingernails, which all intelligent persons practice regularly. Nothing gives greater indication of body carelessness than the mourning bands carried at the tips of the fingers. This does not mean that everyone must have a professional manicure at frequent intervals. The cuticle may be pressed back, perhaps twice weekly, with an orangewood stick and may be softened by the application of some bland oil or vaseline. In all manicuring cleanliness is of the utmost importance. Before receiving the manicure, the person should wash the hands thoroughly with soap with a good deal of lather, using hot water and a nail brush. The manicurist who has just finished a manicure of some other person should treat her hands to the same process. All instruments used in manicuring should be suitably sterilized. When the manicurist cuts too deeply and bleeding occurs, it should be controlled by pressure with dry sterilized gauze and not by the application of a styptic pencil or surgical powder. Suitable antiseptics should be applied under these circumstances.

The nose, eyes, and ears do not demand routine washing with medicated solutions or indeed in any other way except when they are giving trouble. In such cases the attention should be regulated by the doctor.

Cleaning of the ear should never be practiced with a rigid instrument of any kind. Doctors prefer syringing with lukewarm water, directing the stream toward the side of the opening, so that pressure will not be directly against the eardrum.

The care of the eyes is largely automatic, since the eye is self-adjusting and self-lubricating. There is no need for the constant use of eyewashes, eyedrops, eye salves, or any other medicines. The use of such preparations is likely to do more harm than good. Nothing should ever be put into the eye except on the advice of a competent oculist. The popular eyewashes that are advertised, applied in barbershops and beauty shops, represent merely a solution of borax, costing about five cents a gallon to prepare and retailing at one dollar an ounce. Occasionally a few drops of some other medication are added, without, however, producing any effect whose specific virtue is required by the eye.

WORRY—Assuming that a person is in good physical health as shown by a suitable examination, one of the most important suggestions that can be made from the point of view of general health is to keep calm. Without being able to measure exactly the amount of damage that may be done to the human body by worry, high tension, or irritation, the experience of centuries has shown that these factors play a definite part in the onset of disease. Nowadays that branch of medicine which gives special attention to such relationships is known as psychosomatic medicine. Many years ago, however, worry was listed as a contributing cause to high blood pressure, hardening of the arteries, diabetes, and many degenerative diseases. Worry plays a part in the causation of such diseases by the secondary effects that it exerts on the circulation of the blood and on the other tissues of the body.

The expert in the treatment of mental diseases attempts to find out the primary cause of the worry or mental distress, to inform the person about it, and to make him realize its relation to his physical condition. Healers of various faith-healing systems rid the patient of worry by providing him with a substitute or by concentrating his attention on a system. Coué did it by having the person say over and over, "Every day, in every way, I am becoming better and better." The intelligent person, realizing his troubles, will do better to say to himself that he has realized and that he will no longer fear his trouble or avoid it. Nothing is gained by telling a person who worries that he must not worry. Emphasis on the situation serves only to cause such a person to concentrate still more on the problem. In fact a person can get to the point where he worries as much about worrying as he worries about the original cause of the worrying.

As a result of the war people have suffered more mental anxiety than ordinarily. From the point of view of mental health war brings both dangers and comforts. The American people's reaction to war has always been one of confidence and of union and of faith in the future of the nation. The fellowship of a common objective binds people together in courage and resolution. Mental wounds, however, tend to be repressed and to be buried under the surface. Experts in psychiatry are of the firm belief that repression and burying of mental problems do not relieve them but intensify them.

HYGIENE OF CLOTHING (See also *Clothing*)—Few people are enough disturbed about their health to select clothing primarily with a view to its healthful features. Style plays a greater part than any other factor in the selection of wearing apparel. Many of the styles are at times detrimental to health, but people wear them just the same.

From the hygienic point of view clothing should protect against cold and permit diffusion of heat by circulation of air in warm weather. Moisture must not be permitted to collect on the body surface, where it may macerate the skin and open the way for infection. Accumulated perspiration tends to produce a disagreeable odor.

Woolen clothing has the value of warmth and takes up perspiration. Woolens are especially desirable as wear for winter.

Modern women workers seem to make little provision for changes from the hot season to the cold. Hence offices are customarily overheated to meet the needs of women, with the result that men workers, who wear heavier clothing, are more likely to suffer unduly with the heat and the dryness of the atmosphere.

Most unhygienic in relationship to clothing of all types are constrictions of various portions of the body. The garment of primitive man was usually a simple robe that covered the body and was suspended from the shoulders. The garments of modern man are suspended from any point of protuberance on the human body, and this means women too.

There was a time when men wore suspenders regularly to hold their trousers in a position both comfortable and modest. Nowadays belts have largely displaced suspenders, although many a conservative man indulges in both belt and suspenders. Presumably constrictions at the waist are undesirable, although good scientific evidence as to any harm being done by wearing a belt that is tight enough to hold up the trousers is not yet available.

Collars that are worn tight enough to constrict the neck may cause pounding noises in the ear and be associated with headache. Garters worn tight enough to constrict the blood vessels of the leg may be associated with varicose veins, pains in the feet, and swelling of the ankles. Healthful garters are worn loose and are made of a wide web; hence they are not likely to produce any serious harm.

Women have discarded the corsets that used to produce wasp waists. The modern girdle is made of an elastic material and is not unduly constrictive. Constriction is especially not advisable during the childbearing period. Rubber garments of any type which do not permit satisfactory ventilation of the skin may cause maceration and infection.

Especially important also is the wearing of proper shoes and stockings. Stockings which do not fit well cause ingrown toenails, hammertoes, and bunions. Stockings that are too long form wrinkles, an uneven pressure, and irritate the skin. Stockings should always be changed daily. Shoes should fit well because cramping of the feet results in corns, calluses, and bunions.

PUBLIC AND PERSONAL HYGIENE— The hygienic functions that each of us must carry on for himself, such as washing the body and the teeth, using clean cooking utensils, and securing regular action of the bowels, are supplemented by other functions of hygiene that must be carried out by the community as a whole. These include the provision of pure water and food supplies, sewage disposal, education of the public in health, destruction of insect menaces to man, and of rats and other rodents, and the provision of pure air, good light, and safety during working hours. Every person can help the public health agencies in achieving these objectives.

Most of these activities are related to the prevention of the growth and spread of germs. Nobody's germs are his exclusive property. A cough, a sneeze, or a touch of the hand may transfer germs that will initiate epidemics. Each of us must be responsible for keeping his own germs within reasonable bounds.

Several authorities have from time to time outlined for the average person the routine of a healthful day. Here is a schedule which may be followed without developing overemphasis on any single aspect of healthful living.

1. Simple setting-up exercises upon arising to loosen up muscles. Simply bending over eight or ten times or stretching the arms and legs will be sufficient for people of middle age.

2. Attention to activity of the bowels, which should be without laxatives.

3. Thorough washing of at least the hands and face in the morning, cleansing the teeth at the same time.

4. A breakfast, to be followed by at least two other meals during the day which will provide altogether the essentials of a balanced diet. Meals should be eaten with sufficient leisure in a quiet, restful place to provide the maximum of nutrition with relaxation.

5. Enough relaxation at various times during the day to relieve accumulated fatigue.

6. Some daily exercise, at least walking, in the open air.

7. Attention to some hobby or avocation that provides mental relaxation.

8. At least eight hours of sleep or rest in a well-ventilated room.

9. Full use of the week end and other holidays for relaxation rather than work.

10. A semiannual visit to a dentist for attention to the teeth.

11. A physical examination by a competent physician at least once a year.

HYGIENE—children: See INFANCY, article CARE AND FEEDING OF THE CHILD.

HYGIENE—dental: See article ARTHRITIS, RHEUMATISM, AND GOUT.

HYGIENE—foot: See FOOT, article THE FOOT.

HYGIENE—menstruation: See article SEX HYGIENE.

HYGIENE—mental: See MENTAL, article NERVOUS AND MENTAL DISORDERS.

HYGIENE—nails: See HAIR, article THE HAIR.

HYGIENE—nose: See EAR, article THE EAR, TONGUE, NOSE, AND THROAT.

HYGIENE—old age: See article OLD AGE.

HYGIENE—personal: See INFECTIOUS DISEASE, article THE PREVENTION AND TREATMENT OF INFECTIOUS DISEASE.

HYGIENE—women: See WOMEN, article HYGIENE OF WOMEN.

SEX HYGIENE—See article SEX HYGIENE.

SEX HYGIENE—anatomy of reproductive system: See article SEX HYGIENE.

SEX HYGIENE—diseases of genital organs: See article SEX HYGIENE.

SEX HYGIENE—mating period: See article SEX HYGIENE.

SEX HYGIENE—menstruation: See article SEX HYGIENE.

SEX HYGIENE—middle and advanced life: See article SEX HYGIENE.

SEX HYGIENE—plant and animal reproduction: See article SEX HYGIENE.

SEX HYGIENE—reproductive system: See article SEX HYGIENE.

SEX HYGIENE—young married couple: See article SEX HYGIENE.

HYMEN The hymen is a membrane, commonly called maidenhead, at the entrance to the female sex organs. The presence of this tissue is usually considered synonymous with virginity, although it may not be; likewise its absence is not to be considered certain evidence of loss of chastity.

HYMEN—danger of rupture by rough handling: See article SEX HYGIENE.

HYPERHIDROSIS (See discussion under *Perspiration*) This is the scientific name for excessive sweating.

HYPERTENSION (See also discussion under *Apoplexy, Arteriosclerosis, Blood Pressure, High, Eclampsia, Emotions, Goiter, Headache, Insomnia, Nephritis, Noise, Obesity, Sleep, Sympathetic Nervous System, Thymus Gland*) Hypertension and arteriosclerosis or hardening of the arteries are by far the greatest killers of mankind in civilized nations. Within recent years this problem has loomed so largely on the medical horizon that special societies have been formed such as the Council for High Blood Pressure Research and the American Society for the Study of Arteriosclerosis. Out of the stimulus of such organizations have come new researches which are beginning to yield an understanding of these complex conditions.

No longer do physicians believe that simply measuring the blood pressure at the time when the heart contracts and recording this systolic blood pressure is enough for the proper study of the patient. Today a study of hypertension involves a complete survey of the condition of the heart, the blood vessels, the kidneys and the brain with a view to assessing the importance of various factors in causation of the condition. Such a study may involve electrocardiography to assay the action of the heart. functional tests on the kidneys in order to determine the activity of each portion of this complex organ, the use of the ophthalmoscope to detect changes in the blood vessels which may be observed in the back of the eyes. Chemical and physical examinations of the blood are being made to determine the body chemistry in relationship to hypertension. The conception is growing that the psychological factor is one portion of the intricate situation which results in hypertension.

Tumors of the adrenal glands are known to be related to the onset of hypertension and such excess activity can produce symptoms which are indistinguishable from ordinary hypertension. A number of tests have been devised which can detect the existence of such tumors of the adrenal and their part in the excess activity. New drugs have been found which act on the sympathetic nervous system and through that on the adrenal glands. These are used in evaluating the mechanisms that may be involved.

TREATMENT—Hypertension was once regarded as a change in the pressure of the blood necessary to maintain blood flow through vital tissues in the face of narrowing of the blood vessels because of hardening of the arteries. Hence high blood pressure was viewed with equanimity and with the understanding that after all it might even be prolonging the patient's life. Modern concepts completely reverse this view. The changes which have taken place in the walls of the blood vessels are now recognized as the result of prolonged abnormal elevations of blood pressure. In some organs, such as the kidneys, blood flow tends to increase when something is done to return the elevated blood pressure to a normal level. Conceivably the factors that result in hardening of the arteries and increase of the blood pressure have been active in the body of the person concerned for a long time.

During the period of equanimity the customary treatment included rest, reassurance, sedative drugs, the avoidance of red meat, tobacco and alcohol, and a lessening of energetic application to work or to play. Now many drugs have been found which have the ability to lower blood pressure and the new approach to the control of the condition is a total approach from every point of view.

The first step in treating high blood pressure is to make sure of the exact nature of the condition in the patient concerned. A brief rise in blood pressure with a subsequent fall is a quite different phenomenon from a blood pressure that is well above what is considered normal and remains in that area. The sudden onset of high blood pressure in a person under 35 years of age who does not have a family history of the early development of high blood pressure is not the same as that which comes on later in life and which either remains high or continues to rise. The sudden onset of severe hypertension is frequently related to some disorder of the kidney. As previously stated, the first step is therefore to make a complete study of the person concerned, searching his personal and family history, the condition of his blood vessels, the functional ability of his heart, the work of his kidneys and the state of the glands.

Dr. Irvine Page points out the desirability of preventive measures with young people and the avoidance of excessive treatment except when there is evidence of progressive disease of the blood vessels and circulation. Many people with mild hypertension may not require active treatment with drugs or other techniques to lower the pressure. This is especially true among older women who do not have any demonstrable progression of the disease of the blood vessels. Summarizing, he says that such people require reassurance, the establishment of a positive patient-physician relationship, mild sedation, an ordered hygiene of daily life and re-examination at intervals of 6 to 12 months. The treatment of slowly advancing essential hypertension is quite different from the treatment of malignant hypertension. The approach to treatment includes diet and drugs with the possible application of more radical surgical measures on the sympathetic nervous system.

The dietary treatment requires first cutting down the overweight which frequently prevails and also cutting down on the amount of sodium taken into the body usually in the form of salt. A variety of diets have been developed of which the simplest is the rice diet. People get tired of these diets rather soon. However, mild sodium restriction or techniques for avoiding the absorption of sodium in the body are considered by many observers to be expensive and useless.

A considerable number of drugs formerly used still continue to be tried with proper cases. The antipressor drugs include the thiocyanates, the drugs which depress the activity of the adrenal glands, the drugs which act on the brain, the central nervous system of the sympathetic nervous system and the ganglions and newer drugs which seem to have as their primary quality the production of lessened stress. Much research has been done on the thiocyanates which have been especially valuable in eliminating the headaches of high blood pressure. Within the last few years the hexamethonium drugs have had much vogue including also pentomethonium. These drugs presumably act by their depressive

effect on the sympathetic nervous system and have even been referred to as a chemical sympathectomy. Another new type of drug is Apresoline which has had beneficial effects on the circulation and on the work of the heart. Some physicians have combined Apresoline and hexamethonium and claim advantages for such combinations.

Most recent in the treatment of high blood pressure has been rauwolfia serpentina and the various active principles derived from it. This drug was brought from India and the romantic aspect is the claim that it was used for years in the care of Mahatma Gandhi. The use of rauwolfia seems to have been effective in lowering blood pressure in approximately 40% of mild hypertensive patients.

For years drugs derived from veratrum were used in high blood pressure. Now new alkaloids derived from veratrum including the protovarines have been introduced in the treatment of essential hypertension and malignant hypertension and in fact in all of the various forms. This drug is given by mouth or by injection into the veins and the muscles. Apparently the response varies from patient to patient. The use of this drug slows the heart rate and is helpful where the heart is failing in cases of high blood pressure.

DRUGS—Investigations continue for drugs capable of controlling blood pressure. The ganglionic blocking agents already mentioned such as hexamethonium and pentolinium are being widely used. These interfere with the transmission of stimuli which cause the blood vessels to contract. In that way they produce increased blood flow and lowering of the blood pressure. A new ganglionic blocking agent of this type is called mecamylamine and appears to be the first drug of its kind that is completely absorbed from the intestinal tract when given by mouth. This drug is used not only in itself but also combined with other drugs of the type of rauwolfia. Excellent reports have already appeared concerning its use in a considerable number of cases.

HYPERTHYROIDISM (See also, *Goiter; Internal Secreting* or *Endocrine Glands*) Although the condition called hyperthyroidism which is due to excessive action of the thyroid gland was first observed around 1830, a really complete understanding of the condition did not develop until 1890. Excessive action of the thyroid may occur at any age. The condition is much more frequent in women than in men. In areas in which goiter is infrequent, women may have excessive action of the thyroid gland in a proportion of four women to one man.

The exact cause of excessive action of the thyroid gland is not known, but the most frequently accepted view at this time is that the body responds to stress, either emotional, physical, or infectious, by excessive action of the pituitary gland which in turn overstimulates the thyroid gland. If this condition goes on, such symptoms may develop as bulging of the eyes which is a part of exophthalmic goiter, and there may be enlargement of the thyroid gland although there are cases in which the thyroid gland is enlarged without other symptoms. The person who is over-stimulated by thyroid is nervous, irritable and emotionally unstable. He perspires a great deal. Frequently shortness of breath and palpitation occur because of overstimulation of the heart. In every such case the doctor will want to watch the heart carefully. The basal metabolism test usually shows excess consumption of oxygen and is not specifically a test of the function of the thyroid gland. There are other conditions which can cause excess consumption of oxygen besides overactivity of the thyroid. The doctor who finds that

a patient has a large excess of thyroid action will want therefore to make other tests, as of the pulse and the temperature, the manner in which the body uses iodine, and the response of the body to the taking of iodine.

Since excessive action of the thyroid is due to secretion of too much hormone or glandular substance, treatment of the condition includes a number of different procedures. The certain method is removal of a portion of the thyroid gland by surgery, with or without the use of such drugs as propylthiouracil which diminish thyroid activity. In some cases, combined with the propyltiouracil is the giving of iodine which has an antithyroid action.

Radio iodine, which is a radioactive form of this substance, is now used to treat excessive action of the thyroid gland. Formerly similar effects were secured by the use of the X ray but the use of radioactive iodine is now considered to be far more preferable by most experts.

In some cases excessive action of the thyroid may be so great that serious symptoms develop including fever, an exceedingly rapid beating of the heart and even prostration. Obviously this condition is so serious that the patient should be under the immediate care of a doctor since he may require oxygen and prompt treatment to control the heart and the fever.

The bulging of the eye in exophthalmic goiter, or as it is now preferably called—thyrotoxic exophthalmos, is a condition which can be controlled somewhat if recognized promptly but not so much can be done if the person waits until permanent changes have taken place in the tissue around the eye. The bulging may disappear promptly following treatment of the excessive action of the thyroid. In other instances, the condition may be so severe that surgery is necessary to decompress the tissue around the eye.

SIMPLE GOITER—The bulging in the throat that is due to enlargement of the thyroid gland was apparently recognized by the Chinese at least as early as 1500 B.C. Such is indicated by drawings and other historical records. Indeed the people used to overcome the condition in the Middle Ages by eating burnt sponge and seaweed which are rich in iodine. Not until 1916, however, was the evidence accumulated that made it certain that small doses of iodine taken frequently by the patient living in areas in which there are small amounts of iodine in the soil and in the water will prevent simple goiter.

Certain substances have been recognized as having the power to stimulate goiter, but goiter caused by these substances—like thiocyanates or cabbage which cause a lessening of thyroid hormone—is infrequent.

The chief symptoms of goiter are of course the enlargement and bulging in the throat due to the large size of the gland. There are cases, however, in which the enlargement becomes so great that it may even interfere with breathing or injure the voice by pressure on the nerves that go to the larynx. The prevention of such enlargement of the gland by the taking of small doses of iodine regularly during the period of childhood and adolescense is now well established. Iodized salt is now commonly used so that the iodine is taken regularly in this manner. In cases of severe enlargement of the gland obviously removal by surgery is desirable.

PARATHYROID GLANDS—Behind and near to the thyroid gland are other glands which are known as parathyroid glands, their chief function being control of the use of calcium and phosphorus by the body. Apparently this gland responds with secretion of its hormone when the amounts of calcium

and phosphorus in the serum of the blood become insufficient. However, extracts of the parathyroid gland have been prepared and are used in cases when people apparently suffer from a lack of parathyroid hormone. The lack of this hormone is made evident by such symptoms as tremors of the body, called tetany, which occurs also with insufficiency of calcium. The tetany or tremors which are like muscle spasms or cramps are due to extra excitability of the nerves controlling the muscles.

Obviously the condition may be controlled by giving extra calcium directly into the blood or by taking large amounts of calcium by mouth. The condition may also be controlled by direct injection of the parathyroid hormone. Calcium is also controllable through the use of Vitamin D or of a substance like Vitamin D called dihydrotachysterol. The action of this substance is more like the action of the parathyroid hormone than is Vitamin D itself.

In the treatment of this condition, the diet should be one which contains much calcium and relatively little phosphorus. The foods which are rich in calcium are milk and cheese products and the leafy green vegetables. Milk also, however, includes phosphorus as does egg yolk, cauliflower and molasses.

As might be expected, excessive action of the parathyroid glands results in changes of the bones of the body because the bones are largely made up of calcium. Since the parathyroid glands so definitely control the use of calcium by the body, some have thought that kidney stones might be due to some action of the parathyroid glands. This has not, however, been established with certainty. Cases of excessive action of the parathyroid gland can occur without any evident changes in the bones and, in fact, the condition may be more frequent than is now suspected. There may be excessive growth of the tissues of the parathyroid glands which can result in excessive activity.

When large amounts of extra calcium are found in the blood and with that muscular weakness, loss of appetite, and pain in the bones, and not infrequently also excessive elimination of fluid through the kidneys, the physician suspects excessive action of the parathyroid glands. There are many different conditions which can interfere with the growth of bones so that studies of the blood as to the amount of calcium and the manner in which the body handles calcium are fundamental in discovering whether or not disturbance of the bone growth is due to excessive action of the parathyroid gland or to some other cause.

Since Vitamin D has become available as a concentrate and since people have been taking exceedingly large doses of Vitamin D to treat a variety of conditions, difficulty has occurred in recognizing the difference between excessive Vitamin D in the body and excessive action of the parathyroid glands.

In every case of hyperparathyroidism the possibility of surgical removal of excess tissue of the parathyroids must be considered as primary in the treatment

HYPOCHONDRIASIS People who enjoy ill-health are unfortunate for themselves and for those around them. Even doctors, unfortunately, like to avoid them. Hypochondriasis, which is the term used for the condition in which people get pleasure out of ill-health, has been called the most foolish and at the same time the saddest of all diseases.

Seldom, if ever, is a human being perfectly healthy. Even those whose pictures are printed in the physical culture magazines, swelling their muscles, when carefully investigated, are found to have aches and pains. The vast majority of people have thresholds of irritation—that is to say, minor pains and aches do not too much disturb them. They pay little attention to these as long as they can do their daily work and be unaware of their bodies during both work and recreation. The hypochondriac is aware of his body at a threshold much lower than that of the average man. To the hypochondriac every cough is the threat of consumption. To a person who knows, a cough is just a symptom of some irritation in the breathing tract, and the vast majority of coughs, he knows, are not too serious.

Symptoms are the means by which nature warns us that something is wrong. The reaction of a normal person to any kind of symptom is not a reaction of alarm but merely the awareness of a signal for investigation. The intelligent person who hears a noise in the house at night knows in the vast majority of cases it is just the effect of the wind or the weather or the expansion or contraction of the furniture. The alarmist takes every sound as an invasion by burglars or the beginning of an explosion. The nervous system is, therefore, constantly subjected to a series of unhealthful shocks.

Most serious for the hypochondriac is fixation on some one or another organ of the human body. Thus there is a tendency for the person with hypochondriasis to fix the attention on the organs associated with childbirth, on the intestines, on the brain, or on the vision, and to begin to develop symptoms especially related to some one or another organ. The result is likely to be constant consultation with specialists and repeated trials of all sorts of unnecessary treatments. Because the mind is so definitely related to the functions of the organs, the hypochondriac who begins to fix his attention on his gastrointestinal tract can promptly develop such symptoms as loss of appetite, nausea, belching, fullness in the stomach, and distress after meals.

One of the greatest assets in overcoming fear is knowledge. Familiarity breeds contempt. The person who knows and can judge the relative importance of various signs and symptoms is not likely to be too easily alarmed.

HYPOTENSION See *Blood Pressure, Low.*

HYSTERECTOMY The five-syllable word "his-ter-ec'-tome-y" is a technical term that is used by the doctor for removal of the womb. The operation is performed by the gynecologist (a surgeon specializing in conditions affecting women) when he believes that the operation is desirable for the health of the woman or for the relief of conditions which may incapacitate her for her daily life. The operation may be done because of the presence of fibroid tumors, which may be responsible for irregular bleeding or for a variety of other disturbances.

Sometimes the physician at the time of removal of the uterus will also wish to remove either or both of the fallopian tubes, which carry the egg from the ovary to the uterus, and perhaps either or both of the ovaries, depending on their physical condition. If they do not show evidence of disease, the surgeon is not likely to remove them. Certainly he will not interfere with the function of the female sex glands, known as the ovaries, unless they are diseased by infection or by cysts, which are collections of fluid, or by tumors. The ovaries are one of the most important parts of the female glandular chain. Complete removal of the ovaries is followed by an artificial menopause. The symptoms associated with that may make it necessary for the surgeon to give female sex gland hormones for a long time until

the body of the woman has become adjusted to the new conditions.

Several different surgical procedures are used by surgeons for removal of the uterus. Occasionally the operation is done through the lower opening of the body rather than through the abdomen. The decision as to the type of surgery to be done must rest with the gynecologist, who makes his decision on the basis of the conditions that exist in the individual woman.

Removal of the uterus alone will not bring about an artificial menopause, since the uterus is simply the organ in which the child lies before childbirth and is not concerned with supplying materials. Of course removal of the uterus does bring an end to the periodic flow, since the material comes from the uterus.

While many thousands of hysterectomies are now done each year in the United States, the operation is considered a major one in which anesthesia as well as residence in the hospital are necessary. Following the operation, time must be allowed for the tissues to grow together. The convalescence should include plenty of rest, avoidance of fatigue, avoidance of heavy lifting or climbing, and only moderate, light exercise.

Many women ask whether or not removal of the uterus will interfere in any way with the ordinary marital relations. The answer is that it will not interfere in the slightest, once healing has occurred.

HYSTERECTOMY—diabetes tendency great: See article DIABETES.

HYSTERIA For hundreds of years doctors have recognized the nature of the condition commonly called hysteria. The average person believes that an individual is hysterical when he screams, tosses his arms and legs about, or, if it is a woman, breaks into a crying fit. This is not necessarily hysteria but may be simply what is better described as a tantrum. A child who has been frustrated will throw himself on the floor, kicking, hitting, and screaming. While this is not hysteria, it may be the preliminary step to a hysterical attack.

During hysterical conditions various functions of the human body are disordered. Many of the usual activities of everyday life are disturbed. Queer actions take place related to eating, sleeping, working, remembering, listening, or talking. In most cases the basis of hysteria is an emotional situation in which an illness or the imitation of illness is the only way in which the person concerned can get out of his trouble. So-called "shell shock" is a condition in which hysteria may develop. A soldier may, for instance, develop a paralysis that does not actually indicate a disease of the nerves to avoid going back to the front line. This is not deliberate malingering, it is actual mental disturbance. Disappointment in love affairs is frequently the form of emotional upset that brings about an attack of hysteria.

There is hardly any disease that hysteria may not imitate. The degree to which hysteria imitates a disease depends on the knowledge that the person affected has of that disease. Thus friends of the patient or even the doctor himself may suggest that certain symptoms are characteristic of a disease, whereupon the person concerned will promptly imitate those symptoms. Incidentally, a person who has hysteria often fails to go the complete limit in the performance. He may stumble and appear dizzy but will manage to save himself from a fall. A person who actually has dizziness or stumbles because of a tumor of the brain or a real physical condition will not be able to save himself from a fall.

The most important step in the cure of hysteria is the certainty of the diagnosis. Failure to detect a real physical condition and to call it hysterical is exceedingly serious for the patient. By psychologic study, by the use of persuasion and the power of suggestion, the physician is able in most instances to bring about relief from the symptoms of hysteria. Once the patient understands the basis of his disturbance, there is likely to be a sudden and what has sometimes been called a miraculous cure. The physician understands that the cure of a psychologic disturbance in this manner is just as scientific as the cure of a physical condition. He is unlikely to claim a miracle. However, many a charlatan has made a reputation on the sudden cure of blindness, paralysis, loss of hearing, inability to swallow, or some other unusual symptom that was wholly hysterical.

HYSTERIA—tongue inflammation: See EAR, article THE EAR, TONGUE, NOSE, AND THROAT.

ICHTHYOL This is the proprietary name for sulfonated coal tar. It
has been used particularly in the treatment of conditions affecting the skin.
Nowadays it is little used in medicine
because of the development of remedies
known to have specific action.

ICHTHYOL—See SKIN, article THE
SKIN.

ICHTHYOSIS Babies are sometimes born with a skin that is dry,
rough, and scaly like that of a fish. The
condition is also called fishskin disease.
The exact cause is not known. There
is a tendency nowadays to believe that
it is due to deficiencies in the diet.

ICTERUS See *Jaundice.*

ILEITIS. Inflammation of the ileum.
Food enters the body through the
mouth, passes downward through the
stomach into the intestines. The first
portion of the small intestines is called
the duodenum, next the jejunum and
then the ileum. The ileum connects up
with the cecum from which juts off the
appendix. The ileum may become
blocked so that food does not pass
through by masses of indigestible residue, by collections of round worms, by
tumors, by having one part folding into
another called *intussusception*. The walls
may be infected by germs or viruses or
become inflamed with swelling, redness
due to congestion and pain. Such inflammation is called *ileitis*. The doctor
diagnoses the conditions from his examinations including use of the X-ray,
feeling the area, and listening for the
movement of the tissues. According to the

extent and severity of the condition the treatment may be palliative or radical which includes surgery. Surgery may involve removal of portions of the bowel, or by-passing the damaged portion through short circuiting which connects the bowel above the damaged portion to the bowel below it.

IMMUNIZATION During the first six months of his life a child usually has in his blood, derived from his mother, substances which aid him to resist certain infections. After the sixth month, however, the infant stops nursing in most cases. Until this age the baby comes little into contact with other people. After this age he begins to be exposed to the infections that other people have. Therefore, as a means of protecting children against the infectious diseases to which they are so regularly exposed, modern medical science has developed a routine of immunization.

At about nine months of age children should be vaccinated against smallpox. The vaccination is usually made in the upper part of the left arm or on the outer side of the left leg above the knee. Most physicians still prefer to vaccinate on the arm. Occasionally, however, mothers feel that a girl baby is bound to be sooner or later an actress or an opera star and therefore prefer to have the vaccination done where it will not show. In view of the nature of modern swimming and ballroom costumes, there is no certainty that the vaccination will not show except in an exceedingly restricted area of the human epidermis.

By the twelfth month children should be protected against diphtheria. Such protection is achieved by inoculating the child with a substance called diphtheria toxoid. This is usually injected into the loose tissue of the arms or legs, occasionally into the buttocks or the abdominal wall. Most doctors now-

adays use a two-dose toxoid, giving the two injections about ten days apart. Usually a child begins to develop within his blood resistance against diphtheria almost immediately after the injection and after a period of four months will have developed enough of such materials to protect him against diphtheria for some time.

Inoculations are also available against lockjaw, or tetanus. All of the soldiers in the United States Army are inoculated against tetanus and smallpox. Tetanus is so serious that doctors generally recommend the use of inoculation against this condition whenever a child has had a cutting injury or been in some way damaged by fireworks or explosives, or indeed whenever there is the possibility that a cut has been contaminated with soil, clothing, or other materials.

Scarlet fever is another disease against which it is possible to immunize the child. Physicians for the most part, however, do not immunize against scarlet fever unless there happens to be an epidemic in the community or in an institution where the child is exposed to the disease.

Many physicians use blood from persons who have recovered from whooping cough to immunize babies against whooping cough. The most modern approved technic includes the use of vaccines.

A technic has been developed for inoculation against measles, using a substance called gamma globulin. The gamma globulin is derived from the blood, which is made available through the vast amounts of blood now being contributed for blood transfusions. Antisubstances against measles, poliomyelitis, and hepatitis are carried by this gamma globulin.

Immunization against typhoid and the paratyphoid infections can be had whenever there is an outbreak of this condition in any community.

The Salk vaccine is an efficient preparation for raising resistance to infantile paralysis and for maintaining it at a high level.

New technics are also available by which a child can be immunized at one time against several infectious conditions. The decision as to when to use the individual or the combined immunization must be left to the physician who has the responsibility for the care of the child.

IMMUNIZATION—children: See article ALLERGY.

IMMUNIZATION—defined: See CHILD-

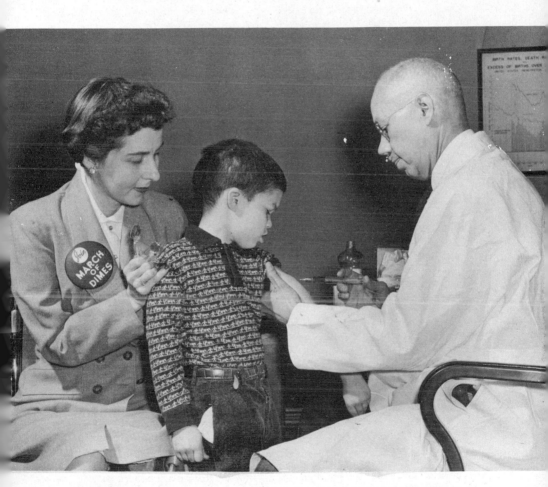

Child getting his inoculation against poliomyelitis. With the discovery of the Salk vaccine has come the hope of abolishing poliomyelitis as a crippling disease.

HOOD DISEASES, article INFECTIOUS DISEASES OF CHILDHOOD.

IMPETIGO Among the contagious conditions that affect the skin impetigo is frequent. In this condition the skin is covered with blisters, often filled with infectious material or pus, intermingled with the dry crusts or other blisters that have broken. Should these crusts be removed, a reddened, moist surface is found below. Occasionally the impetigo spreads from the face, where it is most frequent, to the hands or other portions of the body.

Usually impetigo is transferred from one person to another by the fingernails or hands, which carry the streptococci and staphylococci, both pus-forming germs. The condition is frequently transferred from one child to another during playtime. Women occasionally get the disease from children, but in men the most frequent source of infection is the barbershop. Not infrequently also men get their skin contaminated on wrestling mats or from boxing gloves or other athletic apparatus.

Sometimes the infected spots dry up quickly, but in other instances they become secondarily infected and result in boils or abscesses. After impetigo becomes established, it is much more difficult to treat than when the condition has first appeared.

With proper treatment the average case will clear up in one or two weeks.

For the prevention of this infection it is necessary to avoid the possibility of contamination with infectious material from people who have the disease. People who are infected should always use a separate washcloth, towel, and similar personal articles. If a case occurs in a school child, the child should be excluded from contact with other children until he has recovered. Those who have the condition should always be warned against scratching themselves; they contaminate their fingers. Thus infection is spread from one person to another.

Incidentally, children who happen to be infested with lice or with the itch mite sometimes get impetigo on top of the other condition. This means that both conditions must be treated simultaneously, since the combination causes both conditions to persist.

Formerly impetigo was treated with various antiseptic substances. Nowadays it has been found that the sulfonamide drugs are especially useful in controlling infections with the germs that cause impetigo. Moreover, the latest information indicates that ointments containing penicillin also have an almost specific effect against infections with impetigo. Such materials as the sulfonamides and penicillin must, of course, be prescribed by the physician before they are used.

IMPETIGO—See SKIN, article THE SKIN.

IMPETIGO—scalp: See HAIR, article THE HAIR.

INDIGESTION Among the most common of human complaints is indigestion. It is also a relative term because often symptoms called indigestion represent ulcers of the stomach or duodenum or occasionally disturbances of the gall bladder and in some cases actually difficulty in digesting food. The old term "dyspepsia" really means pain accompanying functioning of the digestive processes regardless of the cause. Of course there may be pain due to arthritis, gall-bladder disease, or other conditions not directly related to the digestion of food. This must be differentiated from dyspepsia.

What happens when food is swallowed? It passes down the esophagus or gullet into the stomach. The stomach was characterized long ago as a mixing vat. Actually digestion begins in the stomach. The saliva that is secreted helps to stimulate digestion. The pepsin and hydrochloric acid of the stomach help to soften the food and then the stomach passes it along into the first portion of the intestines. This is called the duodenum. The name comes from the Latin word for twelve. The duodenum is about twelve finger-breadths long. In the duodenum the food is mixed with bile from the liver and with another digestive juice that is produced by the pancreas. The pancreas also produces insulin which digests sugars. The insulin, however, goes directly from the pancreas into the blood. As the food passes along, digestion is completed and the digested material is picked up by the blood and carried through the body. People wonder why the stomach does not digest itself but there are means by which the glandular tissues on the inside of the stomach are protected against the acid and the pepsin. In cases of ulcers of the stomach, when the living tissues in the inside of the stomach have been damaged the

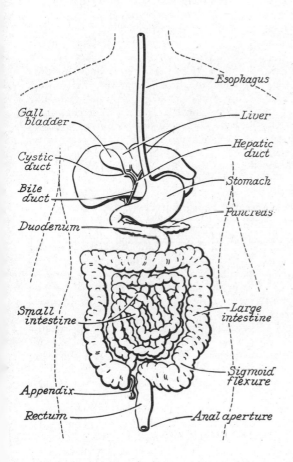

The human digestive system, showing organs and parts of the body concerned with the ingestion of food and the elimination of waste materials. Food goes into the mouth, down the esophagus, into the stomach, small intestine, large intestine, and finally to the anal aperature. The esophagus is ten to twelve inches long and very muscular. Digestion starts in the stomach where the food accumulates. The strong muscles of the stomach grind and mix the food with the stomach secretions and the contents are emptied into the small intestine where digestion is completed. The small intestine measures approximately twenty feet long and occupies most of the abdominal cavity. The small intestine opens into the large intestine which is about five feet long and three inches in diameter. The large intestine gradually narrows to form the rectum and anal aperature.

acid can produce constant irritation and burning.

SYMPTOMS OF INDIGESTION—The chief symptoms of indigestion are pain in the neighborhood of the stomach or in the lower part of the chest and sometimes in the back. There may be belching and even vomiting of food. These symptoms are not due to the fact that the food is failing to be digested. They are actually due to irritation of the lining of the stomach by the acid in the stomach juice. This acid, as has already been explained, will not hurt a healthy stomach. It may seriously damage a stomach in which the lining has been injured. People with indigestion take alkaline substances like bicarbonate of soda. These neutralize the acid and thus help to relieve the pain. The stomach may be emptied by vomiting, thus relieving the stomach of the acid and stopping the pain.

Ulcers of the stomach are exceedingly serious since they may perforate. When an ulcer perforates, a hole is formed in the stomach or duodenum and the material gets out into the abdominal cavity. For perforation of the stomach or duodenum there is just one proper treatment and that is surgical operation to sew up the hole and stop the leakage. Occasionally an ulcer will eat its way into a blood vessel. Then a hemorrhage occurs. The blood may be vomited from the stomach or may pass along through the bowel. Then the material excreted from the bowel appears black and shiny like tar.

Experts in conditions affecting the stomach and intestines recommend that every symptom of indigestion be treated promptly. This is one way to prevent the formation of ulcers. The treatment includes methods that soothe the injured lining and permit the living tissues of the body to heal themselves. If such methods of treatment do not bring about healing of the ulcer, various surgical operations have been developed which permit removal of the ulcer and repair of the tissue. One operation involves the cutting of the nerves that control the movements of the stomach and its activity. This operation is known as vagotomy, since it is the vagus nerve that is cut.

TREATMENT OF INDIGESTION—Recently Dr. C. M. Fletcher, a distinguished British physician who specializes in disturbances of the stomach and intestines, has offered a number of suggestions regarding the diet of persons who have digestive disturbances, frequently called dyspepsia.

These suggestions follow:

1. Have regular meals. The stomach is affected by habit. It likes regular hours. It gets ready for food at the time when the meal is expected. This it does by producing digestive juice and acid. If the meal is delayed, these substances have contact in concentration with the walls of the stomach and may cause harm.

2. Have frequent "snacks." Food, and particularly milk, helps to neutralize the acid in the stomach. That is why the pains of indigestion are lessened by taking a snack. Some people have thought that it is better to avoid food when there is indigestion. A light meal or snack taken at fairly frequent intervals helps to overcome the excess acid in the stomach. Indeed this has become routine advice for digestive disturbances.

3. Avoid big meals. Big meals overfill the stomach and by stretching the tissues may do harm. In general six small meals a day are better than three big ones.

4. Eat slowly and chew thoroughly. Meals that are hurried are not properly chewed. A large mass of unchewed food means that the food will remain a long time in the stomach because it has to be penetrated and softened by the digestive juice. Again there is the danger that

lumps may irritate the walls of the stomach. If your teeth are not good enough to enable you to chew your food sufficiently, you will do well to see a dentist, who will be able to correct the condition. Some foods are hard to chew even with good teeth. A certain amount of hard foods is necessary for health but this can be taken in the form of finely macerated fiber.

5. Avoid irritating stimulants. Physicians are now convinced that tobacco, strong tea, coffee, or alcohol may irritate the stomach. Smoking after a meal is less likely to irritate than before a meal. Alcoholic drinks taken before a meal increase appetite because of the irritation to the wall of the stomach. The investigators are convinced that tea and coffee taken with plenty of milk or cream are less irritating than black coffee or strong tea. Most people have sense enough to realize that a certain food is irritating to them. Certainly one should avoid foods that are known by experience to be irritating.

THE MIND AND THE STOMACH—Research of recent years has shown that the stomach and the digestion of food are greatly influenced by mental factors. People talk of being sick with fright. They say that the stomach turned over. Some people are easily nauseated and vomit when affected by odors or sudden shocks. A sudden shock of fright does not do serious harm. When, however, a person is subjected to repeated nagging, mental strain, anxiety, frustration, or resentment, he is likely to react with a continuous irritation in the stomach area and eventually symptoms of either indigestion or ulcers. The people who get indigestion are often people who worry a lot or who are especially sensitive to criticism. Dr. C. M. Fletcher suggests that such people ask themselves the following questions:

Do you turn little worries over and over in your mind, although you try to appear calm and unconcerned?

Do you brood over bad luck, or when you feel you have been "done"?

Do you resent criticism or worry about what people think of you?

Do people "get on your nerves" easily?

Do you have to drive yourself all day because you have really got too much to do, so that you are always "on the go" and cannot relax?

Are you usually dissatisfied with yourself so that you are always striving to do "one better"?

Do you feel people do not understand or appreciate you enough?

Dr. Fletcher says that if you must honestly answer yes to more than one of these questions, mental strain is playing a considerable part in upsetting your stomach.

People can learn to worry less. Indeed people can learn to take things less seriously simply by constantly reminding themselves that irritation and anger are bad. Someday perhaps we will learn to teach little children early in life that worry and anger and sensitivity are unhealthful. Long ago people learned that it is a relaxation of tension to talk over your problems with somebody else. You may talk about your problems to a religious counselor or with friends whom you can trust or even with members of your family unless they are the cause of your trouble. Of course the doctor is a specialist in listening to people's troubles and worries. He can, moreover, give not only advice but medicines that help to dull the sharp edge of sensitivity and lower the threshold of irritation.

THE HYGIENE OF INDIGESTION—Rest has always been a fundamental remedy for human illness. Nowadays people learn to get up fairly early after surgical operations or after childbirth, but for fatigue and particularly for mental irritation, rest and relaxation are still most important.

Dr. C. M. Fletcher suggests that people avoid exercise either just before or just after a meal because the exercise places a strain on the blood supply and thus takes away from the stomach materials needed to aid digestion. Indeed he suggests that people sit still for at least a quarter of an hour before and after each meal so that the stomach can do its job in peace. For people with serious indigestion or ulcers, a long stay in bed is helpful not only because it gives complete rest but also because it offers an opportunity for control of eating habits. Most restful of all of the procedures in which the human being can indulge is a really sound sleep. A restless night is worse on the stomach than a day full of anxiety. The doctor can always help to overcome restless nights.

People who have serious mental strains at regular intervals should learn particularly to practice good mental hygiene and good physical habits before, during, and after such periods of strain. Among the worst of these periods is the quarterly income tax payment, the period immediately following return from vacation, the rush before Christmas to get the Christmas gift shopping done, and, for many people, any fall in the stock market. Just how to anticipate a fall in the stock market is not yet clear but physicians have noticed for years that any sudden drop in the stock market is immediately followed by an increase or rise in the cases of ulcers of the stomach, diabetes, arthritis, and even colds. Thus the proper hygiene for overcoming digestive disturbances and the onset of ulcers includes, first, a suitable diet with regular, frequent, small, unhurried meals; second, avoidance of all stimulants or other substances that experience has shown will irritate the stomach; third, a calm mind and time to relax; and, fourth, sound sleep. With these practices, Dr. Fletcher says, anyone's stomach will get well and stay well.

The following is the smooth diet that is recommended to people who have nervous indigestion. It is taken directly from the recommendations of Dr. Walter Alvarez.

If you are to give this diet a fair trial, eat no coarse foods with fiber, skins, seeds, or gristle. Avoid particularly salads with celery, tomatoes, cucumbers, and pineapple, many of the green vegetables, raisins, berries, jams full of seeds, nuts, and many of the raw fruits. Beans, cabbage, onions, green or red peppers, melons, cucumbers, and peanuts are notoriously gassy. If you are living in a boardinghouse you can stick to this diet by simply avoiding the forbidden foods and eating more of the digestible ones which are put before you.

Avoid sugar in concentrated form and take no candy or other food between meals. Hot cakes and waffles might not be bad if they were not eaten with so much syrup. Fried foods are not bad if they are properly fried—that is, totally immersed in fat at the right temperature. Avoid eating when in a rush and when mentally upset. Family rows should be held away from the table. Chewing gum may cause distress, as much air is swallowed with the saliva. Digestion is greatly helped by a good chewing surface. If there are any gaps in your teeth, have your dentist fill them with bridges. Purgatives often cause flatulence and distress in the abdomen.

The following are suggestions for breakfast: Orange juice, grapefruit (avoid the fiber in the compartments); cantaloupe and melons are inadvisable. Coffee, if desired, is allowed in moderation; it sometimes causes flatulence. If you are sensitive to caffeine, try Kaffee Hag or Instant Postum. Chocolate, cocoa, or tea, one or two eggs with ham or bacon (avoid the tougher part of the bacon), white bread, toast, or zwieback with butter, any smooth mush such as farina, germea, cream of wheat, corn meal, or rolled oats (a fine oatmeal can be obtained by calling for Robinson's Scotch Groats), puffed cereals and corn-flakes are also allowed. Shredded-wheat biscuits and other coarse breakfast foods are not allowed. Bran is particularly harmful. Graham bread is permitted but not the coarser whole-wheat bread.

Suggestions for lunch and dinner: In fruit cocktails avoid the pieces of orange and pineapple. Broths, bouillon, cream soups, and chowder are allowed, also meat, fish, or chicken, squab, or game, excepting duck (avoid the fibrous parts and gristle). Veal may be tried; it is not digested well by many persons. Eat no smoked fish or pork. Crab and lobster had better be left alone. Oysters and sausage may be tried later.

Bread and butter are allowed, and hot biscuits if they are made small so as to consist mainly of crust. Rice, potatoes—mashed, hashed brown, or French fried —are allowed; and later may be added sweet potatoes, hominy, tomatoes stewed, strained, and thickened with cracker or bread crumbs, well-cooked cauliflower tops with cream sauce, asparagus tips, Brussels sprouts, squash, beets, turnips, creamed spinach, Italian pastes, noodles, macaroni, and spaghetti cooked soft, purées of peas, beans, lentils, lima beans, or artichoke hearts. All skins or fiber should be removed by passing the food through a ricer. Sweet corn may be used if passed through a colander. There are practically no other vegetables that can be puréed to advantage. String beans (large tender string beans which can be used as a vegetable or salad can now be obtained in cans) are allowed if they are young and tender.

No salad should be taken at first. Later you may try a little tender lettuce with apples or bananas, tomato jelly, or boiled eggs. Mayonnaise and French dressing are allowed. Potato salad without much onion may be tried.

Suggestions for dessert are: Simple puddings, custards, ice cream, jello, plain cake, and canned or stewed fruits, particularly pears and peaches. Cottage cheese is permissible; other cheeses often cause trouble. Apple, peach, apricot, custard, and lemon-cream pie may be tried if only the filling is eaten.

In case of constipation stewed fruit may be taken once or twice a day. In winter the dried pared fruit may be used for stewing. Prunes are probably the most laxative of fruits and if eaten every other morning they will relieve the average case of constipation. They should be cooked slowly, until they almost go to pieces. If the skins are still tough, they should be discarded. Apple-sauce is much more palatable if made from unpared and uncored apples. The sauce is strained later. It may be mixed with a little tapioca or sago. The apples may be baked. Apples, even when cooked, often cause distress. Black-berries and loganberries can be stewed and strained and the sweetened juice thickened with cornstarch. This makes a delicious dish with the full flavor of the berries. Later you may try fully ripe pears and peaches.

Make no effort to drink water. Be guided by your thirst. Avoid excessive use of salt or other seasoning. If you wish to gain in weight, eat as much cream, butter, fat, and starch as you can. If you wish to lose or to stay thin, live largely on vegetables, fruits, and salads, with a moderate amount of lean meat.

DYSPEPSIA—See article DIGESTION AND DIGESTIVE DISEASES.

DYSPEPSIA—constipation: See article DIGESTION AND DIGESTIVE DISEASES.

DYSPEPSIA—differentiated from indi-

gestion: See article DIGESTION AND DI-
GESTIVE DISEASES.

DYSPEPSIA—stomach cancer mistaken
for: See article CANCER.

DYSPEPSIA—unscientific word: See article DIGESTION AND DIGESTIVE DIS-
EASES.

INDIGESTION—See article DIGESTION
AND DIGESTIVE DISEASES.

INDIGESTION—appendicitis and gall-
bladder disease often responsible: See
article DIGESTION AND DIGESTIVE DIS-
EASES.

INDIGESTION—cancer danger signal:
See article CANCER.

INDIGESTION—constipation: See article
DIGESTION AND DIGESTIVE DISEASES.

INDIGESTION—diet, smooth: See article DIGESTION AND DIGESTIVE DIS-
EASES.

INDIGESTION—differentiated from dyspepsia: See article DIGESTION AND DI-
GESTIVE DISEASES.

INDIGESTION—stomach cancer mistaken
for: See article CANCER.

INDIGESTION—treatment: See article
DIGESTION AND DIGESTIVE DISEASES.

INDUSTRIAL ABSENTEEISM

The disabilities that keep employees
from their work include the common
cold as the most significant; second are
the disturbances which occur in women
simply because they are women. Third
are disturbances of digestion and, fourth,
mental problems.

No one has yet found a method for
lessening absenteeism due to colds. Routine inoculation of people against colds
with vaccines made from germs or from
the influenza viruses does not do the
job. Some people still believe that exposure to cold while hot and sudden
changes of temperature are important.
Therefore, avoidance of exposure and
elimination of drafts may be attempted.

Physicians in some large industries
report that employees who take shower
baths before going outdoors tend to
fight off colds. This is believed to be
part of a hardening process. In some
industries it is believed that prompt
attention to colds in the factory dispen-
sary will lessen the number. Measures
instituted include such treatments as
the use of alkaline powder and, in other
places, drugs like aspirin.

Most important probably is a study
of the industrial plant with relation to
the departments in which colds are most
prevalent and an attempt to find out
why colds spread more rapidly and
more frequently in those departments.
Certainly overcrowding of personnel
aids transmission of infectious germs.
Moreover, it has been proved that germs
may float for an hour in the air, held
by drops of moisture due to coughing
and sneezing.

In plants where great numbers of
women are employed, investigators
divide women into those who work
through their periodic disturbance without complaint, those who begin work
but sooner or later show up in the rest
room, and those who invariably stay
home a full day or longer.

Disturbances of digestion are more
likely in men than in women in industry.
They occur more often in the summer
months. In plants where employees lose
much time because of digestive disturbances an investigation will frequently
show that the disturbances are associated
with hurried eating, use of eating places
that are not quite suitable, and complete failure to understand the simplest
facts about nutrition.

INDUSTRIAL HEALTH

Sickness
causes approximately twenty times more
cases of absenteeism in industry than
are caused by accidents and about seven
times the total loss of working days.
The sicknesses which are mostly responsible include the common cold, diseases
of the stomach, pharyngitis and tonsillitis, functional nervous diseases, men-

strual disorders in women, rheumatism, arthritis, and gout. While colds are responsible for more absences than other diseases, the severity of this type of absenteeism is low. Functional diseases of the nervous system actually cause the highest average working days lost per case.

There are very few strictly occupational diseases, although some industries give rise to certain kinds of disability. Examples are exposure to silica dusts, which produce silicosis, or to the inhalation of lead, which produces lead poisoning, or the breathing of carbon monoxide gas, which produces carbon monoxide poisoning.

Especially frequent nowadays are inflammations of the skin due to irritation from various chemicals to which the worker may be exposed. The experts have listed hundreds of different types of chemical substances which may cause inflammations of the skin. Certain industries by the nature of the work produce constant pressure against various portions of the body, so that calluses form or swellings of protective oil sacs take place. Such swellings are called bursitis. Housemaid's knee is an example of this kind of occupational disease. Fatigue or strain from certain movements that are often repeated, as in sewing, writing, holding a pneumatic hammer, operating a telegraph key, can also produce conditions which are classified as occupational disorders.

Some occupations expose the worker to certain kinds of infections. The worker with infected cattle may get undulant fever. Anthrax is contracted from contact with infected hides or wools. Machinists get serious inflammations and infections due to irritations from oil and cutting compounds. In other industries the worker may be exposed to such hazards as ultraviolet light or constant glare, so that conditions occur like electric ophthalmia, glassworker's cataract, nystagmus of coal miners (which is a shifting of the pupils due to working under irregular light). There is also the kind of inflammation of the eye called conjunctivitis which happens to movie stars who are not protected against the light. Laundry and kitchen workers may suffer from severe heat exhaustion from abnormally high temperatures, and workers in cold storage plants suffer with disturbances due to exposure to cold. Boilermakers have disturbances of hearing associated with noise, and workers in tunnels and those who fly at high altitudes develop conditions like caisson disease and altitude sickness. Certain monotonous jobs expose the worker to the double danger of fatigue and functional nervous disturbances.

Care and Feeding of the Child

BY

PHILIP C. JEANS, M.D.

Head Pediatric Division, University Hospitals and Prof. of
Pediatrics and Head Dept., State University of Iowa College of Medicine, Iowa City, Ia.

INTRODUCTION

INVESTIGATIONS INDICATE *that the boys and girls entering college these days are on an average two inches taller and from seven to ten pounds heavier than their parents and grandparents who entered these same institutions at the same ages in the previous two generations. The fact is significant because it shows what preventive medicine and hygiene have done to build better bodies. In an earlier day children just "growed" like Topsy in* Uncle Tom's Cabin. *Nowadays the diets are regulated, as well as the hours of sleep, the hours of exposure to sunshine and fresh air, the clothing, and all of the other factors of the child's hygiene.*

The reason for such regulation lies, of course, in the change in the habits of civilized man. In a previous generation, children were raised largely in rural populations where they had plenty of sunshine and fresh air, plenty of fresh vegetables and milk, and all of the circumstances combined to promote the growth of a healthy little animal. As human beings moved into great collections of humanity in cities, the sunlight and fresh air began to be shut out. Because of the difficulties of transportation, it became necessary to depend largely on food from cans and on materials transported over many hundreds of miles before they were used by the consumer. The more food and milk are handled, the more likelihood is there of contamination from the hands of those who bring them to their final market.

In order to know whether a baby is normal and developing as he should, it is necessary to have certain standards for judgment. In setting up any such standards, it must be remembered that individual babies will vary somewhat from the average. To say that a baby should weigh seven pounds at birth is stating an approximately average value which everyone knows is strictly true for only a few babies. Babies at birth may weigh six, eight, or nine pounds and be perfectly normal. Extreme variations from the average are of significance. A baby weighing five pounds or less at birth must be classed as a delicate or premature baby requiring special care. Similarly moderate variations from the average in all of the other criteria of growth and development are not to be taken seriously in themselves. The weight or development at any particular period is not of as great significance as the progress which the baby makes from time to time. The infant should show constant and steady progress as indicated by the various standards.

A baby of average weight at birth should double the birth weight by five to six months and treble it by one year. These are average values. A baby who is well fed with ample food will grow faster than this. If the diet has been a balanced one, it is probable that the larger baby is physically superior. The baby may be expected to gain six to eight ounces a week in the first six months and four to six ounces a week during the second six months. After this time the weight gain is much less.

The body length of the baby is also a criterion of growth, but it is not always used in routine evaluation of progress, because of the greater extremes of food quality and quantity required to affect growth in length.

The head grows rapidly in size during the first year, increasing two and one-half inches in circumference in this period. The bones of the skull are relatively soft and may be moulded easily by permitting the baby to lie in the same position. Many infants' heads have become permanently misshapen because the mother did not take care to see that the baby's position was changed frequently. A good practice is to turn the baby on the left side after one feeding and on the right side after the next one. The soft spots or fontanels of the skull represent areas which have not yet calcified. The small one at the back of the head is usually hard by three months. The large one in front should close by eighteen months, but in many vigorous, well-nourished babies, the anterior fontanel has disappeared by one year of age.

The first or deciduous teeth are twenty in number. These begin to erupt at about six months of age and should be completely erupted by two and one-half years. They tend to erupt by pairs, the lower central incisors coming first, then the two upper centrals, followed by the upper lateral incisors. These six incisor teeth should be erupted by one year of age. Moderate variations in the time of eruption of teeth may indicate nothing abnormal.

The muscular movements soon after birth are few, but activity increases rapidly, although in the beginning the movements seem purposeless. By three months the neck muscles are strong enough to support the head. At three months the infant will attempt to grasp objects although with poor muscular control. The grasp becomes accurate at five to seven months. Vigorous well-nourished babies sit alone at six months with occasional falls: they usually sit securely at eight months. Although babies may stand awkwardly earlier, they usually are able to stand well when supported at nine months. The usual time of first walking is sometime between twelve and fifteen months. Between the ages of sitting and walking, most babies accomplish progression over the floor by creeping or otherwise, although a few normal babies do not.

Babies are able to laugh and coo sometimes at two months, sometimes not until several months later. They do not say understandable words until the latter part of the first year. By the end of one year usually several simple words are in the vocabulary. By two years simple short sentences are used. Many entirely normal children are late in talking. In a few instances this delay is of several years, often it seems because a child has felt no necessity for speech, in that all desires are anticipated. Parents should not use baby talk to children, as they learn only that kind of speech which they hear.

The infant's vision seems very imperfect in the beginning. It is not until five or six weeks of age that he pays attention to objects held in front of him. He does not follow with his eyes until he is three to four months old, at which time, or soon thereafter, he makes combined purposeful movements of head and eyes and recognizes people and objects familiar to him. At about this time, or a little earlier, he will turn his head toward a sound and be able to recognize voices.

The mental development of the infant in the first year or two is judged largely by the criteria of physical development which have been discussed. A baby may be slow in sitting, standing, and walking, for the reason that he has been ill or has been poorly fed; or it may be because he is mentally backward. With good food and in the absence of illness, mental backwardness should be suspected when purposeful motor behavior of all types is abnormally delayed or when the infant is inattentive to familiar sights and sounds.

Physical Care and Hygiene

The baby should always have his own bed. Whenever possible he should have a room exclusively for his own use. The room which he occupies should be well ventilated or the air changed frequently. During his waking or play hours the temperature should be in the neighborhood of 70 degrees F. During sleep time the temperature can be 10 to 30 degrees lower than this, depending upon the age, size and vigor of the baby. When the room is kept cold for sleep it is advisable to have available a warm room to which he can be taken when necessary. When properly supervised and protected, a baby can spend much of his time out of doors after two weeks in summer or after three months in winter. Common sense must be used in putting the baby out of doors, particularly in winter. One criterion for the winter is the baby's reaction to cold; if his face becomes pale and blue and his hands and feet cold, he should not be left outside. The baby must be provided steady warmth and fresh air; if this cannot be done out of doors, the baby must be kept indoors. In the summer babies placed out of doors in the shade usually present no special problem. Several precautions are necessary, however, for sun bathing. Sunstroke from excessive heat is possible. The eyes should be protected from direct sunlight. In the beginning only a limited area of the skin should be exposed; usually the feet are exposed first and the area gradually increased. The first exposure should be not more than 5 minutes. Exposure time is increased gradually until the skin is tanned.

In the first weeks after birth the infant will sleep practically all of the time except when he is bathed and fed. At two to three months he sleeps fourteen to sixteen hours daily, and lies quietly for possibly two hours more. At six months the average baby sleeps about fourteen hours and at one year very little less than this. After eighteen months one expects a twelve-hour sleep at night with an additional daytime nap. Although sleep requirements are stated rather definitely here, there are found to be individual differences in sleep needs. The criterion as to adequacy of sleep should be the health status of the infant or child. One who is getting enough sleep should have a good color and show no undue fatigue, should be bright-eyed, happy and not irritable. If no undesirable symptoms are evident and yet the amount of sleep is minimum for the age, the chances are that the sleeping time is adequate.

The daily bath should be given before one of the morning feedings. After the cord comes off, this should be a tub bath. The room should be warm, not hot, and without drafts. The temperature of the bath water is best at about 100 degrees F. for the young baby, gradually decreased to 90 degrees F. at one year. Unnecessary exposure is to be avoided, especially for the young or delicate infant. Avoidance of exposure may be accomplished by lifting the baby directly from the tub onto a large bath towel. Whether the baby is dried on the mother's lap or on a table matters little, although usually the procedure is more quickly performed on a table. The use of talcum powder is not a corrective for poor drying. Babies would be fully as well off without this accessory. In very hot weather it is often advantageous to give the baby one or more sponge baths in addition to the morning tub bath. Routine care concerning the eyes, ears, nose, mouth, and other details of body cleanliness, is given at the time of the morning bath. The only care needed for the eyes is possibly the cleaning of the inner corners. In cleaning the ears there is no need and some danger in entering farther than the tip of the canal. Nothing should be inserted into the nose. Any crusts or secretions in the lower part of the nostrils may be removed with absorbent cotton. The mouth ordinarily needs no attention until the teeth appear. Then all that is required is to keep the teeth clean. While the teeth are few, this can be done easily with cotton on a toothpick, perhaps with the aid of a toothpaste (not powder). While the baby is young the hair and scalp are washed daily at the time of the bath. This is done with soap and water, as for the remainder of the body. In case there is a "milk crust" on the scalp, some simple oily preparation, such as mineral oil or vaseline, may be placed on the scalp at night and the scalp washed as usual in the morning. At the time of the bath also the genitalia should receive attention. Boys are prone to have adhesions of the foreskin to the glans, and a material known as smegma accumulates back of the glans. If the foreskin is retracted each day and a small amount of oil applied, the part is kept desirably clean and adhesions are prevented. If the foreskin retracts with difficulty, a physician should be consulted in order that the difficulty may be corrected. Smegma accumulates also in the vulva of girls, and this part should be cleansed daily. Cleaning is desirable only of the visible parts.

Very young babies often have a small amount of milk in their breasts. The only importance in this fact is that it be recognized as normal, and all that is required is to let the breasts alone.

It is desirable that the baby's buttocks be washed with soap and water after each stool. Occasionally the buttocks become reddened or even excoriated. This is due to one of two causes. One of these is the strong acid present in diarrheal stools; the other the formation of ammonia from the urine as it remains for a period in the diaper. In either case it is useful to keep the baby's skin protected with some simple ointment. When due to diarrhea the trouble will cease as soon as the diarrhea is controlled. Since the ammonia is formed by the growth of certain bacteria in the urine as it is kept warm next the body, and since it is not possible always to change a diaper immediately it is wet, the management of choice is to place some antiseptic in the diaper which will prevent bacterial growth. Several effective antiseptics are available. Those belonging to the safest and least harmful group are known best by their proprietary names. A good example is Diaparene chloride. For use, one commercial tablet (0.09 gram) of Diaparene is crushed and dissolved in 2 quarts of water, making an amount of solution that will take care of 6 diapers. The solution is used in the final stage of laundering the diapers, after they have been freed from soap and wrung out. The diapers should be allowed to soak in the solution for at least 3 minutes, then wrung out and dried without further rinsing.

In the care of the diaper much has been said against the use of laundry soaps and washing powders, because it was felt that these were instrumental in causing ammonia formation and excoriations. Since these are not the cause of such difficulties, diapers may be washed in the same manner as all other clothes, and then should be well rinsed.

CLOTHING

Lists of clothing for babies and children can be found in many books; probably no two lists are alike. Customs in clothing change. Clothing lists of a few years ago are outmoded now to some extent. The gertrude and petticoat of former lists have now disappeared. Selection of clothes for a baby should be guided by experience and common sense. The baby should be clothed for comfort and health and not primarily for the gratification of the mother. The clothes should be simple and easy to use. Most of the clothes for the young baby are outgrown by six months. After this age, when the baby is more active, a different type of clothing is used.

A list of clothes for a young baby could include diapers, shirts, night gowns and possibly sweaters. Small blankets also should be added to the list. Stockings and dresses could be added, depending on circumstances.

Shirts can be long sleeved or short sleeved, depending on the temperature. On very hot days no shirt is worn. Night gowns for the young baby should be long enough to reach well below the feet; in such case usually stockings are unnecessary. In very hot weather no gown is needed.

It is obvious that wide variation exists in the choice of clothing. The chief objective is comfort of the baby. He should be dressed warmly enough in cold weather and lightly in hot weather. Too often babies are dressed too warmly; they perspire and become restless. If they should kick off the bed covering, they may become chilled.

CRYING

A certain amount of crying daily serves a useful purpose. It is a form of exercise and constitutes a large part of the exercise a young baby gets. Also, in the very young, crying helps to expand the lungs and keep them expanded, overcoming the state of collapse which is normal before birth. However, crying is sometimes excessive. Such crying is usually due to discomfort, which may be from hunger, extremes of temperature, colic or other pain. Although babies cry from fright and anger, these are not causes of habitual crying. It must be admitted also that babies cry sometimes in order to get the attention which they find that crying brings them.

EXERCISE

Exercise is essential for good development. In the early weeks, when the infant is relatively helpless, sufficient exercise is obtained by the usual carrying around of the baby by the mother, although some mothers have been taught to leave their babies too much alone for fear of spoiling them. As muscular development progresses the baby gets his exercise by kicking and other movements while lying unrestricted on his bed. Later he sits, plays, creeps, and walks. After the first few weeks, if permitted, the baby usually will obtain sufficient exercise for himself, but care must be taken that he is at liberty to do so. In addition to permitting the baby to exercise himself while lying unrestricted on the bed, certain formal exercises may be given. After 5 months the baby may be pulled to a sitting position by his hands; while holding his feet gentle resistance can be given to his kicking movements; his straightened legs can be bent upward at the hips until the thighs are on the abdomen. For the runabout child, two hours' exercise in the open air, preferably playing with other children, may be regarded as an average daily requirement.

TRAINING

The training of children begins in early infancy. Babies are born without habits, and those which they get are either accidentally acquired or are taught to them. In infancy small things lead to habit formation. Regularity in feeding and ·in everything done for the baby is conducive to good habits. The baby should become accustomed to going to sleep without the presence of the mother, and certainly he should not be rocked to sleep. He should become accustomed to sleeping without a light at night and if he should awaken at an unusual time and cries, he should be allowed to "cry it out," if it is reasonably certain nothing serious is wrong. The age at which babies can be trained to the toilet is early in proportion to the amount of teaching energy spent in this direction. At three to four months of age, sometimes sooner, the bowel movements tend to occur at rather regular times each day, viz., immediately after the morning bottle. It is a good plan to place the baby over a small vessel regularly at this time after he is mature enough to be held comfortably in this position. In this early period of training the baby should not be held over the vessel for long and no special measure should be used to induce a movement. Although encouragement in developing a regular habit is useful, the baby should not be expected to be reliable for many months. Reliability as to wetting is even slower in development. A good degree of reliability by day may be expected by 18 months and many children have dry beds by 2 to 2½ years.

Thumb sucking of a happy, well fed baby can be disregarded, so long as it occurs only in the period of infancy. Most babies suck their thumbs for a while and then cease as they find other satisfying things to do. Persistent thumb sucking may be associated with malocclusion of the teeth. Moderate thumb sucking in early infancy is normal. Persistent thumb sucking usually represents a feeling of insecurity or other emotional disturbance. In management, preference should be given to efforts at proper education using rewards for compliance rather than to mechanical devices for the thumb.

NUTRITION OF THE INFANT

INTRODUCTORY DISCUSSION

Nutrition deals with the food we eat and the structures which the body makes of it. A diet which is adequate to maintain the body in good nutritional health must include the essential food materials. These essentials are protein, carbohydrate, fat, mineral salts and water.

The body needs all of these various food materials at all ages of life, although the amount and the form in which they may be offered vary according to the age. The infant, the child, and the adult need exactly the same essential food elements. The foods chosen to supply them must be adapted to the digestive capacity and the relative need of the individual. Many foods as prepared for the adult are not in a suitable state for digestion by the infant. Because milk is so easily digested by the infant and because it is so nearly a perfect food, it is commonly the basis on which the infant's diet is constructed.

In the life processes of the body, certain materials are constantly being broken down to simpler ones; the process is comparable in some respects to the burning of fuel in a furnace. This combustion takes place even when the body is in complete repose, and it is increased by activity in proportion to the degree of muscular exertion. In the process of combustion, heat is liberated. This is what keeps the body warm. Heat produced in this manner can be measured. The measurements are made in heat units or calories. A known amount of food will give rise to a definite amount of heat, which can be calculated. Thus it is that food is often measured in terms of calories. If insufficient food were furnished, the body would consume itself to the point where life would be impossible. It is necessary therefore to supply energy (food capable of producing energy) to the body for the purpose of maintaining life. In order that the infant may grow and develop properly, it is necessary to supply energy in addition to that which will only maintain life. Growth takes place only when food is supplied in excess of the amount needed to replace that which is burned to maintain the body. The infant's need for energy is relatively (per unit of body weight) far greater than that of the older child or adult and the effects of an inadequate supply show themselves more quickly. Between 85 and 90 per cent of the infant's energy needs are supplied by fats and carbohydrates, this being the chief function of these two food materials. The remainder of the energy is derived from protein.

Protein is an essential part of all cells; without it, life would be impossible. Plants can form protein from substances which they are able to obtain from the soil and the air. Man and the animals cannot do this but must have the constituents of protein supplied to them either from plants or from other animals. For existence a certain amount of protein must be supplied in the diet, and for body increase (growth) an increased amount is necessary. Since no other food material can replace it, protein is an essential part of the diet. A sufficient amount may readily be supplied by the milk of the infant's diet provided the amount of milk offered is adequate. A moderate deficiency of protein causes slow growth and feeble musculature. Gross deficiencies will eventually lead to death. Proteins from different sources differ in their chemical structure. When a protein has all the components necessary to build the kind of protein needed by the body it is called a "complete" protein. Milk protein may be considered as complete. It is characteristic of the vegetable proteins that they are not complete and as a consequence are not as adequate for producing good growth as are the proteins from animal sources.

The food materials that have been discussed (fat, carbohydrate and protein) are present in the food in relatively large amounts. Other food essentials are present only in small or even minute amounts. The latter group includes both the minerals and the vitamins that are necessary for growth and the maintenance of health. The materials that have been grouped under the general term of vitamins differ widely from one another, yet some similarity exists in that they all are organic substances similar to enzymes and hormones. Formerly they were designated exclusively by letters of the alphabet, but as their structure becomes known their chemical names are used.

Vitamin A is necessary for growth, for a normal state of the skin and the various mucous membranes, for ability to see in a dim light and for certain other functions. While some vitamin A is present in milk fat, egg yolk and in the glandular organs (such as liver) of animals, the largest part of the vitamin A of the diet is in the form of the yellow pigment carotene, which is of vegetable origin and which is changed into vitamin A in the body. Any diet of the infant or child that is considered good from all other points of view contains also adequate amounts of vitamin A or carotene. Additional vitamin A from sources such as cod liver oil, although unnecessary, serves as a safeguard against possible deficiency. A large excess of vitamin A is toxic.

The vitamin B complex is composed of a group of vitamins which tend to occur together, although the relative proportions of each vary in the different foods. Deficiencies of a single member of the group are thus improbable, although deficiencies of one vitamin may predominate. Thus, beriberi is chiefly a thiamine deficiency disease, pellagra results from a shortage of niacin, and a shortage of riboflavin causes sores about the corners of the mouth and disturbances of twilight vision. The B complex occurs in the embryos of seeds, in meat, milk, eggs, fruits and vegetables.

The amount of the B vitamins in human milk depends in a large measure upon the amount in the diet of the mother. The diet of many mothers is so incomplete that the B in the milk is often dangerously low. For this as well as other reasons the diet of the infant is advantageously supplemented at an early age with B containing foods. Although a deficiency of B leads to a loss of appetite, not all babies have their appetites improved by addition to the diet of vitamin B preparations, for the reason that other causes for poor appetite are also common. If fruits, vegetables and egg yolk are included in the infant's diet at an early age it is rarely necessary to give special vitamin B preparations.

Vitamin C also is present in fruits and vegetables. For the young infant either orange juice or tomato juice is relied upon as an adequate source, and the diet should be supplemented early with one of these foods. Deficiency of vitamin C in the diet leads to the disease scurvy. As with vitamin B, the amount of vitamin C in human milk depends on the amount in the diet of the mother. When the mother's diet is good, her milk contains enough vitamin C to meet the needs of the baby. Even so, it is good practice to have the baby accustomed early to orange juice in preparation for the time when he is no longer breast fed. The amount of C in fresh cow's milk may be sufficient to protect the artificially fed infant, but this never should be relied upon, as vitamin C disappears rather rapidly from milk with the lapse of time and especially when milk is pasteurized or kept hot for longer than a few minutes. It is not advisable to feed to an infant fresh cow's milk unless it has undergone some heat treatment. It is a good general rule, therefore, to supplement the diet of every infant with vitamin-C-containing foods, such as orange or tomato juice. If necessary, pure vitamin C (ascorbic acid) can be given as a medicinal preparation.

Vitamin D is essential to the body for the proper use of calcium and phosphorus with which to build bone and teeth. A deficiency of this vitamin in infancy leads to rickets, a condition in which the bones become soft and often crooked. Vitamin D is present in any common food in very large amounts. A well-known and moderately concentrated commercial source is cod-liver oil. Other fish liver oils (percomorph) supply vitamin D in greater concentration. Fat-like substances (sterols) which are normally present in the body may be converted into vitamin D by the action of ultraviolet energy. The common source of ultraviolet energy is sunshine, which explains the infrequency of rickets in the summer and its prevalence in the winter and spring. The very short energy waves which are classed as ultraviolet are easily filtered out of sunshine by clouds and dust, and they do not pass through ordinary window glass. Special lamps have been devised for the production of ultraviolet energy, some of which give off this energy in an amount considerably greater than that obtained from sunshine. Ultraviolet energy converts certain sterols into vitamin D wherever it may come into contact with them, whether it be in the body, in food material, or in some concentrated state. Ergosterol and dihydrocholesterol are the two sterols used for manufacturing vitamin D by irradiation. These two forms of vitamin D can be prepared in a pure crystalline state; they are highly potent in minute amount and are diluted in a solvent for distribution, sometimes in oil, sometimes in a water dispersible solvent. In many communities milk fortified with vitamin D is available. All evaporated milk is fortified. The standard amount used for fortification of milk is 400 units to the quart, or in the case of evaporated milk 400 units to the reconstituted quart. A supplement of vitamin D is highly desirable throughout the growth period, particularly in infancy. Many preparations of vitamin D are available. So far as effectiveness is concerned, little choice exists among them. An appropriate amount of vitamin D is 300 to 400 units a day. When nutritionally adequate amounts of fortified milk are taken, no additional supplement of vitamin D is needed.

Vitamin E is unimportant for the infant because of its wide distribution and the improbability of any infant's receiving an inadequate supply.

Vitamin K may be given to the infant at birth when there is bleeding because of a disturbance of the clotting mechanism.

Under usual circumstances it may be considered that all of the mineral salts necessary to the body, with the exception of iron, are supplied by the milk of the diet. Normally the infant is born with a store of iron which will serve his iron needs for several months. Certainly not later than six months after birth, and preferably sooner, iron or iron-containing foods should be added to the diet. The addition may be by means of egg yolk, strained meats, ground boiled liver, vegetables and fruits, or if desired by iron salts used as a medicine.

Babies born prematurely do not have the usual iron stores at birth, and babies who are ill during the early months may have their iron stores exhausted sooner than the normal expectation. Calcium and phosphorus are essential minerals which are supplied by milk in relative abundance, but are markedly deficient, as compared to milk, in all other foodstuffs. This is important when in later infancy the baby refuses milk.

Water is essential for the storage and combustion of food, for the excretion of waste products, and for many other life processes. The baby's needs for water are relatively much greater than those of the adult, and he shows the harmful effects of deprivation or loss much more quickly and more seriously. This fact becomes important in certain illnesses, such as diarrhea with marked water loss in the stools, and vomiting with failure of water retention. Sometimes a baby becomes so dehydrated (dry) that its life is threatened for this reason alone. In health and with a good diet the amount of water ingested usually need be no cause for special concern since the infant's diet normally contains such a high proportion of water. Water, in addition to the regular diet, may be indicated in hot weather or in case of sweating from any cause. Because of the difficulty of determining when a baby is thirsty, water can be offered regularly at suitable intervals as a routine measure, but frequently it will be found that the baby will refuse it.

Digestion

It is common knowledge that the digestive capacity of the infant is limited. Many foods served to adults would cause digestive disturbances if fed to an infant. The basic food of an infant's diet is milk. The stomach of the new-born baby seems to have acid and digestive juices adequate to digest human milk without difficulty. Unmodified cow's milk tends to cause more or less digestive difficulty in the early months of infancy. The common modification of cow's milk, such as boiling, acidification, or dilution, makes it better adapted to the digestive capacity of the infant.

The young infant has relatively little capacity to digest starchy foods. Babies who are fed cereals or other starches in the early weeks usually have no difficulty from them, as the undigested part of the starch merely passes through as a harmless foreign body. Only occasionally are fermentative processes set up with their consequent distress.

Other foods commonly offered to infants (fruit juices, fruits, sieved vegetables, cod-liver oil) usually cause no digestive difficulties, although sometimes the coarser parts of some of these foods are not digested and are passed in the stools.

The emptying time of the infant's stomach is of some importance. The stomach usually is empty in from two to three hours after a feeding of human milk; and two and one half to three and one half hours are required for cow's milk in the usual modifications. It is inadvisable to feed babies at such short intervals that the stomach at feeding time still contains some food from the last feeding. Too frequent feeding leads to digestive disturbances. Illness from any cause tends to delay the emptying of the stomach and to affect the digestive capacity sufficiently to cause digestive symptoms. Sometimes when the digestive symptoms (vomiting or diarrhea) are prominent and the responsible illness somewhat obscure, the illness is attributed erroneously to the digestive tract.

Stools

The first passages from the bowel after birth are dark green. As soon as food is given, the character of the stool begins to change and usually by the fifth day it has assumed the type characteristic of infancy. When the baby is breast fed the stools are usually passed two to five times daily; they are soft, bright yellow, acid in reaction, and have a slightly sour cheesy odor. The stools from cow's milk are less frequent (one to three daily), somewhat firmer, a less brilliant yellow, and with a more disagreeable odor than those from human milk.

When milk is the principal food, the color of the stool depends in a large measure upon the speed of passage through the bowel. If the passage is rapid, as in cases of diarrhea, the bowel movements do not have time to turn from their normal green to a yellow color, and the stools then are green. If the rate of movement of the intestinal contents is very slow, the stools may become gray or white in color. These various colors are of no significance except as indicators of the speed of movement of intestinal contents. If for any reason the baby is deprived of food, the stool color becomes brownish and increasingly dark and finally dark green, depending upon the degree of starvation.

Probably much more attention is paid to curds in the stools than their importance deserves. The curds most frequently observed are composed of soaps which have been derived from the fat of the food. A moderate amount of these curds may be considered normal for the baby receiving human milk. Usually with cow's-milk feeding, the intestinal contents are moved along more slowly, and the soaps are drier from absorption of water and are pressed more firmly together so that they do not appear as curds. Anything which causes diarrhea or increases the frequency of stools allows the passage of soaps in the form of small masses or curds, so that usually their presence has no greater significance than an indication of more rapid movement of intestinal contents.

The significance of mucus in the stools is also commonly misconstrued. Mucus appears in the stools when the intestinal tract is irritated for any reason. Diarrhea is commonly associated with irritation and consequently with increased mucus. Most cathartics are irritative and are productive of increased mucus, and the common idea of continued catharsis for the purpose of getting rid of mucus is absurd, for the reason that the greater the amount of catharsis, the greater the amount of mucus.

BREAST FEEDING

It seems unnecessary to present arguments that every mother who can should nurse her infant, and most mothers can, at least for the first few months. It is in these early months that natural feeding is of greatest importance. Despite the fact that human milk is such an excellent food, it must be recognized that the milk varies in quality with the diet and habits of the mother. For example, the various vitamins cannot be present in the milk unless they have been taken in adequate quantities by the mother. In order that her milk be at its best and serve well its intended purpose, the mother must observe the common rules of good hygiene and diet. These rules are fully as necessary for her own health as for that of the baby. Mothers frequently develop cavities in their teeth during lactation, because they secrete more calcium in the milk than they ingest. It is desirable also that the mother have sufficient sleep and moderate exercise but never to the point of fatigue. Worry and other nervous states often have a harmful effect which may be reflected in the quality of the milk.

The diet of the mother may be quite varied, and any food is permissible unless it causes digestive disturbance. The avoidance of acid foods is a fallacy. Examples of a well-balanced diet for the pregnant and nursing mother are given in the preceding chapter.

Sometimes it is found that the mother is unable to secrete adequate quantities of milk. If the mother's diet already is good, the milk supply cannot be increased by increasing the diet, although the milk may be increased by improving the diet when this has not been satisfactory. The best stimulus to maintaining or increasing the milk is regular and thorough emptying of the breast. When milk accumulates in the breast because of incomplete emptying, parts of the breast tend to become hard and painful from the pressure of the retained milk. This condition is often called caked breasts. The surest way to decrease the milk is to permit the breasts to become and remain caked.

There are very few good reasons for the mother not to nurse her baby. She should not nurse it if she has tuberculosis or a serious chronic illness. Nursing should be suspended temporarily during a severe acute illness. Menstruation is not a good reason for weaning, even though the baby may be uncomfortable for a day or two. Should the mother become pregnant the baby should be weaned gradually to avoid overtaxing the mother. Medication taken by the mother need not constitute a reason for weaning, for no drugs given in customary doses are secreted in the milk in harmful amounts.

TECHNIC OF NURSING

It is customary to place the baby to the breast six to twelve hours after birth and every six hours during the next twenty-four hours and every four hours thereafter. During these first few days little is obtained by the baby, but the nursing helps to stimulate the flow of milk. Water or 5 per cent sugar solution is offered every four hours. The milk usually is secreted after the third or fourth day. The nursing interval then should be either three or four hours, depending upon the quantity of milk available. More milk is obtained with the shorter interval, and this is usually the better choice in the beginning. The baby should be nursed at one breast at one nursing and the other breast at the next. If the milk supply is not fully adequate, the baby can be fed briefly from the second breast. The average time at the breast is about fifteen minutes. More than half of the milk is obtained in the first five minutes, and the greater portion of the remainder in the next five minutes. Usually something is wrong when the baby nurses longer than twenty minutes.

All babies swallow some air with the milk. This may be a cause of vomiting or of discomfort. It is desirable therefore to hold the baby upright after each nursing and to pat him gently on the back until eructation of the air occurs.

The care of the mother's nipples is important. They should be bathed before and after each feeding. A fissuring of the nipples may occur. This is always painful and sometimes leads to breast abscess. Fissuring of the nipples has the same cause as chapped hands, and can be prevented in the same manner, viz., keep them as dry as possible as far as milk is concerned, and if necessary keep them greased with some simple ointment such as vaseline or cold cream.

DIFFICULTIES

The difficulties encountered in breast feeding are few. Some babies are overfed. This may be evidenced by a large weight gain and intestinal discomfort often of a colicky nature. There may be unusual regurgitation of food and increased frequency of stools. Since most of these symptoms may be produced by other causes as well, it is desirable to make certain of the diagnosis by weighing the baby before and after nursing. The remedy for overfeeding is simple. The baby should be placed on a four-hour schedule. Usually this is sufficient. If it is not, the time at the breast should be shortened. Another measure is to give the baby water immediately before nursing so as to satisfy his hunger sooner.

Relatively large numbers of babies are underfed. This often happens in milder degrees without the mother being aware of it. The chief symptom is a slow or negative weight gain. There may be evidence of hunger, or intestinal discomfort, colic and regurgitation from swallowed air. Air swallowing tends to be greater in underfed babies. Weighing before and after nursing to determine the amount of milk taken will disclose the difficulty. The remedy in underfeeding is to give food in addition to the breast milk, and not to wean the baby. A suitable formula prepared from cow's milk should be given after each breast feeding. In some instances enough human milk may be obtained by feeding the baby at both breasts each nursing.

Whenever the baby becomes ill from any cause, he is likely to have gastrointestinal symptoms, even though no primary disease exists in the intestinal tract. Thus, one should not be too ready to blame these intestinal symptoms upon the milk and to overlook the real causative factor. So often when the milk "disagrees," the difficulty is entirely unrelated to the milk.

WEANING

In general it is the choice of wisdom to wean the baby from the breast at the age of six to nine months. This may be done gradually by substituting an increasing number of bottle or cup feedings. If the baby has reached the weaning age without being accustomed to a bottle or cup, it often happens that he will refuse it as long as he can get the breast. Thus abrupt weaning is necessary at times. In the case of abrupt weaning, when the baby is unaccustomed to cow's milk, it is usually preferable to have the formula slightly weaker for a few days than it would be normally for the baby's age. Weaning in the summer is still feared by many mothers. There need be no such fear if the milk formula and other foods are appropriate for the baby and are properly prepared.

ARTIFICIAL FEEDING

Human and cow's milk are similar in many respects. They have the same constituents, but the proportions are different. It is chiefly because of these differences in proportion that digestive difficulties occur when unmodified cow's milk is fed to young infants. The milk of all cows is the same except for the quantity of fat. For infant feeding it is generally advisable to use milk of medium or low fat content. Holstein milk or milk from a mixed herd is preferable. Milk from Jersey or Guernsey cows should be partially skimmed.

Milk is easily contaminated in the milking and handling and is an excellent food for the growth of bacteria. All harmful bacteria and most of the others are killed by pasteurization. Boiling milk for several minutes also kills the bacteria and in addition alters the milk in such a way that the casein forms a finer curd and is thereby more easily digested by the infant. For this reason it is generally preferable to use boiled milk, and when this is done pasteurization is unnecessary.

Evaporated milk is ordinary fresh cow's milk which has been concentrated to slightly less than half of its volume by the evaporation of the water. It is then sealed in cans and sterilized. It has been shown to be an excellent, safe, and convenient food for the artificial feeding of infants. For use it may be diluted back to its original volume with water and used in the same manner as fresh milk. The sweetened varieties of evaporated milk (condensed milk) are not suitable for the routine feeding of infants, as the protein content of such milk when diluted for use is so low that it does not permit proper growth of muscle tissue.

Dried milk is milk which has had practically all of its water removed. It is useful in infant feeding, although usually more expensive than fresh or evaporated milk. Some dried milks are prepared from skimmed milk instead of from whole milk. Dried milk is used frequently in communities which cannot obtain fresh milk and for other special reasons. To obtain a product similar to whole milk it is necessary to add one part by weight of the dried whole milk to seven parts of water.

SUGARS AND CARBOHYDRATES

Milk alone is not a suitably balanced food in early infancy without the addition of sugar, and when the milk has been modified by dilution sugar is necessary to satisfy the energy requirements of the infant. Thus some variety of sugar is usually used in the milk formula. The sugars commonly used are lactose (milk sugar), cane sugar (table sugar), and derivatives of starch (dextrin, maltose, dextrose, and mixtures of these). All of these serve the baby equally well after they have been absorbed from the intestinal tract. The choice of sugar is based upon its cost and upon its behavior in the intestinal tract of the infant. Certain sugars are more laxative than others. For example, lactose is absorbed relatively slowly and usually passes far down the intestinal tract before complete absorption. This long presence in the tract has a laxative effect. At the other extreme is dextrose, which is absorbed quickly and consequently is a good sugar to use in cases of diarrhea. Corn syrup is a mixture of dextrin, maltose and dextrose and has found favor because it is inexpensive as well as useful, although it is less convenient to handle than the dry sugars. Dry dextrin-maltose mixtures are extensively employed.

DILUENTS

One of the chief objects in the modification of cow's milk to make it more suitable for young infants is to alter the casein in such a manner that it forms a fine curd in the stomach. This object is very commonly achieved by dilution with water. Sometimes cereal water, usually barley water, is used for this purpose. Such diluents do no harm but provide little food value. Lime-water, so commonly used in the past, is now seldom employed as a diluent.

SYNTHETIC FOOD MIXTURES

Several manufacturers have prepared mixtures of milk and sugar in proportions thought to be suitable for infant feeding, and these may be obtained in a dry or liquid form. All that is required for use is the addition of water in specified proportions. All of these mixtures are relatively expensive. In most instances an attempt has been made to make these synthetic foods similar to human milk. Because of their low protein content, many such milks are not well suited to the rapidly growing infant. Malted milk and sweetened condensed milk are examples of milk and sugar mixtures which are quite ill suited for infant feeding, because of their high sugar content.

FORMULAS FOR WELL BABIES

Milk satisfies the need of the infant for most of the nutritional essentials when at least 1½ ounces for each pound of weight is given each twenty-four hours. By the time the baby is taking a quart of milk a day, other foods may be added to supplement the diet in such a way that more milk is unnecessary.

The amount of sugar added to meet the total food requirement is usually one ounce daily during the first two months and one and a half ounces during the succeeding four months. More or less than this may be indicated under special circumstances.

The amount of diluent (water) used should be sufficient to bring the total volume to that which the baby will take conveniently in twenty-four hours. In general it may be stated that a young baby should take at a single feeding two to three ounces more than his age in months. Seldom is it desirable to give more than seven ounces at a feeding at any age, for by the time the baby is receiving seven ounces he is taking also foods other than milk.

As an example, a baby four months of age weighing 14 pounds might do well with a formula containing twenty-four ounces of milk, one and one half ounces of sugar, and water sufficient to make five feedings of six and one half ounces each, or six feedings of six ounces each, as seems best suited to the individual baby.

During the first two weeks after birth the milk dilution usually should be a little greater than that which has been specified until the baby becomes accustomed to the cow's-milk feeding. The original mixture should never be less than half milk, and this should be used for only a few days. It is frequently customary to start with two thirds milk and one third water.

A feeding schedule which will be found suitable for the majority of well babies is as follows:

Age Months	Weight Pounds	Milk Ounces	Water Ounces	Sugar Ounces	Feedings Number	Ounces
½	7	11	7	1	6–7	2½–3
1	8	14	10	1	6–7	3½–4
2	10	18	12	1¼	5–6	5–6
3	12	21	9	1½	5–6	5–6
4	14	25	10	1¾	5–6	6–7
6	16–17	28	7	2	5	7
8	18–20	32	8	1½	5	7
12	22	32	—	—	4	8

If corn syrup is used as the sugar, an equal volume of water is omitted.

Sugar Equivalents

1 ounce by weight of cane sugar = 2 level tablespoons.
1 ounce by weight of lactose = 4 level tablespoons.
1 ounce by weight dried malt sugar = 4 level tablespoons.
1 ounce by volume of corn syrup = 2 level tablespoons and contains 1 ounce of sugar.

It must be remembered that the formulas and schedules given are calculated for the average baby and that adjustments frequently will be necessary for any individual baby. A baby who is hungry, not gaining as he should, and who is having no digestive difficulties should have more food than is indicated in the schedule. Often minor adjustments in the quantity or type of sugar will make the difference between constipation and loose stools. For these and many other reasons it is highly advisable to have the infant's feeding under the supervision of one who is expert in such matters.

FORMULAS WITH UNDILUTED MILK

Cow's milk may be altered in other ways than by dilution so that it is readily utilized by the infant. One of the methods of accomplishing this is by the addition of an acid in carefully regulated quantities to milk which has been previously boiled. Lactic acid (the acid of naturally soured milk) and citric acid (the acid of citrous fruits) have been used extensively for this purpose. Milk which has been soured by bacterial growth under laboratory control is excellent when it is available. The feeding of undiluted acid milk permits a greater food intake and thus a more rapid growth is brought about. These babies exceed the averages in height and weight. In the light of some of our more recent knowledge this would seem to be an advantage. The following table gives an approximate feeding schedule for the average well infant using undiluted acidified milk:

Age	Milk oz.	Sugar oz. (wt.)	Feedings oz.
1 wk.	12	½	6 x 2
2 wk.	15	1	6 x 2½
1 mo.	18	1½	6 x 3
2 mo.	25	2	5 x 5
4 mo.	30	2	5 x 6
6 to 10 mo.	35	2	5 x 7

If corn syrup is used as the sugar, an equal volume of milk is omitted.

THE PREPARATION OF FORMULAS

Sweet Milk Dilutions

The milk, sugar, and water should be mixed and then boiled from one to three minutes with constant stirring. It should be poured immediately into boiled nursing bottles, stoppered and cooled rapidly, and placed on ice until ready for use.

Lactic Acid or Citric Acid Milk

The milk and sugar should be mixed and boiled for two minutes while stirring. It should be cooled rapidly; when quite cold the acid is added slowly while constantly stirring. It should then be poured into nursing bottles, stoppered, and placed on ice.

The amount of citric acid required is usually two grams to the quart of milk. Citric acid is purchased as a powder, of which one teaspoonful weighs approximately two grams. It is dissolved in a small quantity of water and the solution stirred into the milk.

Lactic acid is purchased as an 85 per cent solution. One teaspoonful or one hundred and twenty drops is required for each quart of milk.

Sometimes orange juice is added to the milk. The amount required to bring a quart of milk to the proper acidity is about two ounces.

The amount of lemon juice required is about two-thirds of an ounce.

Evaporated Milk

Evaporated milk is sterile and further heat treatment is unnecessary. For the preparation of a formula the mixture of water and sugar is boiled and added to the evaporated milk. To prepare an acidified formula only two-thirds as much acid is required as for fresh milk.

CHOICE AND CARE OF BOTTLES AND NIPPLES

It is preferable to have as many nursing bottles and nipples as there are feedings in the day. Both the bottles and the nipples should be of such a type that they can be readily and thoroughly cleaned. The bottles and nipples should be washed with soap and water and boiled for five minutes. The bottles are then ready for filling and the nipples for clean storage.

Any funnels, spoons, pans, etc., used in the preparation of the formula should be boiled each time before use. If possible it is advisable to have one set of utensils for use in the preparation of the baby's formula only.

TECHNIC OF FEEDING

For feeding, the milk should be warmed to body temperature by placing the bottle in a vessel of hot water. Care should be taken not to heat acidified mixtures much above body temperatures for the reason that the curd is likely to clot and settle out. The size of the hole in the nipple should be such that when the bottle is inverted the milk drops out rapidly but does not flow in a steady stream. The baby should be fed in arms and in a position in which the shoulders are higher than the buttocks. Any milk refused should be discarded. After feeding and before being put to bed the baby should be held in a position which will permit regurgitation of any swallowed air. Gentle patting on the back will assist in eructation of the air.

ADDITIONS TO THE MILK DIET

Neither human nor cow's milk is a perfect food. Babies fed exclusively on either for a long period will develop certain nutritional diseases. Iron and vitamins C and D and possibly some of the B vitamins are likely to be deficient. Foods which supplement the milk diet in these respects should be given early.

Orange juice should be started early in the first month. Two tablespoons of orange juice should be diluted with an equal quantity of water and given once daily. This amount is gradually increased to the juice of half an orange at three months of age and then to that of an entire orange daily. In some instances it is advisable to substitute tomato juice for orange juice. When this is done a somewhat greater quantity of tomato juice should be used.

Vitamin D should be started early in infancy. If cod liver oil is used, the amount in the beginning can be one half teaspoonful daily and gradually increased until one teaspoonful is given. One teaspoonful daily of a high-grade cod-liver oil will be found sufficient for most babies. It is probable that the baby needs cod-liver oil in the summer as well as in the winter, for during the hot summer months it is not always possible to give him sufficient sunshine. Iron in some form should be given the baby before he is six months of age. Although it may be given in the form of medicinal iron, it is usually preferable to administer it in some iron-containing food. Egg yolk, green vegetables and fruits are the foods commonly chosen for infants. They are offered to babies at increasingly earlier ages and are of value not only for their iron, but also for their content of B and other vitamins and minerals.

It is customary to give various cereals to infants beginning at about 3 months. Cereal is entirely satisfactory as an infant food, although it is probably not as important as are the fruits and vegetables and egg yolk. Consequently it seems more advisable to have the infant well established on these other foods before cereal is started, unless a fortified proprietary cereal food is used.

CARE OF THE SICK INFANT

The illnesses of an infant are usually of an acute rather than of a chronic nature, and the general care is very similar for all illnesses. The infant should be allowed to lie quietly in bed, and the feedings, treatments, etc., should be spaced at as long intervals as possible. There is often a strong tendency to keep doing things to and for the patient, with the result that little of the much needed rest is obtained, and the baby becomes exhausted. Excitement should be avoided and unnecessary entertainment reduced to a minimum.

An effort should be made to have the air of the sick-room fresh at all times, but this does not mean that it need be raw, cold winter air. No illness of infancy requires any special type of clothing. The clothing should be that to which the infant is accustomed during sleep in health. Except in the case of premature and very delicate infants, the patient should have a cleansing bath (at least one) daily. There is no acute illness in which bathing is harmful. The feeding of the sick infant is discussed subsequently.

Infants have higher body temperature from the same or less important causes than do adults. A temperature of 104 or 105 degrees in an infant does not demand any measures for relief unless it is of considerable duration or unless it is associated with such nervous symptoms as restlessness and inability to sleep.

A common and effective method of reducing high temperature is bathing. A bath of the type designated as a sponge bath is satisfactory.

At times definite indications for the use of drugs are encountered in infancy, but in general, drug treatment plays a relatively minor rôle. The measures which assume greater importance are diet, hygiene, and general nursing care.

COMMON ILLNESSES AND ABNORMALITIES

JAUNDICE IN THE NEWBORN

Icterus or jaundice occurs in newly born babies with considerable frequency and in the vast majority of instances is without significance for the health of the infant. When jaundice is present the white part of the eyeball is yellow, and in the more marked cases the skin also has a definitely yellow color. It appears in the first two or three days after birth, and its persistence varies from a few days to several weeks. No treatment is indicated for this common form of jaundice.

HERNIA OR "RUPTURE"

The most frequently encountered hernia in infancy is at the navel or umbilicus. At this point the usual finding is a weak place in the abdominal wall, which upon finger pressure is felt as a hole, usually smaller than the end of the finger. With the intra-abdominal pressure produced by crying a protrusion is to be observed at the site of the hernia. Umbilical hernia usually causes no discomfort or other difficulty. With the wearing of some device which effectively prevents protrusion of the hernia, the defect nearly always disappears in the course of some months. The simplest method of controlling the hernia is to cover it with a tightly drawn strip of adhesive tape. No device should be used which keeps the defect open by pushing inward through it.

The inguinal hernia occurs with considerably less frequency. In this condition the protrusion is on one or both sides of the lower abdomen (the groin) immediately above and to either side of the genitalia. The general principles of management are the same as for umbilical hernia. Adhesive tape cannot be applied effectively, and the simplest truss is made from a skein of yarn.

COMMON COLDS

The symptoms of the common cold are well known to everyone, and it is unnecessary to enumerate them. Some of the consequences of this infection are very important for the infant. An infant cannot suckle satisfactorily when the nose is obstructed. Difficulty will be encountered in the feeding, with the possible result of marked underfeeding. In infancy some vomiting and looseness of the stools frequently accompany a cold. In general, colds affect infants much more seriously than older persons, not only by producing more marked symptoms, but also by having a greater frequency of complications. Secondary inflammations in the ears, bronchi, and lungs are not infrequent.

In the endeavor to prevent colds it is important to realize that they are infectious and contagious. They are readily contracted from others. Exposure to drafts and low temperatures can be of no significance unless infectious material is present also. The difference between those who are subject to frequent colds and those who seem relatively immune is not known with exactness, but in general those who have good hygienic care, receive a complete diet, and are in a good state of nutrition, have fewer colds than those who are lacking in these factors.

A measure important in the management of a cold in an infant is an endeavor to keep the nose open sufficiently for breathing and for drainage. Oil preparations, particularly those containing such substances as camphor or menthol, should not be used in infancy. Frequently physicians prescribe a drug, such as a solution of ephedrin or neosynephrin, to be sprayed or dropped into the nose for the purpose of reducing the swelling and thus producing a larger breathing space. Often free drainage from the nose is a great aid in the prevention of a complicating ear infection.

OTITIS MEDIA

Otitis media is inflammation within the cavity of the ear immediately behind the eardrum. This cavity is connected directly with the throat by what is called the eustachian tube. Thus infections in the nose and throat have a more or less direct path to the ear. It is the rule in infants that otitis media produces a relatively high fever, pain, restlessness, and often general constitutional symptoms among which may be vomiting and diarrhea. A few babies sometimes have otitis media with only a part of these symptoms or even none of them, and the otitis is diagnosed only by examination of the ears.

Otitis media occurs in varying degrees of severity and may be seen first by the physician in different stages of development or subsidence. The treatment to be instituted depends upon these various factors. With a severe inflammation and bulging of the eardrum, the drum should be incised to permit drainage of the pus lying within. In cases of moderate or early inflammation the proper treatment may be to let it alone and observe its progress. If there seems to be pain, the physician often advises the dropping into the ears of certain pain relieving preparations. Often also one of the antibiotic or sulfa drugs may be prescribed.

The bony cavity of the mastoid connects directly with the middle ear and consequently is inflamed in every case of otitis media. In most instances the products of inflammation drain by way of the middle ear, and the mastoid inflammation subsides along with that of the ear. In a few instances the mastoid inflammation causes sufficient swelling about the opening into the ear that drainage is not possible. The mastoid inflammation then assumes increased importance and is designated mastoiditis. In many of these cases it becomes necessary to make a surgical opening into the mastoid from the exterior. Mastoiditis is even more likely than otitis media to produce constitutional symptoms, and sometimes in infancy the resulting vomiting and diarrhea constitute a grave menace to life. Often the gastro-intestinal symptoms completely overshadow the slight or even negative external evidences of mastoiditis.

CROUP

The term croup has been used to designate inflammations in the larynx which give rise to difficulty in breathing. The term "membranous croup," now being used decreasingly in the interest of more exact diagnosis, has been applied to the obstruction of the larynx produced by inflammations associated with exudates in a form resembling membrane. Membranous croup is practically synonymous with diphtheria of the larynx.

The less serious form of croup, and the form which is usually implied in the term croup, is known also as spasmodic or catarrhal croup. In this condition a relatively mild inflammation of the larynx leads reflexly to a spasm of the muscles of the larynx. During a period of spasm the opening through the larynx is almost completely closed, and air is drawn into the lungs with considerable difficulty and with a plainly audible noise. No difficulty exists in expiration. The attacks of spasm, which are often alarming but rarely serious, tend to recur for a period of about three days, when the inflammation and its symptoms usually subside. The attacks are more frequent at night, the days often being entirely free from them.

The attacks may be relieved by breathing air containing warm-water vapor (steam), and for this purpose croup kettles have been devised. A less troublesome, effective method is the administration of certain antispasmodic drugs, with which the attacks may be forestalled and prevented as well as relieved. In using croup kettles be sure to avoid turning them over and burning the child.

PNEUMONIA

Pneumonia may be primary or secondary. By secondary is meant that the pneumonia occurs as a complication or an extension of some other disease, such as a common cold, bronchitis, measles, influenza, etc. Primary pneumonia occurs in a manner similar to other contagious diseases, being contracted from one who has the disease or a carrier, and not ordinarily secondary to or complicating some other disease. In many respects the general nature of the illness is much the same in these two types of pneumonia. Both types of pneumonia are serious, but the primary type is much less so.

The fear of pneumonia has been removed to a great extent by the use of sulfonamide drugs and the antibiotics, and the course is greatly shortened. The treatment in infancy is much the same in the two types of pneumonia. In addition to the treatment mentioned, other treatment is given according to the symptoms present. Sedatives are indicated for severe and constant cough; bathing for high fever accompanied by nervous symptoms; oxygen for breathing if the baby should become blue; stimulation in case of failing vital functions. Babies with secondary pneumonia, babies with any considerable degree of bronchitis, and delicate infants should not be placed in cold air, but should be given warm moist fresh air. Babies with pneumonia should have their position changed frequently. Pneumonia is one illness in which it is of advantage to hold the infant in arms, because of the frequent change of position that this causes. The administration of considerable amounts of water or fluid is especially advantageous in pneumonia.

THRUSH

Thrush is the result of the growth of a specific fungus on the mucous membrane of the mouth. The fungus in its growth forms small slightly elevated white plaques which are difficult to remove. Thrush, as it usually occurs, causes no symptoms. The treatment consists of local applications made gently by means of cotton on the end of an applicator. Roughness in treatment tends to spread the infection. The preparation to be used as a local application depends upon the preference of the individual physician. Several preparations are about equally effective.

INTUSSUSCEPTION

Intussusception is a condition almost exclusively of infancy, in which one part of the bowel enters and becomes infolded in the part of the bowel in immediate contiguity to it. The blood supply of the invaginated bowel becomes cut off and in the course of a short time that part of the bowel dies and becomes gangrenous. The condition is characterized by an abrupt onset, associated with vomiting, sharp pain, and increasing prostration. At the onset there may be one or two small bowel movements, usually with some evidences of blood. After this time nothing is passed by the bowel. If an enema is returned it will usually contain blood.

Intussusception demands immediate operation for its relief. Early operation has a low mortality, while delay increases the seriousness of the condition.

RECTAL PROLAPSE

Rectal or anal prolapse is a protrusion of the mucous membrane of the anus or anus and lower rectum which occurs usually only at stool. It is possible for this to occur occasionally in a normal infant when the stool is large and hard and is passed with much straining. However, it is more frequent in babies who are poorly nourished and as a consequence have relaxed muscles about the anus. In these prolapse may occur either with constipation or with diarrhea; occasionally when the prolapse has recurred over a long period, it may occur with more or less normal stools.

Three factors should be considered in the treatment. The prolapse should be replaced whenever it occurs and some means should be used in an endeavor to hold it in at all times. For this purpose the buttocks can be strapped tightly together with adhesive tape or a pad should be worn which makes pressure at the anus. If either constipation or diarrhea is present it should be corrected by appropriate means. The stools should be made of such a consistency that they are passed with a minimum of effort and without straining. The general nutrition should be improved, thus improving general muscular tone. It is seldom that the proper application of these measures fails to be effective.

PYELITIS

Pyelitis is an inflammation of the pelvis of the kidney. It may occur at any age, but is much more common in infants and young children, and more frequent in girls than in boys. The infection may ascend the urinary tract to the kidney from the exterior, or perhaps more frequently the bacteria causing the inflammation are carried to the kidney by the blood. The bacteria most often responsible are normal inhabitants of the intestinal tract. The intestinal wall seems more permeable to these bacteria in the presence of diarrhea or marked constipation. In infancy the tendency to intestinal disturbances as a result of colds and respiratory infections increases the frequency of pyelitis during the existence of these head infections.

The symptoms of pyelitis in infancy are usually general rather than local. Fever is the most constant symptom, and this tends to be very irregular. Sometimes fever is the only definite symptom, or perhaps fever and irritability. Because of the lack of localizing symptoms, the diagnosis is not made except by examination of the urine. The urine shows evidence of inflammation, chiefly pus cells and bacteria.

These urinary infections usually respond promptly to treatment with sulfonamides or antibiotics. In the few instances in which the inflammation recurs frequently or becomes chronic special examination is necessary; usually some urinary obstruction is present which requires relief.

VAGINITIS

Inflammation of the vagina or of the vulva and vagina as it occurs in infancy and childhood is chiefly of two varieties. The most frequent of these is due to lack of cleanliness. In general mothers seem very hesitant about the detailed cleansing of the external genitalia of their children, and later about teaching the children to cleanse themselves. Secretions accumulate, decompose, and not only give rise to an unpleasant odor, but actually set up inflammatory processes. Usually these are of mild degree, but they can be severe enough to cause an active discharge. This variety of vaginitis can be prevented and usually cured by ordinary cleansing measures.

Less frequently is encountered vaginitis due to a specific bacterium, the gonococcus. Among adults this variety of infection is looked upon as a social disease. Among girls, however, it is contagious, and it is nearly always innocently contracted. It is distinguished from other varieties of vaginitis chiefly and definitely by identification of the specific bacterium in the discharges. Bacteriological examination of the discharge is usually the first measure undertaken by the physician. This variety of vaginitis responds promptly to penicillin or other antibiotic treatment.

CONVULSIONS

The common type of convulsion is a condition in which the child loses consciousness, becomes rigid and then has spasmodic jerking movements of the face and extremities. They may be very brief, may last several minutes, or occasionally a longer time. They may be repeated, the child having a series of short convulsions.

A convulsion is merely a symptom and the possible disease causes are many. Infants have convulsions more easily than do adults. Sometimes convulsions usher in some acute infection such as pneumonia. In fact, the onset of some acute infection with rapid rise in body temperature is perhaps the most frequent cause of convulsions. A convulsion is very alarming to the parents, but in itself it is not serious except as the underlying cause may be serious. Sometimes the underlying cause is not readily found. In the case of pneumonia, for example, several days may elapse before the diagnosis can be made with certainty. Whether or not the diagnosis can be made at once, the indication is to bring the convulsions under control and take measures to prevent their recurrence. The most effective remedies are sedative drugs, and these must be administered or prescribed by the physician according to the individual indications. A hot bath is often used in an endeavor to control a convulsion. Wrapping the baby in blankets and applying a hot-water bottle or electric pad to the feet is equally effective and considerably less disturbing.

The foregoing discussion concerns chiefly those convulsions associated with fever. Those occurring in infancy without fever are most frequently a symptom of tetany, a condition caused by changes in the calcium and phosphorus content of the blood. The relief of convulsions of this type is most readily and advantageously brought about by the use of certain mineral salts. These and the method of their administration would be chosen according to the preferences of the physician.

Convulsions which occur without fever and which recur from time to time and for which no definite cause can be found are usually classified under the term epilepsy. These require prolonged treatment with drugs under the management of a physician.

FEEDING IN ACUTE ILLNESS

It has been mentioned previously that any acute illness lowers the digestive capacity of the infant and consequently may be a cause of vomiting, or diarrhea, especially when the usual type of feeding is continued. It has been mentioned also that the underlying infection may be obscure, and the difficulty erroneously attributed entirely to the gastro-intestinal tract. Because the continuance of the usual diet is so likely to lead to disturbance in the presence of acute illness, it is desirable to make certain alterations.

It is often beneficial to remove some or most of the fat from the milk and to discontinue the more solid and less easily digestible foods. If the illness is prolonged it will be found necessary to continue to give fair amounts of food, even though a certain amount of digestive disturbance is present, for otherwise the general nutrition will suffer greatly. The baby must be given enough food to keep up his resistance in order that he may be aided in overcoming the disease.

VOMITING

Vomiting may occur in infancy from many causes. The most frequent cause in the otherwise normal baby is some factor which produces distention of the stomach. This may be produced by too large a feeding or by feeding at such short intervals that the stomach is only partially empty when the next feeding is given. The stomach may be distended by the presence of a large amount of swallowed air in addition to the usual feedings. The effects of distention are obtained with tight clothing or abdominal bands. Occasionally the infant has a small stomach capacity, and the feeding of the usual volume of food causes distention. The remedy for all of these distention-producing factors is obvious, once the cause is determined.

The next most frequent cause of vomiting is illness. Almost any acute infection in the infant will produce this event. Vomiting in the acute infections is largely the direct result of irritation of the stomach by the fermentation of food which lies in the stomach unusually long because of the impaired emptying power of the stomach. An excess of fat in the diet may act in this same manner, by delaying the emptying of the stomach. Other less common causes of vomiting depend upon stomach irritation or the ingestion of spoiled foods or inappropriate foods.

A few babies vomit merely because of an apparent desire on their part to do so. This is spoken of as "rumination" in certain instances in which the food is voluntarily brought up for no good reason. In occasional cases babies seem to vomit as a defense reaction against certain foods or against forced feeding. In cases of voluntary vomiting a change in the method of management is indicated. A temporary complete change in environment including caretaker often is all that is necessary.

Any obstruction in the intestinal tract leads to vomiting. The varieties of obstruction are numerous, and all are serious. Some of these seem to have a gradual beginning, as in the obstruction at the lower end (pylorus) of the stomach, which is noticed in the first six weeks after birth; and some may have a sudden onset associated subsequently with evidence of great prostration, as in cases in which one part of the bowel becomes looped into the part immediately next to it.

This is not a complete enumeration of the causes of vomiting, but the discussion includes the most important causes from the standpoint of frequency.

Thus, vomiting may be produced by such simple and easily remedied conditions as overfilling of the stomach, or it may be a symptom of some very serious condition which demands immediate medical attention.

COLIC

In practically all instances intestinal colic in infancy is associated with the presence of gas in the intestines. This gas may have either one of two sources. It may be air which has been swallowed and which has passed beyond the stomach, or the gas may be the result of fermentation of sugar within the intestinal tract. For permanent relief of colic the cause must be abolished. Swallowed air should be made to pass upward after each feeding. Since underfed babies are more likely to swallow air, one should make certain that the food supply is ample. Fermentation may be the result of overfeeding or of the presence of a large quantity of sugar. The correction of overfeeding at the breast has been discussed. When colic occurs in the breast-fed baby in the absence of overfeeding, often the giving of an ounce of boiled skimmed cow's milk before each breast feeding will bring relief. In the artificially fed baby the sugar may be reduced in quantity or altered as to variety. It should be made certain that the baby is receiving sufficient food.

Effective simple measures for temporary relief are enemas or hot applications to the abdomen. In cases of severe colic sometimes an opiate (paregoric) or other drug is required temporarily to give relief.

CONSTIPATION

With the rare exception of certain congenital defects, the causes of constipation in infancy can be classified chiefly into two groups. One group includes those instances in which the residue of food left for excretion is too small to constitute sufficient stimulus to intestinal movement. A small residue is usually the result of underfeeding, though it may also be due to the giving of a type of food which is absorbed to an unusually high degree. The other group includes those instances in which the fecal mass becomes so firm or putty-like that it is moved along with difficulty. This type of constipation is not seen in the naturally fed infant. In the artificially fed infant it is dependent chiefly upon the relative proportion of milk to sugar. A high-milk, low-sugar diet tends to produce the dry type of stool, and thus this kind of constipation; whereas a low-milk, high-sugar formula is laxative.

In the treatment of constipation in infancy drugs ordinarily should not be used except as a temporary measure, pending dietary adjustment. When a drug cathartic is considered necessary, milk of magnesia is usually satisfactory in doses of one to two teaspoonfuls. Instead of drugs it may be preferable to use enemas or suppositories also as temporary measures. In practically every case it will be found that constipation can be relieved by appropriate alteration in the diet, and an earnest attempt to establish a regular habit.

In cases in which the food residue is small it is desirable first to make certain that the food intake is adequate. Additional measures are the feeding of fruits and vegetables somewhat earlier than the customary age, or if these are already being given, to increase the amount. Strained orange juice is not laxative, but prune juice is.

In cases in which it is desirable to alter the nature of the fecal mass a favorable result often may be achieved by increasing the amount of sugar in the formula. If moderate and reasonable increase in the sugar does not give relief, a change in the type of sugar is advisable. Certain sugars are more laxative than others. Milk sugar is more laxative than some of the malt sugars, although the syrupy malt sugars (malt soup extract) are the most laxative of all the sugars. Although constipation may be relieved by decreasing the amount of milk, this should not be done unless the quantity taken is well above the requirements which have been stated previously.

DIARRHEA

In general it may be considered that diarrhea is the result of irritation or abnormal stimulation of the intestinal tract. Because of the unusual stimulus the intestinal movements are increased in intensity, and food material is passed along at a rapid rate. Because of this rapid rate of passage some of the food and much of the water are not absorbed, and as a consequence the stools are fluid and often contain a fair proportion of undigested food.

The increased stimulus may be caused by infection and inflammation of the intestinal tract. In this group belong bacillary and amebic dysentery and typhoid and paratyphoid (salmonella) infections. With better hygiene and improved care of milk and other food these infections are much less common than formerly. In each of these infections the stools show evidence of the disease. In the dysenteries pus and often blood are present. In all the infections the cause can be determined by bacteriologic examination. Prompt determination of the cause is important in order that appropriate treatment may be given. Bacillary dysentery responds promptly to sulfonamides and antibiotics. Typhoid infection responds to chloromycetin. We have very useful remedies for amebic dysentery.

A type of diarrhea difficult to manage is one that occurs epidemically among newborn babies. Many of these diarrheas, if not all, are the result of a virus infection for which we do not yet have a specific remedy. Most of the babies recover if expert medical and nursing care is given.

Diarrhea, often accompanied by vomiting, may occur as a complication of infection elsewhere than in the intestinal tract, such as an inflammation in the ears. In these instances the diarrhea responds to treatment of the infection and to appropriate changes in the diet.

Diarrhea may occur as a result of taking improper food or food that has been contaminated by bacteria which produce toxic products in their growth.

Even perfectly proper foods may be a cause of diarrhea if they are given in excess of the infant's ability to digest and absorb them. For example, almost any infant can be made to have diarrhea by increasing sufficiently the amount of sugar in the diet.

In many instances the cause of diarrhea can not be determined. In such cases response may be expected to appropriate dietary changes.

Some food loss occurs in diarrhea, but the most serious effect is water loss. In the usual mild diarrhea the baby is not particularly ill and the water loss seldom becomes important. However, when diarrhea is severe and prolonged, severe and even fatal dehydration occurs unless measures are taken to keep the body supplied with fluid.

Even though the diarrhea may not be primarily dependent on the diet, certain alterations in the diet are desirable when the diarrhea has occurred. First, it is desirable to allow the intestinal tract to empty. It is customary for some physicians to give a cathartic to hasten the emptying, but this is not necessary. During a brief period, when the tract is emptying, water but no food should be given. The fasting period need not be more than a few hours, in cases of mild diarrhea, although its duration depends upon the severity of the diarrhea and the general condition of the infant. In a few cases of severe diarrhea fasting may have to continue for several days. The first food after the fast may advantageously be one which is high in protein and low in sugar and fat. Boiled skimmed milk is a customary means for fulfilling these requirements. As the diarrhea improves, sugar and fat are gradually replaced in the diet.

MALNUTRITION

Malnutrition may be due to a low food intake, or to failure of absorption. A common cause of malnutrition is failure to offer the infant sufficient food. The body continues to burn food materials whether or not sufficient food is given. If the ingestion and absorption of food are inadequate, the body burns its own tissues. It is thus possible for extreme malnutrition to occur even to the extent of causing death. Malnourished infants are more susceptible to infection than are the better nourished. These infections only add to the difficulties in improving the nutrition.

Another common cause of severe malnutrition is loss of food by chronic or frequently recurring diarrhea together with the underfeeding so often employed in the treatment of diarrhea. Chronic infection anywhere in the body tends to decrease the appetite and to increase the tendency to diarrhea and increase the food requirement.

When malnutrition is caused solely by underfeeding, the remedy is obvious. When it is caused by diarrhea, which in turn is dependent upon infection, the management is more difficult, but even so, careful treatment will usually bring about recovery.

RICKETS

Rickets is a disease of nutrition in which the chief fault lies either in a deficiency of calcium and phosphorus in the diet, or an inability on the part of the body to make proper use of these materials. If the infant receives sufficient milk, the amount of calcium and phosphorus will be adequate. The proportion of these two substances relative to each other affects their absorption. However, when the intake of vitamin D is adequate or with a sufficient amount of sunshine or ultraviolet energy, calcium and phosphorus are well utilized from a customary diet regardless of their proportion. The greater frequency of rickets in late winter and spring is explained by the small amount of available sunshine.

The most striking effects of rickets are seen in the bones because bones have such a large proportion of calcium and phosphorus in their structure. The mineral deficiency associated with rickets causes them to be softer than normal and more easily bent and deformed. When the minerals are not being laid down in the bones, the softer tissues (cartilage) continue to grow at the ends of the long bones; this enlargement develops at the wrists, ankles, and at the points of growth of the ribs. As a result of rickets the skull is often late in closing, the teeth delayed in eruption.

The effects of rickets are seen also in the muscles, which become more lax and weakened. Infants with rickets are likely to be delayed in such muscular acts as sitting, standing, and walking. Infants with rickets are subject to profuse sweating and often to restlessness.

The symptoms which have been enumerated are chiefly those of the well advanced disease. The milder disease is much more frequent than the severe. The same changes take place in the milder disease, but these changes are more difficult to detect. The accurate diagnosis of rickets in the mild disease is made easier by X-ray examination of the bones.

In a few cases of rickets very marked and alarming symptoms appear which are associated with a decrease in the amount of calcium in the blood. When these symptoms occur, the condition is termed "tetany," or "spasmophilia." Tetany may exhibit itself in the form of convulsions or as a spasm of the larynx which causes obstruction and difficult breathing; or as a peculiar spasmodic state of the hands and feet. All these symptoms subside promptly with suitable medical treatment and their return is made impossible by the effective application of the same measures as bring about the cure of rickets.

Rickets is a disease which is easily prevented and easily cured. Prevention is preferable. Any infant who receives the amount of milk that he should is thereby receiving sufficient calcium and phosphorus. If he receives a teaspoon of cod-liver oil daily or 400 units of vitamin D from some other source, the chances are that no rickets of any significance will develop. The same factors that are effective in prevention are equally effective in bringing about the cure of this disease.

INFANTILE PARALYSIS Most terrifying of all the diseases which attack children is infantile paralysis, sometimes called poliomyelitis. There are other diseases that constitute a double threat to mankind—the threat of crippling and the threat of death—but infantile paralysis is the most visibly crippling.

In the schools for crippled children and in the hospitals and institutions that care for them, the great majority of children with paralyzed legs are there as a result of what infection with the virus of infantile paralysis can do to the human body.

Infantile paralysis is caused by a virus. A virus is living material, previously characterized by the fact that it is so small that it can pass through the pores of a clay filter. However, we now know that there are germs that pass through such filters. Viruses differ from germs mainly by the fact that germs can multiply in cultures or tubes outside the human body, or outside of any living host, but viruses cannot. Viruses cannot move by themselves; they cannot reproduce themselves. Therefore the investigators who study viruses in the laboratories grow them in the bodies of animals or on the embryo chicken in the shell. The viruses of infantile paralysis have been grown best outside the body on the tissue of the kidneys of monkeys.

The virus of infantile paralysis is one of the smallest of the known viruses. It does not seem to affect many animals. Man is the favored host for this agent of disease. A few of the monkeys can be infected. Quite recently some rats have been found which can be inoculated successfully with this virus. In the United States the virus of poliomyelitis occurs in three types known as Lansing, Brunhilde, and Leon types.

Simply because of its dramatic and terrifying character, scientists have concentrated greatly on this disease in recent years; we have learned much about it and its method of spread. Each year in the United States since 1940 some 25,000 to 30,000 cases are reported annually. Non-paralytic poliomyelitis is now more frequent than the paralytic form.

The development of a successful method of vaccination against infantile paralysis means that eventually this condition will occur infrequently. The inoculation of some 30,000,000 children may require ten years or more. By early 1956 20 million doses of the vaccine were ready but priorities had to be maintained for children up to the age of 15 years and for pregnant women. The first two doses were given two to four weeks apart and the booster dose ten months later.

Quite possibly, however, far more people have infantile paralysis than are recognized as cases of the disease. The reason is, of course, that many people who become infected do not get paralyzed. Perhaps the vast majority of those who get infected do not get paralyzed. There are some who think that just as many people have infantile paralysis as get measles. Few of the people who get measles—speaking proportionately—get an earache and a running ear. If we could recognize measles only by an earache or a running ear, we would probably miss many of the cases. If there were a rash on the skin in infantile paralysis, we would probably recognize many more cases. It is fortunate for mankind that everyone who becomes infected with infantile paralysis is not paralyzed. If he were, the crippling might constitute an intolerable burden to a weary world.

These facts indicate some of the lines of study that are still needed in order to bring about complete control of this infection. We need a test like the Wassermann test for syphilis or like the examination of the throat in diphtheria, which

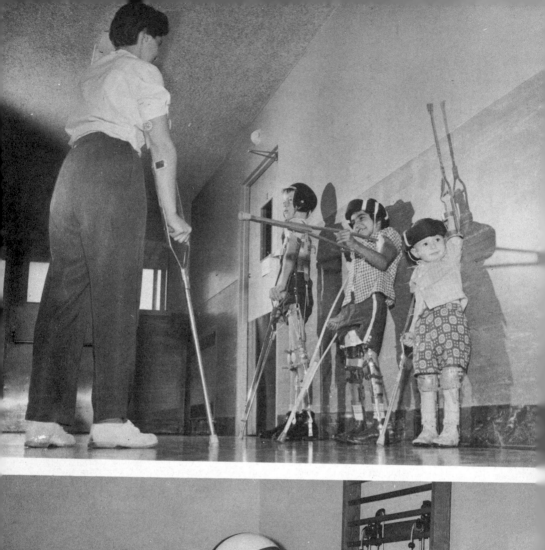
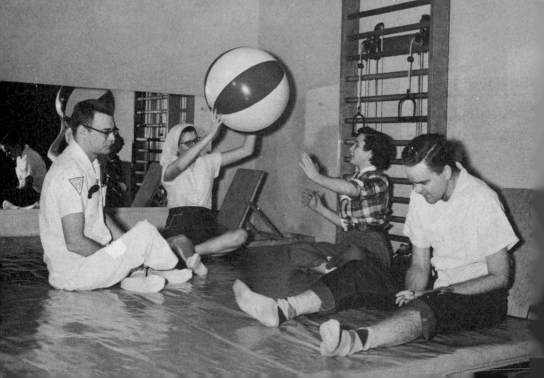

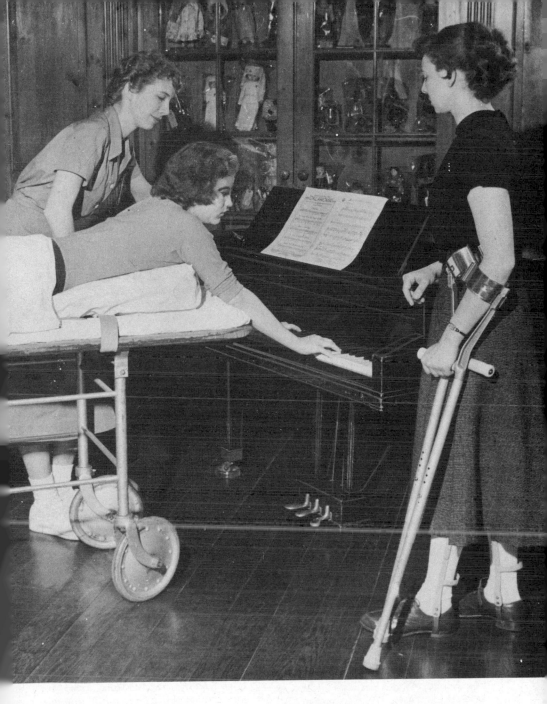

Polio victims at play. With the aid of wheelchairs and crutches many patients are able to engage in amusing activities with their playmates.

National Foundation for Infantile Paralysis

would make possible the identification of infantile paralysis in every instance. We need a method of determining how the infection actually passes from one person to another. We need to know why some people do not get the disease and others fall ill. We need to know why some people who get the disease become paralyzed and others do not.

All of these questions are now being investigated by workers in clinics and laboratories throughout the world. We have actually made great progress. No doubt more progress will be made as time goes by. When an outbreak of crippling infantile paralysis strikes fear in a community, mothers ask first of all what they can do to help their children escape the disease. Dr. Philip M. Stimson summarized a few suggestions which everyone should keep in mind. Here they are with my explanations:

1. We do not know that infantile paralysis is spread by water. We do know, however, that the virus is found in sewage and that sewage can carry the virus for considerable distances and for a long time. Therefore avoid the use of water that may possibly be contaminated with sewage either for drinking, for swimming, or for washing dishes.

2. Experience in a number of epidemics has shown overexertion and chilling during the period when the virus is in the body and before the person becomes paralyzed seem to augment the effects of the virus on the body. The time that passes between entrance of the virus into the body and the development of the first symptoms may be as short as four or five days; it may be as long as ten days or two weeks. Therefore, in times when there is an outbreak in the community, do not permit children to become exhausted from exertion. Do not permit them to become chilled from swimming too long in pools, rivers, or lakes.

3. There are records of cases of infantile paralysis following removal of the tonsils during the period of an epidemic. Apparently the removal of the tonsils leaves open pathways in the throat whereby the virus may get into the nervous system and pass perhaps to the higher areas of the nervous system, which are those that control the vital activities of the body. This produces the bulbar type of infantile paralysis, in whicn paralysis of the breathing comes early. In several outbreaks there has been a relatively high percentage of bulbar cases; therefore avoid injury to the membranes of the nose and throat. Unless necessary because of serious infection, operations on the tonsils and adenoids should not be performed during the time of the outbreak.

4. The earliest symptoms of infantile paralysis are like those of many other infectious diseases. During the time of an outbreak every minor illness should be considered as a possible case of infantile paralysis, and particularly if there is fever, headache, or spasms of the muscles of the neck, the spine, or the thighs.

Any child suspected even slightly of having been infected should be kept quiet for several days in bed and should not get up until the doctor says that he may do so.

5. Flies and other insects may carry the virus of infantile paralysis and thus contaminate food or water used. The insect, in contact with sewage or filth, picks up the virus and perhaps deposits it on food, milk, or water that is going to be taken by a child. Therefore screening of the house against flies and mosquitoes may be important in keeping away infection. The best evidence shows that insect transmission is not the common method of spreading infantile paralysis. In any case it is good sanitation to destroy flies and their breeding places.

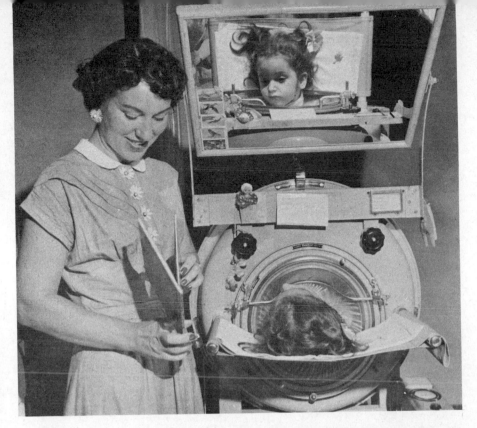

Although these children are physically handicapped, they are able to enjoy their books and keep up with their studies.

National Foundation for Infantile Paralysis

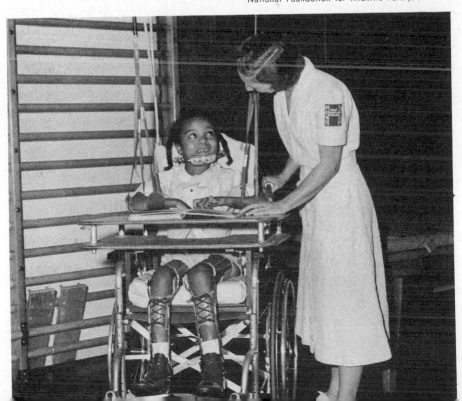

Even though it has not yet been proved in any single place that flies actually carry enough virus from infected sewage to produce the disease definitely in any human being, the path of safety is to avoid the danger.

6. Most infectious diseases are spread from one person to another. Therefore in times of outbreaks of infectious disease unnecessary physical contacts with other people should be avoided. Wash the hands carefully before eating. Do not put unclean objects in the mouth. Certainly it has been proved that people who have been infected with the virus of infantile paralysis can continue to pass it from their bodies by way of the bowel for several months although they themselves are well. Proof seems available also that the usual way for the virus to get into the human body is by way of the throat and stomach.

7. We now have gamma globulin and a vaccine that have been shown experimentally to be able to protect a child against infantile paralysis. Controlled studies have been made on thousands of children in many different states with gamma globulin. This affords about thirteen weeks of protection. The vaccine as now prepared uses the three types of virus which are grown artificially outside the body. All the results were achieved through research supported by the National Foundation for Infantile Paralysis. Most experts believe that abolition of poliomyelitis as a crippling disease is now possible.

Usually when the child gets infantile paralysis there is a period called the preparalytic stage. Such children have fever, sometimes a sore throat, a cough, or a cold, a headache, nausea, or vomiting. These symptoms occur in practically all infectious diseases. Many times there is diarrhea. In some instances there may be pain or distress in the abdomen so severe that the parents fear appendicitis. Some children seem to be fatigued to the point of exhaustion and so apathetic that they have apparently lost interest in what is going on, yet others are nervous and irritable, indeed frightened out of all proportion to the severity of their symptoms.

Important and alarming symptoms include trembling of the hands or other parts of the body and pain or stiffness in the neck and back. Difficulty in moving the back, such as would be involved in putting the chin on the chest or the head between the knees, is an indication that something is wrong. The child may perspire a great deal and his face may flush with a minimum amount of exercise. These symptoms are, however, still such that the diagnosis of infantile paralysis cannot be made with certainty even when all of them are present.

Sometimes the symptoms are so mild that the first one noted is actual paralysis. This, however, is unusual. Most commonly for anywhere from a few hours to several days the early signs of the illness are detected. If any of these signs appear, call a doctor at once. Another serious symptom of the early stages of this disease is pain. The muscles are sore, the pain gets worse when the legs and arms are moved, the muscles are tender if anyone touches them. In many instances even when these symptoms are present paralysis does not follow and recovery is rapid and complete. Some patients—the exact percentage varying, however, from one epidemic to another—proceed and develop definite paralysis. This early stage of the disease is the time when the services of the doctor and the trained nurse may be most important. The extent of the permanent paralysis may depend a great deal on what is done at this time.

The detection of the muscles that are involved at this time demands a careful kind of study that only a physician trained in observation of infantile paralysis can give. As everyone knows, the number of muscles that may be involved vary from case to case and from epidemic to epidemic. Seldom are all of the muscles of a leg or an arm incapacitated. However, groups of muscles in various portions of the body may become paralyzed. Usually from two to three days after the first signs of paral-

ysis appear all of the damage that is going to be done will have occurred.

Thus far, particular mention has been made of the muscles. However, infantile paralysis is not a disease of muscles, but a disease of the nervous system. The virus gets into the nervous system and attacks the cells in the front part of the spinal cord that are responsible for

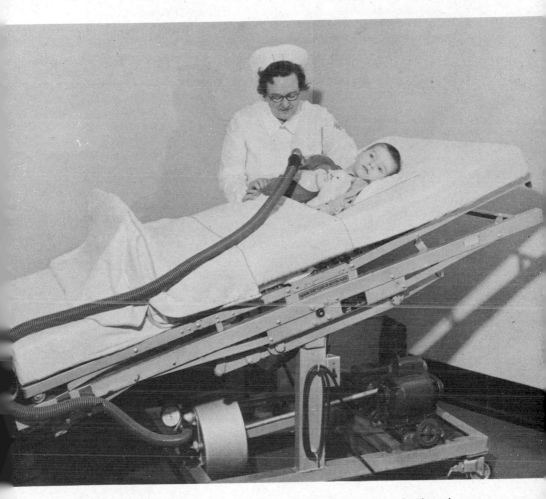

Young polio victim breathes with the help of a rocking bed and chest respirator.   National Foundation for Infantile Paralysis

carrying the impulses to movement along the nerves to the muscles. If the nerve cells are damaged but slightly or if only a few nerve cells are destroyed, the muscle weakness will be temporary. If many nerve cells are killed by the infection, the paralysis may be extensive and it may be permanent. Nerve cells, unlike many of the other tissues of the human body, do not easily grow back again after they have been destroyed. In fact nerve cells are so delicate that they are more easily destroyed than other cells of the body. These are just some of the reasons why early competent attention may be so vital in the control of infantile paralysis.

Frequently there are changes in the spinal fluid which bathes the spinal cord and the nerve cells as an early sign of this disease. Hence the doctor may want to put a needle into the spinal column in order to get out some of the fluid for examination. If this can help him diagnose the disease earlier and thus be helpful in controlling it, the measure is more than warranted. Once infantile paralysis is diagnosed, the case should be reported immediately to the health official. The family should be willing to keep the infected child absolutely quarantined so as to prevent as much as possible spread of the condition to other children.

During the early stages of infantile paralysis, when the muscles are tender and painful, the doctor, the orthopedic surgeon, and the nurse must co-operate in doing the utmost possible to prevent extensive paralysis. A few simple suggestions have been prepared for nurses by the National Foundation for Infantile Paralysis. It is well that every mother should be familiar with these suggestions given to nurses.

1. Keep patient in a quiet room out of drafts.

2. Handle the patient as little as possible. Touching and moving the patient aggravate spasm.

3. Always be sure hands are warm before touching patient.

4. Warm bedpan or urinal before giving to patient.

5. Omit baths during stage of painful spasm. When baths are given, handle patient gently. Blot up moisture with towel. Don't rub.

6. Omit alcohol rubs.

7. Allow patient to assume any position which is comfortable but, as painful spasm is relieved, gradually bring the body into normal alignment.

8. Use an air ring instead of a pillow under the head during the time there is difficulty in breathing and swallowing.

9. In turning the patient, give support to joints and avoid touching muscle bellies.

10. Never tire the patient by care being given. Stop care before patient shows signs of fatigue.

11. Observe and report promptly to physician any of the following symptoms:

a. Retention of urine.

b. Constipation.

c. Difficulty in breathing, swallowing, talking.

d. Accumulation of mucus.

e. Increase or recurrence of spasm. Some of the signs which indicate presence of spasm are shortening of muscles, causing the body to be pulled from its normal position, presence of abnormal skin creases, sulci, or bony prominences, absence or diminution of skin folds, prominence of muscle tendons, and flatness of muscle bellies, pain.

The following list of rules is especially directed to parents:

1. Keep the covers from touching the patient's body by draping them over the

footboard or using a bed cradle or other support.

2. Allow patient to lie in the position which is most comfortable for him. As the pain is relieved, the nurse will teach you how to place him in the normal position.

3. Scrub your hands thoroughly after giving any care to the patient. The nurse will show you how to protect the patient, your family, and yourself in giving care. This instruction will include method of disinfection of stools and disposal of stools and nasal discharges in accordance with directions given by your physician.

During the acute stage of infantile paralysis many parents become alarmed and are willing to try any kind of massage, manipulation, pulling, heating, freezing, or any other treatment that almost anybody will suggest. Actually there is no disease in which so much harm can be done in the early stage by the wrong application or the unnecessary application of such methods.

Modern investigations and particularly the Kenny method have shown that control of the pain, the tenderness, and the spasm by that technic do much to relieve pain and spasm, maintain the function of the tissues, and save life. However, even these methods demand application by persons who have been trained in the technic. Long before Sister Kenny, some doctors advocated warm baths for this stage of the disease. Others had developed other technics. However, as Dr. Frank R. Ober points out, Sister Kenny's treatment combines good nursing and common sense.

The problem in the early stage is expert nursing, expert application of the hot packs, gradual controlled movement within the range of discomfort in order to prevent stiffness of the muscles and joints, and controlled active exercises of groups of muscles as soon as the spasm and soreness have disappeared.

We do not know of any drug or serum that will cure infantile paralysis. Already the sulfa drugs and penicillin have been tried and have not seemed to be more promising than other drugs in their attack on this virus condition.

This means, therefore, that the doctor who treats the patient with infantile paralysis will be responsible for the methods that are used to control the pain, the tenderness, the fever, and the other symptoms. He will want the advice of an orthopedic surgeon who specializes in nerves and muscles, bones and joints, who will use all that that special branch of medicine provides to prevent deformities and disabling injuries.

The use of splints, frames, and plaster casts in the care of early cases of infantile paralysis has been largely replaced by the so-called Kenny method. Not all patients recover completely even with this method. Apparently many more recover completely with the Kenny method than used to recover when the affected parts of the body were kept almost wholly under the control of splints, frames, or plaster casts early in the disease.

The National Foundation for Infantile Paralysis, 120 Broadway, New York, N.Y., has up-to-date books and pamphlets for doctors, nurses, and the public generally that they gladly send on request.

Under the auspices and with the assistance of the National Foundation for Infantile Paralysis, research on infantile paralysis has been intensified throughout the world. Under grants made by the Foundation the care of the patient with acute infantile paralysis has been greatly improved. Several drugs are now known that control muscle spasm. Physical therapy technics have been introduced that maintain the tone of the tissues until the greatest possible recovery of the nervous tissues has occurred.

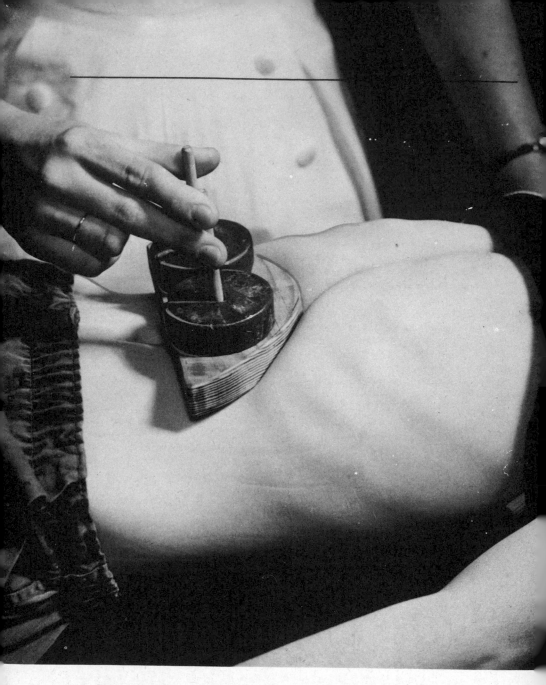

Exercising the muscles of the abdomen and diaphragm is an important part of treatment for infantile paralysis. Patient undergoing underwater treatment is kept afloat by means of floats at the head, hips and right ankle.

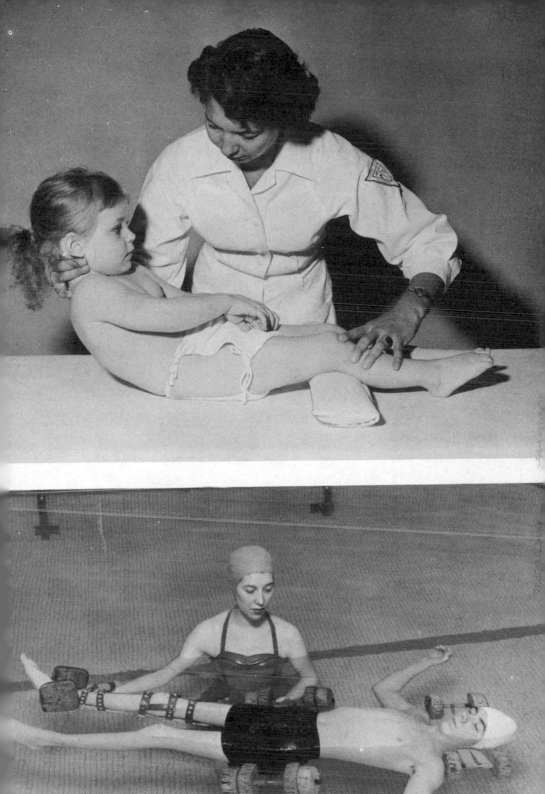

The latest development is the recognition of the need for scientific rehabilitation of the handicapped patient. Many special services are integrated around the patient including orthopedics, physical medicine, psychiatry, nursing, occupational and recreational treatment, and resettlement. Departments of rehabilitation and centers are being established.

Usually the patient with infantile paralysis is seen first by the family doctor. Then he calls as a specialist the pediatrician, who takes care of children, the specialist in nerve conditions, or the orthopedic surgeon. Since the attention of all of these may be helpful or most

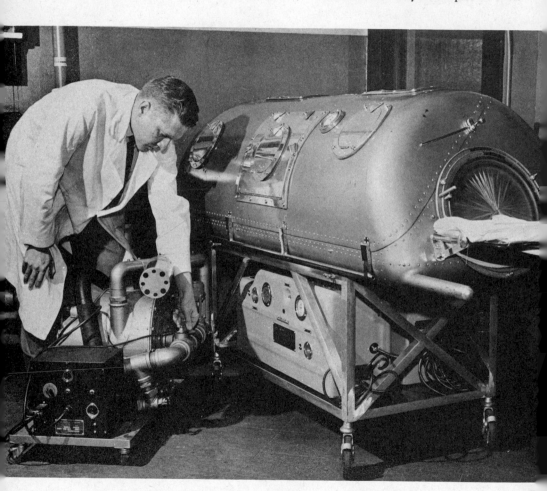

A self-operating respirator together with the newly developed Portolung. Without the assistance of these machines many patients with respiratory difficulties would find it difficult to survive.

desirable in most cases, it is probably best for the infected child to be taken promptly to a hospital. In the hospital the toxic symptoms of infection may be overcome. Frequently the child will be found depressed because of a lack of fluid in the body. Doctors may inject a 10 per cent solution of dextrose directly into the veins in order to overcome these conditions. Remember, however, that all these children should be subjected to a minimum amount of handling until the initial painfulness and tenderness have disappeared.

Naturally such troubles as difficulty in swallowing, breathing, or urinating must be given the immediate attention of the doctor. Anyone with infantile paralysis who has trouble with breathing is likely to be put immediately in a respirator or breathing device. The National Foundation for Infantile Paralysis has established twelve centers in the United States where patients who require treatment in a respirator may be given care by trained teams. New types of respirators which fit like a jacket are now available.

Most important in the control of infantile paralysis is the maintenance of the morale, not only of the patient but of the patient's parents. There are few illnesses which so greatly shake the courage of parents as does this disease. The use of the Kenny method helps morale because it gives visible evidence that a great deal is being done.

The final steps in the care of a patient with infantile paralysis are usually carried out by the physical therapist and the surgeon. It is in these stages of the disease that the underwater treatment or swimming-pool technic is particularly valuable. A pool itself is useless unless there are available competent teachers who encourage the use of weakened tissues, control the amounts of exercise and rest, and aid in developing properly those muscles that are

capable of being developed. The surgeon can transplant muscles so that parts of healthy muscles will take the place of those that are not able to carry on their work. By the use of braces and supports the weakened tissues may be helped in carrying the weight of the body. Joints can be made to bear weight, and walking power can be restored. These braces and supports are used, however, only until healthy muscles can be made to take over the functions of those that have been damaged or destroyed by disease.

Certain patients in spite of everything that can be done remain crippled. For these patients modern civilization pro-

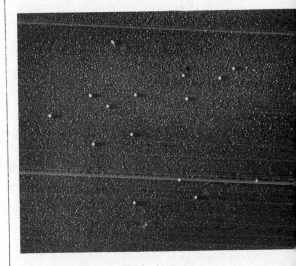

The human polio virus magnified 100,000 times by the electron microscope. The viruses in this photograph were obtained from tissue cultures of monkey kidneys. The particles are about 28 millimicrons or one millionth of an inch in diameter.

vides schools which can help to improve the physical condition and help to readjust the mental state. Many a child who has had infantile paralysis recovers and goes on to lead a successful life. Wherever patients crippled by infantile paralysis assemble, one sees the great boost to their morale that has come from the notable example of famous persons who have been crippled and who made successful careers despite their handicap. As was said by Violet Storey in her beautiful poem:

Milton, the blind, who looked on Paradise!
Beethoven, deaf, who heard vast harmonies!
Byron, the lame, who climbed toward Alpine skies!
Who pleads a handicap remen..bering these?

Most notable was, of course, the example set by President Franklin Delano Roosevelt.

INFANTILE PARALYSIS—childhood disease: See CHILDHOOD DISEASES, article INFECTIOUS DISEASES OF CHILDHOOD.

INFANTILE PARALYSIS—deaths: See CHILDHOOD DISEASES, article INFECTIOUS DISEASES OF CHILDHOOD.

INFANTILE PARALYSIS—diagnosis, early: See CHILDHOOD DISEASES, article INFECTIOUS DISEASES OF CHILDHOOD.

INFANTILE PARALYSIS—exercises: See CHILDHOOD DISEASES, article INFECTIOUS DISEASES OF CHILDHOOD.

INFANTILE PARALYSIS—foot deformities may result: See FOOT, article THE FOOT.

INFANTILE PARALYSIS—hiccups: See article FIRST AID.

INFANTILE PARALYSIS—incubation period: See CHILDHOOD DISEASES, article INFECTIOUS DISEASES OF CHILDHOOD.

INFANTILE PARALYSIS—lymph glands swell as in German measles: See CHILD-

HOOD DISEASES, article INFECTIOUS DISEASES OF CHILDHOOD.

INFANTILE PARALYSIS—prevention: See INFECTIOUS DISEASE, article THE PREVENTION AND TREATMENT OF INFECTIOUS DISEASE; CHILDHOOD DISEASES, article INFECTIOUS DISEASES OF CHILDHOOD.

INFANTILE PARALYSIS—proportion of non-paralytic to paralytic cases: See CHILDHOOD DISEASES, article INFECTIOUS DISEASES OF CHILDHOOD.

INFANTILE PARALYSIS—Sister Kenny treatment: See CHILDHOOD DISEASES, article INFECTIOUS DISEASES OF CHILDHOOD.

INFANTILE PARALYSIS—symptoms: See CHILDHOOD DISEASES, article INFECTIOUS DISEASES OF CHILDHOOD.

INFANTILE PARALYSIS—treatment: See CHILDHOOD DISEASES, article INFECTIOUS DISEASES OF CHILDHOOD.

INFANTILE PARALYSIS—water exercise: See CHILDHOOD DISEASES, article INFECTIOUS DISEASES OF CHILDHOOD.

INFANTILISM Sometimes because of the failure of development of certain glands the characteristics of childhood persist into adult life. The condition is called infantilism and is marked by mental retardation, underdevelopment of the sexual organs, and sometimes diminished stature.

INFECTIONS AND IMMUNITY
When living organisms such as germs or viruses invade the human body, the tissues of the body undergo changes which help them to resist the poisons of the invader. By this reaction the tissues become immune to the poisons. Much depends on the virulence of the infections, the total number of germs invading, the place where they enter the body, the tissues or structures where they settle and grow. If you are susceptible to the infection it will attack you; it may even overcome you. If you are resistant, the

tissues of your body may develop antibodies which will overcome the germs or viruses or their poisons.

Certain environmental conditions may increase or lower your resistance to infection. Chilling of the body, excessive fatigue, absence of some essential nutritional substance as proteins, or mineral salts or vitamins, or the presence of another disease at the same time may modify the resistance of the body to an invader.

The chemical composition of the invading organism may be significant in the way in which the body responds to it. An invading substance is known as an antigen. Usually the response of the body to an invading germ is specific against that germ or against that type of germ. Bacteria may contain a number of antigenic substances against each of which the body will rebuild resistance. An example of an antibody against infections is the immune globulin. This is a protein substance found in blood in which we now know are accumulated substances that help to resist various infections such as those of measles or poliomyelitis. In man most of the antibodies are found in the immune globulin of the blood. The amount of antibody that develops is also governed by such factors as the amount of infectious material that gets into the body. The doctors find that they can help you build resistance by repeatedly injecting small doses of an infecting substance. We know that a child gets resisting substances from its mother in her blood at the time of birth and in the first material that comes from the breast when the child begins to nurse. This is called colostrum. The amount of antibodies may be unfavorably affected by starvation, exposure, reduced protein intake, alcoholism, or other poisoning.

TYPES OF INFECTION—For certain diseases there are certain specific types of causative germs such as the viruses of measles, smallpox, infantile paralysis, or the germs that cause diphtheria, typhoid, gonorrhea or meningitis. The total number of germs, viruses, rickettsia, amebas, spirochetes, or other parasites that may infect the body reaches into thousands. Many germs have been described in groups according to their appearance under the microscope such as the streptococci that grow in chains or the staphylococci that grow in clusters. The streptococci and the staphylococci may invade any portion of the human body and set up infection.

HEMOLYTIC STREPTOCOCCUS INFECTIONS—The streptococcus is one of the most widely distributed and variable organisms that attacks mankind. Such conditions as sore throat, sinus infections, scarlet fever, erysipelas, puerperal fever, or lymphangitis may be caused by streptococci. Other conditions associated with such streptococci include acute rheumatic fever and acute inflammations of the kidney.

Such infections are found in all races, in both sexes, at all ages, and they come on at any time of the year. Scarlet fever is said to be rare in the tropics. Very small babies, under three months of age, seldom have streptococcal infections because they get some immunity from their mothers at the time of birth. Tonsillitis, pharyngitis, and scarlet fever are more frequent up to ten years of age. Streptococcal infections can result from contaminated food, milk, water but most frequently pass from one person to another with coughing, sneezing, spitting and what are known as hand to mouth infections.

Tonsillitis and pharyngitis are usually streptococcal infections which begin with sore throats. When there is a rash, the rash is said to represent sensitivity of the skin to the products of the streptococcus; this condition is scarlet fever. Infections of the sinuses usually follow infection of the tonsils and throat. Ear infections occur in many cases and the streptococci are said to be responsible for ten per cent of ear infections. Specific methods of inoculation against streptococci are difficult because of the many different varities of the germ. The Dick test will indicate whether or not a child is susceptible to the streptococcus of scarlet fever and there are methods of building resistance against these streptococci by inoculating small doses of the toxin.

Regardless of the portion of the body that is attacked by the streptococci, the control of the condition is now possible through the proper use of the sulfonamide and antibiotic drugs that have been mentioned. Streptococci are especially susceptible to attack by the sulfonamide drugs. The complications of infected throats are more important than the sore throat itself. Penicillin is the antibiotic drug most frequently used in treating throats infected with streptococci. Penicillin is especially beneficial in laryngitis, pharyngitis, tonsilitis and scarlet fever. The complications of scarlet fever have in the past done more harm than the disease itself. In severe cases of scarlet fever convalescent serum may be used, and good results have been reported from use of the antitoxin.

Saline gargles and irrigations of the throat help to wash out the by-products of throat infection. One of the most significant advances is the use of sulfonamide drugs to prevent streptococcal infections. When there are outbreaks in large homes, in barracks, in asylums, or places where great numbers of people assemble, the sulfonamide drugs may be taken as a means of preventing infection with the streptococci. All sorts of attempts have been made to cut down respiratory diseases by the use of ultraviolet light in the air, by the spraying of medicated vapors or aerosols and by other technics for keeping the germs from floating in the air. These, in general, have not been successful.

THE COMMON COLD—Almost anyone can tell you right off when they have a cold and yet there is no real agreement in the medical profession as to just what a common cold is. No single germ has yet been incriminated as the causative factor nor has any group of germs or viruses been established as responsible. At present the sequence of events seems to include a first period when the lining of the nose and throat seems to respond to some foreign invading substances by reddening and congestion and a profuse flow of mucus. With this may be frequent sneezing, stuffiness, difficulty in breathing, perhaps some fever, a feeling of lassitude, and some aching of the limbs.

Colds spread rapidly from one person to another and the resistance established by having a cold lasts a very short time. Some people have many more colds than do others and the average for the country as a whole seems to be about four colds a year. Chilling, exposure to damp, sudden changes from a dry hot air to a cold damp atmosphere, sitting in a draft, getting the feet wet, and particularly working or playing in crowded rooms with others who have colds seem to be important factors in the spread of respiratory diseases.

The suggestions as to how to prevent frequent colds are numerous but some doubt prevails as to whether or not any of them really work. You may try to keep away from contact with others who have colds, but under the crowded conditions of our civilization this is well nigh impossible. People have tried wearing face masks of gauze or paper during epidemics but they permit contamination. Use of ultraviolet in the air has seemed to be useful but carefully controlled experiments with this technic and with spraying medicated vapors in the air have not yielded conclusive results.

Mothers have tried to harden children by frequent cold baths, going without stockings, and hats and similar methods. These methods do not work and the unnecessary hardship makes the children unhappy.

Most colds get well in from five to ten days. Complications are fortunately now controlled by the use of the sulfonamides and antibiotic drugs. Some claims hold that colds can be cured by taking an antihistaminic drug during the first twenty-four hours of invasion; most experts doubt that this is specifically helpful. The congestion in the nose is relievable by the use of decongestant preparations such as menthol, camphor, privine, amphetamine and other preparations which the doctor must prescribe. People feel more comfortable if they go to bed, take some aspirin, or a small dose of an alcoholic drink. Frequently a hot bath and plenty of fluids such as citrus drinks secure relief. Secondary coughs are controllable with a variety or remedies. Particularly feared as a complication is secondary pneumonia. The doctor watches for signs of this in rising temperature, congestion and pain in the lungs, signs of congestion which he hears with his stethoscope, or can detect by percussion, or see certainly with the X ray. Fortunately again such secondary infections are now controllable with the new drugs.

INFLUENZA—Influenza is an acute infectious disease caused by a virus. It comes on suddenly with fever, muscular aches, chilliness, and a cough. After an attack serious weakness is common for some weeks. Although outbreaks of influenza have occurred for centuries only in recent years have the different forms of virus associated with epidemics been isolated. Two forms known as influenza virus. A and B have been isolated since 1933. Vaccines for inoculating against these forms have been developed but routine immunization is not advised because the uncomplicated disease is rarely fatal and because the type or nature of the virus varies from one epidemic to another.

The virus of influenza is transmitted from one person to another by droplets of fluid coughed out of the nose, throat, and lungs. An epidemic usually reaches its peak in two or three weeks and then subsides in from four to eight weeks. The worst period of the year is winter and early spring. The influenza virus seems to be constantly present among human beings and epidemics occur under the specially favorable circumstances that aid spread of the virus and lessen resistance.

Influenza comes on suddenly after an incubation period of a few days. The common complaints are headache, drowsiness, fatigue, and chilliness, but there may also be general illness with nausea and vomiting. The fever starts to rise and usually hangs around $102°$ F. but may get up to $104°$ F. A cough with dryness and irritation of the throat and tightness across the chest are common. A running nose is not nearly as frequent as with the common cold. The person with influenza feels really sick and is disinclined towards work or amusement or even reading. Pain in the eyes with some redness may occur. The disease itself is uncomfortable but not too serious but secondary complications through invasion by other germs causing pneumonia, ear infection or even inflammation of the brain may make it dangerous to life.

The sulfonamides and antibiotic drugs can prevent secondary complications of influenza but do not act specifically against the viruses. Most doctors recommend rest in bed, plenty of fluids, aspirin or other salicylates, codeine to quiet the cough and if necessary drugs to help the patient sleep. The condition must be watched most carefully when it affects the very old or very young who are more likely to get secondary infections and to be less able to resist the wear and tear that influenza causes.

BRONCHITIS—Any of the germs that get into the nose and throat may secondarily invade the lung or the bronchial tubes and set up the inflammation called acute bronchitis. This usually starts gradually with frequent coughing that is more severe at night. Slight fever may be present. If the amount of debris and infected material is profuse the coughing will raise a thick material that has to be expectorated. Young children do not spit but swallow the material and then frequently vomit to get rid of it.

Bronchitis is not really a disease in itself but far more often a complication of a common cold, influenza, measles, rhinitis, diphtheria, scarlet fever or rickets. Prompt attention to these conditions with special consideration for the inflammation that has extended into the lungs will help to prevent acute bronchitis and may do much to stop its becoming chronic. Bronchitis is chiefly dangerous to little children and continuous inflammation with much coughing may make desirable removal to a warm climate to help the child get rid of the infection.

Since inflammation becomes worse when tissues are irritated people with chronic inflammation of the bronchial tubes should avoid contact with irritating dusts, fumes, gases, or paints. Tobacco smoking must be stopped. The infected individual does better in a clean atmosphere where the air is neither too cold, too damp, too warm nor too dry.

All sorts of cough mixtures are known that will increase the flow of mucus and make the raising of the sputum easier. Inhaling steam seems to help many people. If there is sensitivity the use of antihistaminic drugs may be helpful and may aid also by a sedative effect.

MEASLES—Measles have been one of the most frequent of the childhood diseases. The condition is quite infectious, and is accompanied usually by a rash, with fever, cough, and inflamed eyes. Measles are caused by a specific virus which spreads easily from one person to another.

From ten to fourteen days after a child has been in contact with another who has had measles, symptoms like those of a severe cold develop. The child becomes drowsy and irritable. The eyes water and look red and the child avoids light. The appetite is poor. By the end of the third or fourth day the rash appears with individual spots that are at first pinhead size and pale red but then enlarge, become elevated and a darker red. The eruption is seen first usually on the face, scalp, and behind the ears, but then gradually covers the whole body. The fever increases as the rash breaks out. After the second or third day the rash begins to fade, the temperature falls and after seven days usually the patient is on the way to complete recovery.

During the first few months of life the child often has immunity from measles by antibodies derived from its mother. As the immunity wears off the child becomes susceptible and most cases occur to children three or four years old. The child may be injected with globulin which provides immunity against measles.

Since the development of antibiotic drugs secondary complications of measles are more easily controlled. During the acute illness the child is kept at rest, given plenty of fluids such as citrus drinks, a soft diet and good nursing. For itching of the skin a calamine lotion is used. The eyes are protected against irritation. For more severe cases convalescent serum or gamma globulin may be used. Measles are not a serious disease except for very small babies. Prevention and control of pneumonia at the earliest sign is most important.

CHICKEN POX—Another common childhood disease caused by a virus is chicken pox. From ten to twenty days after exposure the symptoms begin with mild headache, loss of appetite and fever. hen after thirty-six hours the eruption appears. The rash usually is seen on the body and later on the face, neck, and extremities. Little red pinpoints enlarge to papules which change to blisters or vesicles. After a few days these break and are covered by dark brown crusts. The spots may become secondarily infected from scratching and pus infection will leave scars.

Chicken pox requires little treatment except to keep the areas free from secondary infection. The fingernails of children should be kept trimmed short. The itching is controllable by a calamine lotion containing one per cent of menthol or of phenol. If secondary infection occurs antibiotic ointments will stop the spread. Chicken pox seems to be related to the nerve conditions causing blisters known as herpes zoster. The common name for herpes zoster is shingles.

WHOOPING COUGH OR PERTUSSIS—A germ called the Hemophilus pertussis is now recognized as the cause of whooping cough. The germ is spread from one person to another by direct contact or through coughing, sneezing, or talking.

The attack of whooping cough is usually divided into four parts, one stage running into another. About seven to fourteen days after exposure the condition begins with symptoms like those of a cold, such as sneezing, running nose, and hoarseness. The fever is mild. In the second stage a cough gradually becomes hard, dry, and annoying; it is more severe at night. The exudation makes this known as the catarrhal stage. During the third stage whooping develops with a wheezing inhalation of breath.

The face becomes swollen and red, the tongue protrudes and the eyes water. After a whoop there may be a pause followed by another spell of whooping and coughing. The difficulty may result in vomiting. During the fourth stage there is a gradual lessening of whooping and paroxysms of coughing. The total duration of the condition may be six to eight weeks or more.

Nowadays inoculation against whooping cough is possible with good vaccines. Children should be protected as they are protected against diphtheria.

In the treatment of whooping cough the new antibiotics have been found effective and the disease is now much less feared. Streptomycin, aureomycin and terramycin are effective. The cough is controlled with suitable medication and sedatives. The nutrition of children must be watched carefully as severe coughing with prolonged paroxysms may seriously interfere with taking and retaining food. Food can be given frequently and in small quantities.

DIPHTHERIA—Diphtheria is caused by a germ called the diphtheria bacillus and known scientifically as the Corynebacterius diphtheriae. The disease is transmitted by droplets thrown into the air by coughing or sneezing. Children who have recovered from the disease may carry the germ. Indirectly the condition is transmitted on books, toys, clothing, and eating utensils.

Diphtheria develops usually from one to four days after exposure. The first signs are chilliness, slight fever, and loss of appetite, sometimes accompanied by vomiting and headache. Within twenty-four hours, sore throat occurs and a membrane or yellowish white deposit is seen in the throat and over the tonsils. Membrane may also form in the nose or larynx. The symptoms become more severe, as the lymph glands in the neck enlarge. The fever may go to 102° F. or higher and is generally highest at the beginning of the disease. Often there is cough and with severe infection, some prostration.

All children should be inoculated with antidiphtheria toxoid as soon as possible after reaching six months of age. The power of the toxoid is well established, and now there are many cities in the United States which haven't a single death from diphtheria in a year.

The treatment of diphtheria is of the greatest importance since the prompt giving of enough antitoxin will prevent spread to important nerves or other tissues of the body. Most dangerous is spread of the membrane into the larynx and serious interference with breathing. Recent research has shown the ability of penicillin to control the growth of the diphtheria germ and conceivable antibiotic treatment may eventually replace other forms of treatment.

ROCKY MOUNTAIN SPOTTED FEVER—Rocky Mountain spotted fever is a severe infectious disease with chills, fever, prostration, and a hemorrhagic rash. It is caused by a rickettsial organism and is transmitted by wood ticks. A disease called Brazilian typhus is identical, as are Mediterranean fever, South African tick bite fever and Kenya fever.

Rocky Mountain spotted fever is largely a rural disease; it has been found in every state in the United States except Maine and Vermont. It occurs chiefly during the warm months of the year when the ticks are active. Indeed the only insects known to spread the disease are the ticks. These include the wood tick, the dog tick, the lone star tick, and the rabbit tick. The tick attaches itself to an infected animal and transfers the infection to man.

Two to fourteen days after being bitten, the illness comes on abruptly with chills, fever, severe frontal, or occipital headache, pains in the muscles and joints and sensitivity of the eyes to pressure and to light. Nausea, vomiting, constipation, nosebleed and a mild cough and similar symptoms appear along with a fever which will rise rapidly from 103 to 105 degrees.

A rash is characteristic. It develops two to six days after the onset of the illness, usually first around the wrists and ankles and then spreading to involve the entire body surface. Several crops of the rash may appear, one after the other. Sometimes the rashes become hemorrhagic. The damage may be so great that gangrenous changes occur in the skin on the tips of the fingers, the toes, the earlobes and even on the soft palate. Secondary to these infections may be pneumonias, hemorrhages of the stomach and intestines and kidneys and serious inflammations of the eyes.

Vaccines have been prepared which are used to immunize people against Rocky Mountain spotted fever. Fortunately chloromycetin, aureomycin, terramycin and para-amino benzoic acid have proved to be beneficial in Rocky Mountain spotted fever. The condition was formerly much more severe than since the new antibiotics have been developed. Once from 12 to 25 per cent of those infected died of the condition but it seems likely that with the new antibiotic drugs something less than 5 per cent of deaths will occur.

Q FEVER—Q Fever is an acute illness often accompanied by pneumonia which results from infection with a form of rickettsia. The first human cases of the disease were observed in Australia in 1933. Since they originated in Queensland, the infection was named Q fever. Now a similar organism has been isolated from ticks captured in Montana and cases have been found in other areas of the United States.

Human beings are highly susceptible to Q fever; from 25 to 40 per cent of those exposed may be attacked by the disease. The condition was found much more often in Australia among people exposed to cattle. Before 1946 the disease was rare in the United States but has now been found particularly in epidemics in stockyards such as the one in Amarillo, Texas, in Chicago, and among dairymen in Los Angeles county. Workers in research institutes have frequently been infected.

From twelve to twenty-six days after being exposed, the disease comes on with symptoms like those seen in other rickettsial diseases. The two striking features that make Q fever different from other infections with rickettsia is the absence of any characteristic rash and the almost invariable presence of pneumonia. However, pulmonary symptoms are often mild or absent. About one-half the patients have aches in the chest. X ray of the chest shows that the lungs have been infected in at least 90 per cent of the cases.

Q fever may be confused with primary virus pneumonia, with tuberculosis, with psittacosis or infected bird fever and must also be distinguished from ordinary influenza, sinusitis, undulant fever, dengue, and other rickettsial infections.

Here again aureomycin, chloromycetin, and terramycin have been found useful in treatment. Relapses are rare. Most of the patients recover. Thus far only some eight or ten deaths have occurred among perhaps 1,000 cases that have been reported in medical writings.

GERM INFECTIONS — PNEUMONIA — Pneumonia was once one of the most feared of all human diseases. Its death rate was about a third of all of those whom it attacked. The germ that caused it is one called a pneumococcus which lives ordinarily in the noses and throats of anywhere from five to sixty per cent of people. The condition comes on most often in the winter months and can affect people of all ages.

The pneumococcus gets down into the lungs and there sets up a severe infection which follows a typical course. For a few days the symptoms are like those of an ordinary respiratory disease. Then comes the sudden hard, shaking chill, rapid rise in temperature and pulse rate, with a severe pain on one side of the chest that the doctor recognizes as the beiginning of pneumonia. The cough comes on painfully and with small amounts of pink or rust colored sputum. Breathing is rapid, shallow and painful. There may be blueness because the blood is not getting enough oxygen.

The doctor, by the use of his stethoscope and by watching the motion of the chest, by thumping to discover areas of consolidation, recognizes that the lung is congested and unable to function. Usually after seven to ten days a crisis occurs. The body temperature falls to normal in from six to twelve hours accompanied by profuse sweating and the pneumonia as such is over.

The development of the new antibiotic drugs has changed the whole picture. Now following the administration of penicillin the pain in the pleura which lines the chest disappears in a few hours and the temperature, pulse, and respiration fall to normal in twelve to thirty-six hours. The spread of the inflammation can be stopped even before a single lobe is involved. This change in the nature of pneumonia is one of the most dramatic occurrences that has ever taken place in medicine and represents one of the greatest accomplishments of the present century.

For the treatment of pneumonia nowadays the chief reliance is on the drugs. The patient is kept in bed in a position in which he is most comfortable. He is given considerable rest but is permitted to sit up for examinations and for any other necessary procedure. He usually has little appetite and need not be urged to eat but within a half a day after the specific treatment has been begun, he may be hungry and can take a soft diet.

Formerly great efforts were made to keep the bowels moving; that too is no longer a serious problem for the doctor. If there is a real shortage of air and the person seems blue, oxygen can be given. It is customary to give oxygen now as soon as it is needed and not to wait until the patient seems actually to suffer from oxygen lack.

The pain in the chest can be controlled with suitable drugs. It is also possible to relieve severe pain by the injection of local anesthetic drugs or by strapping or wrapping the chest wall to prevent unnecessary motion.

The doctor is alert for complications. If penicillin is not as effective as seems to be desirable, aureomycin, the sulfonamides, such as sulfadiazine, and other methods may be tried. Particularly, however, the doctor must look out for complications such as secondary formation of pockets of infected material at the bottom of the lung.

The former fatality rate of 25 to 30 per cent has now dropped to less than 5 per cent. Pneumonia is still a particularly serious disease to those who have been long weakened by some other disease such as cancer or alcoholism or malnutrition or some other serious complication involving the heart.

BRUCELLOSIS OR UNDULANT FEVER— The brucella germs are the cause of brucellosis or undulant fever. Undulant fever has been known also as Malta fever. The condition is far more widespread now than formerly although methods of prevention have been developed based on our knowledge of the fact that the disease is spread through drinking milk from infected cattle and through contact with the meat of infected animals.

Aureomycin has been found to produce prompt improvement in the symptoms of undulant fever with a lowering of the fever, a reduction in the size of the spleen and the other general symptoms of this disease which are so unpleasant. Streptomycin and sulfadiazine employed together are especially effective in controlling the organisms of undulant fever. Aureomycin seems to be preferred, however, to this combination of drugs because later reports show more satisfactory results and less of the toxic reactions that accompany the use of the other antibiotics that have been mentioned. The results with terramycin appear to be about as good as those with aureomycin.

Before the antibiotic drugs were discovered and found to be so useful in brucellosis, patients were usually put to bed and given proper diet. Under these circumstances they seemed to recover gradually although relapses were exceedingly frequent. Brucellosis is a rather chronic disease which may last for several months—even years—and be quite weakening. After the infection is over, people are weak, fatigued, nervous and often depressed. Loss of ambition is one of the most prominent symptoms of people who have had undulant fever.

Because the emotional reaction to the weakness may be so great, doctors are warranted in assuring patients that with proper treatment, complete recovery may occur and they can eventually regain their strength. In order to enable the person who has been weakened by a chronic disease to regain strength, rest, sunshine and a good diet with plenty of protein and vitamins is of the utmost importance.

POLIOMYELITIS OR INFANTILE PARALYSIS—In the summer season poliomyelitis rates begin to rise. People become more and more anxious about what they ought to do in presence of the threat of infection. The magnificent work of the National Foundation for Infantile Paralysis has made it possible to put most of the people who get poliomyelitis in hospitals where the diagnosis may be made positively and where new methods of treatment may be applied. Unfortunately we do not have at this time a specific method of treatment that will quite certainly destroy the virus of infantile paralysis or control its spread inside the body. New investigations are being made using the gamma globulin derived from serum, also convalescent serum in large doses, but the evidence is not yet sufficient to warrant the belief that these methods can either stop the disease or control it.

For many years, mild, nonparalytic cases of infantile paralysis have been cared for suitably in the home. Unquestionably, however, the patient who has paralysis is far better off in the hospital than at home. In the hospital modern methods of treatment with hot packs, control of distortion due to weakened muscles, encouragement of recovery after paralysis and particularly the use of the respirator are made available. These may mean the difference between life and death.

Not much seems to be gained by isolating every patient with infantile paralysis. Such patients can be cared for in general hospitals as well as in hospitals devoted exclusively to infectious diseases.

Since the virus of infantile paralysis seems to be spread by excretions from the bowel, the excretions of patients should be considered infectious and should be disposed of with precautions that they do not spread contamination. Little seems to be gained by adding antiseptic substances to the excretions but disposal of the material in a suitable toilet and thorough cleansing of vessels, such as bedpans, are important.

Because infantile paralysis is so widespread, particularly in the nonparalytic form, any disease with fever occurring to children and young adults in the summertime must be regarded with suspicion, particularly in times of epidemic. A competent doctor can diagnose the disease and suitable care during the early stages is significant. Far too often patients in the early stages are submitted to pulling, manipulation, rubbing and all sorts of energetic treatments which are likely to do more harm than good.

As soon as there is a question that the patient may have poliomyelitis, bedrest is important. The patient without paralysis must be confined to bed for at least three or four days after the temperature has returned to normal.

Most orthopedic specialists recommend the firm, hard bed from the beginning. The muscle tightness and paralysis can be helped by a suitable bed. The bed should be fitted with a footboard which is placed several inches beyond the mattress and allows room for pressure by the heels or toes of the patient when the patient lies on the back or on the stomach. This foot-board also protects the legs from the pressure of bedclothing and gives opportunity to avoid muscle weakness by such use as can be made of the limbs. If the legs are weak, the knees are usually supported in a slightly relaxed position.

Since poliomyelitis is such a frightening disease, the doctor must do everything that he can to prevent fear and terror on the part of the infected child or of the parents. Early in the disease the whole family must be adjusted to the fact that there is a medical problem. Such attention given early in the condition is likely to avoid nervous and psychotic disturbances at a later date.

In the early stages, infantile paralysis is treated exactly as one would treat other infectious diseases like measles, scarlet fever, or whooping cough. The treatment is usually rest in bed with a light diet but particularly with good nursing care.

During the early stages of inflammation, the patient must be provided with relief from pain. The use of moist heat is now considered most effective, including the application of hot baths for small children or for older ones, hot packs applied for thirty minute periods every four to six hours. The extreme ritual developed by recent technics is not absolutely necessary. If patients revolt against hot packs, they should be discontinued.

EPIDEMIC ENCEPHALITIS—Epidemics of brain fever are not an excessively large cause of disability and death in the United States. There have, however, been outbreaks such as the one which occurred in St. Louis in 1933 in which there were more than 1,000 cases. In the St. Louis epidemic there were 100 cases for every 100 000 population and 20 per cent of those who were infected died. In various epidemics the number of cases varies from two cases for every 100,000 people to as many as 22 for every 100 000 people.

Now it is established that the cause of epidemic encephalitis is a virus and that the outbreaks in human beings are closely related to certain similar conditions attacking animals, particularly an epidemic of a similar condition which concerns horses.

In several regions domestic birds such as chickens have been associated with the spread of the condition. In a California outbreak, the English sparrow and several species of blackbirds were involved. Research has also shown that various mosquitos and mites as well as ticks may be associated with the spread of this virus.

In the prevention of encephalitis, control of the mosquitos is of the utmost importance. Vaccines have been developed which may be used in outbreaks among horses. The condition is so serious that its appearance in any community should involve immediate investigation by competent health authorities.

INFECTIOUS DISEASE (See also discussion under *Carriers of Disease, Coughing, Immunization*) The outstanding feature of the progress of medicine since sulfonamides and antibiotics were introduced, has been the decline or disappearance of infections which used to devastate communities throughout the world. Typhoid fever and the dysenteries, which still plague the Latin American countries have become minimal in the United States and in most of the large countries of Europe. Malaria which is still in many parts of the world a scourge that destroys hundreds of thousands of people has practically disappeared from the United States and the well developed areas of other nations. We hear nothing of cholera, bubonic plague, yellow fever or typhus as threats to the health of the American people. Diphtheria and smallpox are now controllable. Today hundreds of communities in the United States go through a year without a single death from diphtheria. Most of these results have been brought about by greater knowledge of the cause, the methods of transmission and methods of control of the infections that have been mentioned. Vaccination is available against typhoid fever, cholera, whooping cough, yellow fever, typhus, smallpox, diphtheria, lockjaw, mumps, and more recently against infantile paralysis. The sulfonamides gave rise to the age of the wonder drugs. With these drugs and antibiotics such as penicillin, streptomycin, aureomycin and terramycin, many infectious diseases are being eliminated. Death rates have fallen at a speed which approaches the perpendicular.

The Prevention and Treatment of Infectious

Disease

BY

MORRIS FISHBEIN, M.D.

Former Editor, *Journal American Medical Association,*
Chicago; Editor, *Excerpta Medica, Bulletin World Medical Assn.; Post-graduate Medicine.*

ABOUT ONE HUNDRED YEARS have passed since it was first shown that germs actually cause disease. In the intervening period hundreds of germs have been identified definitely as associated with certain diseases that attack human beings. In 1880 the germ associated with typhoid was isolated. Since that time such important diseases as tuberculosis, diphtheria, glanders, pneumonia, cholera, lockjaw, undulant fever, meningitis, dysentery, plague, syphilis, whooping cough, gonorrhea, leprosy, and many other specific infections, have been definitely related to invasion of the human body by specific germs or viruses or other living organisms.

ABOUT GERMS

Few people really know what a germ looks like or how it invades the human body. Germs are so small that it takes three hundred billions of an average germ to weigh a pound. They multiply rapidly under favorable conditions. One germ can produce two new ones in twenty minutes. Anyone who has tried to estimate how much money he would have by beginning with a penny and doubling his fortune every hour can realize how rapidly germs multiply. If a germ divided and made two new ones every hour it would, at the end of a day, have sixteen and a half billion descendants.

Doctors identify the germs that cause disease in various ways. First they take some of the material from the infected saliva or from the discharges or from the blood of the person who is infected. They examine this under a microscope. The germs are seen as little round dots, or as rod-shaped organisms, or even as long, slender filaments when they are greatly magnified under the microscope. Like human beings, the germs tend to live preferably in certain forms, sometimes two together, sometimes a group of many, sometimes a chain. Some germs are surrounded by capsules, usually a sort of fatty envelope that enables the germ to resist attacks in the body or in the blood of the animal it invades. Other germs have little tails like fins which enable them to move about.

There are still people foolish enough to talk about the germ theory. Germs are no more a theory than are plants, birds, and other living things that live and reproduce. The power of most germs to cause disease can be tested on animals. When the germs are injected into animals they produce changes in the tissues of the animal which are specific for the germs concerned. A pneumococcus in the lung of a man produces pneumonia; first a consolidation of the lung due to invasion by red blood cells and other material and later a softening of this mass and a clearing up of the lung if the patient lives.

When the typhoid germ gets into the human body it produces ulcers in the intestines, and germs are found in the ulcers. When the meningococcus gets into the linings of the spinal cord and brain it sets up an inflammation of these linings, which are called meninges; then the person has meningitis, an inflammation of the meninges. When the spinal fluid is examined the germs can be found in the fluid.

These tests which were developed by the great Robert Koch, with Louis Pasteur, a founder of modern bacteriology, constitute the acid tests for determining with certainty that any germ is associated with the production of a certain disease. If the germ can be found in the infected tissues, if the germ can be artificially grown outside the human body, if the germ can then be injected into an animal like the monkey and produce in that animal a condition like that in the human being from whom the germ was originally taken, it is the cause of that particular disease. Anyone with a reasoning mind should be willing to grant that the germ actually causes the disease.

INCUBATION PERIODS

The common contagious diseases include measles, scarlet fever, diphtheria, whooping cough, mumps, chicken pox, and German measles. The best way to avoid these diseases is to keep away from people who have them. However, this is not so easily done, since many parents do not feel their responsibilities greatly and do not see to it that their children, when ill, are kept away from other children. Really the chief responsibility rests on the parents of the sick child for the prevention of infectious diseases rather than on the parents of the well child.

Most of the common infectious diseases are caused by organisms which get into the body and then begin their action. A certain amount of time elapses between the period when the germ first gets in and when its visible manifestations appear. This is known as the incubation period, and it varies with different diseases. For instance, in meningitis it is from two to four days, in erysipelas from one half to three days, in measles from ten days to two weeks, in German measles from five days to twenty-one days, in scarlet fever from a few hours to a week, in smallpox from ten days to two weeks, in typhoid fever from six days to twenty-five days, and in chicken pox from four days to sixteen days.

In most of these diseases an eruption occurs in the surface of the body. These eruptions have characteristic distribution on the skin, so the physician asks particularly as to whether the redness first began on the face, the neck, the hands and feet, the abdomen, or the chest. The eruptions also differ greatly in their appearance: from tiny red spots to large red patches, from tiny pimples to crops of blisters.

Practically all of these conditions are likely to begin with a mild cold. In some of them the sore throat is severe; in most of them there is fever, slight headache, dizziness, nausea or vomiting. Obviously it is not safe to disregard any of these symptoms, particularly when they appear in a child.

The excretions which carry disease include the material that is coughed from the throat, that is spread by spitting, by sneezing, or that may pass from the body in the form of discharges of one kind or another. Therefore, mothers should guard particularly against contact of a well child with one that is coughing, sneezing, spitting, or that manifests any of the other signs of infectious disease that have been mentioned.

RESISTANCE TO INFECTIOUS DISEASE

Four factors are chiefly responsible for infection of the human body: First, the presence of a germ with sufficient toxic power to grow in the body; second, a sufficient number of these germs to overcome attacks by the body against the germ; third, some special condition in the body that makes it possible for the germ to live and grow; and fourth, some method of getting the germ into the body.

Were it not for the fact that human beings develop within their bodies conditions which make it difficult for germs to live and grow, the human race would long since have been destroyed by the bacteria. However, the resistance which the human being has is not absolute. The constitution of the human body changes from time to time. Resistance is decreased when the body is greatly undernourished, when a person is exceedingly fatigued, when he has been exposed to sudden severe changes of temperature, or in several other ways.

Therefore, the line of defense varies in its intensity from time to time. When the enemy is sufficiently numerous, or sufficiently strong, it breaks through. For this reason, even in the most severe epidemics, some people escape, although there are conditions in which practically everyone attacked is unable to resist. Such conditions occur, for example, when a population among whom a disease has never previously appeared suddenly comes in contact with it. This occurred in the Faroe Islands when measles was brought by a ship carrying white men; at that time more than half the population of the islands died of that disease.

Sometimes the resistance of the body to one disease is broken down by a mild attack of another previous disease. For instance, a person who has had influenza, diabetes, tuberculosis, or some other chronic disorder, may thereafter develop pneumonia, typhoid fever, rheumatic fever, or tuberculosis much more easily than he would have previously.

CARRIERS OF DISEASE

Frequently people who are healthy carry about in their bodies germs which do not attack them but which have sufficient virulence, toxicity, strength, or poison to invade the body of another person and in that person to cause disease. A person who carries the germs about is called a "carrier." Should the carrier suddenly have his own resistance lowered by any of the factors that have been mentioned he might suddenly be invaded by these germs, although previously they had not been able to set up infection in his body.

There is no doubt that all of us are constantly being invaded by germs in contaminated food and water, in breathing, in touching infected items with our hands, which are then conveyed to the mouth and nose. Germs occur on money, in clothing, and on various other objects. However, the dosage of germs received through such contacts, or the virulence of the germs, may not be sufficient to bring about disease. The exposure of the germ to fresh air and sunlight, and the fact that it is trying to live on a substance not suitable to it as a habitation, may prevent its multiplying and may cause the germ itself to lose its strength.

Under other circumstances, germs multiply in tremendous numbers, so that the human being who comes in contact with them sustains a massive assault. For instance, an infected fruit peddler may use saliva to polish the fruit, and the germs might grow well on the fruit thus polished. Germs may be deposited with sewage in running water and multiply tremendously in the sewage. When the water from the contaminated stream is drunk by a human being he gets in enough germs to cause prompt infection. Sometimes an infected food handler is employed to mix a potato salad, to bake a custard, or to make a pie which is then kept under insanitary conditions before being eaten, so that the germs multiply profusely. When this occurs anybody who eats the infected food may become seriously infected, as occurred recently at a picnic when eight hundred people became sick from eating infected potato salad.

PATHS BY WHICH GERMS INVADE

Germs can get into the body in all sorts of ways: with food and water, by inhaling, through open wounds on the skin, by the bite of an insect, as occurs with mosquitoes in malaria and yellow fever, ticks in Texas fever, fleas in plague, and tsetse flies in African sleeping sickness.

When the means by which the germs get into the body are understood, scientific medicine develops methods for keeping them out. When the means are not fully understood, as occurs, for instance, in infantile paralysis, prevention is difficult.

Often the germs produce disease by developing a poison which is then absorbed by the body. After absorption, the poison acts on the nerves or the muscles or the blood vessels. Sometimes the germs themselves gradually break up, and the products of their disintegration are poisonous. Again clumps of germs float around in the blood and cause death by developing in overwhelming numbers in the blood. On other occasions the germs may attack certain organs of the body and so injure these organs that death ensues.

It has been said that the germs like to pick out certain places in which to live under the conditions which suit them best. This happens, for instance, with a germ called the pneumococcus which settles in the lungs and produces pneumonia, but which also may infect the eye or the spine. It occurs with the germs of meningitis, which practically always settle on the coverings of the spinal cord and of the brain, the typhoid germ which settles in the intestines, the germs of lockjaw and of hydrophobia and of epidemic encephalitis which attack the nervous system. There are some germs, like those of tuberculosis or syphilis, which may affect any tissue in the human body although preferably entering by way of the lungs or mucous membrane. There is tuberculosis of bones, of joints, of the eye, and of the nervous system. The organism that causes syphilis actually attacks every organ and tissue in the human body.

RESPONSE OF THE BODY TO GERM INVASION

When germs get into the body and release their poisons the tissues react usually in definite ways. One of the reactions of the body is fever. This is apparently due to the effects of the poisons of the germs on the nervous mechanism of the body which controls the body temperature. Associated with the fever there is speeding up of the chemical changes that go on in the body, so that there may be perspiration and, as a result of the increased activity, a loss of weight. For this reason it has become customary to feed fevers rather than to starve them.

Associated with the disturbance of the nervous system there may be dizziness and loss of appetite, also vomiting and an increased activity of the motion of the bowels. This helps to cause loss of material from the body. Due to accumulations of fluid or swelling of tissue there may be aches and pains in the joints and in the muscles. The interference with the action of the kidney may cause fluid to be retained in the body. The blood usually responds by an increase in the number of the white blood cells, but there are some conditions in which the number is decreased, notably influenza and typhoid fever.

Because the fever is considered to be one of the mechanisms of the body in defense against the attack of germs, scientific medicine does not always attempt to reduce the fever too suddenly or too rapidly by the use of drugs. A fever that is not exceedingly high or prolonged for any length of time is not especially harmful to the body, particularly if the amount of fluid in the body is watched and enough of the right type of food is put into the body to prevent too great a wastage of the tissues.

A normal temperature is 98.6 degrees F. A great many investigations indicate that temperatures over 100 degrees F. are unfavorable to the growth of bacteria and may inhibit the action of some of the poison developed by the bacteria. As will be shown later in the discussion of many of the infections which attack human beings, it is much better to prevent infections than to endeavor to treat them after they have been established.

STAMPING OUT DISEASE

By scientific methods applied since the nature of the germs and their methods of attack on the body have been discovered, certain diseases are now practically eliminated as of exceeding danger to mankind. Yellow fever occurs now in only a few isolated spots throughout the world. In the United States the number of cases of typhoid fever has been so greatly reduced that many young physicians never see a case even in the hospitals where they take their training. Cholera and plague are limited to the remoter areas of China and India and are seldom if ever seen in the United States.

Mankind has undergone progressive changes from the beginning of time; the diseases of man, particularly such as are caused by living organisms, likewise undergo such changes. True, some diseases have been overcome and eliminated, but new diseases constantly appear and demand consideration. The development of new methods of transportation and conveyance, such as the airplane and the ease of intercommunication between various portions of the earth, have brought into the temperate zone the diseases of the tropics which were formerly limited to such areas.

Many a great civilization has fallen because of the development, endemically or epidemically, of diseases that were previously under control, or because of the introduction of some new disease that had previously been considered a rarity. The great civilizations of Greece and Rome fell because of epidemics of malaria. In the United States today certain forms of infections of the glands, certain forms of infestation by tapeworms, and similar disorders, are seen with comparative frequency, whereas formerly they were practically unknown.

The time will never come when man will be free entirely from the fear of disease. The battle is unending, but more and more mankind can celebrate the fruits of victory. As diseases change and as new diseases appear, scientists observe them in their earliest stages, determine their causes and their modes of transmission, and prevent their development.

PREVENTION OF INFECTION

The prevention of disease must be related to our knowledge of the way in which infectious disease gains entrance into the body. Everything possible must be done to see that the germs in the person who is infected do not get out and thus get into contact with other people. If this could be done in every case, many infectious diseases would probably disappear.

If everything possible is to be done, all of the sheets, pillow cases, clothing, handkerchiefs, and, in fact, everything touched by a person who is infected, will have to be sterilized by boiling or by steam under pressure before being permitted in contact with other people. All of the excretions from the body of the infected person must be disinfected by proper antiseptics or by burning. The person with a discharge from the nose, such as occurs in the common cold, might at all times wear a face mask. To carry out completely these procedures would mean such an obstruction and hampering of the usual routine of existence that it not likely to be generally adopted.

The next step is to do everything possible to prevent infected material from being passed from one person to another. This means complete control of food, drink, and air, also the earliest possible detection of human beings, animals, or insects which carry disease, the control of such carriers and their possible elimination.

A human being who is carrying typhoid cannot be eliminated but must be controlled. Since there are millions of persons who carry disease constantly, it is not likely that this source of infection will ever be brought completely under control. Moreover, there are some diseases of which the cause is not definitely known, and it is unlikely that healthy carriers of such diseases will ever be controlled until the cause of the disease is known.

PERSONAL HYGIENE

The best step that the average person can take to prevent infectious disease is to raise his individual resistance by practising the best possible personal hygiene. This means the eating of a suitable diet, the securing of sufficient exercise and sunlight, and enough rest to give the tissues of the body opportunity to recuperate from fatigue.

Moreover, it is possible to aid resistance to certain infectious diseases by injecting the human being either with blood that has resistance, such as the blood from a person who has recovered from the disease, or by injecting serums from an animal which has been infected with the disease and which has in its serum substances opposed to the disease. A considerable number of such specific preventive serums and vaccines will be discussed under each of the infectious diseases as it is considered.

INCIDENCE OF INFECTIOUS DISEASE

The number of cases of the various infectious diseases varies from time to time. There have been great epidemics of influenza such as the epidemic of 1918, in which tremendous numbers of people were involved, whereas there have been minor epidemics in which relatively few people were concerned. Cases of influenza are difficult to differentiate from the common cold. The reports of the United States Public Health Service indicate about 700,000 cases of influenza in 1929, but if all of the conditions resembling influenza were included, the number would be many millions.

The figures for such conditions as measles (about 366,000), chicken pox (216,000), scarlet fever (182,000), mumps (103,000), and whooping cough (197,000) are relatively accurate, since the large majority of such cases are reported. Everyone knows that the rate of incidence of tuberculosis has dropped greatly. The number of deaths from this disease has dropped from 275 per hundred thousand people in the United States to around 12.5 in 1953.

Notwithstanding that typhoid fever can be completely controlled by proper measures, thousands of cases of typhoid fever still occur annually in the United States. Notwithstanding that we have in vaccination and in isolation certain methods of controlling smallpox, a considerable number of cases and deaths from this disease are still reported.

CLEANLINESS AND INFECTION

If infectious disease is to be prevented and brought under control, people must learn to know the nature of disease, the method of its spread, and the methods of prevention. They must do everything possible to keep themselves in such fit condition that infectious disease will not readily attack them.

Much infectious disease can be prevented by keeping as clean as possible, including frequent bathing with plenty of soap and water. Thorough washing of the hands with plenty of soap, particularly before eating, will destroy millions of germs which may otherwise infect human bodies. Vaccination against smallpox is important for everybody. Children should be protected against diphtheria by the use of diphtheria toxoid or toxin-antitoxin. When there are epidemics of typhoid or of other infectious diseases, physicians should be consulted as to the desirability of using other specific vaccines, serums, or antitoxins. Remember that most infectious diseases are spread by contact with persons who have the disease or who may be recovering.

TREATMENT OF INFECTIOUS DISEASES

In the treatment of most of the common infectious diseases, rest in bed is absolutely necessary. The diet should invariably be mild and bland, depending largely on milk, but supplemented with well-macerated vegetables and occasionally with enough thoroughly macerated liver or lamb's kidney to supply the necessary iron and vitamins that are needed in the diet.

For many of the specific infectious diseases there are now specific methods of treatment. For example, there are serums, vaccines, or antitoxins available in scarlet fever, measles, diphtheria, whooping cough, tetanus, meningitis, erysipelas, and undulant fever. In some of the conditions, moreover, the blood serum taken from a person who is convalescing from the disease has been found to have virtues in certain instances.

Typical of the treatment of most of the infectious diseases is the usual method of handling measles. Every child with this disease should be put to bed and kept there, with light covers, as long as it has any fever and for a few days thereafter. If the eyes are irritated, they may be treated with iced cloths soaked in a cold solution of boric acid. The doctor may prescribe the application of an ointment which will keep the lids from getting sticky. The itching and burning of the skin which frequently occurs in the infectious diseases is often relieved by bathing with a simple solution of bicarbonate of soda or a calamine lotion.

The doctor will treat the cough, if it is distressing, by small doses of sedative drugs. The restlessness, headache, and general discomfort may also be relieved by small doses of aspirin or similar remedies, as the doctor prescribes. When, however, any patient develops serious complications or symptoms, such as dullness, stupor, or convulsions, whenever he breathes rapidly or turns blue, it is well to have the physician in immediate attendance. Under such circumstances, the application of a bath, a pack, or a proper remedy may mean a turning between the tendency toward recovery or the tendency toward a more serious condition leading to death.

The details of the treatment of infectious diseases are discussed much more fully in the chapters dealing with individual diseases. The sulfonamide drugs and the antibiotics have revolutionized the treatment of all infectious diseases. Penicillin, aureomycin and terramycin are most widely used with chloramphenical or chloromycetin in typhoid. Thus far specific substances are not available for poliomyelitis, chickenpox and measles. The forms of sulfonamides most widely used are sulfadiazine and gantrisin. Even when not specifically used sulfa drugs and antibiotics control secondary infections such as those of the throat, sinuses or meninges.

INFERTILITY Infertility means inability of any species to conceive and to reproduce its kind. In general, the words infertility and sterility are used interchangeably. Estimates indicate that approximately 10 per cent of married couples are unable to reproduce or have children. The reasons vary according to many different aspects of the problem.

The difficulty may be due to inability of the sperm cells of the male to travel into the female tract because of some obstruction in either the male or the female. Obviously studies must be made as to this condition on both husband and wife before any positive decision is reached. Difficulties with glands are relatively insignificant because they are exceedingly uncommon. Psychologic and emotional disturbances may lead to complete disorganization of both the male and female sexual activities. Certainly emotional causes may make it impossible for a man to be potent sexually.

There are of course cases in which either the male or female sex glands may be deficient in their reproduction of the necessary cells. Before a doctor will give a definite diagnosis he must make extensive and careful studies as to the marriage relationship, the general physical and mental conditions of both husband and wife with particular attention to the sex organs and glands. He will have to study the question of dietary, glandular, or other disturbances. He may find it necessary to call in psychiatric consultation when the preliminary studies indicate the difficulties are chiefly mental or emotional.

In many instances physicians have found that detailed sex education is all that is necessary because of some wrong sexual pattern that a married couple may have adopted. In the treatment of such conditions the use of both male and female sex glandular materials has been helpful in a few instances. Some-times the difficulty is in the pituitary gland or in the ovary or in the male sex gland. In some instances even the giving of thyroid extract has been helpful as a sort of general glandular stimulation. Study of the sex cycle is also important since there are certain periods when the woman is much more fertile than others, and the intensive efforts towards having a child may be concentrated in this period.

INFLUENZA Differentiation between the common cold and influenza is a job for an expert and even many an expert has some trouble making this fine distinction. However, influenza is likely to occur in epidemics whereas the common cold goes on all the time. Influenza spreads rapidly, usually beginning with a sudden fever, marked prostration, pains in the back and legs, redness of the eyes, and some inflammation in the throat.

The first epidemic of influenza carefully recorded was in 1510, and there have been at least eight instances when influenza spread throughout the world. At first these outbreaks seemed to come about fifty years apart, then forty years apart, and nowadays about twenty-five years apart. However, there is no exact regularity in this matter. Frequently small waves of recurrence will follow a great epidemic.

Several viruses have now been isolated when epidemics of influenza have occurred recently. Viruses, it must be remembered, were only discovered and seen in recent years. Two of the forms of virus associated with epidemics recently are called influenza A virus and influenza B virus. However, when influenza occurs, many other germs are likely to invade the infected and swollen tissues. These others include the germ of pneumonia and several different forms of streptococci and staphylococci. The combination of an influenzal infection with a streptococcal infection may be particularly deadly.

Usually from one to three days after a person has been exposed he comes down with the disease. The fever lasts from one to five days, in the majority of cases about three days. The symptoms related to the nose and throat are worse at the end of twenty-four hours and then in general get better. Most serious is a secondary inflammation of the lungs, so that there is a constant harassing cough.

Following influenza there is usually a period of depression and weakness which, for many people, is far more serious than the acute disease itself. In fact it is the secondary depression and weakness and the complications which make influenza a serious disease. The majority of people with influenza get well promptly but a considerable percentage develop the secondary complications (particularly pneumonia) which are responsible for death.

Recently vaccines have been developed which are known to be especially useful in preventing influenza. They have been tried in some outbreaks in colleges and universities. The influenza virus is classified as virus A, A^1, and B.

If an influenza outbreak is exceedingly serious, it is now customary to try the antibiotic drugs as a means of preventing secondary complications, including the invasion of the pneumococcus and the streptococcus.

The best advice of the doctors for the person with influenza is to go to bed until convalescence is well established and the danger of complications is passed. Take plenty of fluids, including citrus drinks, which have a tendency to alkalinity. The diet is usually light. Various remedies are prescribed to relieve any pains or headaches or symptoms that might cause sleeplessness.

INFLUENZA—cold differs greatly: See RESPIRATORY DISEASES, article THE RESPIRATORY DISEASES.

INFLUENZA—cyclic recurrence: See RESPIRATORY DISEASES, article THE RESPIRATORY DISEASES.

INFLUENZA—death rate: See article DIABETES.

INFLUENZA—decrease in number of white blood cells: See INFECTIOUS DISEASE, article THE PREVENTION AND TREATMENT OF INFECTIOUS DISEASE.

INFLUENZA—encephalitis mistaken for: See article TRANSMISSIBLE DISEASES.

INFLUENZA—endocarditis may occur: See HEART, article DISEASES OF THE HEART AND CIRCULATION.

INFLUENZA—epidemic of 1918: See INFECTIOUS DISEASES, article THE PREVENTION AND TREATMENT OF INFECTIOUS DISEASE.

INFLUENZA—epidemic sore throat mistaken for: See EAR, article THE EAR, TONGUE, NOSE, AND THROAT.

INFLUENZA—gall bladder may be affected: See article DIGESTION AND DIGESTIVE DISEASES.

INFLUENZA—incidence in 1929: See INFECTIOUS DISEASE, article THE PREVENTION AND TREATMENT OF INFECTIOUS DISEASE.

INFLUENZA—inflammation of colon: See article DIGESTION AND DIGESTIVE DISEASES.

INFLUENZA—hair loss may follow: See HAIR, article THE HAIR.

INFLUENZA—leukopenia: See BLOOD, article THE BLOOD AND ITS DISEASES.

INFLUENZA—pandemics: See RESPIRATORY DISEASES, article THE RESPIRATORY DISEASES.

INFLUENZA—pneumonia cases increase when influenza epidemics strike: See RESPIRATORY DISEASES, article THE RESPIRATORY DISEASES.

INFLUENZA—reduces resistance to other diseases: See INFECTIOUS DISEASE, article THE PREVENTION AND

TREATMENT OF INFECTIOUS DISEASE.

INFLUENZA—undulant fever less serious: See article TRANSMISSIBLE DISEASES.

INFLUENZA—viruses: See RESPIRATORY DISEASES, article THE RESPIRATORY DISEASES.

INGROWN TOENAILS (See also, Feet)

When stockings are too long or too short pressures occur on the sides of the toenails, with overgrowth of the tissue around the corners of the nail. Eventually the nail grows into the tissue forming an ingrown toenail. The nail on the large toe is the one usually involved. Usually the person who suffers with ingrown toenail tries all sorts of poultices, antiseptics, and ointments on his toe, in addition to a little home surgery, before he limps into the doctor's office. The doctor finds the toe red and swollen and often with pus oozing from under the nail onto the stocking or the cotton the patient is using for protection. People seldom sterilize the scissors or even the razor blades they use at home for first aid to afflicted feet.

One surgeon has suggested the following procedure for the cure of ingrown toenails. It is necessary to cause the middle of the nail to catch up with the corners. He therefore cuts a small V or U in the center of the nail. This slows the growth at the side of the nail and takes the pressure off the corners. If the foot is kept scrupulously clean, if stockings are worn thick enough to afford protection, if the shoes are loose enough to prevent pressure but not so loose as to cause rubbing, and if the toenail is kept properly trimmed during the process of healing, the nail will gradually become normal. Proper foot hygiene will keep the nail in normal condition.

INHALING OF DANGEROUS SUBSTANCES

SILICOSIS—Perhaps the most dangerous and disabling of the diseases that come from inhaling foreign substances is the one called silicosis. This results from the presence of particles of silicon dioxide in the air. The condition was first discovered from an examining of the X-ray plates of workers in industries using silicon. First came the fibrous changes in the lung and then small nodular infiltrations appear. Later there may be large masses in the lungs as a result of formation of fibrous fluid.

The occupations in which silicosis occurs most frequently are mining, sandblasting, foundry work, the prolonged use of polishing and cutting wheels composed of sandstone and, finally, stone cutting and polishing. Because the condition is one that affects the lung primarily, the changes that occur are related to the respiration, including some blueness, clubbing of the fingers, perhaps an increase in the total number of red blood cells. As soon as the condition is discovered, the patient, if a young person, should be immediately removed from the job. Men of advanced age who have taken many years, perhaps more than twenty to develop the condition, may be permitted to continue at their work since the condition is not likely to become worse. The person with silicosis who subsequently develops tuberculosis has a difficult time.

ASBESTOSIS—Workers may inhale other substances than silicon and develop changes in the lungs. Asbestosis which comes from the inhaling of asbestos fiber is one. These people, in addition to the lung changes, expectorate brownish formed material which contains the fibers and spicules associated with asbestos.

SIDEROSIS—Another condition called siderosis results from deposits of iron in the lung. This is seen in such occupations as those of the acetylene welder and workers with the electric arc.

BAGASSOSIS—Bagassosis is the name given to the results of inhaling bagasse dust. Bagasse is the name of pulverized and dried stalks of sugar cane. Bagasse is much used in manufacturing insulating board.

BERYLLIUM DISEASE—Beryllium disease of the lung is a new condition resulting from inhaling beryllium in the manufacture of fluorescent lamps. Most of the cases so far reported have occurred in women. The lungs in this condition when observed with the X ray are found to have what has been called a sandpaper appearance.

ALUMINUM DUST—The employees of smelters dealing with bauxite are found to suffer with the results of inhaling aluminum dust which produces the formation of tissue in the lung. Another complication is a condition called bissynosis which is ascribed to the inhalation of cotton fibers. The condition is known to workers around cotton gins as gin fever and "Monday morning fever." The inhaling of almost any substance may have serious effects on the lungs and among the latest noted is cadmium workers' disease which brings about lung changes. Finally those who work with severe irritant substances like sulphur dioxide and other substances used in refrigeration may have damage to the lung resulting finally in secondary chronic infections from the inhaling of various irritating gases.

INHERITANCE OF DISEASE (See also, *Heredity*)

Customarily we say that disease is not inherited by people, but that the body constitution which makes people susceptible is inherited. Structural disturbances may be inherited. Red-green color blindness affects males who transmit the condition only to their daughters—who do not have it—but transmit it to their sons in about half the births. The response of our bodies to any infection or other trauma or stress depends to a large extent on the nature of our constitution.

Many disease conditions seem to occur more often in some families than in others. Hardening of the arteries, diabetes, rheumatic diseases, and some forms of cancer are conspicuous examples. Tuberculosis, goiter, ulcers of the stomach, and even appendicitis seem to be related to body structure in ways that make a hereditary factor a possibility.

In addition to red-green color blindness, hemophilia—the tendency to bleed—is passed from males through females. Baldness is another condition which is related to the genes that determine characteristics. Strangely the experts in genetics are now convinced that a large amount of head hair is not correlated with virility. Instead, once the baldness gene is present, the excess of male hormone associated with virility is the likely additional factor for baldness. Degrees of baldness and the pattern of distribution are also regulated by hereditary factors.

Absence of certain teeth, deformities in the growth of the jaws, sweat gland deficiencies, albinism—or lack of pigment in the eyes, skin and hair—and extra breasts or nipples as well as extra fingers and toes may also be inherited. Difficulties of vision, and of hearing, taste, and smell occur in families. Finally, heredity also plays a part in determining intelligence or the lack of it.

INSECT PESTS

The number of insects that disturb human beings is legion. Most common of those that attack the body directly are the lice and the itch mites. Less frequent are bedbugs and spiders. In the woods and in tropical areas chiggers and mosquitoes, ticks and the biting flies annoy mankind.

Among soldiers in the armed forces

insects are so serious a menace that special divisions of the department of preventive medicine are concerned with the control of insects.

Chiggers are known scientifically as *Trombicula irritans*. They hook themselves onto the skin; the skin becomes irritated, and an intolerable itching begins. Red blotches appear, and blisters form. The chiggers do not burrow into the skin, but they inject a substance which dissolves and softens the tissue, and this causes the itching.

Infestation with chiggers can be prevented by putting flour of sulfur on the stockings or underclothing when going into tall grass or weeds. Soldiers are protected by wearing leggings and closing off the bottom of the trousers.

If one has been seriously bitten by chiggers, it is customary to wash the skin thoroughly with soap and water and allow the lather to remain on the skin ten minutes before removing. Then any of the anti-itch preparations can be applied to keep the itching under control until healing has occurred.

Recently insecticide and insect-repellent mixtures have been developed, based on the use of freon, containing pyrethrum, and there is also the new insect repellent called DDT. These are efficient in controlling not only chiggers but mosquitoes, moths, and many other types of insects.

The louse is an annoying inhabitant of the human body. In the armed forces and wherever great numbers of people are assembled, delousing technics have been developed for ridding the body of this unwelcome visitor and also for removing both the lice and their eggs from clothing. Usually live steam is used for disinsectization.

Following is the advice circulated by the health department of the city of Chicago:

Articles Needed—Kerosene oil; olive oil (sweet oil), half pint of each.

To Kill Vermin—Mix the kerosene and sweet oil and rub this mixture well into the scalp. Then with a piece of muslin cover the hair for at least two hours or, better, overnight. Do not bring the head in contact with a lighted gas jet or flame of any kind. When the muslin cover is removed, wash the hair and scalp with soap and hot water and rinse well with clear water. Repeat this procedure as often as live vermin are found in the hair.

To Remove Nits—Wet the hair thoroughly with hot vinegar, and comb with a fine-toothed comb. Repeat this daily until all nits are gone. Always dry the hair thoroughly before going out.

A product called Kwell is efficient and not as disagreeable to use as kerosene.

Scabies is a disease caused by the itch mite, which burrows under the skin. It causes what is called the seven-year itch. Usually it is controlled by sulfur preparations or Eurax.

The only venomous spider in the Western Hemisphere is the black widow. When a person it bitten by a spider, the first step is to prevent absorption of the poison into the circulation. The wound can be disinfected with tincture of iodine or any other good antiseptic.

Finally, the housefly is under suspicion not only of being an annoying insect but also one capable of menacing health by carrying filth and germs from one person to another. The common housefly spreads disease as do also the tropical flies and fleas.

In Africa the tsetse fly spreads African sleeping sickness. Texas fever and Rocky Mountain spotted fever are spread by ticks. Indeed any insect that sucks blood or that injects poison into the body is a menace in relation to the spread of disease.

INSECTICIDES—See article OCCUPATION AND HEALTH.

INSECTS—allergy caused by: See article ALLERGY.

INSECTS—bites: See article FIRST AID; INFECTIOUS DISEASE, article THE PREVENTION AND TREATMENT OF INFECTIOUS DISEASE; SKIN, article THE SKIN; EAR, article THE EAR, TONGUE, NOSE, AND THROAT.

INSECTS—ear entered by: See article FIRST AID; EAR, article THE EAR, TONGUE, NOSE, AND THROAT.

INSECTS—encephalitis: See article TRANSMISSIBLE DISEASES.

INSECTS—psittacosis carried by: See article TRANSMISSIBLE DISEASES.

INSOMNIA Failure to sleep at any time when sleep is ordinarily expected is called insomnia. Very few, if any, people have complete insomnia. That ocurrs only when pain is continuous and unrelieved or when there is mental disease. However, partial inability to sleep is a frequent condition and may be due to a variety of causes.

Sleep may be so disturbed as to be inadequate, so that when one awakens he is not refreshed but tired.

Regardless of the vast amount of study that has been conducted in laboratories of physiology all over the world, the exact mechanism of sleep is not yet fully understood. Since certain forms of disorder in the brain may produce inability to sleep, there seems to be reason to believe that some portion of the brain is involved in the mechanism by which sleep is induced. However, there are many contributing factors which have to be considered in insomnia, and allowance must be made for people's peculiarities and habits.

People who are especially sensitive to noises will awaken much more easily than others. There are light sleepers and heavy sleepers. Some people get along with just a little sleep—say, six hours a night—whereas others require from eight to ten hours each night.

When a doctor treats a person with insomnia, he tries to determine whether or not the insomnia is associated with any mental or physical condition in the brain, whether or not it is associated with high blood pressure, hardening of the arteries, whether or not there are infectious conditions or poisoning due to various drugs. He will try particularly to find out whether or not the person has anxieties about his family relationships, his money, or his career.

If the insomnia is due to anxiety, sleep is likely to be disturbed and fitful. The person with insomnia goes to sleep but shortly thereafter awakens and is often unable to get back to sleep. As a result he gets up in the morning tired and with the feeling that his brain has been working all night. Sometimes indulgence in hard mental work just before going to sleep will keep the mind so active that it is difficult to go to sleep in the first place.

Physical discomforts of all kinds, such as coughing, difficulty in breathing, indigestion, overactivity of the bladder, or ringing in the ears, may also produce sleeplessness. The treatment of insomnia is obviously directed in such cases to the physical condition that is responsible. Insomnia is not a disease but a symptom. The treatment is directed to the cause when that is found.

Today there are innumerable drugs which tend to depress the activity of the brain. These drugs are known as hypnotics, and very strong ones as narcotics. People can very easily get into the habit of taking some hypnotic drug just before going to bed. However, preparation for sleep without the taking of a hypnotic often enables one to do without the drug. A walk outdoors for fifteen to twenty minutes may be good preparation. A light massage with a genial masseur often produces both a physical and mental frame of mind conducive to sleep. A heavy meal should not be taken within four hours of the time of going to bed, but a snack including hot milk, cocoa, or any similar drink just before going to sleep is sometimes helpful. Difficult study should not be practiced within an hour of going to sleep, but reading of a relaxing book—that is, one which does not induce mental tension—also aids sleep when the habit of reading before going to sleep has been formed.

INSOMNIA—encephalitis: See article TRANSMISSIBLE DISEASES.

INTELLIGENCE Probably there are in the United States about 500,000 people who are mentally defective. These have been classified as including 30,000 idiots, 100,000 imbeciles, and the remainder morons.

Among the factors related to the failure of a human being to develop intelligence are injury to the brain at birth, infections or inflammations of the brain like meningitis and encephalitis, severe injury to the brain resulting from accident and defective actions of the glands, as well as the effects of heredity.

Intelligence is described as the total capacity of anyone to think rationally, to act with a definite purpose, and to be able to deal effectively with the situation in which he lives. Other factors also are related to intelligence or the intellect, but there is also the possibility of confusing intelligence with education and knowledge. Some people know a great deal about many things and still cannot meet the standards for intelligence. The only way by which we can measure intelligence is to test a large number of different factors which measure the power to reason, the memory, the knowledge, and the experience of the person who is being tested.

Intelligence tests are simpler for children than they are for adults because the amount that a child has ex-

perienced or learned during the short time of his existence is not so great as that of an older person. With very old people, experts who make these tests must take into account the possibility of mental deterioration.

Some of the technics by which we distinguish various grades of intelligence are relatively simple. An idiot will not protect himself against common physical dangers because his instinct of self-preservation is not strong. An imbecile cannot manage his own affairs and cannot be taught to do so. Morons cannot compete with others in earning a livelihood or in protecting themselves from those who would exploit them. Therefore morons require constant supervision and care.

The scientists distinguish between mental defects and mental retardation. A mental defect cannot be corrected beyond the limitations of the brain in the person concerned, no matter how skillful or persistent the treatment may be. If, on the other hand, a child has merely been retarded in his mental development, the possibility for bringing him up to a proper age level in intellect exists. A child may be retarded, for example, because of impaired vision or hearing, or because the people around the child speak a language which is not the common language of the community, so that the child does not get beyond the language and mentality of those who care for him. Finally, anxieties and fears will hold back development, and removal of such anxieties will permit the child to develop rapidly.

Out of a sampling of almost 46,000 registrants examined for Selective Service, 1.9 per cent of white boys had to be rejected because of educational deficiencies, and 12.2 per cent of Negro boys had to be rejected for this cause. Careful analysis has not yet been made as to the causative factors chiefly responsible.

INTERMITTENT CLAUDICA-TION See *Buerger's Disease* and *Limping, Intermittent.*

INTERNAL SECRETING OR ENDOCRINE GLANDS—About one hundred years have passed since a scientist who removed the sex glands of a rooster found that the animal could be restored to its masculine vigor by transplanting into its tissue the glands of another rooster. Later a British doctor named Addison described a disease due to insufficiency of action of the adrenal glands which is now known as Addison's disease. In 1889 a French scientist named Brown-Sequard attracted world attention by the claim that the injection into his own body of male sex hormone had produced a rejuvenating effect. It didn't work with him and it still doesn't work to produce rejuvenation or restore lost sex power, notwithstanding the imaginative and emotional claims of a few too credulous scientists. Nevertheless, the new knowledge of the glands, most of which has developed since 1900, is one of the greatest contributions ever made to human health and happiness.

From the point of view of chemical study four types of hormones are known, including those like insulin, which have large protein molecules, those like ACTH, which are called polypeptides, those like thyroxin and adrenalin, which are aromatic derivatives, and the steroid hormones which include Cortisone and the sex hormones.

Much has been learned about hormones from the study of animals in which the glands can be removed and in which other glands can be transplanted to determine the effects. Similarly glandular materials may be given to human beings and the effects then studied. Sometimes a tumor will cause overgrowth and overactivity of a gland. The results are reflected by various changes in the body and in its functions.

THE PITUITARY GLAND—Perhaps the most important of the glands is the pituitary although disturbance of any of the glands of internal secretion is serious. The glands include the anterior and posterior pituitary, the thyroid, the pancreas, the thymus, the adrenals and the sex glands. Among the hormones that have been identified in the anterior pituitary are a growth hormone which can increase height and raise body weight.

The anterior pituitary also develops substances which pass by the way of the blood to the adrenal gland, the thyroid, the sex glands and the milk-producing glands and influence their function. Recent studies have shown that the pituitary itself may be stimulated to act by adrenalin coming from the adrenal glands and by nervous stimuli coming from the emotional center in the brain. Since so many differently acting substances are developed in the pituitary, disturbances of this gland may be reflected in the body in many different ways.

Lessened activity of the pituitary gland before a child reaches adolescence may be observed as dwarfism and subnormal mentality and sexual development. However, deficiencies of growth also result from deficient action of the thyroid gland and instances are known in which dwarfism is hereditary. The failure of the pituitary gland may be due to deficient development or to infection or to the presence of tumors which may damage the gland. While substitute materials for the whole anterior pituitary have not yet been developed satisfactorily, some of the deficiencies can be corrected by giving thyroid, or sex gland, or adrenal cortex materials. Research has been given such a tremendous push by the discovery of Cortisone and ACTH that the outlook is more bright now than ever previously.

In the pituitary gland lies the function of creating a substance which is known as the growth hormone. This acts directly on the growth of body tissues. A dwarf is a person who is conspicuously smaller than other people of the same age and species. For normal growth a person must have proper amounts of the necessary food substances. The body takes this material and puts it into proper places as new tissue. People may be stunted in their growth from lack of essential foods or lack of oxygen. In addition the body must develop for itself the growth hormone, thyroid hormone and sex hormone. Among other causes of dwarfism are diseases or failure of growth of bones such as may occur with rickets.

Often children have been much smaller than others all through the period of childhood. When they pass into adolescence the body fails to make the spurt that is usual. Not only do they fail to grow in height but also they remain mentally and sexually immature. In some instances this is just a delay in action of the interlocking chain of glands that includes the pituitary, adrenal and sex glands.

The treatment of dwarfism depends on the cause. If a deficiency of essential protein and vitamins is responsible a supply of these substances will bring about growth. Similarly, thyroid deficiency can be met by giving thyroid extract. Pituitary growth hormone has not yet been developed for general use. In many cases of delayed adolescence doctors can now prescribe certain of the sex hormones with excellent results. The determination of which to give and the time and duration of treatment must be decided for each patient according to the conditions found when the patient is studied.

If an excess of growth hormone develops in childhood before the centers from which bones grow have ceased to function, the child becomes a giant. If the excess of growth hormone comes after this time, the condition called acromegaly develops. At the beginning the giant may be strong, alert, and intelligent, but in most cases as the giant growth continues the pituitary functions lessen; then the giant becomes weak and slow. Giants naturally attract much attention. Several cases have been recorded of growth over eight feet.

Usually in acromegaly excessive glandular tissue is found in the anterior pituitary gland. Such people may have enlargements of the lungs and liver and other organs as well as general increase in growth. Acromegaly is a relatively rare condition. Attention is called to it first by the increased size of the head, hands and feet. Fatigue, headache, and muscle pain may be noticed. Among the most observed signs is the enlargement of the lower jaw. The features become larger and coarsened, the skin gets rough and the ridges above the eyes become prominent. A voracious appetite is often noticed and sometimes is blamed for the growth changes.

Acromegaly is not a fatal condition and many of these patients live to advanced years. Some of the people developed diabetes because of changes in the glands. Formerly operation on the pituitary gland was recommended for most of these patients but more recently the overgrowth of glandular tissue has been found to be susceptible to the X ray. Often exposure of the tissue to X ray will stop the progress of the acromegaly.

Since sex gland disturbances are frequently associated with acromegaly the provision of male or female sex hormones as needed may be most helpful. Altogether much more may now be done for such people by giving proper amounts of the glandular substances available.

While the front portion of the pituitary gland provides a number of hormones—substances circulating in the blood—which stimulate the thyroid, the adrenals and other glands to perform their functions, the posterior or back portion of the pituitary gland has quite different effects. When injected into the body extracts similar to those provided by the back portion of the gland act to stimulate the muscle in the walls of the intestine, the muscle of the uterus and that in the walls of the blood vessels. Hence the bowel is made active, and the blood vessels contract. Thus this substance is used to stop hemorrhages after childbirth. The substance also has a profound effect on the action of the kidneys, controlling the way in which they eliminate water. If, therefore, there is a deficiency of the substance that comes from the posterior portion of the pituitary gland, people develop a condition called diabetes insipidus in which large amounts of fluid are poured out of the body. This condition is rare; in fact, a large clinic found only about twelve such cases in 100,000 patients.

The chief symptoms of *diabetes insipidus* are the pouring out of great amounts of water from the body and, naturally associated with it therefore, the taking in of tremendous quantities of water. The amounts may reach fifteen to twenty quarts a day. Because of the excess elimination of fluid, these people have a dry skin and an insatiable thirst. Under the circumstances, the condition is usually treated by giving the substance which is known as "pitressin." Two different substances have been isolated, one of which has the power of contracting the muscle of the intestines and uterus as its chief function and the other which controls the elimination of fluid.

THYROID—The activity of the thyroid gland is apparently controlled by the hormone that comes from the pituitary gland. For a variety of reasons the thyroid gland may be inactive or excessively active. Inactivity of the thyroid may result in the condition called cretinism which is associated with a deficiency of the thyroid gland in early childhood and the condition called myxedema which comes on later in life. The person with myxedema has a typical face with puffy eyelids and an apparent lack of interest in what is going on. The skin is dry and rough, the hair coarse, brittle and dry. Because the tongue and throat are swollen, the speech is slow and slurred. With all of this there is a tendency to slowing of all of the functions of the body and because of the deficiencies of the blood and the circulation, the person with myxedema is sensitive to cold.

Since the condition is so certainly due to a lack of thyroid material, the treatment includes the giving of thyroid and the dosage is adjusted according to the need of the patient and his response to the drug. Customarily doctors will begin with exceedingly small doses because the thyroid is a potent material and overdosage may result in a rapid heart, sweating, loss of weight, and diarrhea. The maximum effect from any dose is not apparent until seven to ten days after the use of the drug is first begun and the action will persist for one to three weeks after the drug is discontinued. The dosage of thyroid needs to be taken only once a day since usually nothing is gained by dividing it over the day.

THE PANCREAS—DIABETES—The pancreas is a gland which lies near the liver, stomach, and duodenum. It has a number of secretions, some of which go directly into the intestine and are concerned with digestion. One secretion goes instead into the blood and is intimately concerned with the way in which the body uses sugars. This substance is called insulin. A deficiency of insulin in the body results in a chronic disease called diabetes mellitus. Diabetes has been known for thousands of years and was described by ancient Greek and Chinese writers who were principally concerned with the large amounts of fluids excreted by the body in this condition. The fact that the urine contained sugar was first noted in the seventeenth century. Not until 1889 was it proved that diabetes results from failure of the pancreas. In 1921 Banting prepared an extract of the pancreas which is now called insulin. At least a million people now in the United States have diabetes and the number increases because the condition tends to come on with advanced years. More than half the people with diabetes develop the condition before they are fifty years old. Women are affected more frequently than men, particularly in diabetes in advanced years.

Studies of diabetes show that heredity plays an important part. This relationship is becoming more and more clear as people with diabetes tend to live longer and have more children. Once diabetes in childhood was considered invariably fatal. Now these children grow up, marry, and have families. We now know that if both parents are diabetic, the children will most certainly inherit the disease. Overweight is also important in relationship to diabetes. Not everyone who is overweight develops the disease. In fact, diabetes is seen in only a small proportion of the people who are overweight. However, nine out of ten people who develop diabetes are overweight. Among those who are overweight and who develop diabetes, dieting and restoration to normal weight lessens the severity of the symptoms and sometimes controls the condition. The person who is overweight, however, can produce more and more insulin and this may be a factor in exhausting the function of the pancreas. As I have mentioned in previous

articles, both the pituitary gland and the adrenal glands are also related in their functions to the use of sugar by the body. Excessive action of the pituitary gland may result in the appearance of sugar in the urine. Excessive action of the thyroid gland may make diabetes worse by increasing the work of the gland through the fact that the person is taking in large amounts of food.

SYMPTOMS OF DIABETES—Chief among the symptoms of diabetes are general weakness, loss of weight, excessive appetite, thirst and excessive flow of urine. Itching is a much noticed symptom. The first sign of severe diabetes may be loss of consciousness which is called diabetic coma.

Children have the disease more severely than do adults and doctors believe that the greater the age when diabetes begins the less severe is the disease.

Nowadays diabetes is usually discovered by an examination of the urine and sugar is likely to be found most often if the test is made immediately after a meal. When sugar is found in the urine, studies must also be made of the amount of sugar in the blood and particularly after the person has been fasting. A normal person has a blood sugar level when fasting of approximately 70 milligrams per 100 milliliters of whole blood, whereas if the person has diabetes, the figure is nearer 150.

Simple tests have now been developed which people use themselves to get an indication as to whether or not there is sugar in the urine. When this is found, the physician should be asked to make all of the necessary studies to determine the severity of the condition and to prescribe treatment promptly in order to control the disease.

Diet and the use of insulin are the basic steps in controlling diabetes.

Since infections are exceedingly serious for persons who are diabetic, a complete study of the body should be made to eliminate any infections in the teeth, the sinuses, the chest, the gall bladder or elsewhere.

The diet is designed to bring the person to his ideal weight and to lessen the total amount of sugar taken into the body. Many persons do not require insulin immediately or when they are on the reduction diet. When insulin is required, the amount is given in relationship to the diet and the maintenance of normal weight. Patients must co-operate with the doctor in regulating the control of sugar in relation to insulin intake. Emotional stresses are serious. Infection may be severe if not fatal. The diabetic patient must be kept clean. Immediate attention is given to all bruises and cuts of the skin. In caring for the nails the diabetic should avoid cutting or pushing of the cuticle. Most important is proper attention to the feet. These should be washed with warm water and a bland soap every day. They should be dried thoroughly but gently. Injuries to the feet must be avoided and particularly injuries from the cutting of toenails or corns. Stockings should be clean and loosely fitting, but without wrinkles.

EXCESSIVE INSULIN—While deficiency of insulin resulting in diabetes mellitus is far more serious and more common than excessive action of the pancreas, cases do occur in which there is too much insulin with a resulting low blood sugar. The sugar level of the blood is maintained by the body's use of glucose in the muscle, liver, brain, and other organs, and by the way in which the glucose is brought back into the blood from the liver and the muscles, and the secretion of insulin which makes possible the use of sugars by the body.

Following meals or periods of excitement there may be excess sugar in the blood, so that the body puts out extra insulin tending then to lower the sugar below normal. In other instances there may be low blood sugar because of a deficiency of the liver in storing sugar. Other cases are known in which tumors affecting the cells of the pancreas may produce excess insulin and with that a low blood sugar.

Overactivity of the nervous system can cause excessive flow of insulin into the blood. In all of these conditions the blood sugar becomes low; as a result, there is weakness and faintness, a rapid heart, anxiety and palpitation. When the person takes sugar or carbohydrates the symptoms are relieved.

In general, people who have low blood sugar do well on diets that are high in protein and fats and low in sugar. When a high sugar diet is taken, the body reacts by putting out excessive insulin which tends to lower the sugar below normal. Excessive secretion of insulin can be controlled by the taking of certain drugs such as derivatives of belladonna and atropine, but control of the emotional and dietary factors is considered a more satisfactory method of treating the condition.

THE THYMUS—Innumerable experiments have been made both on human beings and on animals to determine the exact functions of the thymus gland. Does it give off some substance directly into the blood—commonly called an internal secretion—which would affect the growth of the body? The thymus is removed occasionally and thus far no recognizable condition has been found which would be exclusively related to removal of the thymus. Neither has there been any effect found from taking large amounts of thymus extract apart from the fact that it contains many important nutritive materials and is therefore helpful in the nutrition of the body.

When a child is born, the thymus is found as a closely packed mass of cells.

This gland is large enough in many instances to occupy much of the space directly under the breastbone. Later in life the size of this glandular material decreases in relationship to the size of the body. Finally the gland disappears and is replaced by fat.

When there is a deficiency of material coming from the cortex of the adrenal gland the thymus is likely to enlarge as well as the lymph glands elsewhere in the body. This has been called *status thymicolymphaticus*. Sometimes these patients die suddenly; death has been attributed to the enlargement of the thymus whereas it was actually due to the deficiency of the secretion of the important material from the cortex of the adrenal gland.

Sometimes people who have a condition called *myasthenia gravis* in which there is the development of serious weakness and incapacity have been found with enlargements of the thymus gland.

It has been thought that removal of this gland surgically or breakdown of the gland by exposing it to X-ray would be helpful in such cases. While some of the patients seem to improve, others have not. One is not quite certain whether the improvement was merely a coincidence and would have occurred anyway or is in some way related to the treatment. Recently attempts have been made to treat this condition with ACTH. Some have said that great benefit has been brought about but others indicate that cases have become worse. This would indicate that ACTH does have an effect in changing both the mental attitude of these patients and also perhaps the general constitution. The drug does not appear to be a specific drug for the treatment of *myasthenia gravis*.

Physicians now believe that the thymus, being composed of lymphoid tissue and containing a high concentra- tion of essential substances, is a store- house for aid of the body, which is directly under control of other glands and a part of the interlocking gland system of the body.

INTERTRIGO What the mother usually calls "diaper rash" the doctor describes under the scientific name of intertrigo. The term really refers to any irritation of the skin which develops where two moist surfaces are in con- tact. This roughness and irritation are usually seen in the folds of the groin, between the thighs, between the but- tocks, under the arms, under the neck, or behind the ears.

Not often is there a determinable infection. In many instances the rough- ness and irritation are merely the result of the combination of moisture, rubbing of the surfaces, and want of cleanliness. Crusting and itching are seldom ob- served.

About the worst form of this con- dition is ordinary diaper rash, which affects babies. Sometimes the irritation is due to the use of laundry soap with an excess amount of alkali, which is left on the diaper when the latter is not properly rinsed after washing. In other instances it seems to be associated with the action of germs on the ammonia in the urine. For a while doctors thought that the ammonia was caused by having the baby drink an insufficient amount of water. Now it is recognized that the ammonia results only from bacterial action on the components of the urine.

When the redness occurs outside the diaper area, it can usually be controlled by the use of a good dusting powder. The combination of dryness and clean liness will usually take care of the condition. When, however, the inflam- mation extends into the urinary pas- sages, so that there is burning and irrita- tion, the mother as well as the baby is likely to be seriously disturbed. The strong smell of ammonia makes her more frightened. Under these circumstances she will do well to consult a doctor and to follow some simple precautions in relationship to the handling of the diapers. Burning and irritation on urination or in the area of the buttocks is so uncomfortable for the baby that it should have prompt attention.

In such cases the constant wearing of rubber or rubberized silk diapers may have to be discontinued until the condition is brought under control. Zinc oxide ointment is frequently used to protect the skin. The washing of the diapers with mild soap, rinsing at least three times to remove all the soap, soaking of the diapers overnight or for at least three hours in water containing three tablespoonfuls of boric acid powder to each gallon of water and, finally, the wringing of the diapers lightly and hanging in the sun for drying will overcome the infection in the diaper. If the diapers are lightly wrung out, so that when they dry enough boric acid is left to prevent bacterial decomposition of the urine, the condition is rather certainly controlled.

INTERTRIGO—See SKIN, article THE SKIN.

INTESTINES The intestines of the human being are a long tubular apparatus which includes the small intestine (23 feet long), the large intestine (5 feet long), and the rectum (about 6 inches long). This tube is lined with tissues which have the power in some places to secrete materials used in digestion and in other places to take up material.

The small intestines will hold about 3 quarts. In the small intestines digestion goes on actively in the upper part but absorption takes place throughout the entire length. The small intestines

include the duodenum, the jejunum, and the ileum. Usually it takes about four hours for food to get through the small intestines from the time when the food leaves the lower end of the stomach to the time when the food enters the cecum. The food thereafter moves at the rate of about an inch a minute. The walls of the intestines have muscles, and the food is passed along by waves of muscular action.

The large intestine handles the indigestible material that is left after the food has given to the body what it requires. The food will stay in the large intestine from ten to twelve to forty-eight hours. The large intestine includes various portions: the ascending, transverse, and descending colons. The cells of the large intestine can take up water and sugar solutions.

When the contents of the bowel pass into the rectum, a mechanism is set up which indicates to the person that material is ready to be expelled from the body.

Any obstruction of action of the large or small intestines is a serious matter. Such obstructions may occur from an intussusception in which one portion of the bowel is drawn inside the other like the drawing in of the toe of a sock. This is occasionally due to a tumor, sometimes to the fact that the indigestible material becomes hardened and impacted. Occasionally the bowel is obstructed by a pushing of the portion of the bowel into a rupture.

When such obstruction occurs, the pain is severe and demands immediate attention of a doctor. Since almost any acute condition inside the abdomen may simulate intestinal obstruction by producing pain and vomiting, the doctor must make a most careful diagnosis. If actual obstruction is found, operation is usually necessary. There are instances in which the bowel becomes paralyzed.

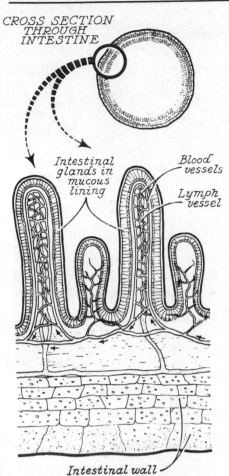

CROSS SECTION
THROUGH
INTESTINE

Intestinal
glands in
mucous
lining

Blood
vessels

Lymph
vessel

Intestinal wall

The intestinal wall is made up of various layers of tissue. Because the intestine is provided with both longitudinal and circular muscle fibres, it is able to constrict circularly and perform worm-like movements (peristalsis) and thus pass its contents on down the tube. Irritation, inflammation and points of weakness in the wall may interfere with the efficiency of the intestine.

This also would constitute a most serious condition.

BOWELS—cancer: See articles DIGESTION AND DIGESTIVE DISEASES; CANCER.

BOWELS—digestive hormones: See article ENDOCRINOLOGY.

BOWELS—dysentery: See article TRANSMISSIBLE DISEASES.

BOWELS—effect of insecurity and anger: See article STRESS AND DISEASE.

BOWELS—hemorrhages: See article TRANSMISSIBLE DISEASES.

BOWELS—pregnancy care: See BIRTH, article CARE OF MOTHERS BEFORE AND AFTER CHILDBIRTH.

INTESTINES—cancer: See article CANCER.

INTESTINES—colic in infants: See INFANCY, article CARE AND FEEDING OF THE CHILD.

INTESTINES—colitis: See article DIGESTION AND DIGESTIVE DISEASES.

INTESTINES—digestive role: See article DIGESTION AND DIGESTIVE DISEASES; DIET, article ADVICE ON THE DIET.

INTESTINES—dysentery: See article TRANSMISSIBLE DISEASES.

INTESTINES—lavage: See KIDNEY, article THE KIDNEY: ITS DISEASES AND DISTURBANCES.

INTESTINES—lymph nodes: See BLOOD, article THE BLOOD AND ITS DISEASES.

INTESTINES—movement of food: See article DIGESTION AND DIGESTIVE DISEASES.

INTESTINES—obstruction: See article DIGESTION AND DIGESTIVE DISEASES; KIDNEY, article THE KIDNEY: ITS DISEASES AND DISTURBANCES.

INTESTINES—parasites: See article DIGESTION AND DIGESTIVE DISEASES.

INTESTINES—skin affected by: See SKIN, article THE SKIN.

INTESTINES—typhoid: See INFECTIOUS DISEASE, article THE PREVENTION AND TREATMENT OF INFECTIOUS DISEASE.

INTOXICATION, CHRONIC AL-COHOLIC (See also, *Alcohol*) The results of chronic alcoholism are physical deterioration, mental disintegration and ultimately death. The border that separates the social drinker from the chronic alcoholic is not easily defined. Most chronic alcoholics drink to escape mental stresses and unsolved social adjustments. They need the help of psychiatrists—but they need also treatment to overcome the nutritional and other physical disturbances that accompany chronic alcoholism.

Persistent drinkers eventually lose their appetite and have stomach troubles with nausea and vomiting. Ordinary foods do not appeal and everything has to be highly spiced. The alcohol damages the walls of the stomach and bowels and interferes with absorption of vitamins. Beer drinkers may take such large quantities as to distend the stomach and bowel.

The picture of a chronic drinker is generally well known. The abdomen is bloated, the eyes and skin reddened with dilated blood vessels. The nose becomes bulbous and as red as a tomato. The injury to the nervous system produces shaky hands and an indecisive balance and gait. Because of the lack of thiamine inflammations of the nerves occur. The emotions hang on a hair trigger. Rage follows giggling and laughter, remorse succeeds a period of exuberance. Judgment disappears and the alcoholic cannot make up his mind to do even things that are important. Finally deterioration becomes complete and delirium tremens may require hospitalization and emergency care.

Chronic alcoholics are now treated by combined physical and mental treatment. Psychiatrists try to find the underlying stresses. Alcoholics Anonymous uses the values of group action to get alcoholics to help each other. Antabuse is a new drug which makes drinking so unpleasant as to condition the alcoholic against drinking.

IODINE Iodine is a medical substance. Usually iodine is applied to the body in the form of the tincture, which is a mixture of iodine with alcohol. There is also a solution of iodine made up with water. When iodine is extremely concentrated, it may blister the skin. Surgeons use iodine to disinfect the skin. It is also employed in various skin diseases to destroy germs. It can induce an acute inflammation of the skin and thus help to overcome disease. Iodine taken internally has a corrosive effect on the mucous membranes and is, therefore, poisonous if taken in concentrated solutions. An antidote in cases of iodine poisoning is a solution of starch.

IODINE—See SKIN, article THE SKIN.

IODINE—allergy to: See article ALLERGY.

IODINE—antiseptic in first aid: See article FIRST AID.

IODINE—deficiency: See WOMEN, article HYGIENE OF WOMEN; article DEFICIENCY DISEASES.

IODINE—dermatitis caused by: See SKIN, article THE SKIN.

IODINE—erysipelas: See article TRANSMISSIBLE DISEASES.

IODINE—function: See DIET, article ADVICE ON THE DIET.

IODINE—goiter: See WOMEN, article HYGIENE OF WOMEN; article ENDOCRINOLOGY.

IODINE—hyperthyroidism treated by: See SKIN, article THE SKIN.

IODINE—infection prevention: See article OCCUPATION AND HEALTH.

IODINE—medicine chest: See MEDICINE CHEST, article THE FAMILY MEDICINE CHEST.

IODINE—poisoning: See article FIRST AID.

IODINE—pregnancy diet: See BIRTH,

IRON and COPPER

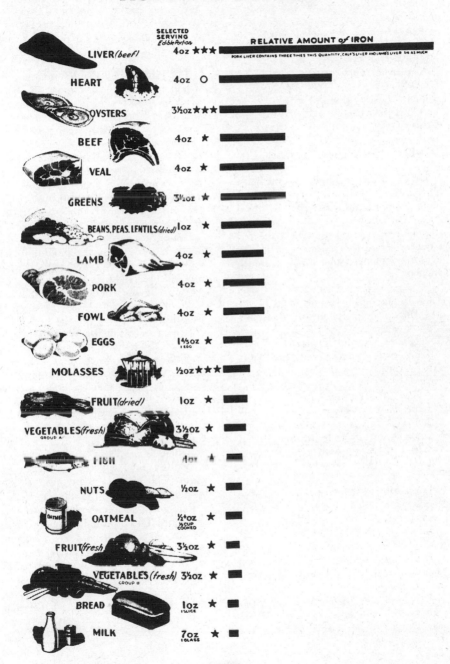

	SELECTED SERVING *Edible Portion*		RELATIVE AMOUNT of IRON
LIVER *(beef)*	4oz	★★★	PORK LIVER CONTAINS THREE TIMES THIS QUANTITY, CALF'S LIVER AND LAMB'S LIVER 3/4 AS MUCH
HEART	4oz	○	
OYSTERS	3½oz	★★★	
BEEF	4oz	★	
VEAL	4oz	★	
GREENS	3½oz	★	
BEANS, PEAS, LENTILS *(dried)*	1oz	★	
LAMB	4oz	★	
PORK	4oz	★	
FOWL	4oz	★	
EGGS	1⅘oz 1 EGG	★	
MOLASSES	½oz	★★★	
FRUIT *(dried)*	1oz	★	
VEGETABLES *(fresh)* GROUP A	3½oz	★	
FISH	4oz	★	
NUTS	½oz	★	
OATMEAL	½+oz ½ CUP COOKED	★	
FRUIT *(fresh)*	3½oz	★	
VEGETABLES *(fresh)* GROUP B	3½oz	★	
BREAD	1oz 1 SLICE	★	
MILK	7oz 1 GLASS	★	

article CARE OF MOTHERS BEFORE AND
AFTER CHILDBIRTH.

IODINE—radioactive: See article ENDO-
CRINOLOGY.

IODINE—stings: See article FIRST AID.

IODINE—tetanus: See article TRANS-
MISSIBLE DISEASES.

IODINE—thyrotoxicosis: See article EN-
DOCRINOLOGY.

IODINE—toxic thyroid: See HEART,
article DISEASES OF THE HEART AND
CIRCULATION.

IRITIS See discussion under *Eye*.

IRON Iron is used in medicine
chiefly for its effect on the formation
of the coloring matter of the red blood
cells. When iron is prescribed properly,
it produces an improvement in the red
blood cells and the red coloring matter
in them. Its chief value is, therefore, in
anemias.

IRON—amount in various foods (fig.):
See DIET, article ADVICE ON THE DIET.

IRON—anemia: See BLOOD, article
THE BLOOD AND ITS DISEASES.

IRON—daily requirement: See DIET,
article ADVICE ON THE DIET.

IRON—deficiency will produce disease:
See article DEFICIENCY DISEASES.

IRON—foods as sources (fig.): See
article DEFICIENCY DISEASES.

IRON—foodstuffs rich in: See BLOOD,
article THE BLOOD AND ITS DISEASES.

IRON—function: See DIET, article AD-
VICE ON THE DIET.

IRON—hemoglobin contains: See
BLOOD, article THE BLOOD AND ITS DIS-
EASES.

IRON—infant's diet: See INFANCY, article CARE AND FEEDING OF THE CHILD.

IRON—measles diet: See CHILDHOOD
DISEASES, article INFECTIOUS DISEASES
OF CHILDHOOD.

IRON—milk diet deficient in: See IN-
FANCY, article CARE AND FEEDING OF
THE CHILD.

IRON—pregnancy requirement: See
BIRTH, article CARE OF MOTHERS BE-
FORE AND AFTER CHILDBIRTH.

IRON—scarlet fever diet: See CHILD-
HOOD DISEASES, article INFECTIOUS DIS-
EASES OF CHILDHOOD.

ITCHING Two hundred years ago
a philosopher defined itching by saying,
"Itching is an unpleasant sensation in
the skin provoking the desire to
scratch." Scientifically itching is a combination of the senses of touch and pain,
since both these sensations must be active or itching will not occur. Incidentally, people can itch while they are
asleep or while they are unconscious, so
that involvement of the brain in this
activity is not absolutely necessary.

Some people itch more easily than
others because their threshold for feeling in the skin is lower than that of
other people. The more you itch, the
more easily you itch. Old people itch
more often and more easily than young
people.

Itching occurs in many different diseases of the skin. It follows sensitivity
to food or drugs when there are eruptions on the skin. Some people itch
particularly after they have had a bath.
Housewives who are sensitive to heat
will develop itching while cooking.
Some parts of the body itch more frequently than others.

Itching is usually associated with infection by fungi of the type of ringworm. The bites of many insects produce itching.

Rarely the whole body will itch at
one time. This is usually due to sensitivity to heat or to cold or to various
chemicals such as may occur in soaps
or bath salts or such as are now used
in the treatment of underclothing.

The sensation of itching is, moreover,
not a single sensation but the blending
of several sensations. In some instances,
for example, the sensation is the same

as that of something crawling on the skin.

Winter itch is about the same in type as bath itch. This is apparently associated with the drying of the skin. It disappears in warm weather because perspiration helps to keep the skin moist and soft.

The control of itching depends on finding the specific cause, as for instance of sensitivity, and removing that cause. If the skin is dry and thin and without moisture, the use of ointments to keep it flexible will be helpful. Solutions containing such substances as menthol and camphor, as well as witch hazel, water, and alcohol, help to control itching. Plain hot water or ice water will relieve the symptoms. Ointments containing tar are frequently prescribed by doctors as especially useful in conditions that itch. The new ointments containing antihistamines are helpful in many cases of itching. There is no routine treatment for pruritus. Itching is no more a single condition than is eczema. Proper diagnosis and treatment related to the cause are the scientific method for control.

Itching has been proved by British scientists to be due to chemical stimuli in the skin. These chemicals are protein destroying enzymes known as mucuain, papain, chymotrypsin. How they produce itching is not established but the evidence shows that the release of these enzymes in the skin, perhaps derived from the cells of the skin, results in the itching symptom.

Itching of the rectal opening and between the buttocks is a symptom frequently reported. In at least 70 per cent of cases, psychogenic factors play a large part. Self-treatment or over-treatment may cause the condition to continue. Several clinics have found that cortisone ointment, which must be prescribed by the physician, is especially helpful.

ITCH—grain: See article OCCUPATION AND HEALTH.

ITCH—jockey: See SKIN, article THE SKIN.

ITCH—mite: See article FIRST AID; SKIN, article THE SKIN.

ITCH—picric: See article OCCUPATION AND HEALTH.

ITCH—prairie: See article OCCUPATION AND HEALTH.

ITCH—threshers': See article OCCUPATION AND HEALTH.

ITCHING—See SKIN, article THE SKIN.

ITCHING—antihistamines relieve: See article ALLERGY.

ITCHING—eczema: See article ALLERGY.

ITCHING—hives: See article ALLERGY; SKIN, article THE SKIN.

ITCHING—jaundice: See article DIGESTION AND DIGESTIVE DISEASES.

ITCHING—leukemia: See BLOOD, article THE BLOOD AND ITS DISEASES.

ITCHING—rectum: See article DIGESTION AND DIGESTIVE DISEASES.

ITCHING—relieving: See MEDICINE CHEST, article THE FAMILY MEDICINE CHEST; INFECTIOUS DISEASE, article THE PREVENTION AND TREATMENT OF INFECTIOUS DISEASE.

ITCHING—scalp: See HAIR, article THE HAIR.

ITCHING—sodium bicarbonate in the bath good for: See MEDICINE CHEST, article THE FAMILY MEDICINE CHEST.

ITCHING—syphilis does not cause: See VENEREAL DISEASES, article THE VENEREAL DISEASES.

ITCHING—uremia: See KIDNEY, article THE KIDNEY: ITS DISEASES AND DISTURBANCES.

ITCH MITE—See article FIRST AID; SKIN, article THE SKIN.

ITCH MITE See discussion under *Insect Pests.*

JAUNDICE Whenever bile circulates in the blood, a condition develops that is called jaundice or icterus. Formerly jaundice was never diagnosed until the skin and the other tissues turned yellow. Nowadays a condition of jaundice is diagnosed by finding excess of bile salts in the blood. After the amount of bile in the blood is reduced to normal, the skin may still remain yellow, requiring some time to return to its natural color.

When red blood corpuscles break down in the blood, that portion which contains iron is used again to produce new red blood cells. The remaining portion is apparently useless in the body and passes through the liver to become a part of the bile.

Whenever the elimination of the bile through the bile ducts is disturbed or whenever the liver fails to carry out its part of the process satisfactorily, jaundice occurs. Sometimes jaundice develops because the destruction of red blood cells is excessive, so that more material is developed than can be eliminated through the liver. If for any reason the liver fails to excrete the bile, it gets into the blood. There are also instances in which the bile ducts are blocked, so that the bile is dammed back. This can be the result of tumors, hardening of the liver, enlarged glands, or similar conditions. Under these circumstances the material excreted through the bowels has a China clay color, is bulky, and has an especially offensive odor. The pale color is due to the absence of the pigment from the bile. The bulkiness and the odor are due to the presence of fats and materials derived from fat which cannot be properly digested because of the absence of the bile acids from the intestines. Under these circumstances the urine becomes dark-colored due to the presence of bile pigments.

There are a number of infectious conditions which so seriously damage the blood as to produce an excessive destruction of blood cells. These include poisonings by various toxic substances including mineral poisons, snake venoms, and the effects of various parasites. Damage to the liver cells may also occur from infectious poisoning with poisons of various kinds including arsenic, phosphorus, and cinchophen. There are also the poisons of eclampsia and similar conditions. There are certain infections with spirochetal organisms which damage the liver and the blood and which are associated with severe jaundice.

The most common type of jaundice is called catarrhal jaundice. This is apparently due to infections by viruses which occur in small epidemics. Such outbreaks are fairly frequent in times of war.

Jaundice is a symptom and not essentially a disease. It is a symptom of damage to the liver in most instances. In order to prevent extension of such damage it is customary for physicians to inject glucose into the body as one of the main portions of the treatment. Because of the damage to the body it is necessary to watch carefully the progress of the condition.

Any patient with severe jaundice should be in bed and all of the necessary tests that can be carried out by the doctor are desirable to determine exactly the nature of the condition and the procedures to be followed in each case.

JAUNDICE—See article DIGESTION AND DIGESTIVE DISEASES.

JAUNDICE—albuminuria may follow: See KIDNEY, article THE KIDNEY: ITS DISEASES AND DISTURBANCES.

JAUNDICE—cancer of bowels: See article DIGESTION AND DIGESTIVE DISEASES.

JAUNDICE—dinitrobenzene may cause: See article OCCUPATION AND HEALTH.

JAUNDICE—familial hemolytic: See BLOOD, article THE BLOOD AND ITS DISEASES.

JAUNDICE—gallstones: See article DIGESTION AND DIGESTIVE DISEASES.

JAUNDICE—hemolytic: See BLOOD, article THE BLOOD AND ITS DISEASES.

JAUNDICE—liver disease: See article DIGESTION AND DIGESTIVE DISEASES.

JAUNDICE—nephrosis: See KIDNEY, article THE KIDNEY: ITS DISEASES AND DISTURBANCES.

JAUNDICE—newborn baby: See INFANCY, article CARE AND FEEDING OF THE CHILD.

JOINT DISTURBANCES (See also *Arthritis, Backache, Gout,* et cetera)

For purposes of action the human body is made with joints which represent the tissues holding together the bones at different points and permitting them to work in relationship to each other. The number of joints in the body is tremendous because there are so many bones. Many people pay little attention to the small joints between the individual fingers and toes or the many bones of the spine, but joint disturbances may affect these joints as well as the very large ones like the knee, the hip, or the shoulder.

A common disturbance of the joints is the accumulation of fluid due to internal irritation. For instance water on the knee is the common name for the flowing of serous fluid into the knee joint following an injury. Sometimes such an accumulation of fluid occurs without any detectable cause. Cases are known in which the knee joint or another joint has filled with fluid which has disappeared within a few days. The scientific name for this condition is intermittent hydrarthrosis, which merely means a collection of fluid in the joint which comes and goes.

People who bleed easily sometimes have sudden pouring of blood into a joint following either an injury or some other disturbance. This condition is called hemarthrosis, which merely means blood in the joint.

Another condition affecting joints that is fairly frequent is the loose body in a joint to which the slang name "joint mouse" is given. Occasionally

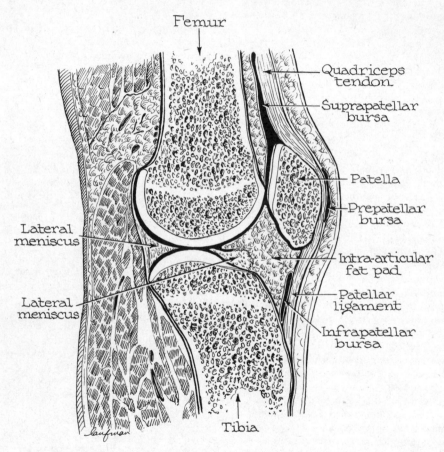

The knee joint is composed of the large bone of the thigh, called the femur, and two smaller bones of the leg, known as the tibia and fibula. The patella is the scientific name for the kneecap.

small pieces of cartilage or bone will break off and get into a joint. Occasionally also such substances as bullets, pieces of glass, or needles will get into a joint, but these are known as foreign bodies and not as loose bodies or "joint mice." The chief disturbance caused by a loose body in a joint is a locking of the joint. The loose substance gets into a place where the bones should come together and acts as a wedge so that they cannot get together. Sometimes pulling the leg will extend it and open the area between the bones so that the joint mouse drops down and out of the way. This will relieve the locking. The joint in which this occurs most often is again the knee joint. Usually one of the semilunar cartilages (which means a half-moon-shaped piece of tissue) will be subjected to an injury by a sudden twist of the leg and a portion of the cartilage will get caught between the bones. This results in locking the knee joint. The injury is seen frequently in football, baseball, basketball, and tennis players. The condition can be relieved by extending the leg and turning it inward. When, however, a locking of the joint occurs so frequently as to interfere with ordinary activities of life, it is customary by surgical operation to remove the torn piece of cartilage and thus to bring about permanent relief.

Another rather common injury to a joint is a pulling away of the ligament which passes from the kneecap to the large bone of the lower leg. When this pulls away, as occurs sometimes when a boy kicks a heavy, wet football, he will be temporarily disabled. The special name of Schlatter's disease has been given to this condition, from the physician who first described it.

Whenever a joint is subjected to severe or sudden strain, the ligaments and the muscles associated with the joint may give way or, as has been mentioned, the cartilage may break or tear loose. Usually muscle tissue will tear first and the ligaments afterward because the ligaments are stronger. The amount of tearing may vary from the splitting of a few fibers to a complete pulling away of the ligament from the bone, sometimes a part of the bone coming with the ligament. This is the condition that occurs particularly around the kneecap and the elbow joints.

The first step to take following any injury to a joint is to make certain that there has been no breaking of bones. An X-ray picture—particularly several pictures taken from different angles—should show whether or not the bone has been broken. Sometimes the X-ray specialist will take an X-ray picture of the joint on the opposite side of the body for comparison with the one that has been injured. If it is found that a bone has not been broken but that the joint has been strained or a ligament torn, it is customary to apply a bandage to make certain that the joint will be protected and properly supported. Sometimes a local anesthetic is injected directly into the joint to relieve pain.

Healing can occasionally be hastened by bathing the affected joint in hot water or by applying heat in some other manner. Occasionally light massage at first and then gradually heavier helps to develop circulation and motion in the joint. As the joint improves, it is moved more definitely.

Sometimes people suffer from what might be called a chronic or frequent spraining of a joint. The accident occurs so frequently and repair takes place so slowly that the joint is constantly in a condition of swelling, inflammation, and irritation. Under such circumstances adhesions and scar tissue may form in the joint. Then it becomes necessary for a specialist in orthopedic surgery to manipulate the joint so as to break up these adhesions and finally to secure healing of the joint with sufficient looseness of movement to enable it to do its work satisfactorily. Adhesions will limit movement and give a feeling of unsteadiness and pain. Many new types of bandages have been developed which are elastic and adhesive and which will aid to hold the tissues in place, at the same time permitting motion of the joint. These have been helpful in treating sprains, strains, and dislocations of joints.

KNEECAP—The kneecap is called by the doctor the patella. If the kneecap breaks following an injury, straightening the leg is difficult. The kneecap will break occasionally from a fall. Many cases have been reported in which the kneecap has been broken following a motorcar accident in which the kneecap has been struck suddenly against the dashboard.

As with other injuries affecting bones and joints, the first step following injury to a kneecap is to have an X-ray picture, so that the doctor will know exactly what the conditions are underneath the skin. If the swelling and pain are not too great, the condition can be determined by feeling with the fingers. However, the X-ray picture taken from several different angles will show exactly how the fragments of the kneecap are distributed. This will guide the surgeon in knowing just what to do.

If the kneecap is broken without wide separation of the parts, the condition is frequently helped by simply holding the leg quiet by a cast or a splint and thus permitting the parts to grow together. If there is a great deal of blood or fluid in the kneecap, the surgeon may wish to withdraw some of the fluid with a sterile needle and syringe.

If the doctor puts on a cast, it may be necessary for the patient to remain in bed for from four to eight weeks, after which the cast is removed. After a cast is removed, it becomes necessary to aid in bending the joint involved. This is helped by the use of hot, wet packs or the application of dry heat two or three times daily and by gradual manipulation or forced movement of the joint.

Sometimes when the fragments of the kneecap are widely separated after a fracture because of the pull of the muscles and the ligaments, a surgical operation is necessary. This is done with an anesthetic. The fragments are drawn together and kept together with stainless steel wire or some similar material which the surgeon may select. At this operation any soft tissues that have been torn are also sewed together by the surgeon. Following such an operation, it is usually necessary to put on a plaster of Paris cast for four or five weeks. When the cast is removed, the patient is permitted to exercise the knee and to bear weight on it with the knee in a straight position. From eight to twelve weeks may be required before the weight can be put on the bent knee. Sometimes six months may have to pass before a knee joint is returned to normal following a severe fracture.

ELBOW (See also discussion under *Elbow*)—The elbow joint moves in two ways: by flexion, in which motion the hand is drawn toward the shoulder, and by extension, in which the hand is drawn away from the shoulder. Two other motions are called pronation and supination. These occur by rotating the elbow joint, moving the palm of the hand toward the body or away from the body.

The elbow joint is often the seat of trouble because it may break following a fall in which the elbow is struck against the ground. It is sometimes injured in throwing a baseball or a football or in playing tennis. Tennis elbow occurs not only as a result of sports which require the use of a racquet such as tennis and squash, it may occur also in golf, baseball, or any occupation which demands lifting and sudden pulling and extending of the elbow joint. These occupations include, for instance, those of the violinist, telephone operators, pressers of clothing, and salesmen who carry heavy sample cases.

In the majority of instances the injury that occurs to the elbow joint is a pulling of the muscles or ligaments with the tearing of some fibers. Occasionally, however, a portion of bone may be broken off from the tip and there is always some pain and swelling. A small sac of fluid that rests over the nodule at the end of the bone may become inflamed. Such sacs of fluid are called bursas. When these sacs become inflamed, the condition is known as bursitis. The pain may be relieved by permitting the excess of fluid to escape. The physician may sometimes press on the point where such a sac of fluid occurs and break it, so that the fluid will escape into the surrounding tissues. Sometimes he will try with a needle and syringe to remove excess fluid. Frequently the application of rest and heat will cause absorption of the fluid. In severe injuries to the elbow it may be necessary to put on a cast and to hold the elbow quiet for a long period of time. Following removal of the cast or sling in which it has been carried, exercise is necessary to restore motion to the injured joint.

JOINTS—aches as result of germ invasion: See INFECTIOUS DISEASE, article THE PREVENTION AND TREATMENT OF INFECTIOUS DISEASE.

JOINTS—allergy sometimes involves: See article ALLERGY.

JOINTS—gout: See article ARTHRITIS, RHEUMATISM, AND GOUT.

JOINTS—pain as symptom of rheumatic fever: See HEART, article DISEASES OF THE HEART AND CIRCULATION.

JOINTS—scarlet fever: See CHILDHOOD DISEASES, article INFECTIOUS DISEASES OF CHILDHOOD.

JOINTS—swelling in arthritis: See article ARTHRITIS, RHEUMATISM, AND GOUT.

JOINTS—tuberculosis: See INFECTIOUS DISEASE, article THE PREVENTION AND TREATMENT OF INFECTIOUS DISEASE.

JOINTS—tuberculosis germ in cattle: See RESPIRATORY DISEASES, article THE RESPIRATORY DISEASES.

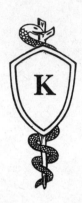

KALA AZAR Along the shores of the Mediterranean, in West Africa, and in southern Russia, also in India, China, and Brazil there appears a tropical disease with fever, progressive anemia, enlargement of the spleen and liver, and filling of the tissues with fluid. This tropical disease is transmitted to human beings by the bite of the sand fly, possibly also by bedbugs and mosquitoes. Some cases have occurred in American soldiers who were stationed in these areas. The condition has also been called Dumdum fever, black fever, and Mediterranean fever.

KELOID Whenever the skin heals with a scar that overgrows considerably, the condition is called keloid. The keloid is actually a fibrous tumor. Usually a keloid develops after a surgical operation but overgrowth of scar tissue has followed even a pinprick, a broken pimple, or a fleabite. Keloids occur to people of all ages but most frequently among young adults.

The exact cause of keloids has never been determined. Some people are particularly liable to develop such growths; others never have them. A morphine addict had over two hundred keloids because he developed an overgrowth of scar tissue every time he punctured himself with a needle. Negroes have keloids apparently more often than people of other races.

Keloids may appear anywhere on the body but are most frequently found on the chest and the neck. When a scar overgrows into a keloid, there is first a rather bandlike mass that rises above the level of the skin. The surface is hard and shiny. The edges at first may be sharp but gradually will extend out into projections into the skin.

Occasionally keloids disappear spontaneously, leaving a depressed scar. However, this is a rare rather than common occurrence.

Usually keloids are quite painless but because of their size or the areas into which they infiltrate, they may become tender or painful. Occasionally people will complain of burning, itching, or pricking sensations. However, there is a tendency, particularly in women, to fix the attention on the scar and to worry about it a great deal, so that the sensations may be exaggerated.

Injection of hyaluronidase directly into keloids and the surrounding area seems to be the first really effective method found for controlling this condition. Attempts have been made to cause the keloids to disappear by electrolysis or by electric injection of drugs into the scar. These methods have also failed to meet with general approval. In some instances very careful plastic surgery, by which the scar is cut away and the tissue sewed together again, has been successful but in most instances surgical treatment is unsuccessful because new keloids form where the skin has been cut and in the stitch tracks.

In old, hard, and stationary keloids which have not changed for a good many years and which fail to respond to treatment with radium or X ray, the surgical removal is sometimes successful. In general physicians today feel that they have discovered the best method of treating keloids by the use of radium or the X ray. Radium is used on small keloids—the amount of the exposure depending on the experience and decision of the specialist in radium treatment. Great care is always taken under such circumstances to protect all of the skin that is normal and to apply the radium or X ray only to the keloid itself. Another technic involves the insertion of radium seeds directly into the keloid.

KELOIDS—See SKIN, article THE SKIN.
KELOIDS—warts treated with nitric acid often result in: See SKIN, article THE SKIN.

KIDNEYS Most of the elimination of substances from the blood that are to go out of the body is accomplished by the two kidneys. They help to keep the material in the blood constant. The kidneys are made of great numbers of little tubes associated with the blood vessels. A complete tubule is about two

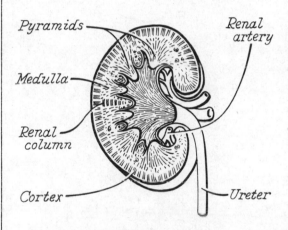

Here is a view of the kidney cut lengthwise to show its structure. An artery enters the kidney and a vein comes out. The ureter carries the urine from the kidney to the urinary bladder. Each kidney is a compact area of collecting tubules and wonderfully small filters. These are found in the cortex of the kidney, from which the fluid passes through tiny tubules to reach the ureter.

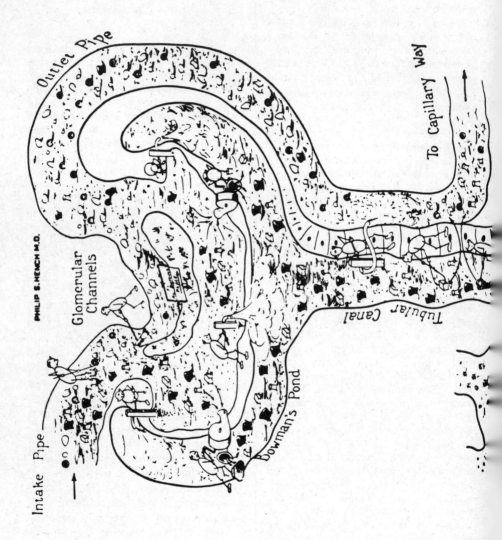

PHILIP S. HENCH M.D.

Outlet Pipe

Intake Pipe

Glomerular Channels

Bowman's Pond

Tubular Canal

To Capillary Way

Cells

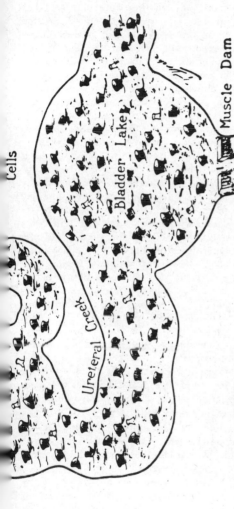

Ureteral Creek

Bladder Lake

Muscle Dam

Urethral River

An animated map showing a little journey through the kidney. Note that the useful substances are reclaimed and return to the general circulation, while waste materials go to the bladder to be expelled through the urethra.

Blood pours through the "intake pipe" (afferent artery) carrying red blood cells ●, white blood cells ○, protein or albumin (egg ◯), sugar ▢ and salt ▨, wastes (urea, uric acid, creatinine, etc.) ▨, and water. Entering the glomeruli all the protein, red and white cells pass on to the "outlet pipe" or efferent artery (with some of the other substances). Large amounts of wastes and water, as well as some useful substances, sugar and salt, escape into "Bowman's Pond" (through Bowman's capsule) and down the "tubular canal."

Through the action of tubular cells useful substances (all of the sugar and most of the water and salt) are normally reclaimed and restored into the outlet pipe to return to general circulation.

Then the urine passes out into "Kidney Bay" (renal pelvis) down "Ureteral Creek" to "Bladder Lake," which collects the final elaboration, a concentrated urine normally containing only wastes, water and excess salts.

1295

inches long. Since each kidney contains about 1,200,000 tubules, the total length of these tubules in an adult man is about seventy-five miles. They are so tiny that they are difficult to see without a microscope. At the end of each of these little tubes is a cup in which the urine to be excreted from the body is collected.

All of the blood in the body passes through the kidneys repeatedly. It has been estimated that more than sixty quarts of blood pass through the kidneys in order to eliminate one and a half quarts of fluid. Fortunately the human being has two kidneys, one of which is sufficient to carry on the work of the body if the other happens to be completely incapacitated.

Various conditions may so damage the kidney that it will not do its work well. An infection of the kidney is called pyelitis. In most instances the germs are brought to the kidneys from other parts of the body and localize there, setting up a secondary infection. When such an infection occurs in the kidneys, the symptoms include fever, nausea, vomiting, occasional pain in the abdomen, and the other changes that are associated with infection anywhere in the body. People with long-standing infections of the kidney show the results by damage to the blood, loss of appetite, headache, loss of weight, and general illness.

Fortunately modern medicine has developed technics for controlling infections in the kidney that are better than previous methods. There are, for instance, the sulfonamide drugs and penicillin, also mandelic acid and furadantin. The drug to be used, however, depends on the nature of the infection, its scope, and the physician who is handling the individual case.

Whenever there is disease of the kidney, determination of the cause is of first importance. The kidneys when damaged may be rested exactly as the heart may be rested when it is damaged. Rest in bed will stop the kidneys from doing much of the work that they generally do. The tissues will form fewer waste products for the kidneys to eliminate. Some of the strain may be taken off the kidney by aiding elimination from the body by the bowels or by perspiration. The diet may be so controlled as to eliminate the substances to be excreted by the kidney.

Some people are born with kidneys of extraordinary shape or size or kidneys that may in some manner have been damaged. Occasionally the two kidneys are joined together, so that they form a horseshoe in shape. This is called horseshoe kidney. Sometimes the tubules are blocked, so that the kidney becomes full of little cavities containing fluid. This is called a cystic kidney. Occasionally people are born with only one kidney. Frequently people with abnormalities of the kidney do not know about them until trouble begins. The doctor can determine the nature of the trouble by injecting into the body fluids which tend to pass through the kidney and which are opaque to the X ray. An X-ray picture taken under these circumstances will show definitely the shape, size, and other structural conditions in the kidney. It is also possible for the doctor to obtain from the bladder specimens of the urine coming from each kidney separately. It is also possible for the doctor to look at the ureters, which are the tubes that carry fluid from the kidneys to the bladder.

KIDNEY STONES—Stones formed in the kidney have now been analyzed by a new method called X ray crystallography. They are found to be mixtures in most instances of various chemical substances chiefly oxalates. Only 6% of 600 stones contained urates. Usually calcium was united with oxalate. This knowledge gave a hint toward prevention of formation of stones. The giving of aspirin or sodium salicylate can do this, by keeping the calcium salts in solution.

NEPHROSIS—The death rate for children with the kidney condition called nephrosis has been reduced from 85 per cent to about 30 per cent by the development of sulfonamides and antibiotic drugs. Formerly most of the fatalities resulted from acute infections rather than failure of the kidneys. Research can now concentrate on the inadequacy of the kidneys. A special foundation has been established to conduct such research.

KIDNEY DISEASE—See KIDNEY, article THE KIDNEY: ITS DISEASES AND DISTURBANCES.

KIDNEY DISEASE—aims of treatment: See KIDNEY, article THE KIDNEY: ITS DISEASES AND DISTURBANCES.

KIDNEY DISEASE—Bright's disease: See entry NEPHRITIS.

KIDNEY DISEASE—causes: See KIDNEY, article THE KIDNEY: ITS DISEASES AND DISTURBANCES.

KIDNEY DISEASE—death rate: See article DIABETES.

KIDNEY DISEASE—diabetes mortality lower: See article DIABETES.

KIDNEY DISEASE—diet: See KIDNEY, article THE KIDNEY: ITS DISEASES AND DISTURBANCES.

KIDNEY DISEASE—eyes may be affected: See EYE, article THE EYE.

KIDNEY DISEASE—forms: See KIDNEY, article THE KIDNEY: ITS DISEASES AND DISTURBANCES.

KIDNEY DISEASE—history before Richard Bright: See KIDNEY, article THE KIDNEY: ITS DISEASES AND DISTURBANCES.

KIDNEY DISEASE — inflammation of colon: See article DIGESTION AND DIGESTIVE DISEASES.

KIDNEY DISEASE — quack remedies: See KIDNEY, article THE KIDNEY: ITS DISEASES AND DISTURBANCES.

KIDNEY DISEASE—symptoms: See KIDNEY, article THE KIDNEY: ITS DISEASES AND DISTURBANCES.

KIDNEY DISEASE—uremia: See KIDNEY, article THE KIDNEY: ITS DISEASES AND DISTURBANCES.

KIDNEYS—See KIDNEY, article THE KIDNEY: ITS DISEASES AND DISTURBANCES.

KIDNEYS—action impeded by germ invasion: See INFECTIOUS DISEASE, article THE PREVENTION AND TREATMENT OF INFECTIOUS DISEASE.

KIDNEYS—amebic dysentery: See article DIGESTION AND DIGESTIVE DISEASES.

KIDNEYS—anatomy: See KIDNEY, article THE KIDNEY: ITS DISEASES AND DISTURBANCES.

KIDNEYS—anemia: See BLOOD, article THE BLOOD AND ITS DISEASES.

KIDNEYS—arteriosclerosis: See article BLOOD PRESSURE.

KIDNEYS—avoided in gout diet: See article ARTHRITIS, RHEUMATISM, AND GOUT.

KIDNEYS—Biblical references: See KIDNEY, article THE KIDNEY: ITS DISEASES AND DISTURBANCES.

KIDNEYS—care during pregnancy: See BIRTH, article CARE OF MOTHERS BEFORE AND AFTER CHILDBIRTH.

KIDNEYS—daily flow of blood: See KIDNEY, article THE KIDNEY: ITS DISEASES AND DISTURBANCES.

KIDNEYS—derivation of word: See KIDNEY, article THE KIDNEY: ITS DISEASES AND DISTURBANCES.

KIDNEYS—effect of overactive parathyroids: See article ENDOCRINOLOGY.

KIDNEYS—enlarged: See KIDNEY, article THE KIDNEY: ITS DISEASES AND DISTURBANCES.

KIDNEYS—examination by modern methods: See KIDNEY, article THE KIDNEY: ITS DISEASES AND DISTURBANCES.

KIDNEYS—functions: See KIDNEY, article THE KIDNEY: ITS DISEASES AND DISTURBANCES.

KIDNEYS—inflammation: See HEART, article DISEASES OF THE HEART AND CIRCULATION. See also entry NEPHRITIS.

KIDNEYS—journey through (fig.): See KIDNEY, article THE KIDNEY: ITS DISEASES AND DISTURBANCES.

KIDNEYS—palpable: See KIDNEY, article THE KIDNEY: ITS DISEASES AND DISTURBANCES.

KIDNEYS—physiology: See KIDNEY, article THE KIDNEY: ITS DISEASES AND DISTURBANCES.

KIDNEYS—polycystic: See KIDNEY, article THE KIDNEY: ITS DISEASES AND DISTURBANCES.

KIDNEYS—scarlet fever: See CHILDHOOD DISEASES, article INFECTIOUS DISEASES OF CHILDHOOD.

KIDNEYS—size: See KIDNEY, article THE KIDNEY: ITS DISEASES AND DISTURBANCES.

KIDNEYS—stones: See article DIGESTION AND DIGESTIVE DISEASES; KIDNEY, article THE KIDNEY: ITS DISEASES AND DISTURBANCES; article DEFICIENCY DISEASES.

KIDNEYS—tuberculosis: See KIDNEY, article THE KIDNEY: ITS DISEASES AND DISTURBANCES.

KIDNEYS—ulcerated: See KIDNEY, article THE KIDNEY: ITS DISEASES AND DISTURBANCES.

The Kidney: Its Diseases and Disturbances

BY

HOWARD M. ODEL, M.D.

Assistant Professor of Medicine, Mayo Foundation. Consultant in Medicine, Mayo Clinic, Rochester, Minnesota.

To THE KITCHEN of a great hotel are brought quantities of food, wholesome and pure, catering to each need and taste. In the preparation and consumption of this food, waste accumulates; useless material in which food has been packed, unused and unusable parts of food itself. Avenues are provided for ready elimination of this waste; boxes and wrappings disappear in fire and in chimney fumes; liquids flow into cisterns; garbage is carted off in wagons of the "reduction company." So too in the organization of human bodies, there are veritable reduction companies.

In the human economy, as has been noted in previous chapters, food is the source of all tissue growth and energy. Yet for all modern laws there is no such thing as "pure food"—at least, in the sense that for the human body there exists no food wholly valuable and completely utilizable. Even from that "perfect product," mother's milk, are formed wastes to be discarded. Men foretell, perhaps not too seriously, the day when a hearty meal will consist, alas, of six courses—each a scientifically compounded pill. Even were the prophecy to come true, waste products would develop from the ordinary wear and tear on tissues. The twitch of the tiniest muscle, the lightning wink of an eyelid, the swift flight of a half-formed thought: each is accompanied by, indeed is the result of, the combustion or reduction of some body substance. In the utilization of food and from the growth and repair of body tissues, end products are formed. Carbon dioxide escapes in the flue of the lungs; food residue is discarded by the bowels; water steams out in the breath, escapes in sweat, and is lost in urine. Daily, about 2 quarts of water are eliminated by the lungs, 1 to 1½ pints in the sweat, and about 1½ to 2 quarts in the urine.

ANATOMY AND FUNCTIONS OF THE KIDNEY

The kidneys, forming urine, are one of the chief organs of elimination. Their function is to keep the body free of an excess of substances derived particularly from protein, albuminous or nitrogenous matter—found, for example, in meats, milk, eggs, and body muscle. When such fuel is consumed by the human engine, the ash or residue consists of certain matters that cannot be eliminated readily or in quantity by means other than in urine. Those about which most is known are urea, uric acid, creatinine, sulfate, and phosphate. Since these substances are not only useless, but also potentially toxic, they must be got rid of; otherwise they would accumulate in the body and be injurious to health and life.

So vital is the need for proper elimination that nature has included the kidneys among those organs of which not one but two seem necessary to provide a safe margin of reserve. Man can live, at least for the time being, even after all of one kidney and about half of the other have been removed or destroyed. Yet nature was not unduly profligate in providing this reserve, for the kidneys are unfortunately called on to excrete not only the natural waste of wholesome foods, but from time to time must hastily and efficiently help rid the body of end products of bad food, germs and their harmful toxins, diseased and dead tissue cells, and chemical poisons.

Every such experience provides a hazard for the kidneys, and little by little tends to lower their reserve. Some insults are borne by them silently and uncomplainingly, without signs or symptoms. To some injurious experiences they temporarily succumb, soon to regain apparently full capabilities. From others they may acquire permanent damage. When the burden is temporarily or permanently too great for the kidneys, when the "threshold of their reserve" is exceeded, when their function is appreciably deranged, a train of events occurs, the symptoms and signs of which indicate what is called "nephritis." Considering the great variations in type and degree of such insults met in the course of a lifetime, different types and degrees of nephritis result. Some forms of nephritis may be the expression of an essentially minor and transient difficulty, a condition about which concern need not be felt, readily amenable to treatment and leaving the afflicted person the happy subject of an early cure. Other forms, however, may signify a grave diseased state fraught with great danger, which may destine its victim to an early fatal outcome.

The term "nephritis" means simply inflammation of the kidneys. While modern medicine recognizes many different diseases of the kidney, each essentially a type of nephritis, the term represents to many people one condition and is synonymous with "Bright's disease." Because the first reports of nephritis, made by Richard Bright, an English physician, in 1827, dealt with one of its most serious forms, to some persons nephritis and Bright's disease remain designations with an evil portent, omens of death. Happily this unfortunate point of view is being abandoned, and modern dictionaries define Bright's disease as "a term of very indefinite limitations, meaning, in general, acute or chronic nephritis," or as "any one of a group of kidney diseases attended by albuminuria" (albumin in urine). Fortunately, modern science has provided ways of differentiating among types of kidney disease and of telling whether a given type is serious or not.

ANATOMY OF THE KIDNEY

The average man has eaten beef or lamb kidneys occasionally, but that is about all he knows of kidneys. The kidneys are so placed that they are amply guarded from injury even during such strenuous exercise as the straining and twisting of an athlete at the hurdles or high jump. Situated in the lumbar region, or small of the back, at about the level of the eleventh rib, they are protected by thick spinal muscles behind them and by the peritoneal cavity in front. Thus they are not in the abdomen but behind it. They are further surrounded by a tough fibrous coat or capsule, around which is packed a considerable amount of fat.[1] The right kidney is usually about a half inch lower than the left, probably because the liver is above it, and is a little lower in children and women than in men; it is often easily felt on examination. Such a "palpable kidney," if smooth and not enlarged or tender on pressure, is perfectly normal.

Each adult kidney is about 4½ inches long, from 2 to 2½ inches wide, about 1¼ inches thick, and each weighs on an average ⅓ of a pound.

---

[1] Placed just above each kidney is the adrenal or suprarenal gland, small organs whose physiologic action is different from that of the kidneys but which sometimes become diseased by extensive inflammations around the kidneys.

In shape it resembles a large kidney bean, being rounded and curved, with a concave area in the middle of the inner border known as the hilus, where the renal[2] artery, vein, and nerves enter the substance of the kidney, and from which arise the ureters, the tubes that carry urine from the kidneys to the urinary bladder.

On slicing the kidney and laying it open, one can see three main areas. The outer zone, the cortex, contains the pinpoint kidney filters, the glomeruli or "little balls." The middle zone, or medulla, is marked by innumerable stripings consisting of microscopic tubules that converge into a number of pyramidal areas. These are connected by many fingerlike projections to a fairly large, smooth-lined, saclike, collecting chamber called the "pelvis." From this pelvis the ureters arise at the hilus. The ureters are hollow tubes about 1/5 of an inch wide, the channel within being only ⅛ of an inch in width. They travel 10 to 12 inches down along the spinal column to the bladder.

Thus each kidney is a tremendously compact area of collecting tubules and of wonderfully small filters, each placed in its minute filter chamber. The filter chambers and tubules are the fundamental anatomic units of the kidney.

Each of these units — or nephrons — begins as a little cuplike chamber, 1/200 of an inch in diameter, comprising the filtration chamber, or Bowman's glomerular capsule, into which are inserted the filters themselves, which are masses of tiny blood vessels (capillaries), the glomeruli. The walls of the cuplike Bowman's capsule are double, with a narrow space between, since the structure is like a round ball pushed in from one side. These small filter chambers are confined entirely to the cortical substance, and from them arise small tubules, which begin meandering courses to end, many of them together, in large collecting tubules that lead to the kidney pelvis. Just after the tubule leaves the filter chamber, it enters a series of convolutions in the cortex ("proximal or first convoluted tubule") and then dips down into the medullary substance as a thin descending limb 1/1200 of an inch thick, which turns as Henle's loop to ascend again into the cortex where, somewhat thicker (1/600 of an inch), it becomes even more convoluted ("distal or second convoluted tubule") before it finally straightens out to join with myriads of others into the collecting tubules, which empty into the kidney pelvis. Despite all this wandering, the tubule has traversed a distance of only about 1½ inches. The purpose of this extreme migration is to permit it to come in contact, in a minute space, with an extensive meshwork of fine blood vessels. It has been estimated by some that there are about 1,000,000 to 1,500,000 of these

---

[2] "Renal" means "pertaining to the kidney." For its derivation see comment on page 1307.

tiny units or nephrons in each kidney. In the adult, therefore, the total length of these tubules in each kidney would be from 1,500,000 to 3,000,000 inches, or the equivalent of a channel about 50 to 100 miles long in both kidneys, compressed into a space of only about 20 cubic inches in volume!

STRUCTURE AND CONTENTS OF FILTER CHAMBER

From the great blood vessel of the abdomen, the aorta, a short, thick, renal artery passes to each kidney, entering at the hilus and carrying a large amount of blood under great pressure. At the hilus this artery divides into several branches, which pass to the junction between the cortex and medulla where each again divides, at length forming a small but stout little vessel, the afferent vessel or arteriole, or intake pipe. This enters the capillary tuft in Bowman's capsule. As it plunges into the cuplike depression constituting the filter chamber, it breaks up into two, then four, and finally into about fifty curling, twisting capillary loops, each about 1/2500 of an inch in diameter, which coil and twine in interlacing fashion and then reunite to pass out of the chamber as the outlet pipe or afferent vessel or arteriole. The latter soon breaks up into fine intertubular capillaries that surround the meandering tubules mentioned above, finally reuniting to leave the kidney as the great renal vein.

The tortuous capillary loops within the filter chambers constitute the glomeruli, or filters, and each glomerulus with its little cuplike room forms a marvelous little filtration plant, the basic unit of the kidneys' excretory system. The reason for such an arrangement of glomerular loops can be understood by visualizing the structure of an ordinary room radiator. The steam enters the room through a single pipe, which breaks up in the radiator into a large number of coils before leaving the room again as a single pipe. The many coils increase by so much the radiating surface of the apparatus. Although the glomerular loops are only 1/2500 of an inch wide, their length totals about 1 inch in each glomerulus. If there are about 1,000,000 glomeruli in each kidney, the surface area of its glomerular capillaries is about 0.78 of a square meter for one kidney, or for both kidneys about 1.56 square meters (15 square feet), the approximate area of the top of a dining-room table.

FUNCTIONS OF THE KIDNEY

In simple terms the function of the kidney is to make urine and get rid of it. The first clue to an understanding of its function is obtained by analysis of what substances are found to be continuously present in normal urine, for such substances obviously are not wanted by the body. The urine contains large amounts of water and urea, smaller amounts of sodium chloride (common table salt), potassium, phosphates and sulfates, creatinine and uric acid, and minimal amounts of several other substances. Some are excreted because they are always and entirely useless; others are got rid of because, while they are ordinarily useful, the body already has enough of them to supply its needs. The functions of the normal kidney are further demonstrated by observing what happens when they go wrong, noting what substances accumulate in the blood and tissues and what deficiencies appear in the urine.

As a result of such analyses, the known functions of the kidney can be summarized as follows:

1. It is the avenue of elimination for 40 to 60 per cent of all water liberated from the body. An excess of this vital substance is always present in healthy bodies, derived from food and drink and from cellular activity.

2. It excretes the waste products of protein breakdown: urea, uric acid, and creatinine.

3. It helps to preserve the normal acid-alkaline balance of tissues by excreting excess acids. The system is never "acid," and by "acidosis" is really meant a reduction in the reserve of alkali. All tissues and fluids of the body except the stomach juices and at times the sweat are faintly alkaline. Although large amounts of acids are eaten in food and more is constantly produced by our normal body processes, the reaction (alkalinity) of tissues remains practically constant. The maintenance of an alkaline reserve is of supreme importance, and the extreme delicacy of this balance is appreciated by realizing that death would occur were the reaction of blood to be altered by the minute change equivalent to that caused by adding one drop of even a weak acid to a quart of water. Blood becoming as acid as distilled water or as alkaline as ordinary tap water would be incompatible with life (Marriott).

4. It helps to maintain that normal physiochemical state of body fluids responsible for osmotic pressure by eliminating just the proper amounts of salt and water. When this balance is disturbed one of two things results: waterlogging of tissues (dropsy, hydrops, edema, ascites, anasarca)[3] or the opposite, a condition of body dehydration,[4] desiccation, or water famine.

5. It has been discovered that the kidneys apparently manufacture small amounts of certain substances found in urine: hippuric acid and perhaps ammonia. All other recognized urinary constituents are brought to the kid-

---

[3]Dropsy means "hydrops" or "water." Edema means "swelling." Ascites ("bag") means "dropsy of the abdominal cavity." Anasarca ("throughout flesh") signifies "general dropsy."

[4]Dehydrate means "to deprive of or to lose water."

ney already manufactured, and the kidney merely excretes them unchanged. Since the synthesis of hippuric acid and possibly ammonia are but steps in the excretion of unwanted substances, it can still be concluded that the known functions of the kidney are chiefly if not entirely excretory.

PHYSIOLOGY OF THE KIDNEY: HOW IT CARRIES ON ITS FUNCTIONS

The striking anatomic arrangement of glomerulus and tubule led early physicians to regard the kidney units as filters and to believe that urinary components passed through glomeruli into tubules by a sort of suction, or a simple process of filtration (resulting from a higher pressure in the glomerular capillaries). Later, others insisted that the cells, or microscopic units of which living matter is constructed, played more than a passive role in formation of urine and that they had an important part in its manufacture, actually pouring out or "secreting" substances into the tubules. Thus a great dispute arose between the "mechanists" and the "vitalists." While the details of this argument need not be considered, a brief statement of the modern view of kidney physiology will aid in gaining knowledge of some of the different symptoms and signs of kidney disease and the rationale of treatment.

It has been estimated that more than 600 quarts (about 20,000 ounces) of blood (some say 1,000 to 1,500 quarts) flow through the kidneys every day, passing through glomeruli at the greatly reduced speed of about 18 inches per hour (Vimtrup). About 90 per cent of it continues on into the efferent arteries and finally back into the main blood stream, but fluid amounting to about 10 per cent of this volume is taken out in the glomeruli and starts flowing down the tubules. The fluid taken out amounts daily to more than 60 quarts (cited by Harvey); others say 170 to 290 quarts (Rehberg, cited by Wilbur; Richards). Were all of it allowed to continue on down the tubules and be lost in urine, there would be an enormous waste of water causing almost constant urination and producing a tremendous thirst to replenish body fluids. In addition to water, this glomerular filtrate includes not only wastes (urea, uric acid, creatinine, and so forth) but also large amounts of useful substances (sugar, salt, and amino acids), foods that the body cannot afford to lose. The tubules, therefore, prevent this waste by reabsorbing through the cells, of which the walls of the tubules are built, all of the sugar and amino acids and almost all of the water and chlorides, at the same time refusing to take back any of the unwanted substances. As a result of this vigorous reabsorption of water (97 per cent or more), the total amount of fluid that finally reaches the bladder to be excreted as urine is only about 1½ quarts a day (instead of 60 or more quarts), in which there is a high concentration of waste products. The latter are not equally concentrated; for example, the amount of urea in a quart of urine is 60 to 100 times that in a quart of blood, but the amount of uric acid is only about 30 times that of blood.

Modern studies indicate, then, that substances pass out of the blood going from glomeruli into tubules in one direction only. Lower down in the tubules some useful materials are restored to the blood by passing through the cells lining the tubules. That the passage of materials through the cells lining the tubules may not be just in one direction, as formerly supposed, is suggested by recent evidence indicating that certain tubular cells may actually take out further waste material from the blood capillaries surrounding the tubules and pour it into the tubules. Thus this waste passes through the walls of the tubules in the opposite direction from the useful substances that are reclaimed by them. By this means, the kidneys are given a second chance to throw off wastes by means of tubular secretion supplementing glomerular filtration.

The co-ordinated activity of the myriad cells in each kidney unit is remindful of a scene in an automobile assembling plant where down along the long runways are placed hundreds of men. Here one is adding a part, there another removing some appliance, until at the end of the runway there rolls off a completed car. As automobiles are thus born at so many an hour, so drops of urine roll out into the bladder at the rate of about four a minute, night and day.

In summary: Both glomerular and tubular cells apparently exhibit definite discrimination in determining just what and how much shall be filtered out of the blood, reabsorbed in the tubules, and eliminated in the urine. By a process of filtration, the glomeruli excrete a filtrate containing substances (except for proteins and cellular elements) in about the same concentration as they exist in the blood, and through the selective reabsorption of useful substances and possibly also some secretion by tubular cells this fluid is further elaborated into the final product, urine.

To demonstrate this graphically, with due apologies for the omission of finer details and at the risk of being taken too literally, I have included a diagram devised in the spirit of modern animated maps by Dr. Philip S. Hench, showing the main essentials of renal physiology.

HISTORY OF KIDNEY DISEASE BEFORE THE TIME OF RICHARD BRIGHT

Almost all information about the kidney and its diseases has been attained in the last century. The term "Bright's disease" is about 125 years old, and previously little indeed was known of the diseases of the kidney. Before that it was not even known that albumin in the urine bore any special relation to nephritis. At the time of the American Revolution, doctors recognized in general only two kinds of kidney disease; namely, stones (*nephritis calculosa*) and suppurative or purulent nephritis (so-called ulcerated or pus kidney). This much had been known two thousand years before, in the time of Hippocrates, the Father of Medicine, when four diseases of the kidney were described, among them calculus (stone) and abscess.

The development of knowledge of the kidney and its diseases and especially of urine, an analysis of which constitutes modern man's commonest medical experience, is an interesting story. Philologists say that the word "kidney" may have been derived from words meaning womb or egg. Its Latin ancestor *ren* (renal and so forth) is thought to have referred to the midriff, the parts about the heart and liver.[5] Hippocrates (460–370 B.C.) believed the kidneys separated out urine, but Aristotle (384–322 B.C.), who was one of the greatest scientists and philosophers of all time and who carried on extensive anatomic investigations, thought the bladder was the chief site of urinary formation. He believed that the kidneys were not essential to life, but "when they are present exist not of actual necessity but as matter of greater finish and perfection." Galen (A.D. 131–201) had no patience with such "nonsense" and considered that the blood serum percolated through the kidneys. A thousand years after Aristotle, errors still persisted in some quarters, and urine was considered by Protospartharius (A.D. 603–641) as a filtrate of the portal vein of the liver.

Long before this, although the ancients knew little or nothing about the kidneys or the source and purpose of urine, much was written about urine itself. Records indicate that Babylonian physicians at the dawn of earliest civilization (around 4000 B.C.) examined it sufficiently to note changes in color, "worms of urine" (casts) and "knots of thread" (albumin). In old Sanskrit writings twenty different diseases were described, each with its characteristic urine, among them "honey urine." Ten of these diseases were said to be due to deranged phlegm, six to deranged bile, and the remaining four to wind. The diagnoses of diseases, as well as prophecies as to their outcome, were made by those ancient worthies from examination of the skin, eyes, and tongue, but "especially the pulse and urine without which all knowledge of physick is obscure, doubtful and uncertain." From observations made on the urine of patients with fever, Hippocrates wrote: "One may judge what is to take place, for

[5]The Bible contains many references to "reins" and kidneys, using the terms literally and figuratively. In a literal sense it refers only to the kidneys of animals offered in sacrifice. By law the kidneys and their fatty covering were Jehovah's special share of sacrificial victims. Their peculiar sanctity arose from the belief that, next to the blood, the kidneys were the seat of life and should therefore be returned to the Author of Life. A natural extension of this idea led to their being considered the "seats of passion," the organs of feeling, or man's conscience. It is used in this latter sense in Psalms 26:2— "Examine me, O Lord, try my reins and my heart"—and not as an appeal for a kidney function test as a recent writer implied when he wrote, "Even the Bible mentions as important 'to test a man's heart and kidneys.'"

if the urine be thick and more yellowish so much the better, but if it be thinner and blacker so much the worse. . . . When in fever the urine is turbid, there either is or will be headache." And again: "The most deadly of all kinds of urine are the fetid, watery, black and thick. . . . If the urine is passed in deficient quantity, with a noise, it indicates either that the man stands in need of purging or that the bladder is diseased."

Urine was held by some to have curative properties, an idea repulsive to others. "It is said that some who have drunk it in the plague have recovered." It was also drunk as a cure for leprosy, putrid ulcers, sprains of the feet, used as antidote for snake bite and deadly poisons and as an application for ery-sipelas! "The urine of mules suits with arthritic remedies, that of goats and camels is laxative of the belly and hence is given in dropsical complaints."

Through the succeeding centuries, uroscopy, the art of inspection of urine, gradually became the greater part of medical practice. Many recall the numerous drawings in European art galleries[6] that depict the physician of the thirteenth to the sixteenth centuries practicing this art, a subject particularly fascinating to Dutch painters. The urine was always contained in a characteristic flask, of transparent "clere glasse," not flat on the bottom, "but the shape of a very bladder (for the urinall should represent the bladder of a man) and so shall every thyng be sene in his dew place and colore." The container being shaped thus, "the urine should be in natural position as in the bladder." With the spherical base the container could not stand alone, and it was therefore always carried to the physician in a basket of cylindrical shape. The gravefaced physician, dressed in doctor's robe and cap, is always represented as inspecting the urine in a most judicial way, sometimes holding the flask in his hand, at other times examining it while it was held in the hand of a patient or servant, as by some a physician was considered too sacred to hold a bottle of urine himself. Near by, the patient silently awaits the verdict, his attentive expression portraying his pathetic anxiety.

A proper light was most necessary, and the urine was held in such a way that no reflection or refraction from the sun's rays would "make the colour more remisse" and thus interfere with a true observation. As many as twenty different colors were described, each of significance. In addition to the color, the urine was studied as to consistency, transparency, quantity, sediment, odor, froth, scum floating at the top, and substances in the watery part. Grave pronouncements followed such inspection. Cloudy urine at the top of the bottle signified disease of the highest parts of the man's body, alterations in the middle part of the urine related to diseases of the spleen, liver, heart, lungs,

[6] I am informed that there are no such originals in the art museums of the United States.

bowels, and stomach, and the urinary sediment showed the condition of the lowest parts of the body. Bubbles and frothing indicated evil digestion.

"In an epoch when all clinical methods and investigation were unknown," as Wellcome has aptly put it, "it is natural that the urine should be expected to indicate the disease and its nature, and so as time went on it is not surprising to find that inspection of the urine gradually became more popular in medical diagnosis, as doubtless it appealed, from the spectacular point of view, as strongly to the patient as to the physician." But as imagination increased, uroscopy became uromancy and quacks flourished everywhere, traveling the land with their flasks, preying on the gullibility of the people, diagnosing all kinds of diseases and prognosticating all manner of events, from the diagnosis of chastity or pregnancy to the sex of an unborn child.

Naturally a reaction was aroused from time to time against such charlatanism, and frequent tirades were made against the "tricks of the water-doctors" who might go to such limits as did "the physician who saw an oat-grain in a urinal and stated the patient had eaten a horse."

Particularly blameworthy were the attempts of physicians to diagnose the ills of an unseen patient from the analysis of urine sent from a distance. This practice in sixteenth-century England caused the passage of statutes forbidding apothecaries from sending such specimens to physicians, and physicians from pronouncing on any disorder from such an uncertain procedure.

Up to this time, the examination of urine was almost entirely by inspection, not analysis. Discoveries in the seventeenth and eighteenth centuries saved it from ill repute and opened the era beginning with Van Helmont's (1577–1644) studies on the variable weight of urine and ending in the epochal work of Bright (1827), which ushered in the modern period in the study of renal disease. Among these were the demonstration of albumin in urine in the presence of acetic acid (Dekkers, 1694), after boiling (Cotugno, 1764), and in dropsical urine in the presence of nitric acid (Cruickshank, 1798); the determination of its water and solid content (Bellini, 1643–1704), its specific gravity (Booerhaave, 1668–1738), and some of its chemical constituents, such as urea (Booerhaave, 1720; Rouelle, 1771), sugar in diabetic urine (Dobson, 1772), and many others.

THE WORK OF RICHARD BRIGHT

Surpassing all these in importance, as previously stated, was the contribution in 1827 of Richard Bright, distinguished English physician of Guy's Hospital, London, whose name will always be associated with kidney disease. The rare and great honor paid by physicians to colleagues who have made outstanding contributions in certain diseases is to designate that disease by the physician's name. Of the thousands of known diseases, less than five hundred are called in modern medical literature after physicians' names. Of all these conditions the layman, happily unacquainted with disease, is familiar probably with the name of hardly a single one save "Bright's disease." (Saints have fared less well, being honored thus only about twenty-five times.)

In retrospect, Bright's contribution seems a simple one, the demonstration that albumin in urine indicated kidney disease. Its importance rested in making with gratifying precision and clarity the differentiation among several diseased states about which there was great confusion.

In Bright's time, the significance of dropsy and of albuminuria was unknown. Dropsy, an accumulation of fluid in the tissues (extremities, abdomen, or lungs), was thought by some to be a disease in itself; by others, it was considered the result of a variety of diseases, among them disease of the liver, ovaries, lungs or heart, or from certain obstructions to circulatory flow. Albumin had recently been found in the urine in dropsical patients (Cotugno, 1764; Cruickshank, 1798; Wells, 1811; Blackall, 1813), but neither dropsy nor albumin was at that time considered significantly related to kidney disease, which was then thought to consist mostly of stones or the inflammation resulting therefrom. This may seem strange when as early as the sixth century a Roman emperor's physician (Aetius) noted the association of dropsy and hardened kidneys. Four centuries later, Avicenna, the doctor of a Mohammedan caliph, commented on the excessive, thin, watery urine in dropsy, and in 1476, Saliceto, an Italian doctor, wrote on the association of scanty urine, hardened kidneys, and dropsy. But this had apparently been long forgotten. Bright first connected these conditions clearly, albuminuria and dropsy, with kidney disease. He showed indisputably that albuminous urine was present in twenty-four cases of dropsy accompanied by kidney disease, but absent in eleven cases of dropsy associated with liver disease and in four cases of dropsy caused by heart disease. Thus he demonstrated that there were different kinds of dropsy, that albuminuria was a sign of nephritis, and that the dropsy resulting therefrom could be recognized by finding albuminous matter in urine.

Although he mentioned several varieties of nephritis of differing severity, Bright spoke of "this most fatal disease"—fatal enough to bring seventeen of the twenty-four patients to the post-mortem table. While he felt that "where the mischief is less rooted we may undoubtedly do much," he admitted that "some cases defy cure." Thus, by the very strength of his observations, both at the bedside and post-mortem, so important to prove the significance of his discoveries, he unwittingly fostered the notion that this new type of nephritis was a hopeless condition. Then began the era when albuminuria doomed many comparatively healthy persons to fear of an early death. So indiscriminately were dire predictions made on the presence of albumin alone that Bright wrote other papers mainly for the purpose of correcting this misconception. He tried to modify the general pessimistic view by stating that "the disease on which the secretion of albuminous urine depends is in the commencement functional, that as long as it continues in this state it is capable of cure or of relief by various means."

His chemist colleagues, Bostock, Barlow, and Rees, further softened the sting of albuminuria by their careful analyses, demanding that laboratory data necessary for a diagnosis of Bright's disease include other tests on urine, such as the nitric acid ring test, in addition to the heat test. While confirming its general importance as pointed out by Bright, they noted cases in which albuminuria was "so trifling in nature as to render it almost a constant occurrence."

MODERN SIGNIFICANCE OF ALBUMINURIA

The development of modern tests of kidney function has extended knowledge of the diseases and disturbances of kidneys so that the finding of albumin in the urine is no longer interpreted as the equivalent of Bright's disease. It is merely a signpost pointing to any one of several different conditions. It constitutes the most readily detected aberration of normal renal function. While it is thus usually the earliest sign of renal disturbance, functional or organic, it may occur in persons who in other respects are apparently entirely normal, or it may be initiated by any one of many conditions that can disturb kidney function, disturbances which are frequently not great enough to warrant the term "nephritis." However, when albumin does appear, it generally indicates a kidney whose function is embarrassed due to some change, slight or great, temporary or permanent, in its cells.

Albumin is a simple protein found in nearly all animal and many vegetable tissues. It is soluble in water and coagulates as egg white (albumin) does on heating. It is formed by the dissolution of dead tissue cells, either of food or from the body, including red and white blood cells. Digested foods form proteins, which are absorbed and circulate in blood to be used in human growth. About two thirds of this blood protein is in the form of albumin. As already noted, healthy kidneys do not allow this useful substance, food albumin, to pass out from the circulation into the kidney tubes and be lost in urine. Hence, the liquid that passes through the small filters of the kidney is normally free of protein or albumin.

There are two additional sources from which albumin may arise to appear in the urine. When tissue cells of the body die, instead of becoming food protein, they occur in the blood as waste protein. Other forms of waste or foreign protein may arise from impure foods or injected proteins. The kidney filters do not try to keep them back, but allow them to pass into the urine as waste in the form of albumin to be excreted. Albumin in urine must come, therefore, either from food or waste proteins in the blood passing through the kidneys or from the breaking down of cells in the kidney itself or along the urinary passages. The loss of food proteins is accidental, that of waste proteins is purposeful.

Because urine from healthy persons is practically free of protein, albuminuria should always be considered an abnormality, even though its significance is exceedingly variable. Found in the course of an examination for life insurance, it serves as the starting point for other than a routine examination.

INCIDENCE

The incidence of albuminuria in a large group of healthy people is approximately 5 per cent. Certain tests demonstrate albumin more readily than others. Various workers using the nitric acid test found an incidence of albuminuria on a single test ranging from 3 to 16 per cent, with 5 to 7 per cent most commonly reported. Albuminuria was noted in about 5 per cent of 60,000 healthy soldiers (MacLean) and in a similar proportion of 5,000 healthy students (Lee). In another series of 20,000 young men (Diehl-McKinlay), 5.3 per cent showed albuminuria on the first examination. In 66 per cent of these the albuminuria was transient, discovered only once; it was occasionally present in 13 per cent, and persistent in 12 per cent, without any other evidence indicating kidney damage. In only 6.5 per cent of those with albuminuria were there other signs indicating probable renal disease. About 3 per cent of 100,924 male life insurance policyholders showed definite albumin in the urine, while slight traces were found in about 19 per cent more (Sydenstricker and Britten). Sudden increases in its incidence may be noted, as in the "epidemics" of albuminuria seen in healthy West Point cadets (Ashburn).

It is found much more frequently in those who are sick or who consider themselves sick and consult physicians. At a large clinic, albumin was detected in the first specimen in 39 per cent of 663 patients seen consecutively (Sanford, Conner, Magath, and Heck). When three different methods were used, albumin was indicated by one or more tests in more than half (59 per cent) of those studied. Further investigations, however, revealed definite kidney disease in less than half (40 per cent) of the 39 per cent in whose urine albumin was found.

Albuminuria bears a definite relationship to age (Calvin, Isaacs and Meyer, Sydenstricker and Britten). Its incidence increases from childhood up to sixteen years of age. From this peak, there is a rapid decline to between thirty and forty years of age, after which a progressive increase again occurs up to seventy years and more.

TYPES OF ALBUMINURIA

When albumin leaks into urine through or from the kidneys, the condition is "renal albuminuria"; when albumin is added to urine in the lower part of the urinary passages below the kidneys, the condition is called "nonrenal" or "postrenal" albuminuria.

Renal albuminuria may be caused by imperfect working of normal kidneys or by actual disease of the kidneys. It occurs (1) when there is disease primarily in the kidneys or when, in a general disease of the body, renal disease constitutes a major part of the disability; (2) from disease primarily arising in other organs but definitely affecting the kidneys and (3) with certain states in which the working of the kidneys is disturbed, thus causing benign albuminuria without other signs indicating disease.

Most important is the first condition when there is true kidney disease affecting either the kidneys themselves, or some other part of the body, with subsequent enhancement of the primary kidney disease. Generally, but with certain exceptions, albuminuria in these conditions is associated with the presence in the urine of casts (plugs of material washed out of the tubules) and sometimes red blood corpuscles but no pus cells and with variations in the amount and composition of urine. There is also a variety of signs and symptoms due to changes in the blood and other organs in addition to the kidneys. The main examples are the various forms of true, acute, and chronic Bright's disease (diffuse bilateral nephritis), cysts or tumors of the kidney, disease of kidneys in pregnancy and in chronic gout, plugging of blood vessels (thrombi) to or in kidneys, and disease caused by the presence of renal stones, tuberculosis, or obstruction to urinary flow. Strangely enough, cases of severe kidney disease without albuminuria are occasionally seen, and then the diagnosis rests on other findings.

Secondly, a large variety of diseases in other regions may affect the kidneys to an extent that albumin appears in urine. Other definite urinary abnormalities are generally not evident. Varying degrees of disturbed kidney function, however, may result. Transient albuminuria may appear in children after a trivial illness, a cold or bronchitis; marked anemia or jaundice may induce it. This type of renal albuminuria may result from almost any febrile condition, especially scarlet fever, diphtheria, malaria, erysipelas, smallpox, and pneumonia; less frequently, from certain drugs, anesthetic agents (ether or chloroform), poisoning with lead, mercury, arsenic, or phosphorus, from alcoholism, burns, toxic goiter, acute gout, from certain diseases of the blood and blood-forming organs and from parasitic infestations and severe burns. It also occurs with disturbances of circulation ensuing from diseases of the heart with heart failure, and with certain vasomotor conditions producing spasm of blood vessels. Many of these conditions produce degeneration of kidney cells, causing a type of kidney involvement, which may ultimately clear up.

The third variety of renal albuminuria is that often called "physiologic" or "benign" albuminuria, arising from a number of conditions producing alterations in the general circulation and corresponding changes in the normal rate and flow of blood in kidneys. They generally result from certain physical or functional states whose influence on the kidney is reflected by a transient, sometimes a rather persistent, albuminuria without additional evidence of renal impairment. The disability produced may be harmless and insufficient to justify the term "nephritis." Thus various amounts of albumin may appear in urine after strenuous exercise, such as rowing, boxing, and running, after sunburn and so forth and in emotional states and malnutrition. This form appears in adolescence, often without apparent cause. It may occur after a cold shower or exposure to cold, in students cramming for examinations, and in football players after a game. Its relation to malnutrition is shown by the fact that more than 60 per cent of poor children had albuminuria, while only 15 per cent of an equal number of children under the best hygienic care demonstrated it.

Some of these benign forms of albuminuria appear only when the person is in the erect position, and hence are called postural orthostatic (cyclic or intermittent) forms of albuminuria. A curious variety, the lordotic type of orthostatic albuminuria, is found occasionally in healthy young persons who have an exaggerated curve in the small of the back. Under these conditions, considerable albumin may be present in urine passed in daytime, but that formed at night while the person is in a reclining position or passed when the person arises in the morning shows none. When the person is up and about again, it reappears. It is thought to be due to pressure of abdominal organs on the vein of the left kidney, causing interference with adequate circulation when the body is upright. As body growth is completed, the condition usually disappears and the patient remains healthy. Some investigators consider it to be caused by mild but persistent kidney damage from an unknown cause.

NONRENAL OR POSTRENAL ALBUMINURIA

Albumin forms on the dissolution of any tissue cells. In the lower part of the urinary tract cellular debris may give origin to small quantities of albumin that are added to urine after its formation in the kidney and its passage into the tubules. The presence of spermatozoa in the male genital tract or of cells from the vagina in women may account for mild albuminuria, because of contamination of an otherwise normal urine. Catheterized specimens are, therefore, sometimes necessary when women are examined. Urine passed by a woman during the menstrual period may be contaminated by large numbers of red blood cells, which invariably give a strong positive reaction for albumin. When inflammation occurs with formation of pus in the urinary tract below the kidneys, such cells may dissolve in varying quantities. Nonrenal albuminuria may thus arise in cystitis (inflammation of the bladder), pyelitis (inflammation of the kidney pelvis), prostatitis, or from stones in the bladder, ureters, or kidneys.

CHEMICAL TYPES OF ALBUMINURIA

The term "albuminuria" is not strictly accurate, for the coagulable protein of urine consists generally of a mixture made up not only of albumin but also of globulin, mucin, and other proteins. In benign albuminuria proteins besides albumin derived from blood serum are prominently present, such as globulin, nucleo-albumin, and mucin. In true nephritis most of the urinary protein consists of serum albumin and globulin, which may be derived from the food proteins in the blood leaking through damaged glomeruli. Occasionally part of the albuminuria comes from proteins other than those normally circulating in blood; one of these is Bence-Jones protein, which will be discussed later. Some evidence indicates that, in the early stages of diffuse bilateral renal disease, at least part of the urinary albumin comes from degenerated liver cells. Later, protein may be liberated from degenerating kidney cells. These, becoming more permeable, then permit the loss of large amounts of serum albumin. Although methods of easily differentiating these chemical types of albumin are as yet not perfected, studies with the microcentrifuge and electrophoresis of proteins have progressed to the point that, before long, these questions, many of which are at present controversial, will be fully elucidated.

CONCLUSIONS REGARDING ALBUMINURIA

Albuminuria has been discussed in some detail because of the importance popularly attached to it. Obviously to determine the type of albuminuria present, a doctor is necessary and not just a microscope or laboratory, as the differentiation between significant and insignificant forms can be made only after a careful history has been taken and physical examination made in addition to chemical studies. It is particularly important to recognize benign, postural, and other forms of functional albuminuria to prevent persons so affected from being limited by unwarranted fears and by needless restrictions in diet and activity, as occurs when such conditions are confused with true nephritis. In such instances the psychic harm from a dreaded diagnosis may be much greater than the physical harm afforded by the condition itself. Thus are created "renal neurotics." It has been said that "frequently the 'disease' occurs only in the physician's test tube and in the mind of the patient" (Calvin, Isaacs, and Meyer).

To the fearful patient, the discovery of albuminuria may be a rude awakening, arousing unduly great concern. Yet even when significant, albuminuria sometimes constitutes a positive advantage, a beneficent warning to slow up, thereby preventing serious illness. From this viewpoint, a great physician once wrote a paper with the paradoxic title, "On the Advantage of a Trace of Albumin and a Few Casts in the Urine of Men over Fifty."

In general, albuminuria in older persons usually represents some organic disease of variable degree, while that in the young is often functional. In many cases either one may be entirely consistent with the prospect of a healthy and active life. When doubts are entertained, prolonged but not too anxious observation is justified, using such supplementary examinations over a period of several months as seem necessary.

The fallacy of placing much reliance on periodic urinalyses without an accompanying history and physical examination seems evident. Of themselves, such analyses are of little value and may do more harm than good. It has been rightfully said that a physical examination with a urinalysis once a year is of far greater value than a urinalysis alone once a week. Yet a mail-order house some years ago offered such service for a short time. The service was catalogued between a bathtub mat and a bottle of milk of magnesia, and an "analysis covering twenty-nine chemical and microscopical tests" was promised.

A woman presented to a great English physician of the seventeenth century a specimen of her husband's urine, requesting a diagnosis and prescription. "Where is he?" asked the doctor, to which she replied, "Sick in bed four miles off." "What is he?" "A boot-maker." Throwing out the urine and substituting a fresh sample, the doctor said, "Take this home with you, and if your husband will undertake to fit me with a pair of boots by its inspection, I will diagnose and treat him by a similar examination."

Shakespeare commented similarly when to Falstaff's inquiry, "What says the doctor to my water?" the page replies, "He said, sir, the water itself was a good healthy water, but for the party that owned it he might have more diseases than he knows for." A modern counterpart is the inelegant but pertinent tale of the canny gentleman who, on receiving a favorable report from a single, but mixed, specimen sent to a laboratory, happily said, "Good! Mama's well, papa's well, the whole family's well."

Modern Methods of Examining the Kidneys

As Bright found more than one test useful, indeed necessary, so benefits are derived by that scientific ingenuity which has provided a number of ways for study of the condition of the kidneys. A routine urinalysis constitutes the first test to be used and affords the chief point of departure, indicating whether other tests are necessary. While it is true that occasional cases of severe nephritis have been found in which the urine was apparently normal, not even containing albumin, generally some abnormality is present. Ordinarily urine is examined for its alkaline or acid reaction, its specific gravity, the presence of albumin, sugar, pus or blood cells, sediment, and casts. The odor and sediment of urine of a normal person can be altered in several ways; by the kind and amount of food eaten, amount of water drunk, length of time the urine has stood, time of day it was passed, and so forth. Odoriferous or cloudy urine, therefore, does not of itself indicate nephritis, nor is clear urine a sure token of healthy kidneys. Casual inspection is valueless and, indeed, may be misleading.

Casts, as has been said, are small masses of protein, cylindric in structure and taking the shape of the kidney tubule. They are of various types. Those most frequently found are the pale, transparent, "hyaline" casts. Others with cellular debris attached to them are called granular, fatty, waxy, epithelial, or blood casts. Their origin is not perfectly understood. Normal persons may pass small numbers of hyaline casts that arise from the same conditions producing albuminuria. When hyaline casts are numerous or when other types of casts are present, the fact usually signifies inflammation or degeneration from renal disease.

The ability of the kidneys to excrete a large amount of waste in a small amount of fluid—in other words, to elaborate a thick or concentrated urine— is one of their most important functions. By the water-dilution and water-concentration tests, it can be determined whether their diluting and concentrating powers are being maintained. On one day a patient is given solid, dry food only; no fluids are permitted. The urine is collected at certain intervals; normally it should become thick and highly colored, with a specific gravity of 1.020 or greater. On another day 7½ glasses (3 pints) of water are given to the fasting patient within a period of one half hour. At least 75 per cent of this water should be passed normally within the next four hours; the urine becomes thin and watery, with a specific gravity as low as 1.002. When the kidney function is seriously impaired, this concentrating and diluting ability is lost and the specific gravity becomes relatively fixed around 1.010. As long as this ability is partially preserved, maximal renal damage has not yet occurred.

The size, shape, and position of the kidney usually can be faintly but unmistakably outlined in an ordinary X-ray picture of the abdomen. The size and shape of the pelvic cavity inside the kidney can be studied also by special means. One of medicine's recent triumphs is the utilization of a harmless substance which, injected by vein, finds its way to the kidneys and becomes concentrated sufficiently to cast a shadow on X-ray plates, thereby in some cases avoiding the discomfort of the cystoscope. This test is termed the "excretory urogram." By means of the cystoscope and ureteral catheters, certain liquids opaque to the X-ray can be made to flow gently up the ureters to fill the renal pelvis, outlining it sharply in the X-ray picture, like a glove with many projecting fingers (a pyelogram). If disease has destroyed part of the kidney substance or its tubular projections, or if a stone is present, blocking all or part of the pelvis or ureter, characteristic alterations from the normal shadow are produced which help the trained eye in diagnosis.

The excretory ability of the kidneys can be tested by injecting into the muscles or veins certain harmless dyes (phenolsulfonphthalein, indigo carmine, or methylene blue) to see how rapidly and completely they are eliminated in the urine. Eight to ten minutes after injection, the dye begins to appear in the urine, and 40 to 60 per cent of the amount injected should appear within the following hour. Disease of the kidneys or any block to the free passage of urine below the kidneys in the tubes or bladder (from stone, adjacent tumors, or enlarged prostate) causes a definite reduction in the amount of dye recovered. Since it is not known just which cells, glomeruli, or tubules have most to do with the excretion of dyes, retention of dye does not imply specifically localizable damage.

By means of dyes and the cystoscope, a trained physician can often determine whether one or both kidneys are diseased and how much. By passage of small ureteral catheters or collecting tubes into each ureter as it enters the bladder, it can be ascertained, in the samples of urine collected separately from each kidney, whether blood, pus, or germs (such as tubercle bacilli) are coming from one or both sides. The importance of this test can be imagined when it is deemed necessary to remove one kidney. The function of the other must be adequately gauged.

Finer details concerning excretory capacity can be determined by giving orally or injecting into veins not foreign dyes but measured amounts of those products which the kidneys naturally handle (urea, uric acid, or creatinine), then studying their concentration in blood and urine and the speed of their elimination. These are called "clearance" or "concentration" tests.

When kidney function is appreciably impaired, waste substances accumulate in the blood so that their concentration may increase from ten to fifty times (urea 40 to 700 mg. per 100 cc.; uric acid 2 to 30 mg.; creatinine 1 to 20 mg. or more, and sulfates from 2 to 40 mg. or more). Since inorganic sulfates are excreted by the normal kidney with maximal difficulty, when the kidneys are disturbed, sulfates are one of the first substances to increase in blood. Urea and uric acid are excreted fairly readily, and the estimation of concentration of urea in blood is the most important and common test of renal function next to a urinalysis. Since creatinine is excreted with great ease, it is an extremely sick kidney that cannot still rid the blood of it; hence it is the last substance to increase. When it increases appreciably and constantly, it is generally an omen of impending death, indicating a kidney too disturbed even to carry on this, its simplest function. Thus it can be appreciated that blood analyses may give information of great value.

As waste substances accumulate in the blood, they begin to adulterate all body tissues and to appear in abnormal amounts in such fluids as saliva, breast milk, bile, and the fluids that bathe the brain, spinal cord, heart, lungs, and joints. They even accumulate in fluids of the eyeballs and are present excessively in tears. Dr. Philip S. Hench showed that when blood tests are inconvenient or impossible because people have small veins or swollen, edematous extremities, a simple estimation of the amount of urea in saliva gives a satisfactory index of nitrogen retention in the body. When disease is serious, nitrogenous waste products and associated poisons are eliminated excessively in sweat and by the bowels and may cause small ulcers of the skin or bowel. In such cases "uremia" is present, a condition to be described later.

The kidneys are not isolated structures, and their disturbances may affect distant organs and systems, especially the heart-blood vessel (cardiovascular) system. Therefore the doctor examines the heart, the blood pressure, the blood vessels in the arms, and, particularly, the smaller vessels in the eye, where at times certain disturbances may be clearly seen with an ophthalmoscope.

KNOWLEDGE DERIVED FROM KIDNEY TESTS

Physicians have gone far—some say too far—from the simple test for albumin in finding ways of diagnosing nephritis. However, no one test tells the whole tale of a kidney's woe. Nor is an elaborate array of expensive tests ordinarily necessary. The intelligent use of four or five (urinalysis, dye test or estimation of urea, water dilution and concentration test, and blood count), along with the patient's story and a physical examination, will give most of the necessary information, at least in so-called medical nephritis. When pus and blood are present or when stones and other surgical conditions are suspected, advantage should be taken of certain additional tests. In many cases the physician from such studies can with remarkable exactness tell the cause and extent of the disease and the exact parts of the kidney affected. He may venture a prophecy on whether or not the patient will recover, and if not how long he may live. Sometimes the information gained from such examinations is limited. While they show approximately how badly the kidneys are diseased, it cannot always be stated that "only the tubules are involved" or "the glomeruli are alone concerned." The kidney filters and tubules work together essentially as units, and when one part is diseased the other part is apt to become disturbed also. Often when the kidney is "sick," it is like the boy with the toothache, "sick all over." At other times, when one part of the kidney is too disturbed to carry on its function, that work is apparently taken over by another part (a compensatory mechanism). Furthermore, invisible lesions are sometimes present that cannot be demonstrated by means of the microscope and test tube. While the doctor cannot see how the kidneys look, he can determine how they are working and act accordingly.

GENERAL CAUSES OF KIDNEY DISEASE

Bright's disease, as the term is used inclusively, is "the response of the kidney to any alteration in its environment, especially to the irritation of toxic substances." As these toxic substances may be numerous, so the causes of nephritis are many. Nephritis may result from (1) invasion of the kidneys by germs (bacteria) of many kinds; (2) poisons either manufactured by bacteria or formed in infected tissues; (3) toxins not of bacterial origin, such as from metals or chemical poisons; (4) infections and intoxications from mechanical interference to the normal passage of urine produced by obstruction (such as from stones or an enlarged prostate gland); (5) abnormalities of growth, such as cysts and benign or malignant tumors, producing interference in the kidneys' function, and (6) by impairment of the blood supply to the kidney as a result of a disease process in the blood vessels themselves.

A large variety of bacteria may be brought to the kidneys and there set up infections that may localize in the kidneys alone or invade surrounding tissues and the lower part of the urinary passages. The commonest bacteria found in such infections are the colon bacillus (the constant inhabitant of the normal intestinal tract), staphylococci, and streptococci. The tubercle bacillus is also an important invader. Some of the bacteria present a curious consistency in the "geography" of their invasion. Thus the colon bacillus usually attacks the interior part of the kidney, its pelvis and urinary tubes, while the cocci fight their battles in the outer part, the cortex and fatty tissues about the kidney. Some bacteria are especially prone to cause precipitation of matter that forms stones. The various bacteria reach the kidney by several routes: through blood vessels (an infected blood stream), along infected lymph channels, or from infected urine dammed back by any interference with urinary flow, such as may be produced by a stone, kink in a ureter, or an enlarged prostate gland. Bacteria that reach the kidneys through the blood arise from an infected focus elsewhere in the body—small collections cf bacteria in infected teeth, tonsils, ears, or other organs.

Some bacteria do not themselves invade the kidneys, but, from a distance, liberate toxins or poisons that injure kidney cells. Toxins may arise in distant infected regions from dying infected cells and injure the kidney tissues as they are being excreted from the blood. Many poisons not of bacterial origin may produce nephritis. Some of them have been mentioned: certain metals, such as mercury, uranium, and lead, and poisons resulting from burns, goiter, gout, and pregnancy.

Some disturbing agents arouse rather individualistic reactions and special types of cellular disturbance identified by signs and symptoms fairly peculiar unto themselves. Such, for example, are tuberculous infections or the manifestation of stones. The majority of such agents, however, initiate changes in function and structure that, at least in the beginning, arouse in their victims more or less identical complaints.

General Symptoms and Signs of Kidney Disease

In the mildest forms there may be no symptoms, and the patient only accidentally learns about his trouble at the time of an examination for life insurance or for some other purpose. The blood pressure may be a little too high, the heart may be a little inadequate, or the urine test may betray its guilty secret—any of these may introduce the unexpected, brutal revelation of the presence of kidney disease. Some patients are aware of vague discomfort; they feel "out of sorts," or "off color," without knowing why. They may complain of an unaccustomed listlessness, unexplainable fatigue, dull headaches, slight puffiness about the eyes, or a poor appetite. Careful parents especially will be alert to such insidious complaints in their children.

As the kidneys become further diseased, a more or less identical train of events often occurs without regard to cause. Slight disturbances of vision may be noted, such as occasional blurring or spots in front of the eyes. There may be disturbances of sleep because of the desire to void urine at night. Wetting of the bed, however, does not necessarily signify nephritis, as it may be caused by a variety of conditions.[7] Dryness of the mouth may appear, with thirst neces-

---

[7]Paulus Aegineta (A. D. 625–690) recommended the following for incontinence of urine (bed-wetting): "Burn the crop of a cock, and give to the patient to drink in tepid water when fasting, or the flowers of the white ox-eye (chrysanthemum) in like manner" (Vol. I, p. 548).

sitating frequent drinking of water. There may be loss of weight, or if water-logging of tissues (edema) occurs, the patient may gain weight as if he were healthy, and thus attain a sense of false security. When stones, abscesses, or inflammations with pus in the lower part of the urinary passages are present, pain may be present, often accompanied by chills and fever. In the majority of kidney diseases, however, pain is not a feature and may be entirely absent. The well-known advertisement illustrating a man slightly stooped with his hand on a painful flank is greatly misleading, inferring, as it does, that pain in this region generally means kidney disease, for which the advertiser has a wonderful medicine for so much a bottle. Most patients who have chronic pain in the flanks are not suffering from nephritis at all, but from some other disease, often some form of rheumatism in the muscles or joints of the spinal column.

As kidney disease progresses, other organs may become disturbed, and a variety of symptoms may arise, such as dizziness, nausea, vomiting, perhaps diarrhea, severe headache, shortness of breath, swelling of feet and arms, enlargement of the abdomen from fluid, and symptoms of congestion in lungs and liver. As the nephritis approaches its most serious phase, unconsciousness may arise from uremic coma, and convulsions may occur.

The general signs of kidney disease may be local or constitutional. Local signs pertain to alterations in quantity, appearance, and quality of the urine. The urine may be pale and thin and voided frequently or in large amounts. In other cases it is dark, cloudy, and markedly diminished in amount. Tests will show alterations in the urine and changes in the amounts of blood wastes present. Signs that reflect constitutional disturbances in association with nephritis may be: increase in blood pressure, an enlarged heart, fluid in the lungs, small hemorrhages in the skin or in the back of the eyeballs, and especially a pale, pasty complexion and anemia. Sick kidneys are truly versatile in the range and scope of their symptomatology.

UREMIA

If both kidneys are removed or both ureters blocked, death results in a few days, as a result of formation and retention of poisons in the blood and tissues of the body. This toxic state is called "uremia," the main characteristic of which is a period of drowsiness interrupted perhaps by convulsions. A similar intoxication may occur in cases of acute or chronic kidney insufficiency. Its first manifestations are often itching of the skin, headache, and cramps or twitchings in muscles. Then intense nausea, vomiting, and shortness of breath may occur. If the condition persists, it may be distressingly punctuated by convulsive or epileptiform seizures, or the patient may lapse into a drowsy state ending in coma and death. There is no more complete nor accurate description of the uremic state to be found in the medical literature than the eloquent words of Richard Bright, written in 1836, to define the characteristics and progress of this unfortunate and pathetic train of events: "Again the patient is restored to tolerable health; again he enters on his active duties; or he is perhaps, less fortunate;—the swelling increases, the urine becomes scanty, the powers of life seem to yield, the lungs become oedematous, and, in a state of asphyxia or coma, he sinks into the grave; or a sudden effusion of serum into the glottis closes the passages of the air, and brings on a more sudden dissolution. Should he, however, have resumed the avocations of life, he is usually subject to constant recurrence of his symptoms; or again, almost dismissing the recollection of his ailment, he is suddenly seized with an acute attack of pericarditis, or with a still more acute attack of peritonitis, which, without any renewed warning, deprives him, in eight and forty hours, of his life. Should he escape this danger likewise, other perils await him; his headaches have been observed to become more frequent; his stomach more deranged; his vision indistinct; his hearing depraved: he is suddenly seized with a convulsive fit, and becomes blind. He struggles through the attack; but again and again it returns; and before a day or week has elapsed, worn out by convulsions, or overwhelmed by coma, the painful history of his disease is closed."

Uremia is not entirely dependent on the duration or amount of kidney disturbance. It may appear as a tragic surprise early in the course of acute and seemingly moderate kidney inadequacy, or it may be postponed for long periods in a patient whose kidneys are known to be hardly functioning at all. It may attack with sudden fury a person in active and apparently healthy life, unaware of impending catastrophe. Nor is uremia dependent on the amount of urea dammed back in the blood, for a marked excess may be long present yet the patient escape its symptoms. It may occur in nephrosis, that form of kidney disease characterized by water and salt retention, when the ability of the kidneys to eliminate toxic waste products fails, whereas it occurs in its most violent form in nephritis without dropsy.

The exact substance responsible for uremic poisoning is not known. When his colleague Babington first noted an increase of urea in the blood of nephritic patients, Bright used the term "uremia," considering urea to be a toxic substance. Recent studies seem to indicate that urea is not sufficiently toxic to account for this profound upset. While various minor disturbances can be produced in the body by feeding excess urea, Hewlett and others noted only slight muscular fatigue, drowsiness, and lassitude after taking sufficiently large amounts of urea to raise its concentration in the blood for several hours to almost ten times the normal amount. The conclusions of such feeding experiments have only a limited application, however, just as symptoms of acute drunkenness cannot be compared to those in the chronic poisoning of habitual alcoholism.

In some illuminating experiments the physiologists, Bollman and Mann, transplanted the ureters of animals into the bowel, thereby causing at least part of the urinary substances to be reabsorbed through the intestine into the blood. The amazing concentration of more than 1,600 mg. of urea for each 100 cc. of blood was reached (at least fifty times as much as is normally present), yet the animals continued to live with no noticeable effect whatever. This seems to present indisputable evidence that urea is not toxic, and physicians must therefore seek to discover and eliminate some far more potent poison.

When uremia begins to occur, that is, when an appreciable and prolonged increase of urea and other waste products in the blood takes place, great caution must be exercised to prevent serious, perhaps fatal, toxicity. A sudden increase of headaches or muscular pains, a rapid increase of blood pressure or blood urea, should warn of impending danger and prompt the physician to initiate the necessary additions to treatment. Unfortunately, in cases of progressively failing kidneys the physician's efforts often only postpone an inevitable tragedy but they do make its coming more bearable.

AIMS IN THE TREATMENT OF KIDNEY DISEASE AND KIDNEY FAILURE

Special treatment is required for such forms of kidney trouble as tuberculosis, tumors, infections, stones, the kidney poisoning that occasionally occurs in pregnancy, and that caused by obstruction from an enlarged prostate gland producing a backflow of urine. What the doctor tries to do in the treatment of nephritis and of renal insufficiency or kidney failure of other types can be discussed together briefly.

There are two aims in treatment: (1) Where possible, to discover and remove the cause of the kidney trouble and (2) to lighten the burden on the diseased kidney while it is damaged. The commonest known causes of nephritis are bacterial and chemical poisons. In nephritis of youth and middle age any chronic source of infection should if possible be removed. If this is impossible, local treatment should be provided for disease such as may exist in tonsils, the middle ears and sinuses, especially in children, the teeth, the prostate gland, and occasionally about the female organs. The time for removal or treatment must be carefully chosen. The habitual use, by susceptible persons, of certain medicines is occasionally found to be a causal factor. "Cleansing mercury douches," for example, may seriously irritate the kidneys, and for this reason their use is to be condemned.

A physician of antiquity (Galen) wrote that "the offices of the kidneys and bladder being incessant, these parts, if diseased, having no rest, can scarcely get well." It has been found, however, that the kidneys as a whole do not work incessantly. Only certain units in a kidney are working at any one time, but when working they do so at full speed. Richards, a physiologist, has proved this by watching, through a special microscope, the glomeruli of a frog's kidney actually working. The glomeruli did not all work continuously but in shifts, some taking time off. Through this wise provision of nature the vitality of these delicate but energetic units is conserved.

The units of a sick kidney need even more rest. For them rest is the great restorer of health and life. It is the one measure that may tide them over until such time as they can recuperate fully, or may conserve their energies so they can carry on as long as possible. The kidneys can be rested in several ways: by not adding to their burdens, by shifting part of their work to other organs, and by helping them carry on such work as is unavoidable. During physical activity body tissues are forming wastes that the kidneys must handle. Rest in bed during the acute stage of nephritis is therefore advisable to prevent avoidable and unnecessary formation of body wastes. Some wastes are excreted through sweat and by bowels. Years ago it was felt that the kidney could be spared considerable work by stimulating the skin and intestines to greater activity. This was accomplished in some cases by the repeated use of mild or strong laxatives, frequent enemas, daily warm baths, and, in some instances, hot packs applied to the entire body to induce sweating. Such measures, for the most part, in recent years have been discarded because of their weakening effect on the patient and because the amounts of waste products eliminated by such means are infinitesimally small. There are, however, three procedures by means of which urea and other waste products can be eliminated from the body across membranes other than the glomerular filter in patients whose kidneys are so damaged that the filtering apparatus is inadequate for this function.

In the first of these methods a tube is introduced by way of the mouth or nose, past the stomach and into the small intestine (intestinal lavage). Introduction of a special solution into the tube causes waste products from the blood to be filtered across the wall of the intestine to be eliminated in the stools. The second method (peritoneal lavage) involves the introduction of tubes through the abdominal wall and filling the abdominal cavity with a special solution of various salts and water, which, as in the former method, causes waste products to be filtered across the peritoneal membrane into the abdominal cavity, from whence they are removed by suction. In the third method (artificial kidney) the patient's blood containing waste products in high concentrations is passed through coils of cellophane tubing immersed in a bath of a specially prepared solution. As the blood passes through the coils of cellophane, waste products are filtered across the cellophane wall into the bath, and the "purified blood" is returned to the patient's body. These three methods of "extrarenal" excretion have rather definite indications for use and have been found to be of great value—indeed, in some instances, life-saving—particularly in patients whose kidney damage is acute, transient, or reversible in nature, when nature will repair the kidney damage present if the functional load on the kidney can be lightened for several days or weeks to allow such repair to take place. However, it must be stated that none of these measures are without some degree of risk, and their use in patients who have far advanced, chronic, irreversible damage to kidney function is debatable if not contraindicated.

Catching cold or the "flu" may add a serious burden to the kidney, and protection from prevalent infections should be afforded, such as avoidance of crowds, keeping away from sick relatives, and so forth.

One of the most important measures is a carefully selected diet. A milk diet is by no means universally adequate. In some types of kidney disease such a diet may provide too much fluid; in another type it may contain too much protein or salt. A proper diet for each patient can be planned only by a physician who has carried out the indicated number of laboratory procedures previously mentioned. Those who have found this necessity irksome will sympathize with Bill Nye. "I have just been sent to the hospital. My physician did it. He did it with an analysis. Anybody who amounts to anything now-adays gets analyzed. Sometimes you find casts, sometimes you find maple sugar and sometimes acids, oxides, paints, oils, varnish, white lead, borax, albumin, lime, hair and cement. In these cases the patient should be placed on a strict diet or he will in the course of his life become a corpse. . . . An analysis today shows more casts, fibrin, gelatin and some zinc and copper. The chemist also discovers that in 1853 I fell from an apple tree and tore my pants in two places. He says I will be unhappy with my third wife. She will be unhappy also."

The important features of diet concern the amounts of salt, water, and protein permissible. When dropsy is present or impending, the amount of salt and fluid allowed must be carefully estimated. When retention of urea and other wastes occurs in the blood, it has long seemed best to restrict the ingestion of proteins. Recently some physicians, as the result of certain experiments, have become more lax, allowing rather generous amounts of protein. Until the effects of such diets are better known, moderate restrictions in meats, eggs, and other proteins seem indicated. A certain amount of fluids and of protein, however, is vitally necessary, and complete abstinence is rarely required. In a form of nephritis known as nephrosis, in which the kidney is adequately able to eliminate urea and other waste products from the body, but in which the content of protein in the blood is below normal, a diet that provides much protein but little salt is called for. There is no essential difference between so-called red meats and white meats as far as nephritis is concerned.

The elimination of wastes by the kidneys can be increased by use of a variety of diuretics, substances which cause these wastes to pass through the kidneys in added amounts.[8] Water itself is a diuretic, and some persons after drinking a quart of water will within a short time eliminate perhaps a quart and a half of urine. Concentrated solution of glucose, coffee, tea, certain mineral waters, beer, and a number of drugs will promote an augmented flow of urine. Some of these diuretics are indicated when dropsy occurs without the increase of wastes in the tissues. Choice of a proper diuretic is important, as the wrong one may irritate the kidneys and add to their embarrassment, thus causing further damage.

The treatment of kidney disease has been made much more successful by the recent discovery of several new and more efficient diuretics. Contemplating the ease of their administration and their efficacy, one can be thankful to live in modern times. Only about two centuries ago an esteemed physician wrote (Pechey cited by Hewitt): "Put washed worms into a curcurbit [flask] so well stoppered that nothing can exhale. Place it to digest either in sea water or in the heat of the sun, that the worms may putrefy and ferment. This fermentation is sometimes so very great that it breaks the glass. The fermentation being over, the earthy part sinks to the bottom, and the skins swim on top, the spiritous liquor is in the middle. Separate this and distill it, and it will yield a spirit; this spirit is an excellent diuretic."

Dropsy or waterlogging of tissues occurs in some cases where too much common salt (sodium chloride) is eaten. However, when a different salt is used (ammonium chloride, ammonium nitrate, potassium nitrate, or potassium chloride), dropsy may be relieved. In cases of nephritis in which dropsy is associated with a decreased amount of protein in the circulating blood (nephrosis), certain substances called "plasma volume expanders" are valuable in promoting flow of urine and reduction of dropsical fluid in the tissues. Acacia, solutions of gelatin, a special preparation of concentrated blood serum, and more recently a substance called "dextran," all have a similar action. In some instances one substance works more effectively than others. In Bright's time mercury in certain forms was used but often was found to be harmful. Newer mercury preparations are now available that are less harmful and often almost miraculous in ridding the body of great quantities

---

[8] "Diuresis" means "to urinate through"; a diuretic is a substance that increases the secretion of urine.

of dropsical fluid rapidly. When necessary, such preparations have been given by injection repeatedly almost weekly for five years without harm. However, mercury in any form must be used with caution in patients suffering from kidney disease, lest the drug, whose effectiveness lies in its property as a mild irritant to the kidney, produce further kidney damage.

If ascites, the accumulation of fluid in the abdomen, is present and cannot be relieved by the use of diuretics, the abdominal cavity may have to be tapped and the fluid removed through a tube (paracentesis). An eighteenth-century physician (Mead) cited the "remarkable case of Lady Page who in seventy-seven months was tapped seventy-six times and had taken away two hundred and forty gallons of water without ever repining at her case, or ever fearing the operation." Fortunately, modern diets and diuretics have largely done away with the necessity for this procedure.

When uremia occurs, drastic measures may be necessary to prevent convulsions and unconsciousness, or even death. Then the resources of the physician are taxed indeed, but sometimes by injections of fluid, transfusions of blood, and other procedures a new lease on life, or at least some comfort, may be provided.

Quack remedies for kidney diseases abound in great numbers. In a recent circular are advertised fifty different "kidney tablets," fifty-one "kidney remedies," and one hundred and twenty-seven "kidney pills," as well as various "kidney-tonics, bitters, cordials, capsules, drops, medicines, treatments and herb teas." Many of them are called "kidney and backache remedies," fostering the classic falsehood of the quacks regarding urinary sediments and pain in the back. The charlatan often recommends a nostrum indiscriminately for nephritis and diabetes, making no distinction between these utterly different types of disease. Scores of them have been analyzed by government and national medical laboratories. Most of them contain drugs that tend to increase the quantity of urine but not the amount of waste excreted. In some cases this is done in a particularly vicious way by including a powerful irritant to the kidney which, though it increases the amount of urine, may cause serious damage. Others are harmless but quite useless. One used to "cure Bright's disease, gravel, all urinary troubles and pain in the back or groin from kidney trouble" was found to contain white sugar exclusively! One widely advertised backache and kidney pill that sells for seventy-five cents for a box of forty pills, and which has been estimated as costing one cent a box to make, was found to contain one harmless and one equally useless but irritating substance. Another well-known diuretic pill, also ineffective, was advertised as worth five dollars a box, sells for twenty-five cents for a box of thirty-five pills, and has been estimated as costing about a quarter of a cent for a full box! Certainly there is no place for alleged cures for the self-treatment of such a potentially dangerous condition as kidney disease.

CLASSIFICATION OF KIDNEY DISEASES: SYNOPSIS OF CHIEF FORMS

None of the many classifications of kidney diseases is entirely satisfactory. Were the cause of each known it would be simple to designate them accordingly, "tuberculous nephritis," "mercurial nephritis," and so on. In many instances the cause is obscure, and classifications are based on the part of the kidney chiefly involved, on what the microscope shows after death: "glomerular nephritis," "tubular nephritis." Others are named from the chief symptoms and signs they produce (or from the main functional derangement): "chronic nephritis with edema," "salt and water nephritis." This presentation permits only a brief mention of the chief forms of kidney disturbance.

They can be divided into four groups. Group I constitutes those diseases which affect primarily the kidneys alone or in which the kidney disturbance becomes the chief cause of ill health. Group II includes different types of toxic or diseased states in which the kidneys are disturbed on account of disease elsewhere and become a secondary cause of ill health. Group III involves certain conditions in which nephritis is absent (the kidneys are relatively unaffected), but in which alterations in the quality or quantity of urine afford important signs in diagnosis. Group IV includes disturbances of kidneys dependent on maldevelopment.

GROUP I. DISEASES IN WHICH NEPHRITIS BECOMES THE CHIEF CAUSE OF ILL HEALTH

The kidneys do not live to or for themselves alone, and nephritis is rarely if ever strictly a disease solely of the kidneys. They become diseased from poisons and bacteria brought to them from some distant site; as a result of the subsequent nephritis, other tissues in turn become involved. The blood vessels of the kidneys may participate with those of other organs in a systemic disease affecting vessels throughout the body. One organ may suffer more than others; when the kidney does so, the nephritis becomes the chief cause of ill health. Kidney damage associated with essential hypertension (high blood pressure) may be an example of the former; acute and chronic glomerulonephritis are examples of the latter. The small blood vessels of many organs, such as heart, brain, muscles, eyes, and liver, are diseased, but the difficulty in the kidney dominates the picture. It is, for example, as if all the pipes in a house become clogged; damage to those in the kitchen where food must be prepared would cause a greater disturbance than to those in the parlor radiator or the bath.

Kidney Disease Secondary to High Blood Pressure

While the blood pressure increases with or as a result of certain forms of nephritis, some types of increased blood pressure (so-called essential hypertension) come at first without nephritis and indeed may never be associated with significant kidney disturbance. As, however, thickening occurs in the walls of the tiny blood vessels in the kidneys (afferent arterioles) as part of the generalized thickening of blood vessel walls throughout the entire body, circulation to the kidney is diminished, and the function of these organs is thereby impaired. By constricting the renal artery, one investigator (Goldblatt) has produced high blood pressure in animals similar to that seen in humans. When the constriction is removed, the blood pressure returns to normal or near normal limits. By wrapping the kidney of an animal in a non-elastic envelope (cellophane), thereby interfering with the normal circulation of blood through the kidney, two other investigators (Page and Corcoran) have found that the blood pressure increases. They have found also that in animals in which high blood pressure has been thus produced, a chemical substance is released into the blood. Blood containing this chemical substance, when injected into a normal animal, causes the blood pressure to increase.

Chronic Renal Arteriosclerosis

Chronic renal arteriosclerosis may occur in elderly persons (more than forty-five or fifty years of age) who have hardening of large arteries elsewhere, at the "temples," wrists, and so on. The condition is often discovered by chance during a yearly checkup or from urinalysis in the course of an examination for life insurance. The larger, not the small, vessels of the kidney are chiefly diseased; hence, a degree of accommodation takes place whereby the patient may not be noticeably incapacitated. The blood pressure increases to force blood through the stiffened vessels. Dropsy is rare. Some anemia may occur, and there may be a lag in ridding the blood of wastes. As a rule, no special cause for alarm need be felt. Under supervision the patient may lead a comparatively comfortable and useful existence for a number of years. Plenty of fluids are required to rid the body of wastes, but because excretion of water is slowed, fluids should be taken mostly before supper to avoid the necessity of arising during the night for urination.

Acute Glomerulonephritis (Acute Bright's Disease)

Acute glomerulonephritis is usually a disease of young people. During World War I it affected many soldiers and acquired the term "war" or "trench" nephritis. Its cause is unknown, but is thought to be due to bacterial infection or to the effect of bacterial poisons on the glomeruli; sometimes it disappears after a focus of infection is removed. The urine is cloudy, dark, and scanty, and contains albumin, casts, and red blood cells and sometimes even visible blood. Wastes do not often accumulate markedly in the blood. Dropsy occurs, and the blood pressure increases. The death rate is low, perhaps 3 per cent. It often clears entirely in a few weeks. Occasionally it progresses into chronic glomerulonephritis.

Chronic Glomerulonephritis (Chronic Bright's Disease)

Chronic glomerulonephritis is perhaps the most serious of all forms of nephritis. It is that form first described by Bright and from which arose the erroneous idea that all nephritis was extremely serious. Its onset is usually before forty years of age and may be insidious or may follow acute glomerulonephritis. It is often part of a general disease of blood vessels. The patient may pass thin watery urine at frequent intervals during the day and night, a total of two or three quarts or more. The urine contains albumin and casts. Dropsy is usually absent or not marked. The blood pressure increases, and the complexion becomes pasty because of anemia. Wastes accumulate in the blood. The heart enlarges and weakens. Vessels in the brain may be affected. Thus death may result from heart failure, a stroke, or from uremia. Some patients live several years, but as chronic invalids. Others are able to lead moderately active lives for many years.

Chronic Glomerulonephritis with Nephrotic Features (Chronic Bright's Disease with Dropsy)

This disease is characterized by marked albuminuria and dropsy, and the presence of peculiar fatty or lipoid bodies in the urine. Anemia, high blood pressure, and involvement of the heart and eyes are not present as early in this disease as they are in the dry form of chronic glomerulonephritis. Kidney function is adequate except for excretion of salt and water, and diets must be arranged accordingly. Diuretics are especially useful in this condition. The edema may clear, and the danger to life may not be great for a long period, although the patient's resistance to infections seems lowered. Health may return, but albuminuria as a rule continues more or less persistently. In many cases a "mixed nephritis" follows, however, in which the symptoms and signs of the dry form of Bright's disease described above are superimposed on the nephrotic picture. This train of events usually is progressive, and the outlook is less favorable.

Conditions Affecting the Renal Tubules (Nephroses)

There are many conditions that produce in kidneys a toxic state affecting chiefly the renal tubules, nephrosis, which affords a secondary cause of ill health. In nephrosis there is usually marked albuminuria, but no increase in blood pressure or generally of waste products in the blood. In some forms dropsy is absent, in others much dropsy occurs. Chemical nephrosis may be caused by certain metals, drugs, anesthetic agents, or food poisons, such as from meat, fish, or mushrooms. The commonest causes are mercury and arsenic. Other responsible substances are phosphorus, chromates, lead, bismuth, uranium, zinc, turpentine, tar, cresol, carbolic acid, certain alcohols, chloroform, carbon tetrachloride, and ether. Toxic nephrosis may be caused, in the absence of fever, by such conditions as jaundice, intestinal obstruction, burns, pernicious anemia, diabetes mellitus, syphilis, and thyroid disease, or by a variety of infectious diseases with fever. Febrile nephroses (febrile albuminuria) may result from pneumonia, malaria, yellow fever, typhoid fever, diphtheria, empyema, blood poisoning, peritonitis, gangrene, or injections of foreign protein. Lipoid nephrosis is a special rare form of tubular disease, the cause of which is unknown.

Mercurial Nephrosis: Excesses of mercury produce serious kidney trouble. The acute form is encountered when tablets of bichloride of mercury are taken by mistake or with suicidal intent. The urine becomes loaded with albumin, casts, and red blood cells. Complete suspension of kidney function with suppression of urine for several days may follow the extensive tubular damage present. Uremia and death may ensue, or slow recovery may follow prompt and vigorous treatment. While the physician is awaited, the patient should be given several raw eggs in milk. Chronic mercurial poisoning is an industrial hazard for the makers of thermometers, barometers, felt hats, and other products necessitating the use of the metal or salts of mercury.

Acute Tubular Insufficiency (Lower Nephron Nephrosis): Mercurial nephrosis, together with tubular damage as a result of several other causative agents, may be classed under the heading of lower nephron nephrosis, or, more correctly, acute tubular insufficiency. This condition is characterized by failure of the kidneys to secrete urine in any appreciable amounts, if at all, progressive retention of waste products in the blood, uremia, and death. It may occur secondarily to any of the systemic conditions already listed, to shock and prolonged decrease in blood pressure associated with hemorrhage or surgical procedures, to transfusion with incompatible blood, and to numerous other situations. The "crush injury" syndrome, frequently encountered in battle and civilian casualties during World War II, is an example. Fortunately, the damage to the kidneys in many of these conditions is self-limiting, reversible, and capable of repair. It is in this group of patients that the three methods of extrarenal excretion described previously (intestinal lavage, peritoneal lavage, and artificial kidney) find their greatest usefulness.

Pyelonephritis

Acute pyelonephritis is caused by bacteria invading the kidneys in the course of infection of the blood stream, or by an infection secondary to obstruction of urinary flow by stones or an enlarged prostate blocking the ureters. Chills, fever, vomiting, and sweating occur, and there may be severe pain and tenderness or merely a dull ache in the kidney region. The urine contains pus, red blood cells, albumin, and bacteria. Wastes accumulate in the blood, but dropsy and high blood pressure are uncommon. When the infection is apparently confined chiefly to the pelvis of the kidney, it is called pyelitis, a condition not uncommon in infants and in pregnant women. It usually clears completely, but sometimes progresses to chronic pyelonephritis and even uremia. When scar tissue forms as the result of chronic pyelonephritis, the kidney often gradually shrinks in size. As this shrinkage occurs, the blood pressure may gradually increase.

[Most infections of the kidney are now treated successfully with sulphonamides, mandelic acid, or one of the antibiotic drugs.—Ed.]

Perinephritic abscess, another form of "pus kidney," is a localized purulent infection in pads of fat about the kidney, usually only on one side. Severe pain in the flanks, chills, and fever are present. An operation to drain the abscess is necessary.

GROUP II. DISEASES IN WHICH THE KIDNEYS ARE DISTURBED BY DISEASE ELSEWHERE AND BECOME A SECONDARY CAUSE OF ILL HEALTH

Renal Lithiasis

A stone in the kidney (renal lithiasis) may give no symptoms, or may produce kidney colic, one of the most agonizing pains known to man. Pain is produced only when a stone tries to pass out of the kidney into the narrow ureter. Small stones traversing the ureters may cause great suffering unless, and until, they pass out into the bladder. Some pass spontaneously or can be removed by instruments. Others must be removed by operation or they may cause obstruction to the flow of urine with resulting pyelonephritis or even complete destruction of kidneys. No known medicines or mineral waters have any effect whatsoever on dissolving stones, the multitudinous promises of quacks, ancient and modern, to the contrary. Stones are of various types, most of which (though not all) cast shadows in X-ray pictures. They consist of urinary salts and albuminous substances precipitated together. The reasons why these salts, normally kept in solution, become precipitated is not known, but such an event is probably induced by chemical alterations and bacterial infections.

Kidney Disturbances During Pregnancy

Most women are able to complete pregnancy with little or no real kidney trouble. In the last three or four months of pregnancy the womb may so crowd the bladder and ureters that free passage of urine is interfered with. When slowing of urinary flow results, a mild bacterial infection of bladder urine often occurs. Occasionally more serious trouble arises, which was formerly called "kidney of pregnancy" or "nephritis of pregnancy" and believed to be essentially one form of kidney disease. Now it is recognized that this term really includes several different disturbances: pyelitis, pyelonephritis, acute or chronic glomerulonephritis, acute nephrosis, pre-eclampsia, or eclampsia. Glomerulonephritis or nephrosis, existing prior to pregnancy but so mild as to go unrecognized, may flare up acutely under the stress of childbearing. More serious are those conditions called eclampsia and pre-eclamptic toxemia, manifestations of a poisoning caused presumably by toxic products thrown out from the uterus or from the growing baby. The manifestations of such a poisoning are headache, disturbances of vision, nausea, vomiting, dizziness, restlessness, dropsy, albuminuria, and high blood pressure. Without convulsions, they indicate pre-eclampsia. "Eclampsia" means convulsions and represents the most serious phenomenon of this condition. It arises more frequently in first pregnancies (about 1 in every 250) and only about once in every 1,200 later pregnancies. In all it occurs only about once for every 500 or 600 births. Generally it is noted during the last three months of pregnancy. Degeneration of the liver and the kidney tubules may be present, and a special form of glomerulonephritis may result. Under appropriate treatment, the pregnancy may occasionally be completed. Sometimes interruption of pregnancy is necessary to spare the patient's life. Thereafter kidney function may be remarkably restored. Obviously it is most important for an expectant mother to co-operate with her physician in routine and repeated examination of urine and blood pressure. It is equally important for a mother, who has experienced eclampsia with a previous pregnancy, to seek competent evaluation of heart and kidney function and advice before attempting further pregnancy.

Tuberculosis of Kidneys

Tuberculosis of kidneys is always secondary to tuberculosis elsewhere—in lungs, lymph nodes, bones or joints. Usually involving both kidneys to a degree at least, it invades one kidney especially and may destroy it entirely. The urine contains albumin, blood, pus, and tubercle bacilli. The latter may be difficult to find, and tests utilizing guinea pigs may be necessary. Tuberculosis in kidneys practically never heals spontaneously, and if the kidney is not removed the disease may invade other tissues and endanger the other kidney. The operation is generally quite safe and the outcome hopeful. Half of a group of patients studied by Wildbolz were found to be apparently completely relieved ten years after operation.

Kidney Disease from Enlarged Prostate Gland

For some unknown reason the prostate gland frequently enlarges in men more than fifty years of age. This may cause difficulty in starting urination, frequent urination, and dribbling due to partial blockage of the urethra. If free flow is not re-established, infection (pyelitis or pyelonephritis) and destruction of kidney tissue may ensue. Ureters and pelvis may be ballooned out with urine (hydroureter and hydronephrosis). Wastes accumulate in the blood and uremia may result. If appreciable urinary retention is present, careful drainage of the bladder and surgical removal of the prostate gland or of a portion of it are generally necessary, despite long-winded and long-distance radio advice otherwise.

Gouty Nephritis (Gouty Bright's Disease)

Years ago a German physician (Hahn) found that when a patient who had gout took small quantities of turpentine, the odor of violets present in the urine of normal persons after taking turpentine was absent. This was one of the earliest tests of renal function. The exact relationship between gout and nephritis is not known, but in chronic gout there is often disturbed kidney function. A mild form of chronic nephritis with manifestations somewhat like those of renal arteriosclerosis may be present. Kidney stones of uric acid salts are not infrequent, and occasionally the actual precipitation of crystals of uric acid salts occurs in kidney tissue.

Scarlatinal Nephritis

In the course of scarlet fever there is usually some albuminuria with no other signs of renal disease. In about 10 per cent of cases, however, definite nephritis develops about the second or third week. If mild, it is signalized by transient dropsy, with albumin, casts, and a few red blood cells in the urine. In other cases considerable dropsy may develop, and the signs of nephritis may last a number of weeks or so and then gradually disappear. In a few patients typical acute glomerulonephritis occurs, which temporarily, at least, may be severe and accompanied by uremia. More or less complete recovery usually follows, but chronic nephritis occasionally results. It is said to occur, however, in only about twenty out of five thousand cases.

Bence-Jones Proteinuria ("White Urine")

Ordinary albumin is invisible in cold urine but becomes apparent as a white cloud after urine is heated. In multiple myeloma, a disease of bones, a special kind of albumin called "Bence-Jones protein" may appear. A patient may pass white urine when voiding outdoors in the cold. The white cloud disappears on heating the urine and reappears on cooling. Early in the disease the kidneys themselves are normal, merely excreting the abnormal substance. However, as the disease progresses, the renal tubules may become blocked with casts of Bence-Jones protein, and renal function may gradually fail, causing progressive accumulation of waste products in the blood, secondary elevation of blood pressure, and death from uremia.

GROUP III. CONDITIONS IN WHICH THE URINE IS ABNORMAL BUT NO NEPHRITIS IS PRESENT

There is a group of diseases in which abnormal substances are present in urine but in which no nephritis exists. The kidneys are merely excreting material present abnormally or in unusual amounts. Alterations in the quality or quantity of urine occur, but renal function is normal.

Diabetes Mellitus

In *diabetes mellitus,*[9] a disease of the pancreas, or human sweetbread, the first symptom generally noted by the patient is the passage of large amounts of urine, usually three to six quarts, sometimes ten quarts or more, daily. In mild cases the output of urine is normal, but in any event sugar is present therein. It has been noted that when blood contains the usual amounts of sugar, the kidneys are able to hold it back and its loss in urine is prevented. When the blood sugar is highly concentrated, as in diabetes mellitus, the excess spills over into urine. Other cardinal symptoms of diabetes mellitus are increasing thirst and consumption of large quantities of water, increased appetite, loss of weight, and itching.

[9]"Diabetes" means "to go through."

Renal Diabetes

In *renal diabetes* there exists an unusual permeability of the kidney to even normal amounts of circulating blood sugar, such that, even without diabetes mellitus being present, sugar (glucose) appears in the urine. The patients are not sick, and no diet or other treatment is necessary except, of course, sufficient observation to make sure that true diabetes mellitus is not present. It is an uncommon condition, and the cause is unknown.

Diabetes Insipidus

In *diabetes insipidus* there is no sugar in the urine and no disease of the pancreas or kidneys, yet the patient passes large amounts of urine that is normal except for its low specific gravity. As a rule, four to ten quarts are passed each day; in severe cases the output may reach from twenty to thirty or more quarts a day. I recall a sixteen-year-old boy who passed thirty-three quarts of urine every twenty-four hours; in forty hours the weight of urine was equivalent to his own body weight. Ten years later he was still passing these enormous amounts. A case is recorded of a twenty-four-year-old man who passed about forty-three quarts in twenty-four hours (Trousseau). Diabetes insipidus is a rather rare disease and usually afflicts children or young adults, probably as a result of disease of the pituitary gland after infection or injury to the brain. It causes intense thirst constantly day and night. Injection of pituitary extract or inhalation of powdered pituitary extract may control the excessive thirst and urination.

"Black Urine"

A curious and rare urinary disturbance is that presented by certain persons who have an inherited anomaly of nutrition producing "alkaptonuria." The infant's urine may stain its linen brown or black. The urine turns dark when exposed to air. In itself the condition is a trifling matter, inconvenient rather than harmful (Garrod). In rare instances the cartilages of the ears and joints also turn dark. There are no symptoms and no treatment is necessary.

GROUP IV. DISTURBANCES OF THE KIDNEY DEPENDENT ON MALFORMATION

This includes such conditions as "single," "horseshoe," "floating," and "polycystic" kidney and certain anomalies of the ureters, such as double ureter and absent ureter. About 1 in 1,800 persons is born with only one kidney. Persons who have this anomaly are unaware of it and there are no symptoms. The kidney present is usually enlarged to compensate for the absent one.

The chief importance of this condition is that when the only kidney is diseased, danger to life is great. A diagnosis of single kidney is, of course, of vital importance when considering kidney removal for any surgical condition.

A bridge of renal tissue may extend across from one kidney to the other, generally at the lower pole, connecting them to form a horseshoe kidney. Such a condition is symptomless and is recognized almost exclusively by means of a pyelogram, an X-ray of the inside of the kidney. When disease is present in one side of a horseshoe kidney, it may spread to the other readily, and thus the union is dangerous to health and life. It may complicate or prevent operation when renal tuberculosis or abscesses are present, and therefore its recognition is important.

The normal kidney can move up and down about an inch, and, as has been noted, the right kidney is lower and more readily felt than the left. Such a palpable kidney is entirely normal. When the kidney moves excessively owing to weakness of its supporting structures, it is then known as a "wandering," "movable," or "floating" kidney and may be felt low in the abdomen or even in the pelvis. It is found low in women six times as often as in men, and generally on the right side in thin individuals. It usually gives no symptoms. Sometimes a dull ache in the flank is present, or, when it moves enough to cause kinking of the ureter, severe pain may result. Operation to secure the kidney should be done only when exercises to strengthen abdominal muscles, the use of supporting belts, and sometimes rest in bed and nutritious diets to replace fat about the kidney have proved unsuccessful.

Certain abnormalities occur in the ureters also, chief of which is the presence of an extra one on either or both sides. These occur in about 1 per cent of people, and when disease is present therein may cause trouble in diagnosis. Special X-rays will reveal their presence.

Polycystic Kidneys

Polycystic kidneys represent a curious congenital anomaly recognized as present in about 1 in every 3,500 patients (Braasch). Often unrecognized, the condition occurs actually much more frequently than this, being found in about 1 of every 1,000 post-mortem examinations. The cause is unknown, but is thought to be related to inadequate fusion of constituent parts of the kidney units during the time the body is developing in the mother's womb. The kidneys swell to various sizes, forming abdominal tumors that are sometimes enormous. A forty-year-old man was found to have such kidneys, each weighing about seventeen pounds! (Normal weight of each is about one third of a pound.) Although both kidneys become enlarged, one is usually felt earlier than the other. The enlargement is due to the accumulation of small and large masses of watery or semigelatinous material in multitudinous pockets or cysts. Symptoms rarely arise before thirty or forty years of age. Weakness appears and a dull ache may be present in the flank. Sometimes blood appears in the urine. A slowly progressive type of uremia develops, and the patient may live several years in relative comfort, even when two to three times the normal amount of wastes are present in the blood.

CONCLUSION

The advice of a fifteenth-century physician (Arderne) on "the governance of nephritics" included the admonition that such patients "should put away anger and all strenuous business and intense occupation and all manner of things that disturb the soul or move it in any way save only joy." Easy words those, but in that day the joyous state of mind must have been indeed difficult of adoption. Today, as a result of the enormous advances of the past century, or even of the past twenty years, it has become possible to remove from many the soul-disturbing fear of nephritis. It has become possible to send many nephritic patients back to their strenuous business. To others more seriously ill, it has become the physician's happy lot to bring a degree of physical comfort undreamed of heretofore.

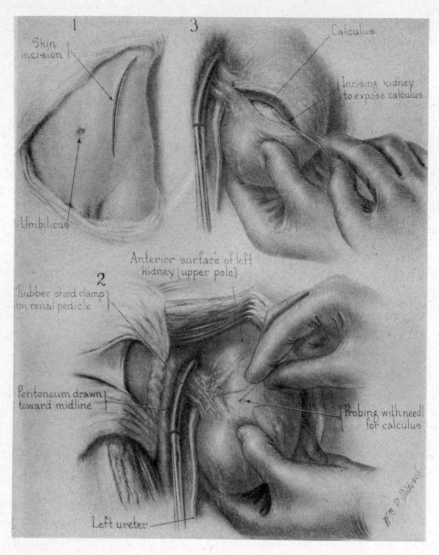

Vertical incision (1) is made on the left side of the abdomen to get to the left kidney which is not functioning properly.

A calculus (stone) is lodged somewhere in the kidney. The surgeon uses a needle to probe the area. (2)

The stone is localized (3) and the portion of the kidney is opened. The stone can be seen through the open wound.

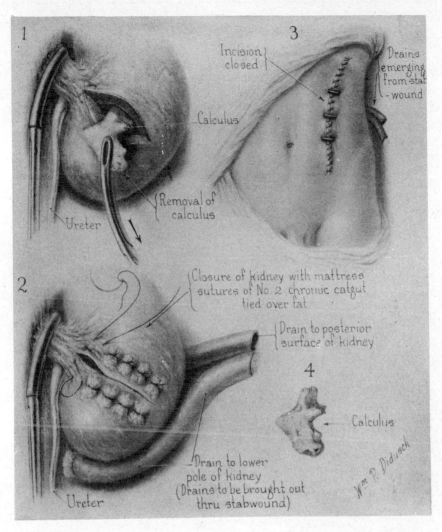

The stone (1) is being removed with a forceps. The ureter is the tube which conducts urine from the kidney to the bladder.

Sutures are used to sew together the sides of the cut surfaces of the kidney. (2)

The incision in the abdominal wall is sewed up and the operation is complete. (3)

Picture of the removed calculus (4) which was causing the kidney disorder.

Postgraduate Medicine

KIDNEY REMOVAL, SURGERY INVOLVING (See also *Kidneys*) When the knowledge of physiology is applied to surgery, new procedures become possible that would formerly not have been attempted. This refers particularly to the necessary removal of what were formerly considered vital organs. Attention is called to the fact that the human body is constructed with factors of safety so that some organs are duplicated and others are of such large mass that sections may be removed without hazard to life. Thus there are two kidneys and one can do the work. The operation for surgical removal of the kidney has been steadily improved. Functional tests will show that the kidney that remains is carrying on the necessary elimination of fluids from the body.

For many years attempts have been made to transplant a kidney into the human body using on occasion the kidney from a person who died suddenly as the result of an accident but thus far failure has resulted in all such efforts. Toward the end of 1955 a successful transplant was made of a kidney from one identical twin into the body of his brother. There seems to be some reason to believe that this type of transplant may be successful.

KNEECAP See discussion under *Joint Disturbances.*

KWASHIORKOR (See also discussion under *Diarrhea, Child Care, Milk, Pellagra*) *Kwashiorkor* is a nutritional disorder found in many countries. The World Health Organization and Food and Agriculture Organization of the United Nations called a conference of experts, which was held in Africa, to consider the problem. The disease is apparently associated with a lack of milk protein in the diet, and a damaging excess of carbohydrates in relation to protein. The name *Kwashiorkor* means "red boy" or "syndrome of the changeling." Signs of the disease appear in infants a few months old, when weaning begins. The symptoms are somewhat like those of pellagra, from which the disease must be differentiated. The child's skin develops an odd appearance, described as "crazy pavement dermatosis." His hair develops a brownish color. And with these symptoms come diarrhea, underweight, swelling of the skin with fluid, weak and thin muscles, anemia, and mental apathy. The child becomes sad and does not smile or play. When the youngster is fed dried skim milk or mixtures of various plant proteins with bananas, he usually recovers.

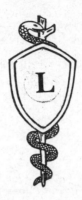

LARYNGITIS (See also *Hoarseness*) Inflammation of the vocal cords may follow overuse of the voice, irritation by chemical substances, or infection.

Men, who are more frequently subjected to exposure to irritant substances in their occupations and who indulge more than women in deleterious habits, suffer more from laryngitis than do women. Contributing causes to inflammation of the larynx include the swallowing of hot or spicy foods, the abuse of alcohol and tobacco and similar irritants. Occasionally the larynx becomes inflamed because there is an infection in the throat or the lungs. In fact any condition that blocks breathing through the nose helps to cause laryngitis because large amounts of air then pass directly to the larynx without having been modified, as is usual, in passing through the nasal tract.

Often laryngitis occurs in such infectious diseases as scarlet fever, measles, chicken pox, and diphtheria as a secondary complication. Eruptions on the skin and mucous membranes may also affect the larynx. Sensitivity to foods which will produce blisters in the mouth and gastro-intestinal tract may also produce swelling and blisters in the larynx. Finally, hemorrhagic diseases, with exudation of blood into the skin or mucous membranes, may cause blood to flow into the tissues of the larynx and thus produce hoarseness.

In serious cases of laryngitis it is customary to go to bed and keep quiet. Nothing helps the vocal cords under such circumstances like continuous rest, speaking only in a whisper. The application of an icebag or ice collar to the throat or of moist compresses is soothing. Some people prefer warmth. This does not seem to make a great deal of difference. A measure which comes down from ancient history is the inhaling of steam to which various aromatic oils can be added. Apparently the chief benefit is derived, however, not from the aromatic oils but from the moisture and the warmth. Nowadays many special devices have been developed, using electrical heat in order to produce such steam for inhaling. These devices are usually much safer than the old-fashoned dish or kettle of hot water. Many instances have been known of severe burns from accidents with open kettles of exceedingly hot water used in this way.

With serious laryngitis, particularly that complicated by inflammation or infection, the physician may prescribe many drugs that are helpful in securing rest and in soothing the area concerned.

LARYNGITIS—See RESPIRATORY DISEASES, article THE RESPIRATORY DISEASES.

LARYNGITIS—adenoidal discharge may cause: See EAR, article THE EAR, TONGUE, NOSE, AND THROAT.

LARYNX The larynx, commonly called the voice box, consists of a number of cartilages held together by muscles and ligaments so as to make a tubular structure holding the vocal cords. At its upper end is a structure called the epiglottis, which serves to keep food from going down the larynx and windpipe and causes it to pass instead from the pharynx into the esophagus and stomach.

The chief purpose of the larynx is to aid speech. However, it also is capable of helping with expectoration. When a moving column of air strikes the vocal bands, it is set in vibration. Speech includes, however, not only the vibration of this column of air but the molding of the column with the help of the tongue, the teeth, the palate, and the lips. If any of these structures does not function properly, the voice can be greatly changed. The adult male possesses a deep voice because of the action of the long vocal cord during its relaxed state. A low-pitched voice is produced by a slow-moving cord and a high-pitched voice is produced by a vocal cord that vibrates with an increased frequency.

The doctor looks at the larynx with several different technics. For the usual examination he wears a head mirror which casts light into the mouth. The person who is going to be examined puts out his tongue, which is held out with a piece of sterile gauze. While the tongue is held gently, the patient breathes through the mouth with short gasps of breath. Then the doctor puts a mirror, which has been slightly warmed to prevent condensation of air on its surface, into the back of the throat and requests the patient to say "Ah." This raises the palate, and the mirror may be passed a little farther into the throat. By regulating the angle of the mirror the doctor can see the vocal cords. If the patient makes various sounds, the doctor can determine whether or not the vocal cords vibrate

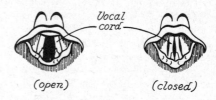

(open)   (closed)

The larynx is the organ of the voice. The vocal cords in the larynx, by stretching and shortening, open and close and give rise to sounds of various pitches.

properly. He can also see whether or not they have been modified by inflammation or swelling or the growth of nodes. For some people who are very sensitive, the use of a local anesthetic may be necessary to permit passing the mirror into the back of the throat. Technics have also been developed which permit the doctor to look directly at the vocal cords with instruments especially designed for the purpose.

One of the first signs of inflammation of the larynx and of the vocal cords is hoarseness, so that hoarseness and laryngitis have become almost synonymous. There are, however, many causes for inflammation.

LARYNX—cancer: See article CANCER.

LARYNX—croup: See INFANCY, article CARE AND FEEDING OF THE CHILD.

LARYNX—diphtheria: See INFANCY, article CARE AND FEEDING OF THE CHILD.

LARYNX—spasmophilia: See INFANCY, article CARE AND FEEDING OF THE CHILD.

LARYNX—tetany: See INFANCY, article CARE AND FEEDING OF THE CHILD.

LARYNX—tuberculosis: See RESPIRATORY DISEASES, article THE RESPIRATORY DISEASES.

LAUGHTER When a human being laughs, he exercises a number of muscles that are not usually put into action. Laughter serves also to stimulate the circulation and for that reason it is a healthy performance. Animals do not laugh but they have other methods of expressing joy.

When a person laughs, his diaphragm moves up and down and the outgoing air stimulates his larynx and produces the sounds that are known as chuckles. Babies laugh very early in life. They respond to tickling by laughter. Women as a rule do not laugh as heartily or easily as men. Experts in etiquette are inclined to rate loud laughter as vulgar. Therefore exuberant laughter by women is not considered refined.

There are still some differences of opinion as to the age at which the baby first laughs. Even tiny babies smile but most scientists are convinced that this is a reaction of some internal mechanism, even "gas on the stomach." Real laughter occurs in babies after they are one month old.

Laughter is seldom followed by any harmful reaction to the body except that occasionally hiccups follow due to the stimulation of the diaphragm. Cases are also known in which excessive laughter resulted in a sudden revulsion of the stomach or contraction of the diaphragm resulting in vomiting. Excessive laughter may also cause loss of control over some of the voluntary muscles of the body so that those which control the bladder and the rectum suddenly relax. This happens particularly to children who soil themselves following excessive laughter. Tickling to excess may produce this kind of reaction.

The chief value of laughter in health is the fact that it is associated with relaxation of the mind and the body, which means a lessening of nerve tension.

While it is true that laughter will exercise the spaces of the lungs that are not easily ventilated, the practice of laughter as a means of ventilation is not helpful. There are other ways of ventilating the lungs. Laughter is then, like every other function of the body, a mechanism that should be used enough but never too much. Overexercise or overuse of any function of the human body is not conducive to its best development.

LAXATIVES See *Cathartics and Laxatives.*

LEFT-HANDEDNESS From the beginning of time left-handedness has had associated with it the idea of evil and right-handedness of good. Man was probably in the first place ambidextrous —that is, he could use both hands with equal facility. The celebrated artist, sculptor, painter, and anatomist, Leonardo da Vinci, according to reports, had equal facility with both hands. It is said that he used to draw with his left hand and paint with the right. It has also been argued that the ancient Semitic peoples were left-handed because they read and wrote from right to left. However, the Bible mentions specifically the fact that David received a company of men who could use both the right and left hands in hurling stones and shooting arrows out of a bow.

Our knowledge of the development of human beings indicates that they gradually tended to become more and more right-handed down to modern times. One suggestion is that man had to face new hazards as civilization developed and that these hazards involved exposure of his vital organs to his enemies. He therefore protected his left side (the side on which his heart lies) and turned his right side toward the foe. Death probably removed those who could not make this adjustment, so that the right hand became dominant. In the modern prize ring it is the custom of good boxers to lead with the left hand so that the left side is the one turned toward the foe.

Attempts have been made to correlate left-handedness with the sizes of various sections of the brain or with various psychological traits. Left-handed pitchers and baseball players generally are supposed to be somewhat bizarre as compared with right-handed pitchers.

Most important about left-handedness is recent evidence to the effect that attempts to cause the right hand to dominate in the child who is normally left-handed are likely to lead to difficulties of mental hygiene. The change from normal left-handedness to right-handedness has been associated with the development of stuttering and awkwardness.

Few people realize that those who are left-handed are also likely to give the preference to the left eye, the left ear, and the left foot exactly as those who are right-handed give preference to the right eye in aiming a gun, turn the right ear when they wish to listen best, and always step first with the right foot. Beyond these facts the normally left-handed child does not differ in any particular of importance from those who are right-handed, so that there would seem to be no good reason to force a normally left-handed child to change to a right-handed one.

LEG ULCERS (See also discussion under *Antibiotics, Edema, Senescence, Ulcers*) As people get older, chronic ulcers of the legs are likely to occur as a result of difficulties with circulation of the blood in the leg. Some drugs introduced into medical practice in recent years have now been combined into a course of treatment for such ulcers. The treatment utilizes methods of overcoming the accumulation of fluid in the tissues, including elevation of the leg and the application of elastic bandages. After the swelling has been lessened, the area is treated with two new preparations. One preparation is plasminogen, derived from the blood, which has the ability to dissolve the accumulated debris. The second preparation is hyaluronidase, which increases the spread of substances introduced into the tissues. Next an antibiotic such as bacitracin is applied. The hyaluronidase permits the penetration of the antibiotic into deep tissues, so as to overcome any latent infections. The Department of Surgery in The New York Hospital—Cornell

Medical Center reports the successful treatment of some cases of chronic ulcers by these methods, most of the patients having been treated entirely as outpatients; the treatment either cleared up the ulcers completely or prepared them successfully for later surgery.

LEPROSY Known to the world since biblical times, leprosy is a chronic transmissible disease due to a specific germ. Characteristic of the disease is the gradual development of areas of tissues without feeling which eventually die and become gangrenous, mutilating the body. In the United States persons with leprosy are kept in colonies—most important of which is at Carville, Louisiana. The condition is directly transmissible and is not nearly so fearsome as its repute would indicate. The condition was without any serious harm to our troops stationed in various portions of the world where leprosy has been more frequent than in the United States.

LEPROSY—cause determined: See INFECTIOUS DISEASE, article THE PREVENTION AND TREATMENT OF INFECTIOUS DISEASE.

LEUKEMIA Leukemia is one of the most fatal of all diseases of the blood. For this condition medicine has not yet established a specific cure. Nevertheless, .technics have been developed which are helpful in many cases; anyone who has the disease or the family of a person who has the disease should not despair, since cases are now known of people who have lived a good many years following the first appearance of the symptoms of leukemia.

Normally a human being has about 7500 white blood cells in every cubic millimeter of blood. In leukemia the white blood cells increase rapidly and may reach figures of from 100,000 to 1,000,000 white blood cells for every cubic millimeter of blood. As the white blood cells increase, the red blood cells and the red coloring matter of the red blood cells break down. This produces a severe condition of anemia and bleeding. The white blood cells are manufactured in the marrow of the bones and in the lymphatic tissues like the spleen, the tonsils, and similar organs. The cells that are made in the bone marrow differ from those made in other places. The white blood cells that are made in the bones have the job of fighting infection whenever germs invade the body.

The sudden tremendous increase of white blood cells which occurs in leukemia has been characterized as a cancer of the blood. The condition occurs not only in human beings but also in horses, dogs, cattle, and other animals. When leukemia develops, the spleen (which is involved in all activities related to the blood) begins to enlarge, and the bone marrow also changes greatly. The doctor makes the diagnosis of leukemia by counting and examining the white blood cells, using a microscope.

A new technic which has given some hope in the treatment of leukemia involves injection into the blood of phosphorus which has been made radioactive with the cyclotron. In twelve cases treated with combined aminopterin and Cortisone benefit was definitely established. New methods of treatment have proved that the life of the patient can be lengthened.

Previously it has been customary to treat leukemia by exposing the spleen and the bones to the X ray. Much depends on the time when the X-ray treatments are given and the extent to which they are capable of lowering the total number of white blood cells. It is also important during the treatment of the patient with leukemia to keep the red blood cells at a proper level by the use of blood transfusions and similar methods.

All studies indicate that leukemia is increasing but the reasons for this are not known. The increase may be related to new conditions of modern life involving exposure to various chemicals, smoke, automobile exhaust, tars in the streets, X ray exposure and dissemination of atomic radioactivity. Drugs have been found such as the nitrogen mustards and a new drug called 6-mercaptopurine which seem to have a definite effect on leukemia. Another new drug which is much used is myleran. These drugs have been so effective in many cases that X ray treatments can be discontinued. Also of use in such cases is an antifolic acid drug called aminopterin. These investigations lead to the belief that science is on the road to a better understanding and control of leukemia.

LEUKEMIA—See BLOOD, article THE BLOOD AND ITS DISEASES; article CANCER.

LEUKEMIA—chemotherapy: See article CANCER.

LEUKEMIA—infectious mononucleosis stimulates: See BLOOD, article THE BLOOD AND ITS DISEASES.

LEUKEMIA—platelet count decreased: See BLOOD, article THE BLOOD AND ITS DISEASES.

LEUKEMIA—radiation may cause: See article OCCUPATION AND HEALTH.

LEUKOCYTES The white blood cells are known technically as leukocytes. They are masses of material seen under the microscope as collections of granular tissue. There are many different kinds of leukocytes, which are classified according to the number and nature of the cells that they contain. In certain diseases, such as granulocytopenia, they may be found almost totally absent from the blood. In other diseases, like leu-

kemia, their number is tremendously increased. Sensitivity to certain toxic drugs like pyramidon may cause a complete disappearance of the white blood cells. Since these cells are necessary in resistance to infection, absence of the cells may result in death.

LEUKOPLAKIA Sometimes great white patches develop on the tongue, the cheeks, and the gums. These patches are separated by little fissures or paths, so that the condition looks like a relief map. Because it has been believed to be related to smoking, it has also been called smoker's tongue and smoker's patches. The exact cause of the condition has not been determined but it is advisable to discontinue smoking. Continuous irritation is sometimes followed by cancer.

LEUKOPLAKIA—See article CANCER.

LEUKOPLAKIA—deficiency of vitamin B complex may cause: See article CANCER.

LEUKORRHEA The word "leukorrhea" comes from two Greek words meaning a white flow. The condition is called in slang "the whites." Usually it represents the excessive formation of mucus and secretion from the cells of the female sex organs. Continued excessive flow means that the physician should be consulted to determine whether or not there is any infection or continued irritation. The repeated use of douches, sometimes containing irritating substances, may make the condition worse rather than better.

LICE The louse is an annoying inhabitant on the human body. Head lice are such a frequent annoyance among children in schools that health departments usually give special instructions for their control. Several specialized mixtures have been developed for getting rid of head lice, body lice, and pubic lice.

To kill head lice ordinary crude petroleum or kerosene mixed with sweet oil or olive oil, half and half, is rubbed well into the scalp. Then cover the hair with a piece of muslin for at least two hours or, better, overnight. Remember that petroleum is poisonous and inflammable. Never let the hair get close to any open flame, such as a gas jet or a lighted match. When the muslin is removed, wash the hair and scalp with soap and hot water and rinse well with clear water. Repeat this process as long as live vermin are found in the hair. The nits may be removed by wetting the hair thoroughly with hot vinegar and then combing with a fine-toothed comb. Always dry the hair completely after such treatments before going out.

For body lice, the body, all clothing, and all bedding may be thoroughly dusted with a suitable DDT powder.

Pubic lice are commonly called crabs. Specialized ointments, including the old-fashioned blue ointment and "Gammexane" ointment, are used, rubbing the ointment thoroughly into the infested areas. If such lice get into the eyelashes they should be picked off, with their nits, by a forcep.

Itching from the bites of lice or other insects is controllable by ointments or lotions containing small amounts of phenol or menthol or camphor, such as 1 per cent phenol or menthol in calamine lotion or phenolated camphor in mineral oil.

Lice—See Skin, article The Skin.
Lice—head: See Hair, article The Hair.
Lice—impetigo: See Skin, article The Skin.
Lice—tularemia: See article Transmissible Diseases.

Lice—typhus fever: See article Transmissible Diseases.

LIGAMENTS Ligaments are the tough fibrous bands that connect bones at the joints and also serve in various portions of the body to support the organs of the body. Ligaments are usually fibrous tissues. They can be torn from the bones at the points where they are joined or otherwise damaged. They may heal by fixation of the part that has been injured. Sometimes a surgical operation is necessary to bring together the torn ends of ligaments. In modern orthopedic surgery motion may be restored when it has been lost by paralysis through the transfer of ligaments from one place to another.

Ligaments—See article Arthritis, Rheumatism, and Gout.

LIMPING, INTERMITTENT Whenever the blood vessels in the legs become obstructed or obliterated by inflammation, by hardening, or by other diseases, there occur symptoms like numbness, tingling, and burning sensations in the toes. Other sensations of deficiency in the circulation include a feeling of heaviness and pain, cramps in the legs, and weakness of the legs and feet.

Before the signs of complete blocking of the blood vessels are apparent, the condition called intermittent claudication, or intermittent limping, may occur. This begins with severe cramping pains in the calf muscles during walking. The pains subside with rest. The symptom is apparently due to narrowing of the blood vessels in the area concerned together with the loss of ability of the body to develop increased blood circulation. People with intermittent limping can regulate the appearance of the symptom by stopping activity of the legs as soon as the sensation appears.

Intermittent limping is particularly associated with a condition called Buerger's disease which is due to an inflammation that blocks the blood vessels. There are other conditions which are much like intermittent limping and which need to be differentiated from Buerger's disease when this symptom occurs. Spasms of the muscles due to difficulties with the nerves that supply the muscles may cause cramplike pains. Lack of suitable balance because of the wearing of the wrong kind of shoes, particularly the wearing of exceedingly high heels by women, may produce trouble in the muscles of the legs and, associated with such trouble, the symptom of limping.

In one case an actor who had been tap-dancing as a job for many years developed a shortening of the tendon which goes to the heel. When he was out of work, he walked a great deal, seeking employment. This overstretched the large muscle at the back of the leg and threw it into spasms so that limping followed. Proper attention to the condition of the muscles and the tendons brought about a cure.

When a doctor is confronted with this condition, his first step is to study the circulation to find out whether or not it is being carried on adequately. The color of the skin is dependent on an adequate supply of blood. In one simple test the leg is raised and then the foot is flexed several times—that is to say, it is bent toward the knee. This will cause the skin to become colorless because of an absence of circulation. When the leg is lowered the color will return if there is adequate circulation. Additional studies are made of the circulation of the blood in the leg. Of course cold will cause the skin to become pale. Therefore it is preferable that the leg be warm and that the air in which the test is performed be warm to prevent disturbance of the test by this factor.

Occasionally limping develops because of damage to the nervous system. In other instances it is associated with dislocations of the hips and still other cases are associated with diseases like infantile paralysis. A child may limp because the foot has been bruised. Adults sometimes limp because of the breaking down of the arch of the foot. A proper study, however, by someone who thoroughly understands the muscles and their functions will reveal the cause of the limping and the steps to be taken to bring about a cure.

LINIMENTS Liniments are usually oily preparations containing irritating substances that are rubbed into the skin with a view to affording relief from pain and to bringing about increased circulation of the blood and thus promoting cure. While liniments are themselves helpful, they are not specifically curative of any condition.

LIPOMA Tumors made of fat are called lipomas. They are usually not malignant and are usually painless. Because of the appearance that they create, they are usually best removed by surgical procedures.

LIPS Lips are essentially muscles covered by mucous membrane.

When the human body is formed before birth, the lips sometimes fail to grow together as they should. The result of such a failure is called harelip. In the more severe cases the palate also fails to grow together, so that harelip is combined with cleft palate. Fortunately modern plastic surgery is able to repair these conditions, frequently with such a high degree of success that the previous existence of the condition is not recognized. Usually the operation is done in early infancy, as it is more easily performed at such time and the possibility of cure is greater.

Another change which occurs in the lips is the development of overgrowth of some of the glandular tissue, so that a gradual painless enlargement (usually of the upper lip) takes place. This condition is also treated surgically with success.

Inflammation of the lips is not infrequently due to irritation or infection. Action of wind, the cold, the sun, or sensitivity to the chemical ingredients of lipsticks may bring about inflammation of the lip with crusting and cracking. Removal of exposure to the cause and application of a protective ointment usually will bring about a cure of such mild inflammations.

More recently there has been recognized a condition in which the corners of the mouth crack with the appearance

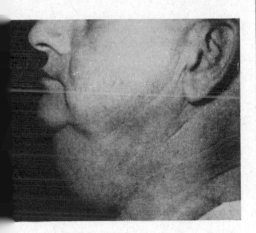

A lipoma is a type of tumor which contains fatty tissue. Lipomas frequently affect the area beneath the chin, and they do not move on swallowing.

Postgraduate Medicine

of blisters. This has been associated with a deficiency of riboflavin. The taking of an adequate amount of this vitamin, together with the practice of scrupulous cleanliness and the application of an ointment to protect the irritated area, usually results in a cure.

Not infrequent also are serious infections of the upper lip of the type of the carbuncle. These are exceedingly serious because the profuse blood supply of the upper lip may cause the infection to extend rapidly to some of the vital areas of the body. Cases are known in which a carbuncle or abscess of the upper lip resulted in death. Infection with the organism called the streptococcus is especially dangerous. Fortunately modern medicine has developed specifics like the sulfonamide drugs and penicillin for infections of this type, so that the danger of death nowadays is much less than previously.

About the most serious condition that can affect the lip is cancer. For years doctors have warned against chronic irritation of the lip. An irritated spot on the lip is much more serious than one elsewhere on the body because cancer of the lip grows more rapidly and spreads faster than does cancer elsewhere. Fortunately there are now excellent methods of treatment, so that early attention to such an irritated area will prevent cancer and bring about a cure. Cancer of the lip is treated by removal with surgery, by irradiation with radium or X ray, by electric coagulation, or by combinations of these methods.

Fever blisters or herpes of the lip are common, particularly in women. They are usually associated with nerve strain, menstruation, or with the eating of substances to which people may be sensitive.

Lips—boils may cause meningitis: See Skin, article The Skin.

Lips—cancer: See article Cancer.

LIVER (See also *Hepatitis, Jaundice*) One of the largest single organs of the human body is the liver. It develops at least a pint of bile each day. Every vein that leaves any part of the digestive tract in the abdomen goes to the liver; these veins carry to the liver in the form of blood the protein, the sweet, and the starchy foods absorbed by the blood vessels of the stomach, the small intestines, the pancreas, and the large intestines. They carry the products of meats, sugars, and starches. The sugar is stored in the liver until it is needed, in the form of a substance called glycogen, which is then used in the muscles when they act.

The liver also acts to break down poisons coming from the stomach and intestines as well as other parts of the body. It helps to remove various foreign substances from the blood. Probably it helps also in regulating the concentration of the fluid material in the blood and in regulating the heat of the body.

So important are the functions of the liver for health that several tests have been developed to measure the scope of its activities. These tests are based largely on determinations of the amount of bile salts regularly developed by the liver, carried in the blood, and excreted in the urine. There are also tests for measuring the ability of the liver to take care of sugar that is put into the body. Tests have also been devised for determining the ability of the liver to get rid of various toxic substances.

When the liver becomes infected or inflamed for any reason, therefore, a serious condition may develop. This is largely dependent on the difficulty in maintaining enough sugar in the circulation to carry on the work of the body. In any instance in which the liver cells have been greatly damaged, the cells react by pouring out their glycogen. Under such circumstances physicians inject extra glucose into the body to meet its needs for sugar and often give insulin as well to help the body take care of the extra glucose. Symptoms indicating a shortage of sugar sometimes brought about by an excess of insulin are abnormal fatigue, sleepiness, apathy, and confusion. There are, of course, many other conditions in which somewhat similar symptoms occur. The diagnosis is made by the physician through actually testing the amount of sugar in the circulating blood.

Fortunately the human being has great factors of safety in relation to the liver. It has been estimated that each of us has about seven times as much liver as is required to carry on the necessary functions of the body. The normal liver weighs three or four pounds.

Among the most serious of the diseases that may affect the liver are cirrhosis, or hardening, and atrophy, or wasting, as well as infection by a wide variety of bacteria and parasites which may cause abscesses. Recent research indicates that vitamin deficiencies, particularly a deficiency of thiamin, or vitamin B_1, may be related to hardening of the liver.

The liver reacts to poisons of various sorts by the disappearance of its functioning cells and their replacement by fat. A high excess of fat in the diet may also tend to produce actual storage of fat in the liver. Drugs particularly harmful to the liver are chloroform, carbon tetrachloride (which is used in dry cleaning), arsenic, and phosphorus.

Most important in relation to the liver is the fact that it can almost completely regenerate itself, if given a chance, after it has been damaged.

People with severe liver disease may have a characteristic odor of the breath variously described as musty or like a mixture of rotten eggs and garlic. Research has shown that this may be due to changes in the chemistry of the blood because of failure of the liver to act on certain protein materials. These substances which may appear in the breath or the urine are sulfides.

LIVER—amebas locate: See article DIGESTION AND DIGESTIVE DISEASES.

LIVER—amebic abscess: See article DIGESTION AND DIGESTIVE DISEASES.

LIVER—avoided in gout diet: See article ARTHRITIS, RHEUMATISM, AND GOUT.

LIVER—cancer of bowels: See article DIGESTION AND DIGESTIVE DISEASES.

LIVER—choline prevents accumulation of fat: See article DEFICIENCY DISEASES.

LIVER—cirrhosis: See article DIGESTION AND DIGESTIVE DISEASES.

LIVER—diabetes affected by: See article DIABETES.

LIVER—disease: See article DIGESTION AND DIGESTIVE DISEASES. See also entry JAUNDICE.

LIVER—dysentery: See article TRANSMISSIBLE DISEASES.

LIVER—function: See article DIGESTION AND DIGESTIVE DISEASES.

LIVER—glandular fever: See article DIGESTION AND DIGESTIVE DISEASES.

LIVER—glycogen stored by: See article DIGESTION AND DIGESTIVE DISEASES.

LIVER—hepatitis: See article DIGESTION AND DIGESTIVE DISEASES.

LIVER—spots: See SKIN, article THE SKIN.

LIVER—sugar stored in: See article DIABETES.

LIVER EXTRACTS Liver extracts are used in the treatment of pernicious anemia. It has been found that the liver contains a substance which stimulates the formation of red blood corpuscles in the blood of people suffering from pernicious anemia.

LIVER EXTRACT—allergy to: See article ALLERGY.

LIVER EXTRACT—gastritis, chronic: See article DIGESTION AND DIGESTIVE DISEASES.

LIVER EXTRACT—pernicious anemia: See BLOOD, article THE BLOOD AND ITS DISEASES.

LIVER EXTRACT—seborrheic dermatitis: See HAIR, article THE HAIR.

LIVER SPOTS Liver spots, scientifically called chloasma, frequently appear without any definite cause. They also represent a deposit of color pigments from the blood in the skin. Liver spots seem to be associated with glandular disturbances. They appear where there is pressure from a pad or belt; sometimes they are associated with the application of light, heat, or perfume. Often they disappear spontaneously.

It is not safe for anyone to attempt to peel away these liver spots by self-treatment because of the dangerous character of the substances that are used.

LIVER SPOTS—See SKIN, article THE SKIN.

LOCKJAW See *Tetanus.*

LOCOMOTOR ATAXIA When syphilis gets into the nervous system, it produces serious changes. By modern scientific technics it has been determined with certainty that two diseases —namely, locomotor ataxia (also called tabes, paresis) and paralytic dementia —are definitely related to syphilitic infection. Locomotor ataxia is the result of infection of the spinal column. Frequently it comes on five to fifteen years after the person was first infected with syphilis.

In locomotor ataxia the tissues of the spine are so damaged that reflexes like the knee jerk disappear. Changes take place in the ability of the pupil of the eye to react as it should. In a typical case of locomotor ataxia the eye will react to looking at a distance and then at a near object with the opening and closing of the pupil. The eye will not, however, in the presence of locomotor ataxia react to dark by closing and opening the pupil. In many cases the pupils are irregular in size and slow to react.

Other disturbances associated with locomotor ataxia are knifelike pains in the abdomen, legs, or face and all sorts of abnormal sensations related to cold and warmth and numbness. Sometimes there is a feeling of tingling and often a sensation that bugs are running on the skin.

One of the most serious symptoms of locomotor ataxia is inability to co-ordinate actions of the muscles. The affected person may not be able to touch the tip of his nose with his finger. His legs get out of order, so that he finds it hard to walk in the dark. His gait may change so that in the late stages his foot seems to be thrown up and then brought down unsteadily as if it were being slapped on the floor. The cast of the legs is somewhat like that in a horse called "string halt."

The sudden severe pains in the internal organs have on occasion been mistaken for appendicitis or inflammation of the intestines.

Without suitable treatment cases of locomotor ataxia get worse but the progress of the disease may be slow, requiring years before the case terminates in death.

New methods of treatment are now being studied with a view to determining whether or not they can control syphilis as it affects the nervous system and thus stop the progress and bring about cure in cases of locomotor ataxia. In some of these studies the drug called penicillin is being injected directly into the spine.

LOCOMOTOR ATAXIA—See EAR, article THE EAR, TONGUE, NOSE, AND THROAT; VENEREAL DISEASES, article THE VENEREAL DISEASES.

LONGEVITY In Sweden in 1755 the average age at death was 34.5 years. In the United States in 1789 life expectancy at birth was about 35 years; in 1955 a child born in the United States can reasonably expect to live more than 68 years. The will to live is deeply rooted in all mankind. From the beginning of time man has sought not only increasing years but increasing years of usefulness. Apparently the older we get, the more anxious we are to keep on living. The person of 85 wants to reach for 90. Those who pass 90 begin to think about reaching 100.

In some families most of the people live to a ripe old age; in others this is the exception. Oliver Wendell Holmes suggested to those who wanted to live long that they select parents and grandparents who live long. In other words, the tendency to live long is to some extent an inherited tendency.

The gag that life in the country is not really longer than life in the city is not based on truth. Of course life in the country may seem longer but the figures show that people who live in the rural districts actually do live four to five years longer than those who live in the cities.

Some jobs are associated with longer life than others. Aviators have a high death rate in contrast even to chauffeurs. The death rate among school teachers is low. Apparently the occupation that is about as safe as any with a view to living longer is that of college professor or president.

Women generally have a better chance of living through to a ripe old age than men. Indeed the largest banks and the insurance companies insist that this tendency is resulting in the gradual concentration of most of the wealth of the nation in the hands of women. It has long been known that retirement not infrequently hastens the death of the aged. A successful businessman when relieved of his usual life tends to degenerate rapidly. Every trifling ailment begins to receive his undivided attention. Dignitaries of the church, chief justices on the Supreme Court benches, prime ministers, and others whose activities may be prolonged to advanced years seem to live much longer than other people.

The common idea that the person who lives long is one of exemplary habits, particularly as relates to the use of tobacco, alcohol, and similar substances, is a false one. An actual study of a considerable number of men who have reached the age of 100 showed that 54 per cent had used alcohol as a beverage during their lives and 46 per cent had been abstainers. Of 26 men over 90 years of age 6 smoked, 5 chewed, and 2 both smoked and chewed tobacco. The remaining 13 (or 50 per cent) had never used tobacco in any form.

Recent figures from the life insurance companies show that a good environment, which means healthy surroundings, is more important in living long than having long-lived parents. One of the reasons why people whose parents have died young also tend to die young is the fact that such people do not have the protection as they grow up which comes to those whose parents live. The child who is an orphan has much less chance of being healthy and of living long than the child whose parents are

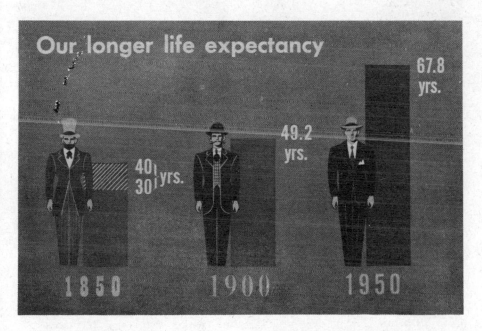

Chart showing the increase in life expectancy since 1850. The increase in longevity points up the great advance in medical science over the past 100 years.

alive. Children from broken families are more poorly housed, fed, and clothed, and receive less medical care than children of families living together with both parents present.

Longevity—See article Old Age.

LOP EARS, PLASTIC SURGERY FOR (See also, *Ear*) There are really few conditions affecting the external ear that are disturbing. Sometimes large portions of the ear may be absent at birth. Occasionally the ears project in an extremely unsightly manner. All these extraordinary appearances are controlled nowadays by the use of plastic surgery. An expert is able to fasten the ear back if it projects exceedingly, to rebuild an ear out of other tissue if portions are missing, and to modify the shape of the ear if it is of extraordinary shape.

Many mothers feel that the ear be-

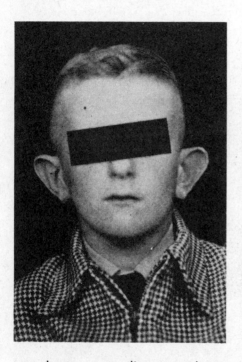 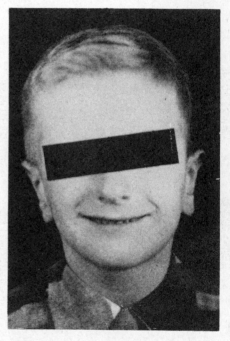

Large, protruding ears do not interfere with hearing but they mar the appearance. A child who is lop-eared should have corrective surgery before school age so he may be spared ridicule from his playmates. Long hair usually hides the deformity in girls, but with modern hair styles correction of the exposed malformed ear is often deemed necessary. Deformities, however slight, may cause psychological consequences, especially in the sensitive child.

Postgraduate Medicine

came a lop ear because the child lay on his ear with the ear crumpled when he was small or because he wore his hat pressed down on the ears. There is no evidence that these factors are really of any importance. The fault is one of anatomical development. Manipulation of and bandaging the ears to hold them against the head will not correct the condition.

Occasionally, small tumors will de- velop on the outer ear; these may be removed if they show the slightest tend- ency to growth or irritation.

The ear may be infected by pimples or boils or by an infection of the type of erysipelas, in which it swells to a tremendous size. Such conditions should have the best available surgical treat- ment, in order to prevent destruction and damage that would require plastic surgery for repair.

CONTINUED IN VOLUME 6

A MODERN MEDICAL AND HEALTH LIBRARY
FOR THE FAMILY . . . INCLUDES ALL THE
CONTENTS OF "THE MODERN HOME
MEDICAL ADVISOR" AND "THE POP-
ULAR MEDICAL ENCYCLOPEDIA"
PLUS ADDITIONAL ARTICLES,
PHOTOGRAPHS AND CHARTS.

ILLUSTRATED

MEDICAL

AND

HEALTH

ENCYCLOPEDIA

VOLUME 6
LOSS AND GAIN OF WEIGHT — PREGNANCY

ILLUSTRATED

MEDICAL

AND

HEALTH

ENCYCLOPEDIA

EDITED BY

MORRIS FISHBEIN, M.D.

EDITOR, MEDICAL PROGRESS; EDITOR, MODERN HOME MEDICAL
ADVISER; MEDICAL EDITOR, BRITANNICA BOOK OF THE YEAR;
CONTRIBUTING-EDITOR, POST GRADUATE MEDICINE; AND
FOR 25 YEARS EDITOR OF THE JOURNAL OF
THE AMERICAN MEDICAL ASSOCIATION

WITH THE COLLABORATION OF LEADING
SPECIALISTS IN MEDICINE AND SURGERY

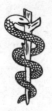

H. S. STUTTMAN CO., *Publishers*
NEW YORK, N. Y.

ILLUSTRATED MEDICAL AND HEALTH ENCYCLOPEDIA
contains new entries and illustrations plus material from
THE MODERN HOME MEDICAL ADVISOR. (Copyright © 1935, 1939, 1940,
1941, 1942, 1948, 1951, 1953, 1956, by Doubleday and Company, Inc.)
and THE POPULAR MEDICAL ENCYCLOPEDIA, revised and
enlarged edition, (Copyright © 1946, 1950, 1953, 1956)
by Doubleday and Company, Inc.

PRINTED IN THE UNITED STATES OF AMERICA
BY ROTARY GRAPHIC PRESS INC., NEW YORK 16, N. Y.

4

LOSS AND GAIN OF WEIGHT

(See also, *Weight, Over and Under*) A careful medical examination always includes a record of the patient's weight and particularly information as to whether he has been gaining or losing weight rapidly. Doctors have tabulations which show the average weight for people according to their age, sex, height, and body build. Some people are tall and thin with light bones and light muscles. Others may be stocky, short, muscular.

Water constitutes about seventy per cent of the body weight. About one fifth of all the water is outside the individual cells. This is found in the blood, the spinal fluid, the lymph and a small amount between the cells. The remainder of the body weight is in solid structures like the bones; most of the minerals of the body are in the bones. Sugars are stored in the body—principally in the liver and muscles—as glycogen.

Fat is an inactive material deposited around the body in storage depots.

Proteins are the chief building elements of the cells. The body needs four grams of water or each gram of protein. The amount of calories taken by the body to maintain its weight depends on the rate at which the body uses up material, and this in turn is related to the amount of activity. Growth requires increased calories. When inadequate amounts of calories are taken into the body the deficit is supplied by using up material from the tissues. The fat is drawn upon but also the carbohydrates. When both fat and carbohydrate are utilized, the protein is taken up. This means the breakdown of some functioning cells.

Conditions in which there is interference with the usual elimination of sodium cause increased water retention and gain in weight. Examples are heart failure, toxemia of pregnancy, hardening or cirrhosis of the liver and congestive heart failure. Elimination of water is improved by stopping salt, improving heart action, or by drugs which increase the action of the kidneys.

Increase of fluid in the body occurs when the protein is inadequate. In such cases restoration of protein results in elimination of water. Excess of sweating or severe diarrhea also draw water from the body and thus lower weight.

The weight of the body is also related to the action of the thyroid gland which has a part in determining the basal metabolism. Fever will increase the metabolic rate. Excess action of the thyroid will also give a rate over on the plus side whereas deficient action of the thyroid moves the rate to the minus side.

Eating is regulated by many factors. Appetite may be part of a habit of large eating. Many families put overemphasis on eating. Grandmothers offer food as cures for most family disturbances.

Sometimes a person who has had an active life with heavy eating changes to a sedentary life. The eating habits persist and he puts on weight. Some people eat as a substitute for satisfactions that they do not obtain through other emotional sources. Incidentally, alcoholics frequently drink because they escape other demands in this way. An unusual cause of excessive eating is overactivity of the pancreas gland in developing insulin. An injury to the brain which affects certain portions of a part of the brain called the hypothalamus may be associated with the development of a voracious appetite. But by far the vast majority of cases of obesity are due to taking too much food in relation to the metabolism and activity of the body.

Loss of weight can be produced by lowering the calorie intake to less than the body requirement. Starvation may result from lack of appetite which is called anorexia. Loss of appetite occurs in acute and chronic infections, in certain forms of cancer and glandular diseases. Loss of appetite may be wholly psychologic or mental, producing a condition called anorexia nervosa.

LUNG CANCER   (See also discussion under *Cancer, Detection of Cancer, Lungs, Research in Cancer, Smoking and Lung Cancer*) The increasing occurrence of primary cancer of the lung has now reached the point where it is second only to the occurrence of primary cancer of the stomach. This is attributed to such causes already mentioned as the use of motor vehicles and tarred roads, exposure to pulmonary irritants from the air and from smoking, the presence of radioactive emanation and increased bacterial and viral infections of the lung tissue. The early diagnosis of cancer of the lung is exceedingly difficult even with the best possible use of the X-ray. Even when the X-ray appearance arouses suspicion, the necessity is still apparent of actually removing portions of the tissue for examination under the microscope. Once the diagnosis of cancer of the lung is made, the only possible chance of cure is a radical removal of the lung which involves at the same time the removal of all possible lymphatic glandular tissue that might be affected. This is a serious surgical procedure but with the great advances in modern surgery, now yields a much higher percentage of success. Radiation treatment helps in occasional cases and the treatment with hormones such as cortisone and testosterone is also palliative.

LUNGS Primarily the function of the lungs is the provision of oxygen to the red blood cells and the elimination of waste carbon dioxide. The lungs are made of tiny spaces, on the surface of which the smallest blood vessels are exposed to the inhaled air. This surface by actual measurement is fifty times larger than the skin of the whole body. In the rest of the body the capillary or tiny blood vessels give up oxygen and take up carbon dioxide. In the lungs the capillary blood vessels take up oxygen and throw away carbon dioxide.

In a period of twenty-four hours an active man can absorb more than twenty cubic feet of oxygen, and the blood will give up more than twenty cubic feet of carbon dioxide. The lungs work like an automatically self-regulating bellows. Seventeen times a minute the bellows take in air and expel waste products. Automatically the bellows will speed up to seventy or eighty times a minute if the need for air is exceedingly great, as during severe muscular effort or in pneumonia.

When we take a full breath, we use every possible means for enlarging the cavity of the thorax, or chest. We lift our shoulders by action of the muscles; we lift the ribs and breastbone. The diaphragm, which is a large muscle between the chest and abdominal cavity, helps lift the ribs and shoves down the abdominal contents. In this way the capacity of the chest cavity can be enlarged more than two quarts above its resting capacity and more than three

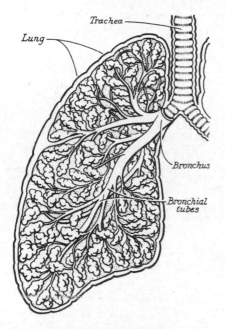

Trachea

Lung

Bronchus

Bronchial tubes

This drawing shows the anatomy of the lung, the most important organ of respiration. There is a right lung and a left lung, with the former being somewhat larger. When the bronchus enters the lung it divides into many small branches called bronchial tubes. The lung is soft and spongy and contains countless tiny air sacs (alveoli). Lung tissue is pink in children and gray to black in adults.

quarts above its capacity at the end of a forced outbreathing or expiration. The mechanism is so complete and so elastic that breathing can go on when the body is in almost any position.

The right lung is larger than the left. It contains three parts, or lobes, whereas the left lung contains two. Sometimes in pneumonia only one lobe will be affected.

Among the diseases which affect the lungs, the most serious are tuberculosis and pneumonia. However, other infections may cause bronchitis or bronchiectasis. All sorts of parasites may affect the lung besides the pneumococcus and the tubercle bacillus. Moreover, the lungs on occasion become subject to cancer. Formerly surgical operations on the lung were impossible. More recently new developments in anesthesia and new methods of surgery have made it possible to operate on the lung. In a period of ten years the surgeons in one hospital did 218 operations on the lungs, removing either an entire lobe or an entire lung, with a total death rate of only 30 deaths out of 218 operations. In a previous century every one of these patients would have died. In 172 cases one lobe was removed, and in this group there were only 9 deaths. In 46 cases an entire lung was removed, and in this group there were 21 deaths. In another hospital an entire lung was removed in 19 cases, and 10 of the patients recovered. Fifty-five per cent of patients who had an operation on the lung because of the presence of cancer recovered. Of course not all cases of cancer can be operated on. The cancer must be localized and accessible, without the possibility of harming other vital organs like the heart.

LUNGS—beryllium poisoning produces changes: See article OCCUPATION AND HEALTH.

LUNGS—bleeding: See article FIRST AID; RESPIRATORY DISEASES, article THE RESPIRATORY DISEASES.

LUNGS—blood circulation: See HEART,

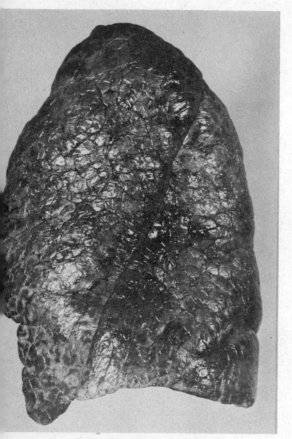

A section of dried lung. In the healthy state the lung is never completely deflated. It may, however, collapse by accident through a puncture wound. In cases of tuberculosis the doctor may collapse a lung as a therapeutic measure. Cleveland Health Museum

article DISEASES OF THE HEART AND CIRCULATION.

LUNGS—bowel cancer: See article DIGESTION AND DIGESTIVE DISEASES.

LUNGS—cancer: See article CANCER.

LUNGS—lymph nodes: See BLOOD, article THE BLOOD AND ITS DISEASES.

LUNGS—periodic examination for cancer: See article CANCER.

LUNGS—pneumococcus: See INFECTIOUS DISEASE, article THE PREVENTION AND TREATMENT OF INFECTIOUS DISEASE.

LUNGS—pneumonia: See RESPIRATORY DISEASES, article THE RESPIRATORY DISEASES.

LUNGS—psittacosis: See article TRANSMISSIBLE DISEASES.

LUNGS—silicosis: See article OCCUPATION AND HEALTH.

LUNGS—tuberculosis: See INFECTIOUS DISEASE, article THE PREVENTION AND TREATMENT OF INFECTIOUS DISEASE.

LUNGS—whooping cough: See CHILDHOOD DISEASES, article INFECTIOUS DISEASES OF CHILDHOOD.

LUNGS—X-ray examination for tuberculosis: See RESPIRATORY DISEASES, article THE RESPIRATORY DISEASES.

LUNG, SURGERY OF THE (See also discussion under *Lung, Tuberculosis, Bronchiectesis, Empyema* and *Pleurisy*) Recent advances in the treatment of tuberculosis have greatly broadened the scope of surgery in that condition. Drugs have been developed such as streptomycin, paraminosalicylic acid and isoniazid which can control infections in many instances. However, the ease of removal of portions of diseased lungs has made it possible to excise such portions. Surgeons believe that lung tissue should be saved whenever possible to avoid complete removal of lobes or whole lungs. The surgeon makes an appraisal of the amount of lung to be removed by the use of x-ray films and the improvements in x-ray have made possible accurate appraisal in three dimensions of the tissue that may be diseased.

Some twenty-five years have passed since a successful removal of an entire lung was accomplished. Among the names which prevail as innovators in this field are those of Rudolph Nissen now of Basle, Switzerland and Evar Graham of Washington University, St. Louis. Today great numbers of thoracic surgeons operate on the chest removing one lobe or several lobes of the lung or an entire lung and these operations have been successful in cases of abcess of the lung, of tumor of the lung and of tuberculosis and many other conditions. In some clinics thousands of such operations have been performed with a

high degree of success. The success of such operations depends naturally on control of bleeding, on devices for maintaining respiration during the operative procedure which may be done in a negative pressure chamber, on the use of anesthesia which is of a type that keeps the breathing out of the picture.

LYMPH In addition to the arteries and the veins, most of the tissues of the body are connected with the lymphatic system. The lymphatic vessels contain a transparent, slightly yellow fluid that is called lymph. When red blood cells get into the lymph, it may have a light rose color. The lymph helps to maintain the fluid state of the tissues. The lymph

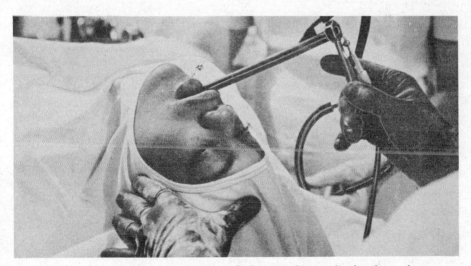

A tube-like instrument with a light on the end, the broncho-scope, is passed through the throat down to the lung. The bronchus and lung area can be visualized and a piece of tissue obtained for microscopic study. The bronchoscope is a valuable aid in diagnosing lung abscesses, cancer and in localizing foreign bodies. The patient is conscious during the procedure but there is a loss of sensation in the chest area because of local anesthesia.

Postgraduate Medicine

channels serve to carry away infected material from the tissues.

LYMPH—See article DIGESTION AND DIGESTIVE DISEASES.

LYMPH NODES—breast cancer spreads to: See article CANCER.

LYMPH NODES—chemotherapy in Hodgkin's disease: See article CANCER.

LYMPH NODES—enlargement: See BLOOD, article THE BLOOD AND ITS DISEASES; article CANCER.

LYMPH NODES—German measles causes to swell: See CHILDHOOD DISEASES, article INFECTIOUS DISEASES OF CHILDHOOD.

LYMPH NODES—glanders: See article TRANSMISSIBLE DISEASES.

LYMPH NODES—"glands" a misleading name: See article ENDOCRINOLOGY.

LYMPH NODES—silicosis: See article OCCUPATION AND HEALTH.

LYMPH NODES—syphilis causes to swell: See VENEREAL DISEASES, article THE VENEREAL DISEASES.

LYMPH NODES—tetanus: See article TRANSMISSIBLE DISEASES.

LYMPH NODES—tularemia causes to swell: See article TRANSMISSIBLE DISEASES.

LYMPH NODES—white blood cells manufactured by: See BLOOD, article THE BLOOD AND ITS DISEASES.

LYMPHOPATHIA VENEREUM

Among the conditions that can affect man and which are spread widely by sexual relations is one called scientifically lymphopathia venereum but known also throughout the world by a wide variety of other names, including climatic bubo and tropical ulcer. It has also been called the fourth venereal disease, the other three being gonorrhea, syphilis, and chancroid.

This venereal disease is caused by a filtrable virus—one of those agents so small that it cannot be seen with an ordinary microscope. Most significant of its symptoms, as suggested by the name, is the swelling of the glands following infection by sex contact. Usually a few days after contact with a person who is infected, a small ulcer will appear on the organs. Often this heals without very much trouble, but occasionally it becomes secondarily infected and becomes a large ulcer. The infection spreads, however, along the lymph channels and reaches one of the large lymph glands after ten to thirty days.

The first symptoms are stiffness and aching in the groin, followed by swelling. After the swelling has been large and hard for a while, it breaks down, frequently leaving an opening with an abscess. The breaking down and gradual healing may take anywhere from two months to two years. In very severe cases the infection may spread from the original gland to other glands, may cause a secondary infection of the veins of the leg with great swelling of the tissues, and may, in fact, involve the whole body in a general disease.

About twenty years ago a diagnostic test for this disease, like the skin tests that are used in other diseases, was discovered, and vaccines have been developed which are used in the treatment.

At first it was thought that this condition affected only males because those who suffered from it were chiefly sailors, but more recently the condition has been found also among women all over the world. The condition can be spread from one person to another by the use of nozzles of syringes and in other ways when strict sanitation is not properly practiced.

Usually the first spot of infection will disappear if simply treated with alcohol and antiseptic dressings, but when the glands swell and are infected, other treatments are tried, some of which seem to have yielded success. A vaccine made from the material taken from an infected gland has been reported by many physicians to be especially useful in controlling the duration of the disease.

LYSOL Lysol is the proprietary name for the compound solution of cresol, an antiseptic solution which is also caustic and poisonous in high concentrations.

LYSOL—irritating as vaginal douche: See article SEX HYGIENE.

LYSOL—poisoning: See article FIRST AID.

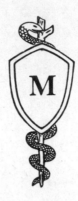

MADURA FOOT In 1898 a Boston physician reported the occurrence in the United States of a peculiar disease usually found only in the tropics. Another case was reported from Galveston in 1921, and a third from Cleveland in 1925.

In this condition a parasitic type of organism gets into the tissue through an opening in the skin, usually an open wound, and there sets up an inflammation which is associated with granulation and overgrowth of the tissues.

The growth slowly progresses, ulcerates sometimes, and eventually may cause serious disability, if not death. The organisms usually enter through wounds in the feet, so that the condition has also been called Madura foot.

In the most recently reported case a Negro meat packer was involved. He had first injured his foot in 1914 and had suffered intermittently with trouble with the foot for twelve years. He was a common laborer during most of that time, and had never attempted to get good medical treatment but had constantly attempted to manipulate and treat the swelling with simple methods of his own.

As a result the granulation had grown until the lump on his foot was about the size of a hen's egg. Scientific investigation revealed the presence in the wound of the organism associated with maduro-mycosis.

The lump was removed by surgical methods and the resulting wound was treated with special antiseptic solutions which have the power to attack the organism that causes Madura foot. In six weeks the condition from which the patient had suffered for more than twelve years was cured.

Other conditions somewhat similar to Madura foot occasionally occur in the United States, among them being a granulation called actinomycosis, which is caused by an organism similar to the one that causes the tropical disease. However, even actinomycosis is a relatively rare condition.

MAGNESIUM CITRATE This is among the most popular of the mild saline purgatives. It is usually bought by the bottle and taken in the morning on arising in the amounts prescribed by the doctor.

MAGNESIA—citrate of, increases bile: See article DIGESTION AND DIGESTIVE DISEASES.

MAGNESIA—laxative: See MEDICINE CHEST, article THE FAMILY MEDICINE CHEST.

MILK OF MAGNESIA—heartburn relieved by: See BIRTH, article CARE OF MOTHERS BEFORE AND AFTER CHILDBIRTH.

MILK OF MAGNESIA—infants: See INFANCY, article CARE AND FEEDING OF THE CHILD.

MILK OF MAGNESIA—laxative: See MEDICINE CHEST, article THE FAMILY MEDICINE CHEST.

MILK OF MAGNESIA—laxative during pregnancy: See BIRTH, article CARE OF MOTHERS BEFORE AND AFTER CHILDBIRTH.

MAIDENHEAD See *Hymen.*

MALARIA Malaria is the number one menace in the world. This disease was known in the fifth century B.C., and its various types were classified at least three hundred years B.C. Scientific control began, however, around 1880, when a French army surgeon named Laveran found that there were parasites in the red blood cells which seemed to be responsible for the condition. Since that time the nature of the disease has been more thoroughly studied. It has been shown that the disease is carried from one human being to another by the anopheline mosquito. More recently means have been found for preventing the disease through the control of the mosquito and also by the use of preventive drugs.

In the United States there are at least 1,000,000 cases of malaria at all times and about 5,000 deaths occur each year from this cause. Great numbers of our soldiers were infected with the parasite that causes this disease.

The mosquito does not carry the parasite directly from one person to another. Actually the mosquito gets the parasite into its body at one stage of its existence; this parasite must develop

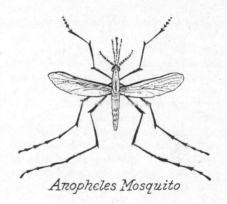

Anopheles Mosquito

An enlarged female malarial mosquito. Malaria is carried from one human being to another by this female Anopheles mosquito. For this reason infected persons should be protected from mosquito bites.

into another stage, which then produces the disease in the second person who is bitten. For the infection to be transmitted, the female Anopheles mosquito must first bite a person who has male and female malaria parasites in the circulating blood. Inside the stomach of the mosquito these parasites undergo fertilization. The male parasite pushes out little filaments which break loose and come into contact with the female form. Exactly as the sperm cell of the male human being penetrates the ovum of the female, so does one of these male parasites penetrate the female and fertilize it. The fertilized forms then push their way out of the stomach cells and gradually enlarge, so that they rupture into the body cavity of the mosquito and make their way to the salivary glands of the mosquito, where they lie. When the mosquito bites an individual, these parasites pass with the saliva and start the development of the parasite in the person who has been bitten. About ten days after the infection has been acquired in this way, the first parasites will be observed in the red blood cells of the person who has been infected. This parasite devours the red pigment and iron-containing material. Then the red cell ruptures and about sixteen parasites are released, each of which attaches itself to a new red cell.

There are various other forms of the parasite which produce different forms of malaria in man. The chief symptoms vary according to the form of the parasite.

The condition begins with backache, muscle soreness, and fever, with paroxysms and chills, about the fourteenth day. When paroxysms occur on alternate days, it is due to the fact that there are two broods of the same parasite developing in the blood. This gives the condition a cold, a hot, and a sweating stage. In the cold stage there are chills

with chattering of the teeth, the skin becoming blue and cold, and, associated with this, an uncontrollable shaking. Then comes a high fever, and after that a sweating stage, when the temperature drops to normal.

In quartan malaria four days intervene between the sets of symptoms, the paroxysms occurring usually every seventy-two hours. In falciparum malaria the temperature is high, the incubation period is about twelve days, the fever is irregular, and bleeding (including blood in the urine) is a frequent complication.

The doctor diagnoses the form of the malaria from the symptoms and the order in which they occur and also, of course, by a study of the blood. Another test involves the giving of quinine, which will control malaria.

Among new drugs are chloraquine, which has advantages over atabrine or quinacrine. For radical cure primaquine is favored. Camoquin is much used for prevention and Daraprim in the treatment of malaria.

Fortunately we have been able to control malaria by the use of quinine and of another form of cinchona known as totaquine, all of which are useful in the prevention and treatment of malaria. About twice as much totaquine as quinine must be given for both prevention and treatment.

One of the most important steps in relation to malaria is the prevention of the spread of the disease through control of the mosquito. This involves cleaning up swamps, removal of excess rain water, and the spraying of areas with oils or insecticides that destroy the mosquito in various stages. People who are constantly exposed to malaria in tropical areas take quinine every day one hour before sunset. They also screen their beds at night and keep the air moving, if possible, by the use of an electric fan. They wear suitable clothing, including leg coverings of soft leather, double stockings, and face nets.

Whereas the mosquito repellents of the past were somewhat ineffective aromatic oils, there are now available powerful insect repellents which are most effective in preventing the bite of the mosquito, the louse, and various other insects.

MALARIA—See article TRANSMISSIBLE DISEASES.

MALARIA—albuminuria may result: See KIDNEY, article THE KIDNEY: ITS DISEASES AND DISTURBANCES.

MALARIA—death rate: See article TRANSMISSIBLE DISEASES.

MALARIA—encephalitis treated with malaria germs: See article TRANSMISSIBLE DISEASES.

MALARIA—enlargement of spleen: See BLOOD, article THE BLOOD AND ITS DISEASES.

MALARIA—epidemics cited as the cause of fall of Greece and Rome: See INFECTIOUS DISEASE, article THE PREVENTION AND TREATMENT OF INFECTIOUS DISEASE; article TRANSMISSIBLE DISEASES.

MALARIA—febrile nephroses may result: See KIDNEY, article THE KIDNEY: ITS DISEASES AND DISTURBANCES.

MALARIA—mosquito: See INFECTIOUS DISEASE, article THE PREVENTION AND TREATMENT OF INFECTIOUS DISEASE.

MALARIA—mosquito (fig.): See article TRANSMISSIBLE DISEASES.

MALARIA—syphilis treated by: See VENEREAL DISEASES, article THE VENEREAL DISEASES.

MALARIA—transmissible disease: See article TRANSMISSIBLE DISEASES.

MALARIA—treatment: See article TRANSMISSIBLE DISEASES.

MALARIA—undulant fever resembles: See article TRANSMISSIBLE DISEASES.

MAMMARY GLANDS The scientific name for the breasts.

MARASMUS Infants are sometimes attacked by an inability to utilize food which produces progessive wasting and emaciation. This condition has been called marasmus.

MASSAGE The word "massage" is applied to any manipulation of the tissue of the body, using the hands or certain special devices that have been invented. Several different movements are used in massage for special purposes.

The simplest form of massage is the superficial stroking movement designed to have a sedative effect. These movements were, no doubt, discovered spontaneously thousands of years ago. Everybody knows that slow, rhythmical stroking will help to relieve pain in various portions of the body and to induce sleep. The chief rules for sedative movement are that it be superficial and rhythmical and that it be done in a manner that is acceptable and not irritating to the person who is receiving the massage. Indeed it is customary to begin over an area that is not sensitive and to continue the massage until it takes in the painful or sensitive area, because only in this way is it possible to find out whether or not the stroking is acceptable to the patient.

A second form of stroking movement used in massage is the deep movement, which is designed to assist the flow of the blood and the lymph through the veins and the lymph channels. Since the flow in these channels is toward the body rather than away from it, it is customary to practice these deep stroking movements toward the center of the body. Such deep stroking tends to relax the muscles and to reduce swelling. Deep stroking over the abdomen will excite the intestines into motion, particularly in a case in which the intestines are sensitive to such stimulation. Actually normal contraction and relaxation of the muscles of the abdominal wall can produce the same effect.

Another movement commonly used in massage is the squeezing movement, in which pressure is applied to the tissues between the fingers or the hands. The tissues may be pulled up and thus pressed between the fingers, or the pressure may be from the outside against the underlying muscles and bones. Such movements help to break up adhesions, to stimulate the circulation, and to induce heat. In these motions there may be friction on the tissues which also increases heat, or there may be vibratory movements which shake and agitate the tissues and thus improve the circulation.

Still another technic used in massage is known as the percussion movement. This is a hammering movement which may be done with the fingers or with various instruments, the effect being, in general, like that of vibration.

Following massage, there should be relief of pain, decrease of swelling, and increase of motion of the parts involved. If, however, the effects are in an opposite direction, it is probable that the massage is not beneficial.

MASSAGE—arthritis: See article ARTHRITIS, RHEUMATISM, AND GOUT.

MASSAGE—foot: See FOOT, article THE FOOT.

MASSAGE—injurious to diseased face: See SKIN, article THE SKIN.

MASSAGE—pregnancy: See BIRTH, article CARE OF MOTHERS BEFORE AND AFTER CHILDBIRTH.

MASSAGE—rheumatism: See article ARTHRITIS, RHEUMATISM, AND GOUT.

MASSAGE—skin: See SKIN, article THE SKIN.

MASTITIS Inflammation of the mammary glands is called mastitis. The condition is usually due to infection with various germs. Infection by the streptococci or the staphylococci produces suppuration. The treatment of mastitis may involve surgical emptying of abscesses and the use of such drugs as the sulfonamides and penicillin, which act specifically against the infecting germs.

MASTOIDITIS Mastoid is the name applied to a portion of the bones of the skull. The cells of the mastoid are behind the ear. When an inflammation occurs in these cells following any infection, the condition is called mastoiditis; this merely means inflammation of the mastoid.

Doctors believe that mastoiditis occurs frequently due to bad habits in blowing the nose. When the little boy with the running nose and sore throat blows his nose vigorously, at the same time keeping both nostrils shut, air is forced from the throat and into the Eustachian tube which passes from the back of the nose to the ear. With the air go the infecting germs that are in the throat. Soon the little boy hears a clinking sound in his ear. Then there is a dull feeling and the ear begins to ache. The doctor finds that the eardrum is quite red and that the boy cannot hear. There is swelling behind the ear and the point is painful on pressure. Usually the doctor will decide to open the eardrum as soon as possible so as to permit infected material to escape and thus to avoid further damage to the mastoid and to the hearing.

The cells of the mastoid are close to the mechanism of the internal ear with which we hear and with which we maintain our equilibrium. They are also close to the outer covering of the brain and to many important nerves. Obviously everything possible should be done to prevent serious damage to these important organs and tissues.

Infection of the mastoid frequently follows such diseases as measles, scarlet fever, and diphtheria. Mastoiditis is a dangerous disease and not to be trifled with.

Fortunately two recent discoveries have done much to prevent mastoiditis as a complication of infectious diseases and also to cure without an operation. The use of the sulfonamide drugs helps to prevent the infections with the streptococcus, which is the most frequent cause of mastoiditis. Quite recently in the more serious cases penicillin has also been found capable of stopping the progress of infections in the ear before the mastoid has become seriously involved.

MASTOIDITIS—See INFANCY, article CARE AND FEEDING OF THE CHILD; EAR, article, THE EAR, TONGUE, NOSE, AND THROAT.

MASTOIDITIS—scarlet fever: See CHILDHOOD DISEASES, article INFECTIOUS DISEASES OF CHILDHOOD.

MASTOIDS—See EAR, article THE EAR, TONGUE, NOSE, AND THROAT.

MASTOIDS—sinus infection may affect: See EAR, article THE EAR, TONGUE, NOSE, AND THROAT.

MATHEMATICAL PRODIGIES

Everyone is interested in lightning calculators and particularly in children who develop unusual gifts in the fields of memory or mathematics. The scientists who study eugenics, genetics and the relationship of heredity to the production of such geniuses have not been able to find quite satisfactory explanations for their appearance in most circumstances.

Popenoe has described some of the prodigies of remarkable ability who have appeared in this country. Thus a nine year old boy from Vermont was able to answer in a minute the question as to the number of seconds in 1 813 years,

7 months and 27 days. His facility was first noted when he was six years of age, at which time he was able to answer immediately such questions as 13 times 97. With a minute's thought he could raise the number eight to the sixteenth power. This boy lived about the time of Napoleon, became a teacher and Methodist preacher, and eventually professor of languages in the University of Vermont. His mental powers declined rapidly and he died at the age of 38 with only ordinary mental ability.

Contests have been held between memory experts. According to Popenoe, a Norwegian philologist, Paula Bergh, learned 408 figures in 104 minutes, thus breaking the world record held by a professor named Diamondi who had learned 200 figures in 75 minutes.

There are many instances of persons mentally defective who developed unusual abilities in memory and mathematics. In an asylum for the insane in Great Britain there was a mentally defective sailor who could read the first page of a newspaper and then repeat it word for word without reference to the original text.

A Florida physician, Hiram Byrd, described a man in Mississippi with a mental age of 8 years who could not repeat more than five digits, a mental task that could ordinarily be accomplished by a six year old child. Nevertheless, this man had committed to memory a large array of facts relating to dates, places and the numbers of locomotives. In the years 1921-1924, given the month, day and year, he could at once name the day of the week, and if given the year and month and asked what day of the month was the second Tuesday or the fourth Friday, he could always give the correct answer. When he was examined by Doctor Byrd, he was extending his ability to the year 1925.

Mathematical talent seems to be

hereditary. Some people are absolutely lacking in any sense of quantity and number. A man in a Pennsylvania family, before he went to work in the morning, had to measure the meat and potatoes that his wife prepared for the dinner. If he left this to her, as she had absolutely no sense of quantity or number, she might cook enough for an infant or enough for a baseball team. In one line of this family the defect has persisted for five generations.

Among famous geniuses who were mathematical prodigies in youth were James Watt, one of the inventors of the steam engine; William Herschel, the astronomer; P. S. Laplace, the astronomer; Isaac Newton, who had mastered differential calculus before he was 24; A. M. Ampere, the physicist, and men who devoted their lives to mathematics, such as K. F. Gauss, L. Euler, Th. Joung, and George Bidder.

MATURITY, MENTAL ATTITUDES TO

People who are infantile in their emotional attitudes are overly dependent on their parents or substitutes for the parents. They expect excessive amounts of services and tolerance from their parents and from others around them. Sometimes this infantile attitude is retained until the death of the parent. The child who has been "teacher's pet" as he grows up will have to be the "boss's favorite" when he gets a job.

A child may develop some sense of personal responsibility but always get rid of it by an excuse. Such children have to trust some other person completely. People who maintain a childish level as they grow up always find excuses for the failures, alibis for their weakness and "pass the buck" in every difficult situation.

Children who reach twelve to fifteen years of age develop secondary sexual characteristics. In early adolescence the child begins to assert itself and begins to resent parental domination. Boys in early adolescence begin to show off and to indulge in contests in which they can demonstrate their superiority. Girls begin to dress up and try to look their prettiest. The boy's room begins to be filled with trophies won at the track or in the swimming pool or at other sports. The girl's room begins to be decorated with programs of dances, souvenirs of parties and knick knacks accumulated on dates.

"Dating" now becomes the most important aspect of life. If this passes on to what boys and girls call "going steady," difficult mental situations may develop. Parents frequently try to dominate the situation because of economic, religious or purely emotional reactions. These situations may lead to emotional disturbances in the young that may mark the life of the growing youth for many years thereafter.

Even adults still need affection, security and well established relationships toward other people. If a person fails to mature and depends heavily on the affection of others, if he requires definite signs of favoritism, he is unlikely to develop satisfactory marriage and may react emotionally to situations which he cannot solve. A good marriage adjustment comes to people who reach mature years after overcoming infantile dependence on affection.

MEASLES

Measles continues to be one of the most prevalent ailments affecting young children. Studies made in our large cities show no appreciable reduction in the number of cases of measles reported each year for the last twenty-five years. However, the ability to control the disease is now greater than ever before. In 1913 there were 12.4 deaths from measles for every 100,000 population in Chicago. By 1940 this figure had dropped to 1 death for every 100,000 persons.

The factors said to be responsible for the decrease in the death rate include improved housing, better medical care, improved nursing, and, above all, the use of drugs which have been found efficient in controlling the complications of measles. It is the complications of measles which primarily cause death in those who are infected.

Today measles is generally considered to be a virus disease caused by an infectious agent too small to be seen with an ordinary microscope. Medicine has developed a number of protective technics which are of great importance in preventing measles.

Among these technics is the injection of serum from the blood of children who have recently recovered from the disease. This is available through so-called serum centers or blood banks which keep such convalescent serum available. The modern technic includes the use of what is called immune globulin. Formerly this immune globulin was developed from the placenta, usually called the afterbirth, the structure by which a newborn child is attached to the body of his mother. More recently it has been found that immune globulin, with all of the virtues for the prevention of disease, can be secured as a by-product of the blood collected through the blood banks. The gamma globulin of the blood contains antisubstances against measles, infectious hepatitis, and poliomyelitis. Globulin is now manufactured by several companies. The amount given depends on the age and weight of the child.

In 1955 John Enders grew the measles virus in pure culture outside the human body. Scientists may soon prepare a vaccine for prevention of measles as effective as that against infantile paralysis.

Following are seven preventive measures recommended in times when an epidemic of measles is prevalent:

1. Don't unnecessarily expose a child to measles. This disease can be very dangerous to young children.

2. Don't permit a child who has been exposed to measles to play with other children for at least two weeks. He may be getting the disease himself, and it might take this long for you to be sure.

3. Don't permit your child to play with another child known to have been exposed to measles within two weeks. You don't want your child to have the disease if you can help it.

4. Don't permit your child to receive repeated exposures to measles. Even if you know he has been exposed, don't let him play with a child sick with the disease or thought to be developing it. Repeated exposures add to the severity of the attack.

5. Don't send your child to school if he is not well. If you think he is sick, call a doctor; if you are not sure, keep him home so you can watch him.

6. Don't let a child who has had measles get out of bed until the doctor says it is all right. Even if he does not appear too sick, the child with measles is very susceptible to such complications as pneumonia and abscessed ears.

7. Don't say, "It's only measles." Measles is a serious disease, and the child with measles requires good medical and nursing care.

The complications of measles are primarily responsible for trouble with that disease. These include infections of the eyes, the nose and throat, the bronchial tubes, and even of the digestive tract. After measles has attacked the body, secondary germs like the streptococcus, pneumococcus, influenza bacillus, and even the organism of meningitis may invade. The complications appear in any stage of measles but are most likely to develop after the eruption has occurred fully.

Once upon a time diphtheria was a frequent complication of measles, but that is no longer the case since we have learned how to prevent the contacts that permit the two diseases at one time. Fortunately the secondary infections of the ear, nose, throat, and glands are controllable nowadays by the use of the new drugs that have been developed, including particularly the sulfonamide drugs and penicillin. These drugs can be given only by the physician, who determines when the drug is to be given and how much is to be administered at any one time.

One of the most serious complications of measles is an inflammation of the brain, which seems to be due, however, not to any secondary organism but actually to the virus of measles itself. We know now that the virus may attack the brain.

Fortunately the secondary inflammation occurs in less than .1 per cent of all cases. Nobody knows just why it occurs in any individual case. It does not seem to be directly related to the severity of the measles.

When death from measles occurs, it is usually among children who are weakened and undernourished. Deaths from measles in children under six months of age are extremely rare because these children carry in their blood the immunity that they derive from their mothers. The maximum death rate occurs among children of preschool age.

Once upon a time tuberculosis was most feared as a complication of measles. Nowadays that also has been greatly decreased because tuberculosis is detected early in children, and with proper care prompt healing is brought about.

The very latest figures show that about .2 per cent of all children infected with measles die, and even this figure is supposed to be too high because it is estimated that at least two or three times the number of children reported as having measles actually have the disease.

MEASLES—See CHILDHOOD DISEASES, article INFECTIOUS DISEASES OF CHILDHOOD.

MEASLES—antibiotics: See CHILDHOOD DISEASES, article INFECTIOUS DISEASES OF CHILDHOOD.

MEASLES—avoidable: See CHILDHOOD DISEASES, article INFECTIOUS DISEASES OF CHILDHOOD.

MEASLES—chicken pox frequently follows: See CHILDHOOD DISEASES, article INFECTIOUS DISEASES OF CHILDHOOD.

MEASLES—childhood disease: See CHILDHOOD DISEASES, article INFECTIOUS DISEASES OF CHILDHOOD.

MEASLES—confused with scarlet fever and smallpox: See CHILDHOOD DISEASES, article INFECTIOUS DISEASES OF CHILDHOOD.

MEASLES—contagious disease: See INFECTIOUS DISEASE, article THE PREVENTION AND TREATMENT OF INFECTIOUS DISEASE.

MEASLES—contagious material: See CHILDHOOD DISEASES, article INFECTIOUS DISEASES OF CHILDHOOD.

MEASLES—deaths annually: See CHILDHOOD DISEASES, article INFECTIOUS DISEASES OF CHILDHOOD.

MEASLES—derivation of word: See CHILDHOOD DISEASES, article INFECTIOUS DISEASES OF CHILDHOOD.

MEASLES—diet: See CHILDHOOD DISEASES, article INFECTIOUS DISEASES OF CHILDHOOD.

MEASLES—diphtheria frequently follows: See CHILDHOOD DISEASES, article INFECTIOUS DISEASES OF CHILDHOOD.

MEASLES—epidemics: See INFECTIOUS DISEASE, article THE PREVENTION AND TREATMENT OF INFECTIOUS DISEASE; CHILDHOOD DISEASES, article INFECTIOUS DISEASES OF CHILDHOOD.

MEASLES—eyes: See CHILDHOOD DI-

SEASES, article INFECTIOUS DISEASES OF CHILDHOOD.

MEASLES—Faroe Islands epidemic: See INFECTIOUS DISEASE, article THE PREVENTION AND TREATMENT OF INFECTIOUS DISEASE; CHILDHOOD DISEASES, article INFECTIOUS DISEASES OF CHILDHOOD.

MEASLES—Fiji Islands epidemic: See CHILDHOOD DISEASES, article INFECTIOUS DISEASES OF CHILDHOOD.

MEASLES—German: See entry MEASLES, GERMAN.

MEASLES—globulin, immune: See CHILDHOOD DISEASES, article INFECTIOUS DISEASES OF CHILDHOOD.

MEASLES—hair fall may follow: See HAIR, article THE HAIR.

MEASLES—immunity induced: See RESPIRATORY DISEASES, article THE RESPIRATORY DISEASES.

MEASLES—incidence: See INFECTIOUS DISEASE, article THE PREVENTION AND TREATMENT OF INFECTIOUS DISEASE.

MEASLES—incubation period: See INFECTIOUS DISEASE, article THE PREVENTION AND TREATMENT OF INFECTIOUS DISEASE; CHILDHOOD DISEASES, article INFECTIOUS DISEASES OF CHILDHOOD.

MEASLES—inflammation of colon: See article DIGESTION AND DIGESTIVE DISEASES.

MEASLES—Koplik's spots: See CHILDHOOD DISEASES, article INFECTIOUS DISEASES OF CHILDHOOD.

MEASLES—mental defectiveness may result: See MENTAL, article NERVOUS AND MENTAL DISORDERS.

MEASLES—pneumonia frequently follows: See RESPIRATORY DISEASES, article THE RESPIRATORY DISEASES.

MEASLES—precautions to prevent spread: See CHILDHOOD DISEASES, article INFECTIOUS DISEASES OF CHILDHOOD.

MEASLES—prevention: See CHILDHOOD DISEASES, article INFECTIOUS DISEASES OF CHILDHOOD.

MEASLES—rash: See CHILDHOOD DISEASES, article INFECTIOUS DISEASES OF CHILDHOOD.

MEASLES—scarlet fever frequently follows: See CHILDHOOD DISEASES, article INFECTIOUS DISEASES OF CHILDHOOD.

MEASLES—scarlet fever spreads less rapidly: See CHILDHOOD DISEASES, article INFECTIOUS DISEASES OF CHILDHOOD.

MEASLES—secondary complications: See CHILDHOOD DISEASES, article INFECTIOUS DISEASES OF CHILDHOOD.

MEASLES—serum: See CHILDHOOD DISEASES, article INFECTIOUS DISEASES OF CHILDHOOD.

MEASLES—specific substance not available for treatment: See INFECTIOUS DISEASE, article THE PREVENTION AND TREATMENT OF INFECTIOUS DISEASE.

MEASLES—spread mostly by direct contact: See CHILDHOOD DISEASES, article INFECTIOUS DISEASES OF CHILDHOOD.

MEASLES—sulfonamide drugs: See CHILDHOOD DISEASES, article INFECTIOUS DISEASES OF CHILDHOOD.

MEASLES—syphilitic rash resembles: See SKIN, article THE SKIN.

MEASLES—treatment: See INFECTIOUS DISEASE, article THE PREVENTION AND TREATMENT OF INFECTIOUS DISEASE.

MEASLES—tuberculosis made active: See CHILDHOOD DISEASES, article INFECTIOUS DISEASES OF CHILDHOOD.

MEASLES—whooping cough frequently follows: See CHILDHOOD DISEASES, article INFECTIOUS DISEASES OF CHILDHOOD.

MEASLES, GERMAN Among the infectious diseases which appear most often in spring and early summer is German measles. Usually it affects children of grade school and high school age and rather seldom those under five years of age. Although the word "measles" is attached to this condition, it is not at all related to ordinary measles.

Apparently German measles is spread as are the other infectious diseases—by material coming from the nose and throat of the person who is infected. Usually about eighteen days pass after a person has been exposed to German measles before he comes down with the disease, although the period seems to vary from nine to twenty-one days. Often the first symptom observed is the rash, although occasionally the usual signs of an infection appear, including headache, runny nose, slight sore throat, and a general feeling of illness. The eruption usually appears on the chest in the form of pale pink spots. It spreads rapidly, however, over the rest of the body, finally producing a distinct scarlet appearance. The fever is not usually high in German measles, nor are the patients so severely ill as they may be with measles or scarlet fever.

One of the special signs of German measles is the swelling of the lymph glands at the back of the head and neck, which most often are about the size of a pea but occasionally may get as large as a hazelnut. Usually the swelling of these glands disappears rapidly, but occasionally it persists for several weeks.

Quite frequently German measles is mistaken for scarlet fever or measles.

Ordinarily a child with German measles is kept at home so as to prevent spreading the infection to other people. The control of the condition, however, is exceedingly difficult because of the long period of time during which it is undergoing development in the body when it is also possible to transmit the disease. Fortunately, however, the disease is not severe and does not last long. In most cases indeed the treatment of German measles simply involves isolating the patient and keeping him in bed with a light diet until the temperature has fallen and the rash has disappeared.

German measles, attacking a pregnant woman during the first four months of pregnancy, may cause a deformed child.

After a child has had German measles, the room is thoroughly cleaned, aired, and sunned, and the linens washed and boiled. No other disinfection is necessary.

Only a few years have passed since the discovery was first made, in Australia, that many deficiencies in a child's vision, hearing, and heart following his birth are related to the mother's having had rubella (German measles) during pregnancy. In Sweden the incidence of rubella was exceedingly high during the years 1936, 1937, and 1941. More than 10 per cent of the mothers of deaf-mutes born in 1937 and 1941 had rubella before their baby's birth. About 2 to 5 per cent of the mothers who had had rubella in the first few months of pregnancy bore deaf-mute children. And deaf-mutism composes only a small percentage of the congenital defects that result from mothers having had rubella while pregnant. Administration of convalescent serum, taken from women who have rubella, as soon as a woman's pregnancy is known is a useful preventive measure.

INFECTIOUS DISEASE; CHILDHOOD DISEASES, article INFECTIOUS DISEASES OF CHILDHOOD.

MEASLES, GERMAN—measles different: See CHILDHOOD DISEASES, article INFECTIOUS DISEASES OF CHILDHOOD.

MEASLES, GERMAN—mild disease: See CHILDHOOD DISEASES, article INFECTIOUS DISEASES OF CHILDHOOD.

MEASLES, GERMAN—secondary complications: See CHILDHOOD DISEASES, article INFECTIOUS DISEASES OF CHILDHOOD.

MEASLES, GERMAN—symptoms: See CHILDHOOD DISEASES, article INFECTIOUS DISEASES OF CHILDHOOD.

MEASLES, GERMAN—treatment: See CHILDHOOD DISEASES, article INFECTIOUS DISEASES OF CHILDHOOD.

MEDICAL REACTOR, FIRST

(See also discussion under *Cancer, Detection of Brain Tumor, Radiation, Radiation in Cancer, Radioactivity, Thyroid and the Heart, X-Ray*) A nuclear reactor is being built as part of the new Medical Center at the University of California at Los Angeles. This is the first reactor designed specifically for use in medical research and treatment.

The device provides two types of radiation—gamma rays and thermal neutrons—which can be beamed selectively at deep-seated cancers, often difficult to treat by surgery and present forms of radiation.

Gamma rays may be used to bombard malignant tissue directly. Thermal neutrons may be used in conjunction with certain injected chemicals to cause powerful but localized secondary release of radiation within the cancer tissue itself.

This use of neutrons, available only in reactor-type therapy, it is thought, has a distinct advantage over X ray and other forms of radiation therapy. There is evidence that a greater selective absorption of radiation by malignant tissue

occurs with less damage to surrounding healthy tissue.

A type of cancer that may be treated by this form of therapy is the glioblastoma, a brain tumor that infiltrates through healthy brain tissue. When borax is injected into a patient with this cancer, boron from the compound concentrates in the tissue. When the cancer area is bombarded with neutrons, the boron captures neutrons. This causes a nuclear reaction in the boron, thus releasing powerful alpha particles. The alpha particles bombard the malignant tissue and destroy it but are absorbed before they reach nearby healthy tissue.

This new reactor, according to Dr. Stafford Warren, will not be available for use until 1957. Physical methods of measuring the neutron and gamma output of the reactor must be developed and also physical methods for measuring energy absorption from the radiation.

The research program will include radiation genetic studies, concerned primarily with mutation effects of radiation. Other studies will include the manner in which radioactive materials are deposited in human bones, and neutron effects on tissue, particularly the lens of the eye.

A wide training program with the reactor will include instruction of medical students, health physicists and others in techniques of reactor operation and utilization of neutrons, gamma rays and pile-produced isotopes.

Simultaneously with clinical uses of the reactor, radioisotopes will be made. Radioactive potassium, sodium and chlorine—short-lived isotopes very much in demand at present—may be made available under Atomic Energy Commission license to appropriate affiliated programs.

MEDICINE CHEST

Most Americans, being independent and individualistic, feel themselves competent to fix defects in plumbing and almost equally competent to take care of their own disturbances of health, as well as to prescribe for more complicated disturbances which really ought to have the prompt attention of a physician.

If one looks over the average family medicine chest, he is likely to find it full of strange concoctions and things of all kinds—an array of disorder which actually endangers the family's health and safety. A survey which I made of the contents of the medicine chests of a considerable number of families brought out some exceedingly interesting information.

Among the strange items found in these medicine chests were old cloths to be used as bandages, cracked atomizer bulbs, horehound candy, shoehorns, curling irons, dried sponges, packages of seeds, hair grease, mange cure, face bleach, shoe polish, empty toothpaste and shaving-cream tubes, fifty different remedies for colds, combs and bobby pins, cuff links, nail polish, bath salts, and discarded sets of teeth. The number of antiseptics found, and their efficiency, varied tremendously. One or two antiseptics were found in some cases, and as many as six different antiseptics in others, individual members of the family having their own likes and dislikes in these matters.

Apparently most American housewives need a lot of education concerning the significance of what are actually effective and useful household remedies. A household remedy should be one with a certain definite action, and usually it should contain but one active ingredient. If the thing is worth keeping in the medicine chest, it should be something which is used fairly frequently.

Dangerous poisons have no place in the family medicine chest. A dangerous poison is one which is likely to produce serious symptoms or death if taken in even moderate amounts.

Prescriptions ordered by the family doctor for a certain illness should never be kept for the future. If any of the material remains in the bottle, it should be poured promptly into a safe place of disposal. Since useful bottles are rare around most homes, the bottle may be thoroughly washed with hot water, dried, and stored away. Few people realize that most drugs deteriorate with age and that a prescription for a certain illness is not likely to be useful for the future.

REGULAR CLEANING—The wise person will go over the family medicine chest at least once every three months and discard all materials not constantly in use. It is also well to have the family doctor take a look at the materials to offer his advice on those worth keeping and make suggestions as to what is needed. Unless measures of this kind are taken, the amount of "junk" that accumulates in the average medicine chest becomes something appalling. Used safety-razor blades are dangerous. A good rule is to put the old blade in the package every time a new blade is taken out. Then when the package is filled with old blades, the box can be thrown in the household rubbish.

ITEMS IN MEDICINE CHEST—Most families want to keep on hand a laxative or cathartic. Under certain circumstances any laxative or cathartic may be exceedingly dangerous. The most conspicuous example is appendicitis. This is at first just an infected spot on a little organ which comes off the large bowel and which apparently has no serious function in the human body. If this infection develops the way a boil develops from a pimple, it is in danger of bursting and spreading throughout the body. Therefore no laxative or cathartic should ever be taken when the abdomen is exceedingly painful.

The most common laxatives used in a family medicine chest include liquid petrolatum or mineral oil, which is a mechanical lubricant without possibility of serious harm. Other common preparations much used include phenolphthalein, castor oil, Seidlitz powders, milk of magnesia, psyllium seed, sodium phosphate, aromatic cascara, and mineral oil mixed with agar.

The next most commonly used preparations in a family medicine chest are pain relievers. Most of these are used for headaches, although sometimes they are used for neuritis, neuralgia, toothache, and other pains of unknown origin, as well as to produce sleep. Most headache powders bought under patent trademarks contain phenacetin or acetanilid, sometimes in considerable dosage. It is not well to experiment with acetanilid because it may, in large dosage, have serious effects on the body, including particularly the blood and the heart. Moreover, there is a tendency to form the habit of taking such preparations. Other drugs much used to produce sleep are derivatives of barbituric acid, of which some of the best examples are veronal, trional, and combinations of barbituric acids with other drugs. The family medicine chest is better off without preparations of this character, as the possibilities for harm are sufficiently great to suggest that these preparations should not be used except with medical advice.

The most commonly used general pain reliever is acetylsalicylic acid, commonly called aspirin So far as is known, aspirin is relatively harmless except for a few people who are especially sensitive to it. Such people cannot take even small doses. One aspirin is as good as another, provided it is up to the standard of the United States Pharmacopoeia.

Among the strongest of medicinal preparations are the narcotics and anesthetics. Narcotics should never be used by anyone without a physician's prescription and, indeed, no drug that has to be administered with a hypodermic syringe should find a place in the average family medicine chest. There are some people with diabetes who have been taught by their doctors to inject themselves with insulin. Even these people should keep their syringe outfit separate from the materials in the family medicine chest.

There are all sorts of antiseptics available for use on the skin, in first aid and also for gargling and for washing various portions of the body.

The most widely known skin antiseptics are tincture of iodine and 2 per cent mercurochrome. The Council on Pharmacy and Chemistry of the American Medical Association permits advertising of recognized antiseptics for first aid, and tincture of iodine and mercurochrome are included among such preparations.

This same Council has concluded that no antiseptic substance is of value when used as a gargle for the destruction of germs in the mouth and throat. If the antiseptic is applied directly on a swab so that the material is held in direct contact with the localized infection, it may have some definite use.

Among the antiseptics approved by the Council on Pharmacy and Chemistry are preparations of hexylresorcinol and preparations of metaphen, also neutral solution of chlorinated soda and hydrogen peroxide. The Council has not approved antiseptics commonly represented as being useful in the relief of all sorts of infections of the throat and also for the prevention of various types of infectious diseases, including colds.

One of the best old-fashioned antiseptic solutions for common use around the home is boric acid solution. Most people prefer to have packages of crystals of boric acid or of the powder and to make up the solution fresh just before use.

First-Aid Supplies—Among the materials needed for first aid are adhesive tape of various widths, sterile cotton, sterile gauze bandages, sterile gauze pads, and scissors, which should be kept in the medicine chest exclusively for such purposes. You should also have the ready-made combinations of a piece of adhesive tape with a tiny piece of sterilized bandage that can be used to cover small wounds after they have been treated with iodine or mercurochrome.

People should know that the proper way to stop bleeding of small wounds is simply to press upon them with a sterile piece of gauze. In case of very serious wounds affecting arteries and thereby difficult to control, it may be necessary to put a tourniquet around the limb. The tourniquet should be fastened just tight enough to stop the bleeding. An ordinary piece of rubber tubing or a narrow towel tied and twisted with a stick will serve most purposes satisfactorily.

The family medicine chest may also contain aromatic spirits of ammonia, which is sometimes given when a prompt stimulant is needed following fainting. Half a teaspoonful in water, for a sudden fainting spell, is a fairly safe thing to give in most cases of this emergency.

The widely publicized milk of magnesia and sodium bicarbonate, or baking soda, are two preparations which can safely be kept in the family medicine chest and which are frequently advised by physicians for alkaline purposes.

Some families keep paregoric as a useful preparation in case of cramps that affect women at periodic intervals.

These items constitute practically all the equipment that need be in any average medicine chest because they are the few materials that can be used safely by most people.

Shaving Materials—Most modern women prefer to keep their cosmetics in their own boudoirs, but the man of the house is very likely to put his into the family medicine cabinet. They should include, in most instances, a razor, which should be kept in its box and not permitted to lie around loosely; also some shaving soap or cream, and some face lotion, which may be either witch hazel or a special lotion which he prefers.

It is not advisable to use a styptic in the form of a stick of alum to stop slight bleeding points after shaving. Much better are any of the astringent surgical powders, of which a small amount may be taken from the box on each occasion and applied directly to the bleeding point. Finally, any good talcum powder may be used after shaving and after bathing, according to the individual preferences of the users.

All such materials should be kept in orderly position and not scattered around the chest helter-skelter, as many men are inclined to do.

Additional Items—It is taken for granted that every modern household has a good clinical thermometer, a hot-water bottle, and an ice bag. These are three exceedingly useful devices in any home, and when they are available in an emergency the comfort they give is tremendous.

In addition to the materials used for first aid, most families will have bedpans for use in cases of illness, glass drinking tubes, syringes for giving enemas, atomizers, and sometimes special devices for creating steam to be medicated with small amounts of tincture of benzoin for relief in various forms of hoarseness or other conditions affecting the larynx and the lungs.

Don'ts—There are certain "don'ts" which should be remembered:

Do not save poisonous preparations of any kind, including particularly bichloride of mercury, pills containing strychnine, or solutions containing wood alcohol.

Do not keep samples of patent medicines of unknown composition recommended beyond their actual virtues.

Never permit any preparation of opium or morphine in the family medicine chest.

Never save any prepared prescription after the specific use for which it was ordered by the physician has disappeared.

MEDICINE CHEST—anesthetics: See MEDICINE CHEST, article THE FAMILY MEDICINE CHEST.

MEDICINE CHEST—antiseptics: See MEDICINE CHEST, article THE FAMILY MEDICINE CHEST.

MEDICINE CHEST—cathartics: See MEDICINE CHEST, article THE FAMILY MEDICINE CHEST.

MEDICINE CHEST—cosmetics: See MEDICINE CHEST, article THE FAMILY MEDICINE CHEST.

MEDICINE CHEST—dangerous poisons excluded: See MEDICINE CHEST, article THE FAMILY MEDICINE CHEST.

MEDICINE CHEST—disorderly (fig.):

See MEDICINE CHEST, article THE FAMILY MEDICINE CHEST.

MEDICINE CHEST—drugs: See MEDICINE CHEST, article THE FAMILY MEDICINE CHEST.

MEDICINE CHEST—equipment: See MEDICINE CHEST, article THE FAMILY MEDICINE CHEST.

MEDICINE CHEST—first aid materials: See MEDICINE CHEST, article THE FAMILY MEDICINE CHEST.

MEDICINE CHEST—items commonly found in: See MEDICINE CHEST, article THE FAMILY MEDICINE CHEST.

MEDICINE CHEST—laxatives: See MEDICINE CHEST, article THE FAMILY MEDICINE CHEST.

MEDICINE CHEST—narcotics: See MEDICINE CHEST, article THE FAMILY MEDICINE CHEST.

MEDICINE CHEST—pain relievers: See MEDICINE CHEST, article THE FAMILY MEDICINE CHEST.

MEDICINE CHEST—sleep producers: See MEDICINE CHEST, article THE FAMILY MEDICINE CHEST.

MEDICINE CHEST—surgical supplies: See MEDICINE CHEST, article THE FAMILY MEDICINE CHEST.

The Family Medicine Chest

BY

MORRIS FISHBEIN, M.D.

Former Editor, *Journal American Medical Association,* Chicago; Editor, *Excerpta Medica, Bulletin World Medical Assn.; Post-graduate Medicine.*

MOST AMERICANS, being independent and individualistic, feel themselves competent to fix defects in the plumbing and almost equally competent to take care of their own disturbances of health, as well as to prescribe for more complicated disturbances which really ought to have prompt medical attention.

A household remedy should be one with a certain definite action; usually it should contain but one active ingredient. If the thing is worth keeping in the medicine chest it should be something which is used fairly frequently. Dangerous poisons have no place in the family medicine chest. A dangerous poison is one which is likely to produce serious symptoms or death if taken in even moderate amounts. Prescriptions ordered by the family doctor for a certain illness should never be kept for the future. If any of the material remains in the bottle it should be poured promptly into a safe place of disposal. Since useful bottles are rare around most homes, the bottle may be thoroughly washed with hot water, dried, and stored away. Few people realize that most drugs deteriorate with age and that a prescription for a certain illness is not likely to be useful for the future.

The wise person will go over the family medicine chest at least once every three months and at that time discard all materials not constantly in use. It might also be well to have the family doctor look at the materials once in a while to offer his advice as to the materials worth keeping.

TAKING MEDICINE

Medicines rightly used can be of immense aid and comfort to the afflicted· wrongly used, they may cause serious damage to the human body. When a doctor prescribes medicines for a patient, they are for that particular patient and not for anybody else in the family. Hence, old prescriptions should not be saved but should be disposed of as soon as possible after they are no longer necessary for the patient for whom they were prescribed.

The doctor usually writes on his prescription, and the druggist recopies on the label, the directions for taking the medicine. It is, therefore, well when giving medicine to a sick person to be sure you know exactly what is on the label of the bottle. If necessary, take the bottle into another room to read the label so as not to be disturbed by conversation with the patient or with anyone else.

Then, when you measure out the medicine, think of what you are doing and pay no attention to anything else. Medicines are usually prescribed in dosages of drops, teaspoons, fractions of teaspoons, and spoons of larger sizes. Because spoons are nowadays in many fanciful shapes and sizes, each family should have a medicine glass with measures of various spoons recorded. When a doctor says any number of drops, the drops should be measured with a medicine dropper and not by guesswork.

If liquid medicine is being prescribed, the bottle should be thoroughly shaken each time before the medicine is measured. When medicine is poured out of the bottle, the cork should be deposited with its top down on the table and immediately put back in the bottle after the medicine has been poured.

Most medicine should be mixed with a little water when taken, but sometimes the medicine may be put in the mouth and washed down with a swallow of water. Pills and capsules should either be handed to the patient from the original package so that he may help himself, putting the pill or capsule on the back of the tongue and washing it down with a drink of water, or else brought to the patient on a spoon so that he may take the pill or capsule from the spoon. In other words, the person who is waiting on the patient should not carry the capsules or pills in the palm of the hand, where they may be softened or disintegrated by moisture or contaminated from the hands.

There are several ways in which medicines of unpleasant taste may be made more palatable. If very cold water is taken, it will serve to cover the taste. It is not advisable to give medicine to children in foods, particularly in milk, as this may create a distaste for the food or milk which lasts for a long time thereafter.

There are very few remedies which should be kept regularly in the family medicine chest. American people suffer today with overdosage of cathartics and laxatives, and with overdosage of medicine to relieve pain and produce sleep. Physicians are beginning to notice some serious results particularly from overdosing with drugs of the last mentioned type. No one should take such remedies regularly without the physician's directions.

Let us consider now the items that are most commonly found in any first-class family medicine chest. Most families want something to use for moving the bowels in the occasional case of temporary obstruction or slowness of action. Under certain circumstances any laxative or cathartic may be exceedingly dangerous. The most conspicuous example is appendicitis. This is at first just an infected spot on a little organ which comes off the large bowel and which apparently has no serious function in the human body. If this infection develops the way a boil develops from a pimple, it is in danger of bursting and spreading throughout the body. When infection is spread in the abdomen the result is peritonitis. Therefore, a laxative or cathartic should never be taken when the abdomen is exceedingly painful.

The most common laxatives found in a family medicine chest include liquid petrolatum, or mineral oil, which is a mechanical lubricant that may interfere with absorption of Vitamin A. Other preparations commonly used include castor oil, seidlitz powders, milk of magnesia, Epsom salts, sodium phosphate, phenolphthalein, aromatic cascara, and bulk formers like cellulose and psyllium seed preparations. For the people who use the medicine chest a large sign should be placed indicating that none of these preparations is ever to be used for abdominal pain of unknown cause.

The next most commonly found preparations in a family medicine chest, aside from the cosmetics, are pain relievers. Most of these are used for headaches, although sometimes they are used for what are called neuritis, neuralgia, toothache, and other pains of unknown origin, as well as to produce sleep. Most headache powders bought under patent trade marks contain phenacetin or acetanilid, sometimes in considerable dosage. Don't experiment with acetanilid because it may, in large dosage, have serious effects on the body. Too large or too frequently repeated doses will poison anyone who uses them. Moreover, people tend to form the habit of taking such preparations, and such habits are dangerous, since they temporize with what may eventually become a serious condition. Least harmful of the pain relievers is aspirin.

Other drugs much used to produce sleep nowadays are derivatives of barbituric acid of which some of the best examples are phenobarbital, nembutal, and ipral. In some states druggists are not permitted to sell such preparations to anyone without a physician's prescription. This should be sufficient indication of their danger as used by many people without medical knowledge. The family medicine chest is better off without preparations of this character. The possibilities for harm are sufficiently great to suggest that these preparations be not used except on medical advice. Thousands of deaths have resulted from accidental overdosage.

The most commonly used general pain reliever throughout the country today is acetylsalicylic acid, commonly called aspirin. It is relatively harmless except for a few people who are especially sensitive to it. Such people cannot take even small doses. One aspirin is as good as another, provided it is up to the standard of the United States Pharmacopeia. Special claims are made for aspirins that dissolve more quickly in the stomach. Old tablets become dry and harden and may not be absorbed.

Among the strongest of medicinal preparations are the narcotics and anesthetics. Narcotics should never be used by anyone without a physician's prescription and, indeed, no drug that has to be administered with a hypodermic syringe should find a place in the average family medicine chest. Some people with diabetes have been taught by their doctors to inject themselves with insulin. Even these people should keep their syringe outfit separate from the materials in the family medicine chest.

All sorts of antiseptics are available for use on the skin, in first aid and also for gargling and for washing various portions of the body. The Council on Pharmacy and Chemistry of the American Medical Association recognizes advertising of recognized antiseptics for first aid to the public, and tincture of iodine and mercurochrome are included among the preparations that may be so advertised. Others commonly used are merthiolates, metaphen, and zephiran.

There is no scientific evidence that any of the widely advertised antiseptic solutions used as gargles, sprays, or in any other manner will prevent the onset of a common cold. One of the best old-fashioned antiseptic solutions for common use around the home is boric acid solution. Most people prefer to have packages of crystals of boric acid, and to make up the solution fresh just before use. Poisoning of children with boric acid taken internally is possible.

The family medicine chest may also contain aromatic spirits of ammonia which is sometimes given when a prompt stimulant is needed following fainting. Half a teaspoonful in water, in a sudden fainting spell, is a fairly safe thing to give in most cases of emergency. The widely publicized milk of magnesia and sodium bicarbonate, or baking soda, are two preparations which can safely be kept in the family medicine chest and which are frequently advised by physicians for alkaline purposes. Some families keep paregoric as a useful preparation in case of cramps that disturb women at periodic intervals. Really these constitute practically all of the drugs that need to be in any family medicine chest because they are the few materials that can be used safely by most people.

SURGICAL SUPPLIES

In these days when everybody takes the chance of needing emergency first-aid treatment because of the common use of the automobile and wide indulgence in sports and gardening, it is well to have a certain minimum quantity of useful supplies around the home.

Among the materials needed for first aid are packages of adhesive tape of various widths, sterile cotton, sterile gauze bandages, sterile gauze pads, scissors which should be kept in the medicine chest and not used for the family sewing or for other emergencies around the home, and the ready-made combinations of a piece of adhesive tape with a tiny piece of sterilized bandage that can be used to cover small wounds or wounds after they have been treated with iodine or mercurochrome.

Most people should know that the proper way to stop bleeding of small wounds on the surface of the body is simply to press upon them with a sterile piece of gauze. In case of very serious wounds affecting arteries, and thereby difficult to control, it may be necessary to put a tourniquet around the limb. The tourniquet should be fastened just tight enough to stop the bleeding. An ordinary piece of rubber tubing or a narrow towel tied and twisted with a stick will serve most purposes satisfactorily. It should be temporarily released every ten or fifteen minutes.

In addition to the materials used for first aid, most families will have bed pans for use in cases of illness, glass drinking tubes, syringes for giving enemas, atomizers, and sometimes special devices for creating steam to be medicated with small amounts of tincture of benzoin for relief in various forms of hoarseness or other conditions affecting the larynx and the lungs.

The final materials to be included are the cosmetics. Most modern women prefer to keep their cosmetics in their own boudoirs or sleeping apartments. The man of the house is likely to put his into the family medicine chest. They should include, in most instances, a razor which should be kept in its box and not permitted to lie around loose; also some shaving soap or cream, some face lotion, which may be either witch hazel or any special lotion that he prefers.

Do not use a styptic in the form of a stick of alum to stop slight bleeding points after shaving. Much better are any of the stringent surgical powders, of which a small amount may be taken from the box at each occasion and applied directly to the bleeding point.

Finally, any good talcum powder may be used with satisfaction after shaving and after bathing, according to the individual preferences of the users.

Every modern household should have a good clinical thermometer, a hot-water bottle, and an ice bag. When these are available in an emergency the comfort they give is tremendous.

WARNINGS

Do not save poisonous preparations of any kind, including particularly bichloride of mercury, pills containing strychnine, or solutions containing wood alcohol. Do not keep samples of patent medicines of unknown composition recommended beyond their actual virtues. Never permit any preparation of opium or morphine to be loose in the family medicine chest. Never save any prepared prescription after the specific use for which it was ordered by the physician has disappeared.

EQUIPMENT OF THE FAMILY MEDICINE CHEST

A fountain syringe: This should be of rubber or of metal. Capacity about two quarts. It will have a long rubber tube and several nozzles of assorted sizes.

A bed pan: In many illnesses it is not safe for the patient to get up even to attend to the usual body needs.

A rubber sheet: This is to be placed under the sheet to prevent soiling of the mattress. A piece of oilcloth will service the purpose satisfactorily for a short time.

Bandages: These are cheaply purchased. They should be in various sizes from one-inch width to three-inch width.

Adhesive tape: This can also be purchased in spools of various widths and lengths.

Scissors: These should always be kept available in the medicine chest.

Thermometer: A good clinical thermometer should be available, and preferably two, one for taking temperature by mouth and another for temperature by rectum.

Ice bag: The ice bag applied to the sore throat is frequently recommended by doctors.

Atomizer: For spraying nose and throat. A graduated medicine glass for measuring dosages.

THE DRUGS AND MEDICAL SUPPLIES

CATHARTICS AND LAXATIVES:

Epsom salts: An old-fashioned remedy with lots of power. Best taken in the morning on arising. About a tablespoonful in a half-glass of warm water.

Citrate of magnesia: A milder saline laxative. Order a bottle from the druggist. Take a half bottle on arising and the rest later if needed. Anywhere from six to twelve ounces of the solution of magnesium citrate is a dose.

Castor oil: An effective and prompt cathartic but likely to be followed by constipation and therefore not indicated in chronic constipation. A dose is four teaspoonfuls. This can now be had in tasteless and flavored forms.

Mineral oil: A lubricant much used in chronic cases of constipation. Dose: One or two tablespoonfuls. Mineral oil should not be used habitually since it absorbs vitamin A.

Other cathartics: Other cathartics and laxatives much used include sodium acid phosphate, phenolphthalein, which is the active substance of such advertised laxatives as Feenamint, Ex-lax, and similar products, also the Hinkle pill, the compound cathartic pill, and other mixtures. Bulk laxatives are psyllium seed, agar, cellothyl. It is not well to develop a cathartic habit. It is not safe to take cathartics in the presence of undiagnosed pains in the abdomen.

GENERAL DRUGS AND SUPPLIES

Glycerine: Useful for many purposes. A few drops warmed and dropped into the ear are frequently advised for earache.

Vaseline petroleum jelly, Cold cream, Zinc oxide ointment: These are useful for abrasions of the skin, chafing, sunburn, etc.

Tincture of iodine: An ideal antiseptic for application to cuts or small wounds of the skin. It is usually painted on, using a toothpick wrapped with cotton.

Boric acid: A concentrated solution is a good home antiseptic solution.

Hydrogen peroxide solution: Diluted about one half with water makes a good cleansing wash for wounds. Diluted one to three with water, can be used as a gargle.

Sodium bicarbonate: Baking soda. Useful as a gargle. Much used for so-called "sour stomach." Good in the bath for itching of the skin.

Aspirin: The great American pain reliever. Much used for headaches. Much safer than pyramidon, barbituric acid derivatives, acetanilid, phenacetin, and all the other coal-tar derivatives. Dosage: one or two five-grain tablets, repeated in about three hours.

Aromatic spirits of ammonia: Used to bring about recovery after fainting spells.

Surgical powder: A styptic powder, best used on small cuts after shaving.

Petrolatum eucalyptus menthol compound: A nice mixture for use in the nose as a spray.

Paper towels, Paper handkerchiefs: Most useful in sickness. Can be destroyed after use.

The medicine chest should always be kept out of reach of the children. Prescriptions in current use may be kept in the chest, but should be destroyed after the patient is well. Every bottle and package should be clearly labeled. Do not stock up with a lot of cathartics and laxatives, cough and cold remedies. Keep only those regularly used and called for by members of the family.

MELANCHOLIA Sometimes with advancing years both men and women tend to develop a mental reaction that leads to melancholia. The symptoms usually come on at what women call "the change of life."

There still seems to be some question as to whether or not men also have a change of life. Certainly they do occasionally develop symptoms following the passing of middle age much like those that women develop under the same circumstances.

At this time the man or woman may find that life is beginning to be more disturbing, the resistance to pressures becomes less capable of meeting the need, the bounce or resiliency that is associated with youth has disappeared, and mistakes are more difficult to correct.

Under the circumstances here described, anxiety, apprehension, and indecision may lead to breakdown. The mental condition that develops represents an attempt to escape from pressure that cannot be overcome. Dr. Edward A. Strecker emphasizes the fact that the increasing likelihood of failure to attain successes that have been sought, financial reverses, disappointments, family worries, and the increasing number of family and friends that are taken by death tend to increase the internal psychic upset.

Women suffer more frequently from this type of melancholia than men—in fact the ratio is about three women to one man. The age range in women is from forty to fifty-five and in men from fifty to sixty five.

Of course inspiration from the lives of others is the answer to the problem for many people. Far too many men and women have made great successes of their lives following the climacteric for anyone to believe that this period represents the end of much that is vital in living.

Moreover, advancement in the care of the human body makes the modern woman realize that one past forty years of age need not necessarily be unattractive. The aids to beauty are sufficient to enable her to be just about as attractive as she wants to be provided she will put in the time and study required.

The chief symptoms, however, are related to the mind and not to the appearance of the body. The woman approaching melancholia tends to blame herself unnecessarily for activities or for lack of action.

Fortunately with the aid of the modern psychiatrist many of these people can be brought to prompt recovery. The treatment includes a study of the mental aspects which can be done only by someone properly trained in this field. The food should be sufficient, and proper sleep must be obtained by the methods that doctors can prescribe.

The glandular preparations which have been developed to replace the hormones (including the estrogenic hormone for women and the testosterone for men) are reported by many to be helpful. Equally important is development of suitable occupations and hobbies so that the mind can be turned to productive purposes.

MELANCHOLIA, INVOLUTIONAL — See MENTAL, article NERVOUS AND MENTAL DISORDERS.

MELANOSIS Abnormal deposits of pigment in various portions of the body are described as melanosis. Since pigment may be involved in all sorts of tissues, the prefix "melano-" may refer to pigment in sweat, melanidrosis; to the pigment in tumors, melanocarcinoma or melanosarcoma; pigment in the menstrual flow, melanorrhagia.

Quite recently reports have appeared in medical writings which indicate a new drug known as monobenzylether of hydroquinone has benefitted areas with excessive pigmentation due to deposits of melanin. A preparation of the drug has now been made known as Benoquin and has been used on some 84 patients with this condition. From one clinic it was reported that 64 of 84 patients had a good response. The method was used particularly on persons with severe freckling, with spots known as liver spots, with darkening of the skin which sometimes follows sensitivity to certain perfumes and with other similar conditions. The method has not been successful however in the treatment of birthmarks in which case there is an excessive amount of blood supply to the area with frequently the deposits of pigment from the blood in the skin.

MELANOMA—See article CANCER.

MEMORY Memory is one of the strangest of all of the functions of the human mind. It has given great concern to the psychologists to determine how it is carried on. Some information has come from experiments on the brain. It is known, for instance, that persons who have tumors of the frontal lobes of the brain complain of loss of memory, particularly for recent events.

Memory is so valuable an attribute to success that its importance cannot be overestimated. We know that hardening of the arteries and diminished circulation of the blood associated with the coming of old age also have an influence on memory.

There are many people who are only apparently unable to remember well. This, however, is the result of absent-mindedness and preoccupation and of the failure to give attention rather than any disorder of memory. Many people have a special faculty for remembering, which can be better developed by training. They are thereby more successful in occupations in which memory is important.

The type of loss of memory that is most serious is that which occurs suddenly and is accompanied by confusion. This may be a sign of disease. However, there is no reason to believe that a gradual failure of the memory indicates the beginning of any disorder of the brain.

Among the most dramatic and impressive disturbances that can affect the human being is the loss of memory called amnesia. This is an inability to remember occurrences that have happened during a certain period of life. Such loss of memory comes on frequently in relationship to a sudden emotional conflict or difficult situation. Usually memory begins to come back when some thread in the past is uncovered. The doctors find it difficult in most of these cases to decide whether or not complete inability to remember anything is actual or simulated. If anyone simply refuses to remember, the diagnosis is difficult. Cases are on record of people who have had as many as five such periods of sudden and complete loss of memory with subsequent recovery.

The psychoanalysts explain this form of loss of memory as a weak attempt of a weak personality to escape conflicts in daily life. Associated with the desire to escape is the fear of punishment, the fear of bodily injury, or the fear of certain human relationships.

MENIÈRE'S DISEASE In 1861 a French physician named Menière described a series of symptoms related to an acute disturbance of a structure in the internal ear called the labyrinth to which the name "Menière's disease" is now given.

Apparently there are several different causes for disturbances of the labyrinth. The chief symptoms are deafness and ringing in the ears associated with dizziness, vomiting, and sudden movements of the eyes from side to side. The attacks come on at regular intervals, and once the condition has started they may return with increasing frequency. Some cases seem to improve without anything special in the way of treatment. Others get better and alternately get worse. Sometimes improvement follows operations on the sinuses, removal of the tonsils and adenoids, treatment of the hearing, the extraction of infected teeth, the blowing out of the Eustachian tubes, and changes in the diet.

It has been thought that possibly the difficulty was associated with a disturbance of the water balance of the body, also that it was associated with a retention of sodium in the body. For this reason diets that are low in sodium and high in protein are sometimes prescribed. Also ammonium chloride is given with a view to preventing salt retention.

More recently a surgical procedure has been evolved. This includes especially operations on the nerve of hearing, also attempts to investigate the area concerned for the presence of infections, tumors, or similar disturbances.

Menière's disease rarely occurs in young people. Most of those affected are between the ages of thirty and sixty.

Dramamine and Bonamine have aided in controlling the dizziness associated with Menière's disease.

MENINGES The coverings of the brain and spinal cord are called the meninges. Inflammation of these coverings is meningitis. A tumor in the meninges is a meningioma. The prefix also appears in many other conditions affecting these membranes.

MENINGES—See INFECTIOUS DISEASE,

article THE PREVENTION AND TREATMENT OF INFECTIOUS DISEASE.

MENINGITIS Meningitis, an infection of the brain and incidentally also of the blood, is caused in most instances by the germ called the meningococcus. It is possible, however, for other germs like the pneumococcus or the streptococcus to cause meningitis and also for viruses to cause inflammation of the coverings of the brain and spinal cord, which are known as meninges.

The doctor diagnoses meningitis not only from the history of the patient, which may indicate that he has been in contact with the infection, and from the symptoms but also by obtaining specimens of the spinal fluid, which are studied for the presence of germs and for other changes which indicate infection and inflammation. In times when epidemics of meningitis are present, doctors examine not only the spinal fluid of those who are sick but also the secretions of the nose and throat of the sick and of those around them to determine whether are not the germs are present. Occasionally examinations are made of the blood to find out whether there is or is not a meningococcemia, which means germs of meningitis in the blood.

The symptoms of meningitis arise from the changes that the germs and their poisons produce in the tissues of the nervous system. During the period of invasion sore throat, dullness, fever, chills, rapid pulse, and a general soreness of the body indicate that an infection is present. Then comes a rash of pin-point-sized red spots or even large spots over the body. In the stage when the infection has spread to the nervous system severe pain is felt, associated with bursting headache, vomiting, and even delirium and convulsions.

Meningitis is particularly a disease associated with overcrowding, so that it appears in wartime when great numbers of men are housed in barracks. Although there had been just a few cases of meningitis in Great Britain up to 1940, the assembling of the army at that time brought about a sudden severe outbreak which affected more than 4000 men in the first six months of 1940.

The way to prevent meningitis is to avoid overcrowding and to avoid contact with sick people. In many of our American camps provision had been made for a cubicle system, so that a curtain or screen comes down at night between the beds of men in barracks. Even without such intervening devices it is possible to decrease the incidence of meningitis by lessening the crowding. In one camp it was found that the carrier rate was 29 per cent when the space between the beds was nine inches, 20 per cent when a foot was allowed between adjacent beds, and only 5 per cent when a three-foot space was allowed.

Before the discovery of a serum which could be used against meningitis, the death rate used to be 80 or 90 out of every 100 cases. There was a severe epidemic in New York in 1904, when there were 2755 cases with 2026 deaths. Following the discovery of the anti-meningitis serum, the rate was greatly reduced. Then came the discovery of the sulfonamide drugs, which were found to have great powers in controlling the germs, and the rate was cut down to much less than 20 per cent. More recently penicillin has been developed. This is injected into the muscles, into the blood, and in fact directly into the spinal fluid. The most recent report on the use of penicillin intensively used in cases of meningitis indicated that there were 75 recoveries out of 76 consecutive cases. Thus the fear formerly associated with this dangerous disease has been lessened. Obviously there are many complications and associated symptoms possible in meningitis which demand the very best of medical attention. Preferably every case of meningitis should be cared for in a good hospital.

Meningitis was always a serious condition. The form caused by the germ of meningitis known as the meningococcus was difficult but other forms caused by the germs of pneumonia, by the streptococcus or by the organism of tuberculosis were considered invariably fatal. The development of the new antibiotic drugs has brought about the possibility of attacking all these infections. The streptococci are controllable by such drugs as penicillin, aureomycin, chloromycetin and streptomycin; tuberculosis is controllable by streptomycin, paraminosalicylic acid and isoniazid; the pneumococcus is also controllable by the antibiotic drugs. The virus diseases of the brain and spinal cord are not amenable to treatment with the antibiotic drugs to the same extent. Therefore the various forms of inflammation of the brain called encephalitis are still difficult to treat by any of the available techniques.

MENINGITIS—arthritis: See article ARTHRITIS, RHEUMATISM, AND GOUT.

MENINGITIS—boils on lip may cause: See SKIN, article THE SKIN.

MENINGITIS—brain: See INFECTIOUS DISEASE, article THE PREVENTION AND TREATMENT OF INFECTIOUS DISEASE.

MENINGITIS—cause: See INFECTIOUS DISEASE, article THE PREVENTION AND TREATMENT OF INFECTIOUS DISEASE.

MENINGITIS—confused with infantile paralysis: See CHILDHOOD DISEASES, article INFECTIOUS DISEASES OF CHILDHOOD.

MENINGITIS—incubation period: See INFECTIOUS DISEASE, article THE PREVENTION AND TREATMENT OF INFECTIOUS DISEASE.

MENINGITIS—lymph nodes swell as in German measles: See CHILDHOOD DISEASES, article INFECTIOUS DISEASES OF CHILDHOOD.

MENINGITIS—rheumatism can result: See article ARTHRITIS, RHEUMATISM, AND GOUT.

MENINGITIS—sinus infection may cause: See EAR, article THE EAR, TONGUE, NOSE, AND THROAT.

MENINGITIS—spinal cord: See INFECTIOUS DISEASE, article THE PREVENTION AND TREATMENT OF INFECTIOUS DISEASE.

MENINGITIS—treatment: See INFECTIOUS DISEASE, article THE PREVENTION AND TREATMENT OF INFECTIOUS DISEASE.

MENINGITIS—tuberculosis: See RESPIRATORY DISEASES, article THE RESPIRATORY DISEASES.

MENOPAUSE Between the ages of forty-five and fifty the average woman undergoes certain physical changes which are grouped by the diagnosticians under the single term of menopause. This is also called by women in general the climacteric, the climax, or the change of life. These changes occur in rare instances before the age of forty and sometimes as late as fifty-five. They are definitely associated with the gradual inability of certain glands to provide the secretions which they provide during youth and maturity.

In some women all of the changes take place suddenly and abruptly and without much trouble. Many, however, go through this period in their lives over a duration of three or four years. Most of the serious symptoms that occur involve the nervous system and the blood. The most common symptom is the appearance of what are called hot flashes, during which the entire body becomes warm and there is excessive perspiration followed by chilliness. The flushes come on at any time, sometimes without any apparent cause and at other times associated with slight excitement. The change in the circulation brings about also such symptoms as palpitation, headache, and dizziness. The symptoms related to the nervous system include irritability, occasionally depression, and quite often insomnia.

The active period of the reproductive system of a woman is about twenty-five years. Then the tissues involved in reproduction gradually become unnecessary and deteriorate. Ordinarily a woman develops once each month an egg cell, or ovum, which is released from the ovary so that she may give birth to a child. The ovaries develop internal secretions, or chemical substances, which go directly into the blood and which govern the condition of the uterus in which the ovum, when it is fertilized by the male cell, comes to rest. If the egg is not fertilized, the wall of the uterus is cast off and washed out by bleeding. This is called menstruation because it occurs about once each month. The Latin term for month is *mensis*. There is no special function for menstruation other than getting rid of this cast-off lining from the uterus Menstruation is not a means of getting rid of body poisons as some women foolishly believe.

Most of the complaints that occur during the menopause are, after all, relatively minor disturbances. In most instances it is possible nowadays to overcome these disturbances by giving the internal secretion that is lacking from the body in the form of a drug. The physician who takes care of a woman under such circumstances is able to determine whether or not the symptoms are the ordinary symptoms of the menopause, also how much of the hormones should be prescribed and when they should be taken. A medical examination at this time is of the greatest importance because there are other conditions which can produce symptoms like those of the menopause. The new drugs that have been developed and the technic of their use represents one of the greatest discoveries of modern times for freeing women from the fear associated with the menopause and for overcoming the disagreeable symptoms.

MENOPAUSE—See WOMEN, article HYGIENE OF WOMEN; article ENDOCRINOLOGY.

MENOPAUSE—age: See WOMEN, article HYGIENE OF WOMEN.

MENOPAUSE—asthma: See article ALLERGY.

MENOPAUSE—devil's pinches: See BLOOD, article THE BLOOD AND ITS DISEASES.

MENOPAUSE—diabetes tendency great: See article DIABETES.

MENOPAUSE—egg cells no longer produced: See article SEX HYGIENE.

MENOPAUSE—glandular change: See SKIN, article THE SKIN.

MENOPAUSE—hair lost: See HAIR, article THE HAIR.

MENOPAUSE—hormones: See WOMEN, article HYGIENE OF WOMEN.

MENOPAUSE—hypertension frequently developed: See article BLOOD PRESSURE.

MENOPAUSE—itching: See WOMEN, article HYGIENE OF WOMEN; SKIN, article THE SKIN.

MENOPAUSE—menstruation ceases: See WOMEN, article HYGIENE OF WOMEN.

MENOPAUSE—mental attitude: See article SEX HYGIENE.

MENOPAUSE—mental depression: See WOMEN, article HYGIENE OF WOMEN.

MENOPAUSE—ovarian hormone: See article ENDOCRINOLOGY.

MENOPAUSE—vascular purpura: See BLOOD, article THE BLOOD AND ITS DISEASES.

MENSTRUATION The average age at which girls in the United States mature varies between twelve and sixteen, although normal girls may mature before twelve or after sixteen. The average interval between periods in women is twenty-eight days, although it may be as short as twenty-one or as long as thirty-five days. Moreover, irregularity may be normal with some women. The length of the periods may vary from two to six days. Slight variations should not cause any mental distress. Physicians should be consulted, however, when there is a sudden change in the regularity or a disappearance of the period.

A disappearance of the period is frequently associated with undernutrition, anemia, wasting diseases, or severe infections. These may not only cause a disappearance of the period but interfere seriously with the regularity, the duration, or the intensity of any particular period. Typhoid fever, rheumatic fever, or tuberculosis may bring about irregularity. Disturbances of the thyroid, pituitary, or the ovarian glands also are responsible for difficulties with the menstrual periods.

If the appearance of maturity should be unusually delayed, a young girl should be taken to a physician for a careful examination so that he may determine whether or not the organs involved have developed as they should. If there is too much delay in making an investigation, changes may occur in the organs and tissues which may ultimately make normal childbirth impossible.

Of course the most frequent cause of failure of the period to appear is pregnancy.

Formerly many girls and young women were incapacitated during the time of the period due to pains in the lower part of the abdomen and the thighs and similar symptoms. When pain is not severe, the use of mild doses of the ordinary sedatives frequently brings about relief. Persistent pain demanding more than such relief means that study should be made as to the cause of the disturbance. Some of the pain-relieving drugs are dangerous to health and life. The use of simple pain-relieving drugs is not harmful but persistence may develop the habit of dependence on the drug even if it does not develop addiction.

Ordinarily the young woman need not change her habits greatly during the time of the period. Most doctors believe that strenuous exercise is to be avoided at this time. Generally it is not considered advisable to take a tub bath for at least the first two days of the period and certainly not to go swimming. When it is realized that the period represents merely the throwing off by the organ concerned in childbirth of excess tissue developed in prepara-

The following charts explain the menstrual cycle, the organs involved, and show what happens when conception takes place. The first day of the menstrual period is the first day of the cycle.

A. THE ORGANS INVOLVED

OVUM
Egg which develops monthly in non-pregnant woman.

OVARIES
Alternate in producing egg each month.

FOLLICLE
Bladder full of liquid which swells and bursts, washing egg out.

UTERUS
Nourishes fertilized egg in its lining. Expels lining monthly (menstruation) if egg is not fertilized.

CORPUS LUTEUM
Gland formed in burst follicle. Promotes growth of uterus lining.

TUBES
Catch egg and transport it to uterus. Meeting place for sperm and egg.

VAGINA
Passage where sperm is deposited to fertilize egg.

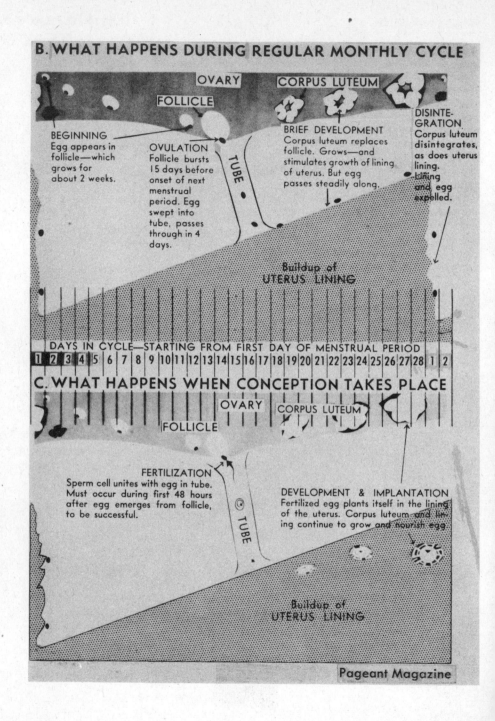

B. WHAT HAPPENS DURING REGULAR MONTHLY CYCLE

OVARY

CORPUS LUTEUM

FOLLICLE

DISINTEGRATION
Corpus luteum disintegrates, as does uterus lining. Lining and egg expelled.

BEGINNING
Egg appears in follicle—which grows for about 2 weeks.

OVULATION
Follicle bursts 15 days before onset of next menstrual period. Egg swept into tube, passes through in 4 days.

TUBE

BRIEF DEVELOPMENT
Corpus luteum replaces follicle. Grows—and stimulates growth of lining of uterus. But egg passes steadily along.

Buildup of
UTERUS LINING

DAYS IN CYCLE—STARTING FROM FIRST DAY OF MENSTRUAL PERIOD

1 2 3 4 5 6 7 8 9 10 11 12 13 14 15 16 17 18 19 20 21 22 23 24 25 26 27 28 1 2

C. WHAT HAPPENS WHEN CONCEPTION TAKES PLACE

OVARY

CORPUS LUTEUM

FOLLICLE

FERTILIZATION
Sperm cell unites with egg in tube. Must occur during first 48 hours after egg emerges from follicle, to be successful.

TUBE

DEVELOPMENT & IMPLANTATION
Fertilized egg plants itself in the lining of the uterus. Corpus luteum and lining continue to grow and nourish egg.

Buildup of
UTERUS LINING

Pageant Magazine

tion for fertilization of the ovum and that this is not concerned in any way with the maintenance of health or with getting rid of poisons from the body, the importance of considering the period a normal physiological reaction is apparent.

LUTREXIN—Lutrexin, a new hormone derived from corpus luteum (the body that develops in the ovary after ovulation), is said to alleviate painful menstruation. The hormone was administered the day before menstruation was expected, before the usual severe cramps and nausea began.

MENSTRUATION—See WOMEN, article HYGIENE OF WOMEN; article ENDOCRINOLOGY.

MENSTRUATION—absence: See WOMEN, article HYGIENE OF WOMEN.

MENSTRUATION—absence does not prevent conception: See BIRTH, article CARE OF MOTHERS BEFORE AND AFTER CHILDBIRTH.

MENSTRUATION—adolescence: See article SEX HYGIENE.

MENSTRUATION—asthma: See article ALLERGY.

MENSTRUATION—bathing: See WOMEN, article HYGIENE OF WOMEN.

MENSTRUATION—beginning: See WOMEN, article HYGIENE OF WOMEN.

MENSTRUATION—breasts should be checked for cancer day following each period: See article CANCER.

MENSTRUATION—cancer possibly indicated by excessive bleeding: See WOMEN, article HYGIENE OF WOMEN.

MENSTRUATION—cotton pads: See WOMEN, article HYGIENE OF WOMEN.

MENSTRUATION—cycle: See WOMEN, article HYGIENE OF WOMEN.

MENSTRUATION—disorders: See WOMEN, article HYGIENE OF WOMEN.

MENSTRUATION—disturbances occasionally due to allergic factors: See article ALLERGY.

MENSTRUATION—douches: See WOMEN, article HYGIENE OF WOMEN.

MENSTRUATION—duration: See WOMEN, article HYGIENE OF WOMEN.

MENSTRUATION—exercise may be continued: See article POSTURE.

MENSTRUATION—exercises: See WOMEN, article HYGIENE OF WOMEN.

MENSTRUATION—fertile period: See WOMEN, article HYGIENE OF WOMEN.

MENSTRUATION—games to be avoided: See WOMEN, article HYGIENE OF WOMEN.

MENSTRUATION—girls' interest in athletics limited by: See article SEX HYGIENE.

MENSTRUATION—herpes: See SKIN, article THE SKIN.

MENSTRUATION—hormones control: See article BLOOD PRESSURE.

MENSTRUATION—hygiene: See article SEX HYGIENE.

MENSTRUATION—iron deficiency anemia: See BLOOD, article THE BLOOD AND ITS DISEASES.

MENSTRUATION—irregular bleeding may indicate cancer of uterus: See article CANCER.

MENSTRUATION—irregularity in fourth and fifth decade: See article ENDOCRINOLOGY.

MENSTRUATION—marriage date: See article SEX HYGIENE.

MENSTRUATION—migraine: See article FIRST AID.

MENSTRUATION—modifications of the glandular mechanism to relieve pain: See WOMEN, article HYGIENE OF WOMEN.

MENSTRUATION—organs involved: See WOMEN, article HYGIENE OF WOMEN.

MENSTRUATION—pains: See WOMEN, article HYGIENE OF WOMEN.

MENSTRUATION—premenstrual tension: See WOMEN, article HYGIENE OF WOMEN.

MENSTRUATION—return after childbirth: See BIRTH, article CARE OF

MOTHERS BEFORE AND AFTER CHILD-BIRTH.

MENSTRUATION—rhythm: See WOMEN, article HYGIENE OF WOMEN.

MENSTRUATION—scanty: See WOMEN, article HYGIENE OF WOMEN.

MENSTRUATION—sterile period: See WOMEN, article HYGIENE OF WOMEN.

MENSTRUATION—swimming: See WOMEN, article HYGIENE OF WOMEN.

MENSTRUATION—vaginal: See WOMEN, article HYGIENE OF WOMEN.

MENSTRUATION—temperature control and rhythm: See WOMEN, article HYGIENE OF WOMEN.

MENSTRUATION—tuberculosis causes cessation: See article SEX HYGIENE.

MENSTRUATION—unusual odors should be investigated: See WOMEN, article HYGIENE OF WOMEN.

MENSTRUATION—urine specimens may give strong positive reaction for albumin: See KIDNEY, article THE KIDNEY: ITS DISEASES AND DISTURBANCES.

Nervous and Mental Disorders

BY

GEORGE K. PRATT, M.D.

Associate in Neuropsychiatry, Bridgeport Hospital, Bridgeport, Conn.

Introduction

About 9,000,000 people in the United States are suffering from mental illness and other personality disturbances—about 6% of the present population, or about 1 in every 16 people. Of this number, about 1,500,000 are suffering from mental illness. About 7,500,000, it is estimated, have other personality disturbances. In addition, there are about 1,500,000 mentally deficient people—conservatively about 1% of the population.

There are about 650,000 patients in mental hospitals. In addition, there are about 120,000 mentally deficient and about 20,000 epileptic patients in institutions for the mentally deficient and epileptic.

Each year about 250,000 new patients are admitted to mental hospitals. In addition, about 100,000 more are admitted who have been in mental hospitals before. Thus new admissions and re-admissions total about 350,000 a year.

About 30% of all the patients who go to general hospitals, and about 50% of all the patients who go to general practitioners suffer from mental illness and *other personality disturbances* or physical illnesses associated with *mental illness and other personality disturbances.*

Mental illness or other personality disturbances are usually significant factors in criminal behavior, delinquency, suicide, alcoholism, narcotic addiction, and often in cases of divorce.

At What Age Do Mental Illness and Other Personality Disturbances Occur?

Mental illness and other personality disturbances occur at all ages. Few cases of psychosis occur before the age of 15. The various psychoses have "preferred" age ranges for their initial development. They do not all affect the same age brackets to the same extent. Schizophrenia (dementia praecox) is the "psychosis of youth and early adult life." This disorder begins as a rule between the ages of 15 and 30. Few people develop it after 50. The most common psychoses of the middle age group—between 35 and 60—are manic-depressive psychosis, general paresis, alcoholic psychosis, paranoia and involutional melancholia. The first three develop most frequently between the ages of 40 and 50. The last two are most common in their initial incidence between the ages of 50 and 55. The "psychoses of old age" are senile psychosis and cerebral arteriosclerosis. The great majority of cases develop after 60.

Emotional Health

Most people have minor emotional disturbances that are not recognized but have medical significance because of their effects on the general health. Many people in industry, in labor and in public life get along although they suffer at all time with difficulties of adjustment to their environment. From 30 to 60 per cent of all the people who come to the doctor as patients come primarily because of complaints due to emotional disorders, which are reflected as physical disorders. Frustrations, anxiety and fear may appear as headaches, ulcers of the stomach, asthma or similar conditions. Treatment is not fully satisfactory unless it takes care of the mental as well as the physical factors.

Our population has become an aging population. People live much longer than was common 50 years ago. As people get older they tend to develop more emotional experiences, and this has greatly multiplied the need of psychiatric help. One out of every twenty people will need advice or guidance from an expert for severe emotional illness at some time during his lifetime. This is proved by the fact that more than one-half of all the veterans in veterans' hospitals are psychiatric patients. Thirty-seven per cent of the men released from the army for medical reasons were for psychiatric disorders. A total of 51 per cent of all medical separations from the military service were due to personality disturbances. In addition people who are mentally disturbed constitute about one-half of all the patients in hospitals in the United States.

Often human beings become mentally and emotionally disturbed because of self-condemnation related to problems which they do not understand. The so-

cial and cultural considerations which regulate human sex behavior are far more rigid than the biological considerations. These considerations define what is moral much more definitely than do biologic and medical science.

In various portions of the United States the attitudes of people vary a great deal as to the ordinary relationships between the sexes. In some portions of the country it would be considered a gross violation of domestic relations for a married man to have lunch with a married woman other than his wife. In other branches of American society, and this refers of course particularly to our larger cities, such ordinary meetings are within the pattern of every day social existence.

When a young man moves in the United States from one community to another he may require several months to find out the restrictions on conduct which are considered suitable to the new community. Up to 1915 people paid very little attention to inhibitions and did not fret much about these matters. Since that time public education on psychological subjects has created fear among many people of being considered inhibited.

People who are infantile in their emotional attitudes are likely to be dependent on their parents or substitutes for the parents as for instance a governess or nurse and to expect infinite amounts of services and tolerance from the parents. Sometimes men and women of advanced years retain this infantile attitude until the death of the parent or some forced separation which may be quite tragic in their lives. Thus a woman 38 years old who was subject to repeated moody spells had that kind of dependence and had to have someone strong on whom to lean in all her difficult situations. The child who has been "teacher's pet" as he grows up will have to be the "boss's favorite" when he gets a job.

The child develops some sense of personal responsibility but can always get rid of it by an excuse. The child still has to have complete trust in some other person. People who grow up and maintain their childish level are people who always find excuses for the failures, alibis for their weakness and who "pass the buck" whenever confronted with difficult situations. The child who passes the period of puberty with its development of secondary sexual characteristics really goes through two periods which may be called early adolescence and late adolescence. The child in early adolescence begins to have a drive for self assertion and begins to resent parental domination. Just as the male animal shows his best characteristics for the attraction of the female, so also the boys in early adolescence begin to show off and to indulge in contests in which they can demonstrate their superiority. The boy's room begins to be filled with trophies won at the track or in the swimming pool or at other sports. The girl's room begins to be decorated with programs of dances, souvenirs of parties and knickknacks accumulated on dates.

As late adolescence develops "dating" becomes the most important aspect of life. If this passes on to what boys and girls call "going steady," difficult mental situations may develop. Parents frequently try to dominate the situation because of economic, religious or purely emotional reactions. These situations may lead to emotional disturbances in the young that may mark the life of the growing youth for many years thereafter.

Finally, adults are supposed to have a balanced perspective and to adjust themselves to various social roles but adults still need affection, security and well established relationships toward other people. If the adult has failed to mature and depends heavily on the affection of others, if he requires definite signs of favoritism, he is unlikely to be able to develop a satisfactory marriage and may react emotionally to situations which he himself cannot solve.

Suitable adjustment of workers to their surroundings is important in establishing a smooth-running condition in any business or industry. Ask the average businessman if he needs a psychiatrist in his business, and he will think you are mentally disturbed. Psychiatrists, most people believe, spend practically all of their time finding people who need to be confined in institutions because they are wholly irresponsible.

Most large industries have employment interviewers who have knowledge of the positions to be filled, of the persons in the department and, therefore, of the kind of employee who will fit best and serve most satisfactorily under the circumstances. Most employment interviewers can recognize easily a prospective employee who is so far "off the beaten path" from a mental point of view as to be unsatisfactory for any job. No one suggests that employment interviewers should be replaced by psychiatrists or psychologists. What a businessman wants is a worker who can respond to the particular problems and procedures of the job for which he is employed. The boss seldom wants to be troubled about the general personality of an employee or the question of how he gets along with his wife. Nevertheless, that very situation may be important in relation to the quality or amount of work. Problems may arise which are due to a neurosis or psychosis in some employee whose mental condition has not been recognized.

Mental hygienists are convinced that training ought to be made available to employment managers or to the workers in the personnel divisions of industries. Workers are frequently transferred into personnel departments because they appear to be able to get along well with other people, but sometimes because they are hard and skeptical. Generally they work out their own technics, whether for the handling of personal problems or for the selection of new employees.

Already there are plenty of reports of instances in which employees who failed to respond acceptably to their executives were given scientific study and *thus saved for the organization. We have learned how to modify the attitudes of parents and to improve their relationships with their children. Similar tactics are needed for executive businessmen to improve their relationships with their employees.*

M. F.

Abnormal mental conditions were not always regarded as sickness. Departures from average mentality in bygone centuries were usually considered to be religious or legal problems. Not until well into the seventeenth century did medicine acknowledge responsibility for "insanity" as a variety of sickness. Not very much was known about its symptoms (except a few of the more violent, spectacular ones) and still less was known about what caused it or how to cure it. For a long time the best doctors could do for mental patients was to see that they were given humane care in suitable institutions and were no longer maltreated or subjected to the abuse that formerly was the lot of the insane in practically every country of the world. For this reason these institutions were called "asylums."

Gradually, physicians came to be interested in the mentally sick people and to engage in scientific research. First it was discovered that mental disease was not just one sickness, but was, instead, a term that applied to a large number of sicknesses; second, these various kinds of mental disease often had quite different symptoms; and third, some cases always seemed mild while others were severe. As a result it became possible to classify the different kinds of mental disease and to pin labels on them. For a long time physicians devoted most of their attention to describing, classifying, and diagnosing the many divisions and subdivisions and sub-subdivisions that were coming to be recognized.

Unhappily for the patients, this describing and classifying failed to do much in a practical way toward getting them well. At last the doctors called to their assistance certain other sciences, particularly psychology and philosophy. Between them they commenced to study the problem of *why* people acted as they did and what it was that made them say the things they said.

Some physicians attacked the problem from the conventional angle of physical medicine. They searched in the physical make-up of the patient's body for the motives that underlay human behavior. In many mentally disturbed people they were able to find physical diseases—or at least disorders of physical functions—that seemed to account for the symptoms. Thus, in that type of mental disease known as general paresis they saw with the microscope and often with the naked eye certain areas in the patient's brain where the consistency of the tissue was altered and partially liquefied. They also discovered (much later) that the cause of all the trouble in these cases was the tiny microorganism of syphilis which had invaded the brain and central nervous system. But when all was said and done, there yet remained a majority of all the known abnormal mental conditions for which the most scientific study failed to find any adequate physical cause.

Other doctors attacked the problem from the functional rather than the organic point of view. If unusual displays of behavior do not seem to have a physical cause, then let us begin with some of the cases in institutions that seem free from any organic disease and see what we can learn by studying, not just the structure and physiology of their organs, including their brains, but also their psychology. In other words, let's study man as a *whole*. This was a novel medical idea in those days, for up to that time most physicians had devoted their efforts to studying anatomical fragments of the patient such as heart or liver or lungs, and what these fragments did and how they acted. Now it was proposed to study, not so much what these special organs did, but what *the whole patient did* who owned these organs. This method finally became known as the study of "total reactions" and is the method that is being given increasing attention today. Essentially this is psychosomatic medicine.

The symptoms exhibited by men and women with various types of mental disorder have a close (if slightly disguised) resemblance to the basic personalities and traits of character that had marked these persons for many years before they became mentally sick. The mental disease symptoms, when properly interpreted, are seen to be but exaggerations of similar symptoms in evidence, perhaps, from childhood, but milder, of course, at that earlier age, and unrecognized then as anything more significant than "queer" or annoying or fussy habits of personality. There usually is a close connection between adult mental disorder and the development of unhealthy "patterns" (or habits) of personality during the plastic years of childhood, when personality is in the process of being molded. Often it is possible today to predict whether a child will grow up to become an adult who develops some form of mental disease, or whether he will go through life with his mental health unimpaired. Thus, a child whose "patterns" of personality are so sound and sturdy that they enable him to meet in a healthy manner disappointment in life, failure, or frustration is the child who will probably become an adult free from mental disorder. But another child may develop patterns that prove feeble reeds on which to lean when disappointment or failure confront him. As a consequence, he is unable to adjust himself in a wholesome manner to these trying experiences and is forced instead to flee into some form of mental disease as a sort of compromise adjustment.

CAUSES OF MENTAL DISORDERS

Why do people behave as they do? One patient was supposed to have become mentally sick because he lost his job and all his money. Another's mental disorder was attributed to a disappointment in love. As knowledge of psychiatry (which is that branch of medicine dealing with nervous and mental diseases) began to grow, it finally became evident that many of these alleged causes were not the real basic causes at all but merely *precipitating* causes. That is, the loss of money or the disappointment in love were only the last straws to break the camel's back—the final strains on an adjustive capacity that had never been strong in the first place. Otherwise, everyone who lost his money or was disappointed in love might be expected to develop mental disease as a result. The great majority of men and women faced with similar difficulties managed to adjust to them. So far as most functional mental disorders are concerned (those in which it is not possible to find a physical cause) the true and basic cause is a failure on the part of the patient to adjust himself to certain of the mental conflicts that beset him.

When a child is born into the world he brings with him a variety of psychological baggage. Part of this consists of his intellectual endowment, but at the moment we are more concerned with another part which might be called certain emotional tendencies inherited from his immediate ancestors—parents and grandparents. Still a third part—one that is beginning to receive a great deal of serious attention nowadays—consists of an assortment of primitive, savage instincts and "drives," which he also inherits as his share of the heritage of all mankind. These might be thought of as racial tendencies which the whole human race inherits from its ancestors of millions of years ago. These primitive instincts or "drives" include the instinct of self-preservation as well as that of race-preservation and many others. In those days, countless ages ago when man was first beginning his long painful struggle toward his present stage of development, there were few niceties. People did about as they pleased. If one cave man was hungry and his neighbor had a fresh piece of bear meat, the first man killed him—if he could—and took what he needed to keep himself alive. If a second cave man took a fancy to the woman of a third, he seized her—if he could—and henceforth she was his, at least until a still stronger cave man took her away from him in turn. Life probably was a pretty simple, crude (according to present standards), direct sort of affair. Men and women did what they wanted to whenever they felt like it with little to hinder them except the one restraint of superior physical strength, and there was scant place in the tribal code of that day for those more civilized feelings of altruism and unselfishness.

But slowly man came to be civilized. Slowly he came to realize that the first stirrings of finer needs within him could not always be satisfied by brute force alone, and that it was to the broader interests of that new, finer part of him, as well as to the interests of his group as a whole, to make a place in his scheme of things for regulations, prohibitions, and self-imposed restraints. This was not accomplished, however, without protests from the other part of him that longed for the "good old days" when there were no restraints and man did as he pleased unless someone stronger prevented. Here, then, developed mental conflict—a conflict between desire versus duty; between the savage, primitive instincts that formerly were expressed in crude, direct form with no pretense at disguising them, and the dawning realization that the demands of individual and social progress called for the repression or the transformation of some of these primitive instincts into more socially acceptable ones.

In the tens of thousands of years that have elapsed since this conflict first began, advancing cultural development has succeeded in annihilating these raw, primitive "drives" whose direct display had become, by this time, quite taboo. But here is where another discovery of modern psychiatry throws an interesting light on human behavior. Doctors know that the human body today harbors several vestigial remains or remnants of organs that have no known function in a 1950 model body, but which are believed to have served a vitally necessary purpose in the human body of millions of years ago. Thus, the human appendix has no known useful function in this day and age, unless, as some wag once remarked, it is to enable surgeons to ride in limousines. But in the psychological field something of the same thing is believed also to have occurred, and psychiatrists insist that modern man carries with him in the unconscious part of his mind certain vestigial remains of ancient instincts and impulses that once served a useful purpose when given frank, direct expression, but which thousands of centuries of civilization now demand be modified.

This is what is meant when we say that a child is born into the world with psychological baggage that includes—'way down deep in his unconscious— the carry-over of some of these primitive "drives." And this is why every modern nursery school teacher will tell you that the very young child is completely selfish (selfish, that is, when viewed from our adult standards) and completely antisocial as well. For the first two or three years of his life the child wants to do what he wants when he wants, without any interference. His tiny mental life for this period is much nearer that of his primitive caveman ancestors than it is of his immediate generation, and at first he tries to act accordingly. He demands immediate gratification of all his desires. If he is hungry for food, he demands to be fed—instantly. If he is hungry for attention, he insists on being cuddled. If he is uncomfortable from a full bladder, he wets himself at once and in any place. He has no consideration for the feelings of others, and his chief aim in life is to get pleasure and avoid pain.

But as he grows older his mother begins to train him in food and toilet habits. She tries to teach him to control his wants, to wait for more appropriate times for their expression. She also, lovingly but firmly, gets it across to him that he can't always have his own way; that self-gratification is only possible through some consideration of others, or is dependent on the will of someone who is stronger. And so gradually he is required to submit to that process known as the "civilization of instinct," and he becomes a more socialized creature. But do not make the mistake of thinking that because he gradually checks some of his primitive desires and shows a willingness to give in to others, he has lost these desires or that he has become altruistic all of a sudden. To be sure, he has learned it is to his advantage to make concessions to this mother-person who has the power to bestow or withhold pleasure; who can approve or punish. And he likewise comes to the conclusion that gratification of his pleasure needs often must come in a roundabout manner, after first placating mother, who stands in the rôle of authority. That is how genuine unselfishness and altruism have their beginnings. The child learns that full gratification requires the coöperation of others, and he becomes altruistic only as he comes to realize that it pays to be altruistic because one gets the most pleasure out of life that way. Nevertheless, while he may submit gracefully to the "civilization of instinct" with a minimum of protest, the savage instincts are always there under the surface of consciousness, and the individual, no matter how old he grows to be, is forever trying to shape his mental life in accordance with what the followers of the school of dynamic psychology call the "pleasure principle." But opposed to this pleasure principle is another called the "reality principle." Both are pulling, in the unconscious mind of the person, in different directions. Swayed by the pleasure principle, he seeks to act in a way that will insure immediate gratification of primitive desires but avoids as much unpleasantness in the process as possible. In the opposite direction he experiences a pull from the reality principle which tends to shape his mental life according to the demands of necessity as personified at first by the stronger power of the parents and later by the customs of society. Dr. Abraham Myerson, a distinguished psychiatrist in Boston, writing about these conflicts, has this to say about them:

> Every human being is a pot boiling with desires, passions, lusts, wishes, purposes, ideas and emotions, some of which he clearly recognizes and clearly admits, and some of which he does not clearly recognize and which he would deny. These desires, passions, etc., are not in harmony with one another; they are often irreconcilable, and one has to be smothered for the sake of the other.

Thus, a sex feeling that is not legitimate, an illicit forbidden love has to be conquered for the purpose of being religious or good, or the desire to be respected. So one may struggle against hatred for a person whom one should love—a husband, a wife, an invalid parent, or child whose care is a burden—and one refuses to recognize that there is such a struggle. So also one may seek to suppress jealousy, envy of the nearest and dearest; soul-stirring, forbidden passions; secret revolt against morality and law which may (and often does) rage in the most puritanical breast.

In the theory of the subconscious these undesired thoughts, feelings, passions and wishes are suppressed and pushed into the innermost recesses of the being, out of the light of conscious personality, but nevertheless, acting on that personality, distorting it, wearying it.

For these reasons we say the real task of childhood is to bring about a balance between primitive, biologic desires on the one hand, and the demands of society as symbolized by mother and father, on the other. If a child can bring about such a balance, we say he is well adjusted and has good mental health. But if he cannot, then the degree of resulting maladjustment depends on the strength of the primitive impulse that grips him, as well as on the severity of the social demands made on him.

Adjustment of Behavior

This ability to adjust one's self to experiences that thwart one's desires or primitive "drives" is an ability partially acquired during childhood. This may sound strange to those brought up to believe that mental disorders or emotional disabilities were a sort of curse visited on the patient through the processes of inheritance by an indiscreet ancestor. There *is* such a thing as heredity figuring in the causation of certain types of mental disorder, of course, and it would be incorrect to assume that the modern psychiatrist wholly disbelieves in heredity. Nevertheless, it has been too great a temptation in the past to attribute practically every display of human behavior we don't happen to like to this factor. Scientists have been forced in recent years to admit that much of the knowledge that exists about the laws of heredity in laboratory white mice and guinea pigs is not necessarily applicable to human beings. Indeed, there are few *facts* about human heredity known to science, and a vastly greater amount of research will be necessary before we will be in a position to say definitely what traits man inherits and what ones he forms after birth as imitations of or reactions to similar traits displayed by his parents.

Modern opinion, therefore, is veering around to the belief that the type of training a young child receives from its parents during the flexible years when its personality is in the process of being shaped determines pretty much how successful he is going to be in harmonizing the conflicts we have just mentioned, and how well he adjusts. For this reason increasing attention is being paid today to problems of mental hygiene and child guidance among normal boys and girls. Mothers, fathers, school teachers, and others may help the child form habits or "patterns" of personality so staunch and sound that these will aid him in meeting and adjusting to the inevitable frustrations in life that come sooner or later to each of us.

The formation of sturdy patterns of personality in these early years helps to explain why one person is able to adjust in a reasonable, healthy way to some distressing experience such as the loss of a loved one, loss of job, or the inability to attain some cherished ambition, while another, faced with a similar experience, cannot adjust to it and expresses his resulting maladjustment in terms of symptoms of some kind of mental disorder. A boy of six is taught by his parents to develop the healthy pattern of making his own tiny decisions and of finding his childhood security in the products of his own accomplishments rather than in having to depend for success on the personal favoritism of others. As this boy grows older and passes into adolescence these patterns remain with him, and he is able to cope with the mixture of adolescent emotions (made up of the desire to grow up and be independent, versus the wish to remain in the sheltered, protected state of childhood) with a minimum of difficulty. This ease of adjustment will likely be true also of his adult years when he will find himself able to meet adult responsibilities, disappointments, and rebuffs without having to run away from them by developing neurotic symptoms.

On the other hand, another boy of six may have a mother whose own emotional satisfaction in life can be gratified only by realizing that someone needs and depends on her. As a result she may develop what has come to be called an overprotective, oversolicitous attitude toward her child which keeps him emotionally tied to her and fails to allow him to become normally independent. As the physical and intellectual growth of such a child continues apace, his emotional growth tends to remain stunted. He reaches the physical age of adolescence, but because his principal patterns of personality are still the dependent childish ones of an earlier age period he is unable to adjust to adolescent demands and produces a variety of symptoms to express his maladjustment. Symptoms of this sort sometimes take the form of quarrelsomeness, defiance, or rebellion; or they may express themselves in the quieter but more ominous form of causing the youth to withdraw into a seclusive, shut-in, and solitary existence in which he forsakes the discomfort of trying to adjust to the world of reality in favor of retreat into a daydream world of fancy and imagination.

Mental Training in Childhood

Proper mental hygiene training in childhood, therefore, becomes extremely important if good mental health is to be maintained and mental disorder avoided. One of the most vital things of all in the process of helping a child form healthy patterns of personality is to assist him in creating a feeling of security for himself. By this is meant, not so much a feeling of physical or economic security as of *emotional* security. To feel emotionally secure a person must develop at least two firm convictions: first, that he is recognized as a person valued by others, and that he really belongs to and is accepted and needed by the group of which he is an intimate part. This means, first of all, by his family, then by schoolmates, next by the neighborhood in which he lives, and lastly, by society in general. The second conviction is that he can be confident of success in doing at least one thing really well. It matters little what this thing is providing the person is able to do it by means of his own efforts and is not dependent for success on the favoritism of someone else. To be able to do this gives a legitimate feeling of accomplishment and provides that poise and self-confidence that are the external signs of security.

Degree of Mental Disorders

At the left-hand end of the line shown below exists a condition of normal or average mental health such as most of us enjoy. As we travel toward the right side of the line some interesting changes begin to appear. For example, somewhere in the vicinity of the point on the line marked (1) we may find that average mental health begins to show a flaw or two in its soundness. This may be manifested by nothing more unusual than the habit of temper tantrums or perhaps of chronic timidity in a child, or possibly by habitual irritability or a feeling of "touchiness" in an adult.

MENTAL HEALTH	(1)	(2)	(3)	MENTAL DISEASE

But as we journey farther along the line toward the right, departures from average mental health become more obvious. At the point labeled (2), for instance, an individual may come to be thought of by his neighbors as "queer" in some way. Perhaps he shows a fanatical streak about religion or politics or some of the healing cults. If it happens to be a woman, maybe she is "queer" about keeping such an immaculate house that everyone in it is uncomfortable; or else she may go around with a perpetual chip-on-the-shoulder attitude, complaining that everyone else is trying to get the better of her. While still retaining more or less of the good mental health they started out with, such persons nevertheless show by their "queerness" that they already have traveled some distance from the left-hand end of our line.

At the point marked (3) mental health becomes unmistakably impaired, and the efficiency of the individual becomes correspondingly lessened. Now the symptoms are much exaggerated. If, previously, these people may have complained that the world has not given them a square deal, now they may develop definite delusions of persecution and arm themselves against their "enemies." Or it may be that other curious notions have crept in. They can't go into closed places or mix with crowds, or else they grow panicky when required to ride on the subway, or are obsessed with distressing ideas that they are going to faint or die.

At last the right-hand end of the line is reached. Here mental health vanishes completely and mental disease reigns supreme. Now the person is "insane," his patterns of adjustment broken down entirely.

There is no sharp or clear-cut line that divides mental health from mental disease. Mental health may be thought of as excellent, good, fair, or poor, grading imperceptibly to the right of this line toward the point where mental disease may be said to enter the picture. This point is extremely difficult to locate on the line because standards differ in different groups, and what might pass for merely a poor or even fair degree of mental health among one group of people or in one section of the world might well be labeled a mild degree of mental disorder in another. Moreover, it is only when mental disease has progressed from mild to extreme that we are justified in calling a person "insane."

INSANITY

"Insanity" is purely a legal term. It has no medical standing. It simply means that a given person's symptoms of mental disorder have grown so serious and his sense of judgment has become so faulty that the law steps in and makes it possible for others to decide for the patient what measures are necessary for his proper treatment and the safeguarding of his property. Although in this country alone there are more than three hundred thousand such "insane" persons in mental hospitals, there are doubtless twenty to thirty times as many others who display some signs of maladjustment or mental disorder of such lesser types as probably will never bring them to a mental hospital. While not in good mental health and often "queer" and hard to get along with, the great majority of these persons are never thought of by their fellow citizens as mentally sick. And yet, according to modern psychiatric conceptions of what constitutes mental disorder, the fears, worries, spells, and what not of these men and women are made of precisely the same stuff, although of course in lesser degree, as that from which definite mental disease is made.

This modern psychiatric conception of what constitutes mental disorder is explained admirably by Dr. C. Macfie Campbell, professor of psychiatry at Harvard Medical School, in the following:

> *A disorder is a mental disorder if its roots are mental.* A headache indicates a mental disorder if it comes because one is dodging something disagreeable. A pain in the back is a mental disorder if its persistence is due to discouragement and a feeling of uncertainty and a desire to have a sick benefit instead of putting one's back into one's work. Sleeplessness may be a mental disorder if its basis lies in personal worries and emotional tangles. In fact, many mental reactions are indications of poor mental health, although they have not usually been classed as mental disorders.
>
> Thus, discontent with one's environment may be a mental disorder if its causes lie, not in some external situation, but in personal failure to deal adequately with one's emotional problems. Suspicion, distrust, misinterpretation are mental disorders when they are the disguised expression of repressed longings into which the patient has no clear insight. Stealing sometimes indicates a mental disorder, the odd expression of underlying conflicts in the patient's nature. The feeling of fatigue sometimes represents, not overwork, but discouragement, inability to meet situations, lack of interest in the opportunities available. Unsociability, marital incompatibility, alcoholism, an aggressive and embittered social attitude; all these may indicate a disorder of the mental balance which may be open to modification.

How different is this conception from the older one that held there were only two varieties of people; the sane and the insane!

MENTAL DEFECT

Before going any further it is important that we digress for a few pages to explain about another kind of abnormal mental condition. This is not a condition of mental *disease,* but instead, of mental *defect.*

After talking with someone who is seriously mentally sick or "insane" many people are astonished to discover that the patient remembers things, knows what they are talking about, and that in general his intellectual faculties are usually not affected by his illness. This is due to the fact that most kinds of mental sickness are disorders of the patient's feeling or emotions and not of his intellect. To be quite accurate, there are a few kinds of mental disease (especially those associated with physical changes in the brain) in which the more advanced stages are accompanied by a lessening of intelligence, but for the most part patients ill from mental disease tend to retain much of whatever original intellectual ability they once possessed.

FEEBLE-MINDEDNESS

With mental defect, however, this is not true. A person who is mentally defective ("feeble-minded" is another term meaning the same thing) is one whose intelligence has never developed properly. Mental defect and mental disease, therefore, are two quite different things and should not be confused with each other. The illustration of two balky automobiles might be used to explain this difference. One auto balks and falters because the driver does not know how to manage its complicated machinery. This might be compared to mental disease where in most instances the auto itself (the human machine) is sound enough, but where the driver has not learned how to coördinate the use of brake, clutch, and gas throttle. On the other hand, a second auto may balk and falter despite excellent driving because there is a defect or flaw somewhere in the original machinery. This is comparable to a person with a condition of mental defect whose intellectual processes have been deficient since birth because of faulty heredity, birth injury, or the onset of infectious disease (measles, scarlet fever, "sleeping sickness," etc.) early in childhood.

In a very simple little pamphlet the late Dr. Walter Fernald, one of the great pioneers in this country in the study of mental deficiency, describes the symptoms of feeble-mindedness as follows:

> The symptoms of mental defect vary according to the degree of defect. In extreme cases the defect is observable in early infancy. The baby does not "take notice" or follow sounds or bright lights, or smile, or grasp objects with his fingers, or have vigorous muscular movements, or nurse properly, and so forth. As he grows older his teeth may not appear at the usual age, or he may learn to walk late and with an awkward, shambling gait, or he may be late in using his hands, or his untidy habits may persist for a long time. He is very apt not to talk until he is three or more years old. In general he remains a baby for a long time.

In less severe cases the above symptoms may be less marked or absent and the defect may not be recognized until the child is found to be unable to learn in school at the usual school age, and cannot be promoted from year to year like other children.

He usually shows his defect in other ways. He may not be able to get along with other children in games and sports. He is often teased and picked on by playmates of his own age, but since they do not regard him as an equal he usually associates with children younger than himself. He is usually easily influenced and shows poor judgment and reasoning power. In general he is not able to meet new situations.

As he grows older he is apt to be led into mischief, since he finds it hard to resist temptation. If neglected or allowed to associate with evil companions they are rather more likely than normal persons to acquire immoral or vicious habits, although this tendency has probably been overstated. Some mental defectives seem innately vicious and troublesome from early childhood, but the majority seem about as amenable to proper associations and proper bringing up as do normal children.

In mental deficiency, whether the cause be inherited or acquired, medical science knows of nothing to do to repair the damage to brain tissue that is responsible for the condition. Consequently, it can never be cured. In this respect, also, mental defect is not like mental disease, where cure is often accomplished. But if mental defect cannot be cured, at least there is much that can be done to help the feeble-minded person make a reasonably satisfactory adjustment to life with whatever limited intelligence he possesses. In the higher grades (there are three recognized degrees of feeble-mindedness: the *moron* who is next to the normal in intelligence; the *imbecile,* who is next lowest on the scale, and lastly the *idiot*); in the higher grades early recognition of the defect will enable parents and teachers to avoid making too many demands that the child keep up to the standards of normal children. This will help him to maintain his morale and prevent him from developing feelings of inferiority as a result of encountering nothing but failure in life. Likewise, he can be trained in good habit formation that will stand him in good stead when his impulsive judgment threatens to fail him. Later, training in simple trades and occupations within their capacity of accomplishment is possible for children of the moron and upper imbecile groups. But like all people with unaverage mental conditions, the mental defective needs *individual* treatment. What works with one fails with another, and each case must be dealt with as a special problem requiring individual methods.

Prevention of Mental Disorder

What can be done about mental disorders? Modern psychiatrists are far more interested in learning why the patient had to take recourse in mental disease, and what his symptoms mean, instead of merely what they are. Instead of talking about the differences in symptoms of dementia praecox, or hysteria, or epilepsy, or some of the many other mental disorders, suppose we review briefly some of the important points already brought out and then proceed to a final discussion of what can be done to prevent or cure mental disorders.

The following outline of important viewpoints already mentioned may help to clarify the situation:

1. Mental health and mental disease blend into one another like the colors in the rainbow, with no sharp line of separation.

2. Since mind affects body, and vice versa, the *whole* patient must be studied, not just one detachable part of him.

3. Mental disorders never come suddenly. Except for those caused by an organic physical disease they have been in the process of making for many years before finally appearing.

4. Symptoms of mental disorders usually are but exaggerations of attitudes or traits of personality present in the patient for many years previously.

5. While there are thousands of different precipitating causes for mental disorders, most of them have one basic cause in common in an inability to adjust to certain inner conflicts or to the demands for conformity of the outside world.

6. This basic cause is practically always in the unconscious part of the patient's mind, and he is, therefore, unaware of what it is about.

7. Mental *defect* should not be confused with mental *disease*. The first has to do with impaired intelligence. The second with mismanaged emotions.

Treatment of Mental Disorder

Now for something about prevention and treatment. To do this it will be necessary to make a rough division in our material between children and adults, but with some inevitable overlapping. In childhood the job has two aspects. One is to help the child's parents help him to build up sound and sturdy mental health. The other consists in helping parents to nip in the bud before they get well established certain traits and attitudes which experience has taught will grow into some kind of mental maladjustment in later years. Please note the difference in the nature of these jobs. The first has to do with insuring mental *health,* while the second is concerned with preventing mental *disease*. One is like building a fireproof house from the ground up. The other is comparable to calling the fire department early before the fire gets completely out of control. The mental hygiene movement in this country has performed a valuable service to parents and teachers in the past with the second aspect of this job, but until very recently no one in the mental hygiene movement has attempted the more difficult task of building health in contrast to preventing disease.

By the time adult years are reached, there is relatively little that can be done by way of preventing mental disorders, except, perhaps, to keep milder ones from growing more serious. The treatment task also grows more difficult as the mental disorder becomes more deeply entrenched.

But to return for a moment to the maladjustments of children. These are expressed in a variety of ways. Temper tantrums, fussy, dawdling food habits, timidity, shyness, overconscientiousness, bed-wetting (in older children), bullying and aggressiveness, stealing, lying, truancy; all these should be regarded as danger signals pointing to some underlying conflict which must be sought out and discovered before anything practical can be done by way of permanently remedying the condition. But unlike the methods of treatment in other branches of medicine, the treatment of behavior disorders and undesirable personality traits in children can seldom be successfully undertaken by directing treatment to the child alone. His annoying behavior is a symptom of maladjustment somewhere within his emotional apparatus and is invariably bound up in some manner with the attitudes and emotional reactions displayed toward him by his parents. The treatment of the behavior problem, therefore, will require that these parental attitudes be taken into account. Indeed, so thoroughly is this believed by mental hygienists that they have created an axiom to the effect that "you cannot change the child's behavior until you first change the parental attitude that caused the behavior." Treatment primarily, then, *is directed toward the parents,* and this treatment consists largely in endeavoring to get them to modify the undesirable attitude that unwittingly and with the best of intentions they have adopted.

But what about the adult? And what kind of treatment is indicated for his mental disorder? Obviously, the answer must depend on the nature of his problem. In general, however, adult treatment can be thought of as comprising two main varieties: treatment of the basic emotional difficulty whenever this proves possible, and treatment of symptoms. One should never be satisfied with restricting treatment of mental disorders to symptoms alone unless there is nothing else to be done. Unhappily, in numerous cases of serious mental disease or "insanity," the case has progressed so far before psychiatric assistance is called that there remains little to do except to treat the symptoms. But with less severe cases—the psychoneuroses, for example, with their many fears, compulsions, anxieties, etc.—it is often quite possible to get at the roots of the trouble and effect a cure by means of a special type of treatment known as "psychotherapy." This method does not make use of medicines or physical kinds of treatment like massage, baths, etc., but relies for its effectiveness instead on a special emotional relationship between patient and psychiatrist. There are several different kinds of psychotherapy. One in particular is called "psychoanalysis" about which a great deal of misunderstanding exists. Only a comparatively few kinds of mental difficulty are suitable, at this stage of our knowledge, for psychoanalytic treatment. Moreover, as yet there are not many psychiatrists in this country who have had the indispensable special training that is necessary before one is competent to use psychoanalysis. But for the particular cases it is suited for, and in the hands of a well-trained psychiatrist, psychoanalysis enables us to explore the unconscious mind of the patient and, after locating the source of the conflict, is a most helpful procedure in the process of emotional reëducation which, if successful, restores the patient to an improved degree of adjustment.

PSYCHOTHERAPY

Other forms of psychotherapy are used for cases that do not require so deep an exploration into the unconscious. Thus, various kinds of suggestion are sometimes made use of, and occasionally even hypnosis, although most psychiatrists have come to the belief that hypnosis at best is of value only in the temporary relief of symptoms and is powerless to bring about a lasting cure. For this reason it is very little used by capable physicians.

The treatment of more serious conditions of mental disorder, like "insanity," where institutional care is required, is very complicated. Suppose we trace the treatment of an imaginary case of "insanity" and see what happens in an up-to-date hospital for mental disease. First of all, the patient has been, in all probability, behaving queerly for some months before the family has gotten courage to seek medical advice. He may have been depressed, or he may have been excited. Perhaps he has had delusions that others are following him, or that something has been placed in his food, or that "voices" speak to him, or what not. It makes little difference. The point is that the family at last recognize he is "not right." The family physician is consulted. He makes a careful examination, both physically and mentally, and either recommends that the patient be treated in a suitable public or private hospital for mental diseases, or, if the case is an unusually puzzling or obscure one, he may ask that the family authorize him to call into consultation a capable psychiatrist.

Some cases of this kind can be cared for at home, but in an overwhelming number of instances it is far better for patient and family alike if the former is removed to a hospital. This is a hard decision for relatives to make, for there still exists a great deal of cruel and unwarranted stigma about people who require mental hospital care. But it is almost certain that much of the patient's underlying conflict—the reasons for his becoming mentally sick—are tangled up in family relationships, and if he can get away from the well-meaning but unwholesome family atmosphere for a time his chances of early cure are improved.

So we will assume that the family agrees to hospital treatment. Next is the matter of commitment. This is merely a legal device to safeguard the interests of the patient. It consists in making application to a court for an order to have the patient admitted to a hospital in order that he can receive the special treatment available at such a hospital. In most states commitment can be made without undue publicity, the judge (unless he be vindictive or a stickler for the letter of the law) waiving the right to have the sick man haled before the court, and accepting the legally sworn-to certificate of the committing physicians who give their professional opinion that the patient is mentally sick and needs mental hospital care.

The patient arrives at the hospital. In modern, well-equipped state hospitals for the mentally sick he is first taken to the receiving ward, where he remains for ten days to several months, depending on the nature of his condition. While in the receiving ward he is examined very carefully by a number of physicians, and treatment for his immediate needs is prescribed. This may be rest in bed, plenty of nourishing food, and an occasional sedative, if sleepless or restless. But sometimes the patient is wildly excited on admission. Then it is likely that a special kind of treatment known as the "continuous bath" will be ordered by the doctor. This consists in greasing the patient's body with vaseline and then placing him in a specially constructed tub through which flows a gentle stream of water heated to whatever temperature is indicated. Usually it is just above body heat. A canvas sheet is placed over the tub to prevent the patient from getting out and an attendant or nurse is stationed near by to see that the sick man or woman does not hurt himself or slip under the sheet.

After a time the patient relaxes under the influence of the warm water. His excitement begins to subside, and he may even go to sleep. The continuous bath is a far more humane method of controlling excitement and violence than any other kind of restraint known, including hypnotic drugs and the strait-jacket. All up-to-date hospitals have them, and in better hospitals of this kind straitjackets, camisoles, and similar devices for confining the arms and legs of patients have been abandoned. Indeed, in many modern hospitals the only place a straitjacket can be found is in the hospital museum.

But perhaps the patient is depressed instead of excited. Possibly he has no appetite and refuses to eat, or maybe he has delusions that he has committed all sorts of fantastic crimes. He may accuse himself of having brought ruin on the family, or of being responsible for all the misery in the world, or of having committed the "unpardonable sin," whatever that may be. At any rate, he is deeply depressed, and the doctors understand that the chances are in favor of his contemplating suicide, if, indeed, he has not already expressed the intention of taking his own life. It is necessary, therefore, to safeguard him from self-injury. Such patients are usually very clever in managing to evade the nurse or others who are on the watch for attempts at suicide, and this is another reason why home care is dangerous, especially for depressed patients. Even under the most constant attention a patient may elude his nurse and dash through a window, or cut himself, or in some other way do away with himself. Eternal vigilance is the price of safety in such cases.

Sometimes the patient won't eat, and then another method of treatment is necessary. If he gets to the point where his refusal to take food threatens to retard his recovery, or if, as not infrequently happens, it comes down to a question of actual starvation, the doctor inserts a soft rubber tube through the patient's nostrils into his stomach and slowly pours down it a mixture of milk and eggs at necessary intervals.

But gradually the patient improves. Now he is transferred from the receiving ward to another. Here he will find other patients whose behavior is like his own and in various stages of recovery. Seeing other patients whose condition has improved is an incentive for our patient to make further progress. Presently he is encouraged to take walks on the ground outside and in company with a nurse or a group of others. He is given an opportunity to visit the occupational therapy department at frequent intervals, where, under skilled supervision, he can get his mind off his troubles and reëstablish habits of concentration and industry.

At last he is well enough to go home. And modern science has another victory to its credit. Unhappily, the hospital course of some patients is not as successful as the one we have described. Some mentally sick men and women are not allowed by their relatives to come to the hospital until their illness has reached such an advanced stage that little but kindly custodial care can be given them. Moreover, some kinds of mental illness seem to be of such a stubborn nature from the beginning that the case is almost a chronic one from the start. Nevertheless, it is astonishing to observe how the rate of recovery is steadily increasing. At the present time about 25 per cent of all first admissions to mental hospitals are completely cured, while an additional 15 per cent are able to return home, after a time, well enough to live in the outside community even though they are not completely recovered.

This recovery rate, however, depends to some extent on the kind of hospital the patient is treated in. Modern, up-to-date hospitals have no difficulty in maintaining this rate, but less progressive ones are usually able to do little more than provide custodial care for their patients. This is why there has come about a technical distinction between *treatment* hospitals and *custodial* ones. In the former every modern form of medical and psychiatric treatment is used to cure the patient. The staffs of doctors are recruited from alert, progressive men and women; the scientific equipment is the last word in efficiency, and the laboratories allow no promising method of treatment to go untried.

COMMUNITY HOSPITALS FOR MENTAL DISORDER

It must be confessed, however, that not all our state hospitals for the mentally sick are of this variety. There still exist backward hospitals where the superintendent is a political appointee whose professional skill has not advanced since his early medical training. In these institutions scientific apparatus is meager, and little or no advantage is taken of recent psychiatric discoveries.

In the last analysis the responsibility for backward mental hospitals rests on the community. It is an axiom as true in this field as in any other that a community gets just about what it is willing to pay for, in the way of public service. If citizens of a community are too negligent to insist on a high quality of psychiatric service, then they must be willing to take what is possible. A well-equipped and modern mental hospital costs money to run, but it also restores a much higher percentage of its patients to health. Any community can have this high quality of service if it wants to.

And now, just a word in closing about state hospitals in contrast to private hospitals or sanatoriums. Any generalizations are sure to do an injustice to certain institutions, but so far as generalizations are permitted, it may be fair to say that a modern *treatment* state hospital is likely to be a more effective place for a mentally sick patient than a *custodial* private one. There are a few private sanatoria not run primarily for commercial profit where some of the best scientific work in the country is being done. These hospitals are at least partially endowed by private funds, so that they are not wholly dependent on patients' fees for support. But if we except these (as well as a handful of commercial ones), then most of the others cannot afford the elaborate and expensive equipment or the legitimately higher salaries commanded by physicians of superior skill.

The modern state hospital, on the other hand, deals with several thousand patients instead of fifty or a hundred or so. It receives its funds from the state government and is thereby enabled to equip itself in the most effective manner. Furthermore, while the salaries of its staff are often lower than those of some private sanatoria, the progressive scientific spirit permeating the whole atmosphere and the opportunity to use adequate equipment tend to attract to it the better medical men and women in the psychiatric field. On the whole, therefore, if expense is a serious matter for the family to consider, it will be well for them to consider the state hospital (but *only* if it is a modern, progressive one) in favor of a small, inexpensive but custodial private one.

This story of mental disorders comes now to a close. Mankind has traveled far since those days, centuries ago, when sufferers from "insanity" were regarded as being afflicted with demons and evil spirits and chained in dungeons. The mystery of mental disease has been stripped away, and now we are able to recognize it as a kind of sickness, often amenable in some measure to psychiatric treatment and curable in an increasingly large number of cases.

Modern psychiatry has new technics like the insulin shock and metrazol shock treatments, which are applied in cases of dementia praecox or schizophrenia and depressive forms of insanity. Similarly, electric shock to the brain has been tried. One of the latest technics is the removal of a portion of the frontal lobe of the brain for depressive forms of insanity. All of these methods are still highly experimental and should be used only by experts working in institutions.

A new apparatus called the encephalograph enables the doctor to determine if the activities of various areas of the brain are proceeding as the normal brain does. Most important is to detect the symptoms of mental disorder early. The earlier treatment is begun the better the chance for recovery.

MENTAL ACTIVITY (See also, *Mental Hygiene*) With the improvement in health our life expectancy at birth has gradually risen. The ancient Greeks apparently lived to an average age of just under 30 years. In 1900 the average age at death in the United States was 45. Now we have raised the average life expectancy at birth to almost 70 years and for girl babies to more than 70 years.

Our mental activities are dependent to some extent on our physical condition. The more any mental activity is dependent on some physical activity of the body, the more that activity is likely to decline with age.

From birth to 15 years the growth of the human being is rapid. Around 25 years of age the human physique reaches its maximum in strength and skill. Most human beings descend slowly from this level until the age of 45, when the momentum of decline increases. Then at about 55 years of age the rate of decline again increases until 70 years of age.

Intelligence, which is the effective organization of mental abilities for a certain purpose, matures quickly, so that by 16 years of age the intelligence of the human being is about at its peak. It remains on this level until the early twenties. From 20 years on, the intelligence decreases. By the age of 55 many human beings have receded to the 14 year old level. Not all of the factors involved in intelligence are lost at the same rate. The voice and the hearing remain efficient until well along in life. The reaction time is, however, likely to decrease more rapidly.

Memory reaches its peak in the late teens and early twenties and declines rapidly with age. The inability to remember recent events is always a telltale sign of senescence. Old people remember happenings of their childhood and forget what happened yesterday.

With senescence they become careless of accuracy, but some youngsters never learn accuracy.

MENTAL DEPRESSION In times of war or of economic disaster there is a tendency for many human beings to be greatly depressed from a mental point of view. This depression is reflected in their attitudes toward other people and in their actions. Depression is a state of mind in which initiative and decision are paralyzed. When people are depressed, they grow too careful. They fear to spend money; they fear to enjoy pleasures and amusements; they hesitate to meet other people. Eventually the person who is depressed becomes on bad terms not only with the world in general but also with himself. Under these circumstances he thinks too much about himself, both physically and mentally. He tends to live in the past and to evade the future. Quite soon his depression reflects itself in his personal appearance. The person who is depressed is slouchy. He permits his clothing to go without suitable attention; he neglects to shave if he is a man or to tend to her cosmetic appearance and her hair if a woman. For this reason people who are depressed come soon to resemble one another.

During a period of depression a man is likely to change his former judgments of other people. Those whom he formerly liked he now finds unbearable; he may actually begin to seek out those whom he formerly hated. His depression makes him irritable, so that he is rude and hypercritical.

Obviously one of the most important steps in overcoming depression if you have it is to understand your own condition. This at least will serve to prevent constant worry and anxiety. People who insist that they never worry have learned to reason themselves, by rationalization, out of anxiety over situations in which they find themselves. Other people develop mental tranquillity or peace of mind by accepting some belief which eliminates from consideration anything that is displeasing. This is not rationalization but may bring about the same effect for a person who is capable of shutting out from his thoughts any problem that disturbs him. Peace of mind is necessary for accomplishment because absence of peace of mind gives a constant feeling of insecurity. Often mental depression is transferred to physical conditions, so that worry may cause a person to have palpitations of the heart or to feel extra beats.

If the nervous condition brings the focus of attention on the stomach and bowels, such symptoms as constipation and diarrhea may occur.

Unfortunately failure to practice good mental hygiene may lead eventually to an attempt to escape from mental disturbance by the use of drinks, drugs, sedatives, or gambling, which in themselves may be worse than the worry that they replace. A restful night's sleep, a vacation, indulgence in outdoor sports, or even frequent use of the radio and the movies are better ways of escape from worry.

People who are depressed have in the past been treated frequently with benzedrine or amphetamine which stimulates but which has the undesirable effect of raising the blood pressure. A new drug called Meratran has little effect on the breathing, the pulse rate, or the blood pressure but does act directly on the brain to overcome depression. If the central nervous system is underactive, this drug seems to restore it to a more normal level of activity. Obviously, drugs of this type are not given to people who are overexcited. The drug has been useful in the condition called narcolepsy in which there is a sudden irresistible desire to sleep.

This condition has also been treated with amphetamine. The new drug is used in cases of fatigue, drowsiness or what is called a low-down-feeling. Another use has been in disorders of the liver, infections, deficient action of the thyroid gland, depression that comes during the menopause, and alcoholic hangovers. The drug does not affect the appetite so that it is given either before or after meals.

MENTAL DISEASE One person out of twenty becomes a patient in a mental hospital at some time during his life. Sooner or later one person out of ten becomes incapacitated by mental disease, at least for a short time. It has been estimated that the national expenditure for hospital care for mental disease approximates at least $200,000,000 a year.

To the expenditure for mental disease must be added the problem of the feeble-minded. Statistics indicate that over 2 per cent of the total population of the United States is feeble-minded. These people are so deficient mentally that they are not capable of supporting themselves or even of guiding their own conduct.

In addition there are the backward children. Of these, perhaps 850,000 are unable to keep up with the courses in ordinary public schools. Special schools must be developed for them. This is the great burden of mental disturbances carried by the American people.

There is hardly a patient of any kind who does not have something of a mental problem. Disease elsewhere in the body is likely to be reflected in the mind or vice versa. Obviously the problem of mental deficiency comes close to the problem of the national defense. Many of our young men were unable to pass the examination of the Selective Service. Some who passed were later found unable to bear the strain of life under military conditions.

Recent surveys of institutions for the care of the mentally afflicted indicate that many of them are overcrowded. Some of them are very old, and the sanitation has not been kept up to date; some represent serious fire hazards. The deficit is estimated by the National Committee for Mental Hy- giene as representing 150,000 beds, with long lists of patients waiting to be admitted. Proper control of mental hygiene would also provide for much-needed research in these fields, with a view to getting patients out of the hospital and back into ordinary life.

Many institutions are now devoting themselves to the study of dementia praecox.

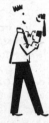

THIS IS WHAT YOU CAN DO

FOR MENTAL HEALTH

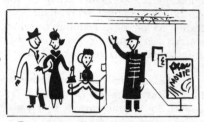

3. Remember that marriage is a partnership.

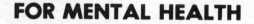

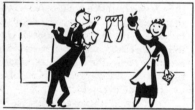

1. Build emotional stability by creating a warm home atmosphere.

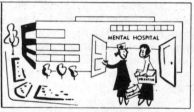

4. Recognize that mental illness can be treated successfully—and YOU can help!

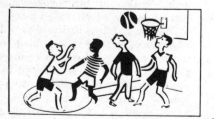

2. Provide satisfying recreation for youth.

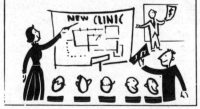

5. Participate actively in your community campaign for mental health.

Insulin and metrazol shock have been used, also electric shock, and more recently surgical treatment of various portions of the brain. Studies are being made as to the extent to which such technics can bring these people back to normalcy and also as to the time they will remain normal after this type of radical treatment.

Special attention is also being given by educators to the problems of the mentally defective. We are moving forward in our control of mental disease, but the field is vast and the conditions of modern life tend to increase the number of persons needing scientific mental hygiene.

MENTAL HYGIENE Health is generally considered to be freedom from disease. However, health also involves a state of mind in which the human being is satisfied with life, in which his mind functions accurately, and in which he possesses enough force, driving power, and impetus to give him confidence in himself and the ability to accomplish his work.

Happiness has been described as a balanced flow of energy and the satisfaction of desires. In other words, you are happy if you get what you want. One of the troubles is that many people do not know what they want and most people differ from other people in the things they want. Everyone who is ordinarily healthful is interested in getting enough to eat, in getting enough rest, and in satisfying the ordinary desire for reproduction. There are, however, different levels in these fundamental desires. Some people get hungry without really needing food; others require far more rest than the average. The nature of any desire is conditioned by experience and knowledge. A person who has never eaten strawberries is not likely to crave them.

Most of the drives of life are concerned with the fundamental things that have been mentioned. An unsatisfied wish is a driving stimulus until it is satisfied. Good mental hygiene requires a certain amount of rationalization. Rationalization is a term used to describe the ability of a human being to satisfy himself with what he gets rather than constantly to be wanting something that he cannot have. For instance every four years several people want to be President of the United States. For many of them this is quite out of the question. Some of them, therefore, satisfy themselves by becoming governor of the state, senators, or even president of a lodge or a club.

Because it is possible to find happiness with less than a maximum of the desires we possess, mental hygienists suggest that everyone develop as a major interest not only a job but perhaps some hobby or game in which he may achieve the success that is not possible in another field. The basic rule for a happy and contented mind is to cultivate certain standards of living against unexpected changes; then maintain a flexible attitude of mind so as not to be incurably depressed when you fail to achieve something you want.

DEMENTIA—pellagra: See article DEFICIENCY DISEASES; SKIN, article THE SKIN.

MENTAL DISORDERS—See MENTAL, article NERVOUS AND MENTAL DISORDERS.

MENTAL DISORDERS—age of onset: See MENTAL, article NERVOUS AND MENTAL DISORDERS.

MENTAL DISORDERS—causes: See MENTAL, article NERVOUS AND MENTAL DISORDERS.

MENTAL DISORDERS—defects: See MENTAL, article NERVOUS AND MENTAL DISORDERS.

MENTAL DISORDERS—degrees: See MENTAL, article NERVOUS AND MENTAL DISORDERS.

MENTAL DISORDERS—feeble-mindedness: See MENTAL, article NERVOUS AND MENTAL DISORDERS.

MENTAL DISORDERS—lobotomy: See MENTAL, article NERVOUS AND MENTAL DISORDERS.

MENTAL DISORDERS—prevention: See MENTAL, article NERVOUS AND MENTAL DISORDERS.

MENTAL DISORDERS—recovery rate: See MENTAL, article NERVOUS AND MENTAL DISORDERS.

MENTAL DISORDERS—shock treatments: See MENTAL, article NERVOUS AND MENTAL DISORDERS.

MENTAL DISORDERS—treatment: See MENTAL, article NERVOUS AND MENTAL DISORDERS.

MENTAL HOSPITALS—community: See MENTAL, article NERVOUS AND MENTAL DISORDERS.

SCHIZOPHRENIA—age at onset: See MENTAL, article NERVOUS AND MENTAL DISORDERS.

SCHIZOPHRENIA—shock treatment: See MENTAL, article NERVOUS AND MENTAL DISORDERS.

MENTAL HYGIENE IN BUSINESS Suitable adjustment of workers to their surroundings is important in establishing a smooth-running condition in any business or industry. Ask the average businessman if he needs a psychiatrist in his business and he will think you are mentally disturbed. Psychiatrists, most people believe, spend practically all of their time finding people who need to be confined in institutions because they are wholly irresponsible.

Most large industries have employment interviewers, who have knowledge of the positions to be filled, of the persons in the department, and, therefore, of the kind of employee who will fit best and serve most satisfactorily under the circumstances. Most employment interviewers can recognize easily a prospective employee who is so far "off the beaten path" from a mental point of view as to be unsatisfactory for any job. No one suggests that employment interviewers should be replaced by psychiatrists or psychologists. What a businessman wants is a worker who can respond to the particular problems and procedures of the job for which he is employed. The boss seldom wants to be troubled about the general personality of an employee or the question of how he gets along with his wife. Nevertheless, that very situation may be important in relation to the quality or amount of work. Problems may arise, which are due to a neurosis or psychosis in some employee whose mental condition has not been recognized.

Mental hygienists are convinced that training ought to be made available to employment managers or to the workers in the personnel divisions of industries. Workers are frequently transferred into personnel departments because they appear to be able to get along well with other people—but sometimes because they are hard and skeptical. Generally they work out their own techniques, whether for the handling of personal problems or for the selection of new employees.

Already there are plenty of reports of instances in which employees who failed to respond acceptably to their executives were given scientific study and thus saved for the organization. We have learned how to modify the attitudes of parents and to improve their relationships with their children. Similar tactics are needed for executive businessmen to improve their relationships with their employees.

MENTAL STRESS AND EMOTIONAL DEVELOPMENT (See also, *Emotions*) During the last fifty years much attention has been given by physicians to the manner in which emotional development affects the general health of people. Almost from the moment of birth a child begins having emotional experiences. Among the first of the child's relationships is that with his mother. From her he gets his food; therefore his early emotions are related to eating and elimination of waste material. Later in life his emotional relationship to his mother may be reflected in gastrointestinal disturbances.

Practically all little children suck their thumbs. I asked one of my little grandchildren why he liked his thumb, "Is it salty?"; "Is it sweet?"; "Are you hungry?" He said, "I suck my thumb 'cause it's mine."

Among primitive people much symbolic magic is associated with eating. People devoured their enemies or portions of the bodies of their enemies to gain strength. They would choose the heart of the lion as a special prize. The most intelligent mother looking at her new baby says: "I would like to eat you." As people grow older these gastrointestinal attitudes are reflected in such conditions as alcoholism, overweight, inability to keep food down, loss of appetite, and ulcers. People reared with ritualistic taboos in their religions against certain foods respond with gastric distress when they violate these taboos after they have become detached from the family shelter.

Babies also react in relation to their habits of elimination and "get even" by refusing to eliminate or by doing so too often. Doctors have related colitis, constipation, and diarrhea to emotional factors.

Modern dynamic psychology also makes much of the family relationships of the older child, including envy of father, mother, brothers, and sisters. Frigidity in women or sexual inability in men may be far more mental than physical.

From the moment of birth the child who has been warm and almost completely protected in the body of its mother becomes subjected to great numbers of new sensations. These may include noises, lights, bruises, hunger, infections, smells, and irritations. While no longer a part of his mother he is still completely dependent on her for food and water and freedom from mental and physical stresses and irritations. Psychologists state that throughout life the individual meets stresses by trying to get back to the security and pleasure of his prenatal and infantile life. If he cannot do it actually in his waking hours in daydreams, he does it in sleeping and dreaming at night. Some people shut themselves off so completely from reality that they show this in hysterical paralyses like inability to speak, to see, to hear, to eat, or to awaken. Again and again we read of patients, mostly young girls, who have slept for weeks or months. Fainting in the presence of any unwelcome sensation is a similar sort of phenomenon.

As the child grows older he learns to reject or spit out what is bad, to eat or assimilate what he likes. The psychologists use the word projection to indicate the way in which a person will project onto someone else their own unsatisfactory feelings or responses. A jealous husband, one authority suggests, is merely projecting onto his mate his own desire to be unfaithful.

As we grow older we learn by imitating others, or identifying ourselves with others or with ideas, to satisfy our cravings for mastery. For that reason generals or leaders who command the admiration of their men get more successful results. We can control feelings of anxiety by translating them into action. Under the threat of bombing in London, those who participated in civilian defense were free from feelings of helpless anxiety. When people become helpless they revert to an infantile state with crying, inability to control elimination and similar phenomena.

METABOLISM In the functions of the human body, it uses up oxygen. The tissues use more oxygen during digestion, during exercise, and during exposure to cold than they do when the human body is resting under conditions of warmth. The rate of use of oxygen to carry on the activities of life and in resting gives a figure which is known as the basal metabolism. Standards have been established for human beings of various weight and size. Infants use up more oxygen for the weight of their bodies than adults. Old people use less. Women use less than men.

The kind of work that a person does determines particularly the use of oxygen for the production of energy. For that reason a person who is in a sedentary occupation like a desk worker or a tailor may require only 2300 calories of food per day, a carpenter may require 3300 calories per day, a lumberman as much as 5000 calories per day. A calorie is also merely a measure of energy. It is the amount of heat necessary to raise a certain amount of water 1 degree in temperature. A woman who is doing practically nothing except a little light dusting can get along on 1200 calories per day. If she eats more, she will get big in all the places where she would rather be little.

The human body has a great many standard factors which indicate to the doctor when he makes an examination that the functions of the body are in the range that is called normal. For instance the basal metabolic rate is generally said to be normal when it is somewhere between plus 7 and minus 7 as measured by the basal metabolic machine. In other words, a standard has been established for the basal metabolism.

The human body needs a certain amount of protein every day in order to provide the body with energy and take care of the waste of tissue and the necessity for rebuilding tissue. The body also requires a certain amount of sugar and a certain amount of fat. It is possible to replace the fat by sugar. Sugar can be taken to spare the necessity of burning protein in order to provide energy. These factors are also concerned in the metabolism of the human body. Metabolism, therefore, represents all of the processes involved in changing the food materials, the oxygen, and other substances taken into the body into the tissues of the body or in converting them into energy.

Chemical tests are possible to check the manner in which the body is using the materials that come in. For instance the chemist can determine the amount of protein in the blood plasma. He can determine the amount of materials eliminated from the body by way of the urine or by the bowels or by perspiration. The level of sugar in the blood is now determined by a number of tests. We know, for example, that the amount of sugar in the blood plasma is reduced when there is exhaustion or when the liver is failing to carry on its work

Chart showing what happens to water taken into the body. The kidneys handle the largest amount in water exchange. However, a certain amount of water is given off by the lungs as well as carbon dioxide. A small amount of water is passed out in the feces. Water also is lost through the skin by perspiration.

Cleveland Health Museum

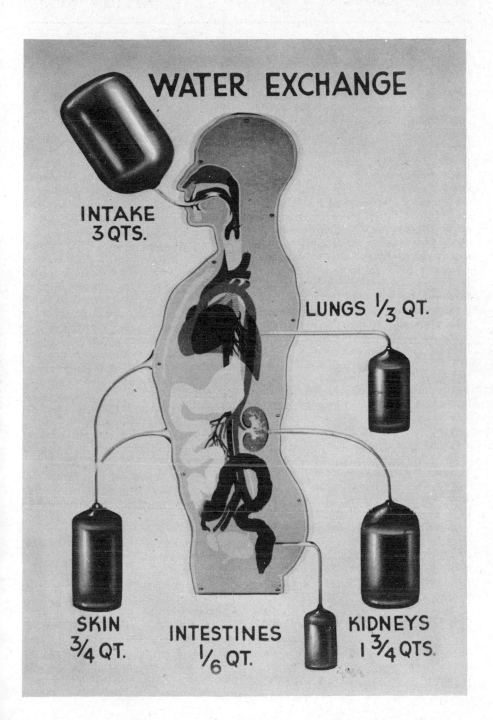

satisfactorily. In order for the various tissues of the body to work as they should, hormones or glandular substances, vitamins and ferments are necessary. All of these substances work together in bringing about a normal state of the body. The failure of any one gland to function may throw an extra burden on others. Some glandular activities are in the nature of breaking down materials; others in the way of building them up. The material from the male sex glands favors the storage of protein in the body, increases muscular development and the growth of hair on the body. Insulin, which is the secretion of the pancreas, helps to develop stores of protein and sugar in the body. Other glandular secretions tend to diminish such storage. Thus the body is in a constant state of balance with these various functions working opposite each other. All of these various activities are included under metabolism.

A number of diseases are definitely related to failure of the body to carry out its chemical functions satisfactorily. Included are particularly gout, diabetes, obesity, and acidosis.

METABOLIC DISORDERS—arthritis or rheumatism may result: See article ARTHRITIS, RHEUMATISM, AND GOUT.

METABOLIC DISORDERS—gout: See article ARTHRITIS, RHEUMATISM, AND GOUT.

METABOLISM—basal metabolism: See entry BASAL METABOLISM.

METABOLISM—hormones control: See article BLOOD PRESSURE.

METABOLISM—tests: See article ENDOCRINOLOGY.

METALLIC POISONS (See also, *Poisoning*) All sorts of metal substances may produce serious poisoning of the human body when these poisons are swallowed or inhaled. Among the most serious are arsenic, cadmium, beryllium, mercury, zinc and lead. Cases of gold poisoning are also seen occasionally since the introduction of the gold treatment for arthritis. Fortunately modern medicine has developed a specific drug called BAL or British anti-lewisite which is now considered to be the most effective treatment of poisoning due to arsenic, mercury, and gold. BAL is also helpful in lead poisoning, silver poisoning, and poisoning due to thallium, selenium and tellurium. Indeed it is of some benefit also in poisoning by cadmium, antimony and zinc.

ARSENIC—Most metal poisoning occurs in industries in which these metals are used. Arsenic is used in agriculture in sprays to get rid of pests; it is also used in copper refining and chemical industries. Arsenic poisoning sometimes follows the use of large doses of drugs which are tried against parasites of one kind or another that invade the human body. Arsenic has been used at times to commit murder and particularly when small doses are added to food so that arsenic poisoning is a favorite among the writers of detective stories.

The symptoms of arsenic poisoning resemble those of a severe inflammation of the stomach with great amounts of gastric distress, associated sometimes with damage to the nerves, rashes on the skin, and similar symptoms.

When arsenic poisoning is suspected, it is customary to find amounts of arsenic in the urine, the hair or nails since arsenic is excreted from the human body in this way. This also adds to the value of arsenic poisoning as a favorite in murder stories. Once a person has been exposed to arsenic, the best treatment is to stop the exposure as soon as possible and to give promptly and continuously BAL until recovery has occurred.

BERYLLIUM—Since beryllium is much used in the study of atomic energy and also as a constituent of the materials in fluorescent lamps, cases of poisoning are now seen more frequently than previously. The workers who are exposed to beryllium dust in their work also occasionally become poisoned. When the dust gets into the lungs, it sets up serious inflammations and reactions, sometimes followed by difficulties with breathing. Cases have also been reported in which beryllium has gotten into wounds when a flourescent lamp broke. A granuloma forms, which is overgrowth of the tissues something like a tumor. Therefore, special preventive measures are now being taken to get rid of old flourescent light tubes without exposing anyone to the danger of injury from them.

CADMIUM—Cadmium seldom causes poisoning but instances are known when acid foods are prepared in containers which have cadmium in the lining. Enough cadmium can be absorbed to cause severe inflammation of the stomach, accompanied by nausea, vomiting and later diarrhea. Serious poisoning can also follow the breathing of cadmium oxide fumes. This happens when cadmium plated steel is heated or welded without adequate ventilation in the room. The inhalation of the fumes is followed by slight irritation of the eyes, dryness of the throat and tightness in the chest. Later the person develops cough, pains in the chest and may ultimately find some blood in the sputum. Cases are reported of fatal poisoning from cadmium. Formerly the only available treatment was rest, oxygen and the usual supportive measures, but now BAL is being tried and presumably is sufficiently effective to warrant its regular use in such instances.

GOLD—Gold is now given in the treatment of a number of diseases and cases have occurred in which poisoning has followed injection of gold salts. The effects are chiefly on the bone marrow, resulting in damage to the blood-form-ing organs. The lessening of the thrombocytes may cause easy bruising and hemorrhages; there may also be damage to the kidney. BAL or British antilewisite has also been shown to be especially effective in poisoning with gold salts.

LEAD—Lead has been for many years known to be a dangerous and insidious metallic poison. Lead fumes may be inhaled or finely divided lead dust may be inhaled and produce serious poisoning. Food and drink may become contaminated with lead from containers. Lead salts are stored in the body and accumulation of small doses may produce serious poisoning. As with other metallic poisons, the first symptoms relate to irritation of the gastrointestinal tract. Later, however, patients develop what is called a lead line—a series of bluish dots occurring along the margins of the gums. Examination of the blood shows characteristic damage of the blood cells. The nervous symptoms are especially important since lead poisoning may damage the brain with mental depression or even severe mental disturbance. Children may develop convulsions. The peripheral nerves—those near the surface of the body—become paralyzed and the characteristic wristdrop of painters, weakness in the shoulder of laborers who use shovels and paralysis in the legs of tailors are known as occupational injuries due to lead. The red blood cells become less in number and examination of the blood, I may repeat, is one of the most important technics in causing a suspicion of lead poisoning in the mind of the doctor. When lead poisoning is diagnosed, the first step is to withdraw the person from all exposure to lead and to promote elimination of lead from the blood. Most persons recover if the exposure is stopped. Calcium gluconate is usually given intravenously to relieve the colic. Salts are given to sweep material out of the bowel. The calcium must be maintained at a high level since this helps to drive the lead out of the blood stream into the bones. Sodium citrate is sometimes given in order to produce a soluble lead citrate which is rapidly excreted from the body. BAL or British anti-lewisite has not been found especially helpful in lead poisoning.

A special warning is needed against the danger of lead poisoning in children. Babies who chew on toys, cribs or window sills which have been painted with lead pigments may be poisoned. Fortunately lead paint is now limited almost entirely to use on the exteriors of buildings. Cases of lead poisoning have also occurred from inhaling the fumes of old battery casings when these are burned as a substitute for other fuel.

MERCURY—Acute mercury poisoning usually happens when a child in a home gets hold of tablets of bichloride of mercury poison which may be used as an antiseptic or for other reasons. No one really needs to keep bichloride of mercury around the house. When it has been used for any purpose, it should be promptly destroyed after that use is ended. Mercury poisoning occurs in industry from inhalation of mercury vapors. This occurs particularly among gold and silver refiners, instrument makers and laboratory workers. The fur and felt hat industry used to uncover cases of mercury poisoning but the material is no longer used to any extent in that industry. During World War II, workers making mercury cadmium dry batteries were found to be suffering with mercury poisoning. The great danger from acute mercury poisoning is the damage to all of the organs that are involved in absorbing and getting rid of mercury from the body. The chief damage is to the kidney with evidence of renal failure and eventually death from uremia. In the bowel, mercury produces colitis and often a severe bloody diarrhea. One form of mercury called calomel has been used as a cathartic for many years.

First aid in mercury poisoning involves giving egg white or milk, washing out the stomach with copious amounts of fluid and finally giving a saline cathartic to sweep the material out of the body. British anti-lewisite or BAL has been found to be a specific antidote against acute mercury poisoning.

Chronic mercury poisoning comes on insidiously with a variety of symptoms. One of those first noticed may be increased amounts of saliva with a metallic taste in the mouth. Associated may be loss of appetite, indigestion, and diarrhea. Finally, such workers may develop tremors. Mental aberrations are seen with excitability followed by periods of dullness. Ulcers occasionally occur on the skin. The one important measure is to withdraw the person immediately from exposure to the mercury and then to sustain him in every possible way with adequate diet and necessary stimulating drugs for the blood.

METRITIS The prefix "metro-" usually refers to the uterus, so that metritis is an inflammation of the uterus. Metrorrhagia is a hemorrhage from the uterus, and metroscope is an instrument used in looking into the uterus.

MIDDLE AGE CHANGE, IN MEN Frequently in the past physicians have suggested the possibility that men also suffered after middle age with symptoms such as those affecting women. (See discussion under, *Menopause*) In women, however, there was visible the definite and gradual disappearance of the periodic functions, whereas in men there was nothing similar which could be definitely traced. Today through new methods of study it has been found that men do develop symptoms as a result of this decline in the functioning of the sex glands. The beginning of this decline in men is usually later in the course of their lives than in women.

Dr. August A. Werner, who has made special study of this subject and written about it in the medical journals, says that the average age for the beginning of the climacteric in women is about 40.8 years whereas for men it is approximately from 48 to 52 years. Of course, the woman no longer has her monthly functions and is then unable to have a baby. This does not mean, however, that she loses interest in sexual activity.

The man who passes 50 years of age begins to lose his ability to fertilize the egg cell of the female, but the exact time when this ability disappears also varies. There are records of a few men who were capable of fertilization up to the age of 80 years. Indeed, a scientific report some years ago indicated the ability of an individual 96 years of age to secrete potent male elements. But the majority of men show a beginning decline of this ability at about 50 years of age and in many instances the power of sexual activity also lessens.

Now that so much more attention is being given to the subject men have revealed the presence of symptoms much like those that occur in women. They become nervous. The irritability which they display in their domestic and business lives is an indication of their emotional instability. They, too, find that their memory for recent events is decreased and indeed also their ability to concentrate seriously on the problems of the day. Especially significant, moreover, are sudden changes of mood and particularly easy weeping so that the eyes become moist under slight emotional stimuli. The man who is hard at work in an outdoor activity may not be as much aware of these changes as the one whose daily work involves mental concentration. The executive at his desk in some great industrial concern, the teacher in a school or university, the engineer, the architect, the lawyer, and the physician are most susceptible. These men observe occasionally the hot flashes, the suddenly increased perspiration, and even occasional attacks of dizziness and palpitation of the heart such as occur in women.

John Smith, about 50 years old, who had always been in good health and who had been most successful in his work, became nervous, irritable and excitable as he approached the age of 50. He noticed that he was mentally depressed and that he cried at times for no good reason. In the midst of the afternoon and especially toward the end of the day when he became fatigued, he would feel exceedingly hot. Sometimes at night while lying in bed, his hands would become numb or there would be tingling in his legs. People in the office noticed that he could remember very well the problems of 1939 but that often he forgot important letters about events that had occurred on the previous day.

His case was typical of the man who is in the climacteric. His case was of the kind in which specialists have found the use of the male sex hormone particularly valuable. It is called by various names, depending on the manner of its preparation and on the name of the company that manufactures the product. Most common is the product testosterone propionate. When this product is given to such cases over a sufficiently long period of time and in sufficient dosage, many of the symptoms seem to improve, the depressed feeling disappears, the man becomes cheerful, and the effects are seen in his work.

While these products are useful for persons who are beginning to have lessened secretion of the hormones, they are especially valuable in those who, because of surgical removal of the sex glands on account of disease or who have lost these organs because of some accident, are wholly without this glandular secretion. These people suffer a true glandular deficiency. Their sexual tissues fail to develop. Men without the functions of the sex glands become wide-hipped, thin skinned, large breasted, and fat. In such cases the use of this material in the proper amounts brings about a remarkable change toward a masculine appearance and a masculine point of view.

THE HYGIENE OF MIDDLE AGE—The man past middle age ought to give special attention to two of the systems which control his body: First, the circulation of the blood, and second, the nervous system. Men who care for themselves properly may well go on into advanced years and contribute greatly for themselves and for the advancement of mankind. But the man past middle age must remember that for him the caution. "moderation in all thnigs" is most important.

The human body is built with great factors of safety which are especially important in relation to circulation of the blood and the breathing apparatus. If your heart breaks down, it is possible for it to recover and to become compensated. By "compensated," I mean, able to do the work that it is called on to do.

Even with a loss of a considerable amount of lung area, because of disease, many people live perfectly normal lives.

Thus a person with organs that have been damaged may yet be considered a healthy human being. When, however, the reserve power of the organs breaks down, the situation is serious and demands attention.

One of the most important changes brought about by modern civilization is the development of systems of transportation which have greatly lowered the amount of exercise available to most people. Fifty years ago people walked a great deal. Today the motor car, the street car, elevators, trains and other means of transportation are making walking a lost art except for those who play golf.

A reasonable amount of exercise is beneficial for health. People whose occupations or the routine of whose lives are such as to interfere seriously with their getting any ordinary exercise, should arrange to walk a little each day to keep their organs at a higher functioning condition. Walking in the open air is best because most of us, especially those who live in cities, do not get enough fresh air. One of the chief values of moderate exercise is to maintain the circulation of the blood and the elasticity of the blood vessels. An old proverb said, "If you rest, you rust."

Modern knowledge of diet makes it possible for any one with reasonable intelligence to assure himself of the daily consumption of all the foods that are necessary to maintain the best of health. These foods include enough fresh fruits and vegetables and enough milk, meat, and eggs to provide the body with suitable nutrition. Moreover, knowledge of calories has become so widespread that any intelligent person with sufficient will power can control his weight.

The spread of information concerning these simple facts of hygiene and the use of modern gland science are certain to add to the efficiency and usefulness of life after middle age.

MIDDLE-LIFE DISTURBANCES

(See also *Menopause*) Men and women tend to develop the same types of emotional disturbances and mental illness in middle life. In men such disturbances usually appear about 10 years later and half as frequently as they do in women. People develop psychiatric symptoms in middle life as a result of a personality predisposed to mental upsets plus the unusual stresses to which people with the responsibilities of middle life are subjected—stresses which seem more serious when people get a feeling that time is running out. Men and women in their fifties often develop psychiatric conditions that range from mild neuroses or depressions to severe mental disturbances. The most common complaints are fatigue, inability to sleep, early awakening, and loss of interest in life. The most serious complaints are irritability and diminished sexual drive. An eminent psychiatrist reports, on the basis of his observation, that the first evidence of trouble is often a newly acquired dependence on alcohol or the seeking of companionship outside the home. All these conditions are not improved by the taking of glandular preparations; they require psychological study and psychotherapy. It is recommended that people with these conditions remain at work; if a change from the usual environment is necessary, the person should not let himself be idle. Major changes in business or family life should not be made until an adequate understanding of the problem has been obtained and treatment has been tried.

MIGRAINE See discussion under *Headache.*

MILK Whereas milk was available in early America only in the form of the fluid taken directly from the cow, modern technology has developed a number of processes for treating milk so that it may be preserved for a long time. In many primitive portions of the world, where such technological developments are not available, American products are shipped.

Dried milk is one of the forms most widely used. When dried milk is shipped, one saves the costs and trouble of handling large amounts of water. Moreover,

dried milk by its method of preparation is free from danger of bacterial contamination, since the bacteria are destroyed in the process. One of the difficulties with dried milk is the fact that some people insist that it does not taste like fresh milk when water is added.

Dried milk is prepared by three main technics. By one method the milk is passed in a thin layer over a heated surface. A second method blows air through layers of partially evaporated milk on drying cylinders. The third method sprays partially evaporated milk into warm drying chambers. The last described is the one most frequently used.

In such milk powder less than 2 per cent of moisture remains. The fat, sugar, and protein of the milk are not changed chemically but are merely dried. The food value, when this form of powder is reconstituted into milk, is just about the same as that of fresh milk except for the vitamin C, which is destroyed by oxidation and much of which may be lost in the drying process. However, vitamin C may be made up by a small quantity of orange juice or any of the fresh fruit juices or tomato juice or potatoes or many other foods.

Dried milk is especially useful in cooking and baking. Today in the United States the production of dried milk is somewhere between 400,000,000 and 500,000,000 pounds per year. In addition to dried whole milk, preparations are also made of dried skim milk, in which the butterfat is much less.

Between fresh and dried milk are such products as evaporated, concentrated, and condensed milk. Evaporated milk is simply fresh milk from which the water has been evaporated to such a point that it contains not less than 7.9 per cent of milk fat and not less than 25.9 per cent of the total milk solids. Concentrated or plain condensed milk is like evaporated milk except that it is not processed by heat, and the container may be unsealed.

Sweetened condensed milk is a liquid made by evaporating a mixture of sweet milk and refined sugar or corn sugar so that the sweetened condensed milk contains not less than 28 per cent of the total milk solids and not less than 8.5 per cent of milk fat. The sugar is used here to prevent spoilage.

When fresh milk is not available, canned milk is obviously preferable to no milk at all. Moreover, in many places the fresh milk that is available is not properly controlled from a sanitary point of view by pasteurizing and sanitary handling. Under such circumstances condensed or evaporated milk is far preferable.

One of the difficulties with the use of sweetened condensed milk is the fact that the large amount of sugar must be considered in calculating the diet. Babies brought up on sweetened condensed milk are likely to be fat babies.

The canned milk industry uses almost 5,000,000,000 pounds of milk a year, which is about 15 pounds of canned milk for every person in the country. About the same amount of canned milk is used by the ice cream industry, and that incidentally is enough to provide 3 gallons of ice cream for each person per year. The chief value of ice cream in the diet lies, of course, in its milk content. Ice cream varies from place to place in quality and in the nature of the ice cream mix. These milk products are exceedingly important, since milk is one of the most nearly perfect foods and should occupy a place particularly in the diets of growing children.

Over a two-year period the pupils in a residential school were given three times as much milk daily as they had previously been given—the increase being from 8 ounces to 24 ounces. During this period many vitamin deficiencies were greatly reduced, the total number of colds and other infections of the respiratory tract decreased, and the pupils performed better and had more energy.

MILK—acidified: See INFANCY, article CARE AND FEEDING OF THE CHILD.

MILK—allergy caused by: See article ALLERGY.

MILK—artificial feeding of infants: See INFANCY, article CARE AND FEEDING OF THE CHILD.

MILK—condensed: See INFANCY, article CARE AND FEEDING OF THE CHILD.

MILK—constipation diet: See article DIGESTION AND DIGESTIVE DISEASES.

MILK—digestibility by infant: See INFANCY, article CARE AND FEEDING OF THE CHILD.

MILK—evaporated: See INFANCY, article CARE AND FEEDING OF THE CHILD.

MILK—food elements in (fig.): See DIET, article ADVICE ON THE DIET.

MILK—food values: See DIET, article ADVICE ON THE DIET.

MILK—fortified with vitamin D: See INFANCY, article CARE AND FEEDING OF THE CHILD.

MILK—goat's, undulant fever spread by: See article TRANSMISSIBLE DISEASES.

MILK—infant's diet: See INFANCY, article CARE AND FEEDING OF THE CHILD.

MILK—pasteurization: See article TRANSMISSIBLE DISEASES.

MILK—pregnancy diet: See BIRTH, article CARE OF MOTHERS BEFORE AND AFTER CHILDBIRTH.

MILK—rickets prevented by sufficient amount in infant's diet: See INFANCY, article CARE AND FEEDING OF THE CHILD.

MILK—scarlet fever spread through: See CHILDHOOD DISEASES, article INFECTIOUS DISEASES OF CHILDHOOD.

MILK—septic sore throat spread by: See EAR, article THE EAR, TONGUE, NOSE, AND THROAT.

MILK—sugar: See INFANCY, article CARE AND FEEDING OF THE CHILD.

MILK—tuberculosis diet: See RESPIRA-

TORY DISEASES, article THE RESPIRATORY DISEASES.

MILK—tuberculosis prevented by pasteurization: See RESPIRATORY DISEASES, article THE RESPIRATORY DISEASES.

MILK—typhoid fever spread by: See article TRANSMISSIBLE DISEASES.

MILK—undulant fever: See article TRANSMISSIBLE DISEASES.

MILK SUBSTITUTE (See also discussion under *Allergy in Children* and *Food Allergy*) Infants are sometimes allergic (sensitive) to milk. For these infants, enriched meat-base formulas seem to be more advantageous substitutes for milk than soy-bean formulas. These meat-base formulas, enriched with calcium, phosphorus, carbohydrates, and vitamins, are nutritionally equal to mother's milk or cow's milk. Generally, meat-base formulas modified according to special needs may also be fed to older children and adults unable to chew, swallow, or digest ordinary meat or for whom tube feeding is necessary. A meat-base formula may be fed alternately with a soy-bean formula in an effort to prevent sensitization from drinking one or the other exclusively. Over 100 infants and children who had eczema, bronchial asthma, and allergic gastrointestinal diseases were given strained-meat formulas for periods exceeding 3 months. Patients experienced no weight loss, and anemia did not develop; actually a rise in the red coloring matter in the blood was usually observed.

MISCARRIAGE See *Abortion.*

MISCARRIAGE, PREVENTION OF Although at least one pregnancy in every ten terminates in miscarriage— most doctors say one in four or five— few married couples know enough about the causes of miscarriage to help the doctor prevent its occurrence.

Yet many miscarriages can be prevented. Today some women who have had two, three or even more successive miscarriages may carry their babies to normal birth. Scientific progress is being made in discovering what causes miscarriages and how they may be avoided. And women themselves have learned the necessity of early prenatal care. That leads to the most important admonition to mothers-to-be—*put yourself in the hands of your obstetrician early.*

In fact, the wise young couple who wish to have a child should both consult the doctor before a pregnancy occurs. If necessary, he will select suitable specialists. Early detection of any abnormality in either the husband or wife may prevent a later miscarriage.

Certainly both the young wife, who has suffered one miscarriage, and her husband as well should undergo thorough physical examinations before another pregnancy occurs. The intelligent woman will have a physical examination of the organs concerned with childbirth even before marriage. What was the reason for the miscarriage? Perhaps the mother's health was below par. Perhaps the father was not in good physical condition. Even minor ailments, such as, anemia, or bad tonsils, or some local infection may be the factor that injured the cells of the growing baby and led to the miscarriage.

A chief cause of miscarriage is defective germ plasm—occurring either in the ovum of the mother or in the sperm cell—spermatozoa—of the father. All too often it is assumed that the mother is responsible for the miscarriage when it may be the father who is producing defective seed.

In many cases unhealthy spermatozoa results in the wife's miscarriage. Spermatozoa are delicate organisms, and disturbances in the male reproductive apparatus may interfere with the delivery of perfect spermatozoa. Men who want children and who wish to spare their wives the suffering and heartache of miscarriage should willingly submit to a check-up in the hands of a competent doctor.

The fate of the ovum is often decided within the first week after conception. If it is fit to survive and prosper, the normal uterus will take care of it. If the fertilized egg is grossly abnormal, it will be expelled from the uterus within two or three months. All the skill of the medical profession cannot save a really defective embryo if Nature has ordained it is not worth saving. Too much stress cannot be placed on this fact: if Nature hasn't disposed of the faulty embryo early in pregnancy, in the vast majority of cases the expectant mother can be confident that she will carry her child to full term and that the child will be normal.

To the mother who has had a miscarriage, the gynecologist says reassuringly: "Don't be discouraged. In the long run you'll be glad you didn't bear the child. If a faulty germ cell was the cause of your miscarriage, you may correct it before another pregnancy. Try again."

Another frequent cause of miscarriage early in pregnancy is some glandular deficiency on the part of the mother. Following conception, chemical substances are sent into the blood stream by such glands as the pituitary, thyroid and ovaries—all organizing energies to support the new life. In particular, an enlargement is noted in the *corpus luteum*—the yellow body in the ovary—which secretes a hormone known as progestin. If progestin is lacking, the egg may be robbed of its sustenance in the wall of the uterus and be expelled prematurely. Or the uterus may not enlarge as it should.

Thanks to modern chemistry, preparations containing progestin are now available and are effective in preventing many of those miscarriages which might be caused by a deficiency of this hormone. Progestin has the virtue of preventing contractions of the uterus by opposing the effects of estrin, which sensitizes the muscle of the uterus.

Certain chronic or acute diseases of the mother may also lead to miscarriages—pneumonia, influenza, malaria, typhoid fever, smallpox. Tuberculosis, incidentally, is seldom a factor in miscarriage, though it may diminish fertility. Syphilis is seldom a cause of miscarriage in the early months of pregnancy but may bring on a premature birth in the second half of the nine months' period. Where syphilis is most prevalent, late miscarriages are most frequent.

What about falls, accidents? Miscarriages rarely result from them. The healthy woman can undergo an amazing amount of physical pummeling without losing her unborn child. Women have carried their babies through train wrecks, mine disasters, bombing attacks. Nature has provided a miraculously protective nest for the dependent embryo, and expectant mothers should have confidence in this fact. If a slight tumble should be followed by a miscarriage, there is usually some more fundamental cause. "Healthy fruit does not fall from the tree until it is ripe."

It is prudent, of course, to avoid taking long automobile trips, lifting heavy weights and playing vigorously such sports as tennis and golf and riding horseback. One New York physician warns against the fatigue of shopping expeditions and apartment hunting. Moving one's home is particularly strenuous and should be done by someone else or preferably postponed. Proper exercise, however, is advisable, and the doctor will usually prescribe the kind and amount that the individual woman requires.

With so many women in industry today, a special warning should be given to working mothers not to overexert themselves, particularly during the first three months of pregnancy.

Many doctors advise against marital relationships in early pregnancy. Others say it is harmless then, while others advise continence on the days when the second and third menstrual periods would have been due.

Miscarriages sometimes follow mental shock. It is no accident that the word "hysteria" derives from the Greek word for womb. There is a close emotional relationship between the psyche and the reproductive organs. The balance beween them should not be rudely jarred. "Bad news" should be broken as gently as possible.

Mental shock can, however, be greatly over-rated as a primary cause of miscarriage. One has only to think of the war-torn countries of today and the amount of shock that prospective mothers have gone through without miscarriage to realize how strong is the mechanism of motherhood. Through hell and high water, through shock and strain, her body and mind instinctively respond to their job of protecting the child-to-be. Severe emotions affect the activities of the glandular organs that are closely related to the mechanism of childbirth. The factors of safety constitute without doubt one of the most awe-inspiring phases in this mystery of life.

There are other causes of miscarriage. In certain cases the uterus may be tilted backward. Persistence in this position results in miscarriage. An early visit to the physician, however, would easily result in the detection of this deformity and its correction by simple measures. After surgery, an appendectomy for instance, a mother may lose her baby. Radiation treatments, if directed to the ovaries, may cause a miscarriage. Recent studies of the blood have shown that in rare cases certain blood groups are incompatible and a woman unfortunate enough to have what is known as an

"Rh factor" antagonistic to her husband's may miscarry.

The mother who is threatened with a miscarriage—symptoms are bleeding or cramp-like pains— should go to bed at once and have her doctor notified. Proper rest and medication may halt the process. The essential treatment for a threatened miscarriage includes absolute rest in bed, the application of an icebag to the lower abdomen, raising the foot of the bed about a foot, complete abstinence from the use of cathartics or enemas for at least three days, the use of suitable sedative drugs as prescribed by the doctor and the use of various glandular preparations to overcome such glandular deficiencies as may be apparent to him. If the miscarriage does continue and the baby is lost, the mother need not fear for her own physical welfare. Deaths or permanent disability seldom result from miscarriages.

The course of pregnancy is charted along a normal path for most women, and they need not fear miscarriage. Nevertheless, this problem should receive more attention. More emphasis should be placed on the father's responsibility so that he will have himself physically checked when looking for the cause of a miscarriage. And the wife should not only be carefully examined early in pregnancy, but she should be taught more of the basic requirements of good health—proper diet, proper exercise, proper rest, proper prenatal care. If precautions are taken, even the woman who has had several miscarriages may be freed of worry and come through safely. Many miscarriages *can* be prevented. More of them *should* be.

MISCEGENATION When two people of different races marry and have children, the condition is called miscegenation.

MONONUCLEOSIS As early as 1889 a German named Pfeiffer described a disease which was called glandular fever. It occurred in children, the chief symptoms being the appearance of fever with general sickness, swelling of the glands in the neck, redness of the throat, and often enlargement of the liver and the spleen. After the passing of some years other doctors began investigating this disease much more carefully, making studies particularly of the blood and of the swollen glands. This has enabled them now to recognize a special disease called glandular fever as a common name but infectious mononucleosis as a name which means much more to the doctor. In it he recognizes two important factors: the first, that the condition can occur as an epidemic or an infection; and the second, that the changes in the blood are especially significant.

The causative organism of this condition is not known, but it is now believed to be a virus—one of those toxic agents so small that it cannot be seen under an ordinary microscope, so small indeed that it can be filtered through the pores of a clay filter.

In the United States the persons most affected with infectious mononucleosis are young people between the ages of fifteen and thirty. Outbreaks have occurred among boys in schools. Rarely have epidemics occurred among adults.

Usually about a week after a person has been exposed to the disease he gets the fever, sore throat, and enlargement of the lymph glands that are significant. Sometimes these are so mild that they are overlooked and the study of the disease is not carried far enough to make a positive diagnosis. Often when there is an infection of the throat with a germ like the streptococcus or the staphylococcus, the glands will swell and even suppurate but the glands in infectious mononucleosis do not suppurate.

When the blood of a child with this infection is examined, the red blood cells and the red coloring matter are found to be normal but the white blood cells vary in number and character during the different stages of the disease. Gradually after six to ten days the white blood cells increase greatly in number and the character changes so that there are a majority of cells with a single central staining spot or nucleus in contrast to having the majority of cells with many nuclei. The name applied to a cell with a single nucleus is mononuclear. The name applied to a cell with many nuclei is polynuclear. Other names given to a cell with a single nucleus are lymphocyte or monocyte.

Usually by the end of the third week the number of white blood cells will have gone back to normal and the characteristic percentage and distribution of the different types of cells will also change.

A blood test has been discovered which makes it possible to diagnose this condition in the same way as the Wassermann test is used to diagnose syphilis or the Widal test is used to diagnose typhoid. Usually these patients get well in three or four weeks with proper attention, although occasionally they may feel somewhat "under the weather" for five or six months.

Thus far ACTH is the only drug found beneficial in treating the disease but of course the sulfonamide drugs and penicillin help to prevent secondary complications which may bring about serious results.

Research carried on by the Army and Navy definitely established prolonged wet kissing as the most significant factor in outbreaks of mononucleosis which have occurred among troops. This means that the virus which causes the condition is not spread through the air but by contamination with saliva.

MORPHINE AND OPIUM POISONING

MORPHINE AND OPIUM POISONING (See also, *Poisoning*) Opium is widespread throughout the world and its many derivatives including morphine, codeine, heroin and other modifications have extensive uses in medicine. Heroin is so addictive that its use is forbidden in the United States but heroin peddlers bring the material from abroad and 1950 saw the beginning of attempts to produce teen-age addicts.

People acutely poisoned with opium or morphine have giddiness, flushing, a lazy feeling and a sort of feeling of well-being, followed, however, by slowing of the pulse in breathing and, finally, unconsciousness. Nausea and vomiting frequently appear; itching of the skin and nose are so common that frequently actors simulate the heroin or morphine addict by their reactions of this type.

Severe poisoning is marked by such signs as constriction of the pupils to pinpoints, blueness, and convulsions. Some people become nauseated and vomit easily, whereas others become agitated with even small doses of the drug. People who are anemic or who have insufficient action of the thyroid gland or of the adrenals are especially sensitive to morphine and respond to much smaller doses than do ordinary people.

When anyone has been poisoned by opium or morphine, the first thing to do is to neutralize the drug and to sustain the patient so that he does not completely collapse. A doctor will pump out the stomach and give materials which will oxidize the opium or morphine in the stomach. The respiratory failure is overcome by giving artificial respiration and by administering oxygen with carbon dioxide. The carbon dioxide stimulates the breathing center in the brain; also stimulating drugs are given to get over the coma and collapse. Benzedrine or amphetamine may also be used to stimulate the higher centers in the brain.

Since people poisoned by sedative drugs often get secondary infection from congestion in the lungs, it is customary to give antibiotic drugs to prevent secondary pneumonias.

All drugs of the opium series can cause addiction and once a person is addicted to the drug, control and treatment are exceedingly difficult. The greatest trouble with opium addiction is the moral disintegration that occurs. Everything is subordinated to the desire to obtain the drug. Morphine addicts lie, steal, cheat and do anything necessary, even to occasional violence, in order to secure the supply of drug for which the craving is completely uncontrollable and constant.

There is much discussion among doctors as to why people get addicted to opium, morphine, and especially to heroin. Unquestionably psychological factors are important. However, there seems to be also something that develops in the body of the person who becomes addicted which continues the desire and even brings about the craving to increase the amount of the drug.

When the drug is withdrawn serious symptoms occur, such as yawning, restlessness and, finally, irritability, loss of appetite, vomiting and diarrhea. Eventually there may be tremors, insomnia and finally prostration and even collapse.

Physicians used to think that the drug could be withdrawn gradually and in that way recovery could ensue. Nowadays the so-called "cold-turkey" treatment is practiced in which the drug is withdrawn completely and immediately and substitutes in the form of barbiturates or less addictive drugs may be used to tide over the serious symptoms. Patients who are undergoing withdrawal treatment need to be kept in hospitals or sanitariums where they are given all of the benefits of what modern medicine can do to avoid serious symptoms and produce comfort. Many physicians are convinced, however, that permanent cure of addicts is difficult, if not impossible, and only a small percentage remain cured for as long as five years. Obviously those who are mentally disturbed or psychopathic are much less frequently cured than are others.

MORTALITY IN CANCER (See also discussion under *Cancer and Research in Cancer*) Each year in the United States about 225,000 people lose their lives through cancer and approximately 700,000 are under treatment for this condition. Cancer is the second leading cause of death. According to estimates by the National Cancer Institute, 32 out of every 100 babies born in the United States will get cancer at some time in their lives. Fortunately, research in cancer is well supported today. Many people are convinced that the funds available are well within what can be successfully used. The bottleneck of insufficient trained personnel must first be overcome; then much more money could be properly used in investigation of cancer. At present about 50 million dollars a year is subscribed voluntarily to such organizations as the American Cancer Society and the Damon Runyon Fund and about twenty-five million is given by the Federal Government. The greatly intensified research of the last ten years is beginning to yield noticeable results.

In 1952 the eminent pathologist, Dr. Paul Steiner, estimated that application of present knowledge everywhere would raise the five year cure rates from five to fifty for some types of cancer; from twenty to seventy-five in others. However, in many types, improvements could not be expected. By the use of surgery and radiology, many cancers can be eradicated from the body of a human being without recurrence at the original site. The chief menace in cancer is often the spread of the cancer to other parts of the body by what is called metastatic growths. Eighty-five per cent is the rate of permanent or complete cure in cancer of the skin simply because this is easily accessible. In contrast the rate for cure of cancer of the pancreas, gallbladder, liver and lymphatic system is only one per cent.

MORTALITY AND OVERWEIGHT—Common knowledge recognizes that any considerable amount of overweight is unhealthy and not conducive to long life. This impression is confirmed by the more rigorous tests of statistical inquiry. These not only substantiate the truth of the general impression, but furnish numerical estimates of the degree of excess mortality associated with various degrees of overweight; more than this, they yield important information regarding the particular diseases or conditions to which overweight persons are more vulnerable than the average.

Relevant statistics come mainly from three sources: first, the experience of life-insurance companies as analyzed by them and by actuarial organizations; second, the records of periodical health examinations made by the Life Extension Institute and other organizations; third, data scattered in medical writings, collected in connection with clinics, and analyzed by physicians who have taken an interest in statistical methods of inquiry.

Those statistics derived from insurance experience present several advantages over those of the others. The examples are great, numbering in some instances in the hundreds of thousands. They represent a fairly extensive cross section of the population, though there is some selection at the time of acceptance for insurance, since definitely substandard risks are sifted out. Data from clinics tend in the opposite direction; from the nature of things they concern essentially persons coming under the doctor's care for some condition sufficiently severe to attract attention.

What is overweight? What is overweight for a given person or, better, for a class of people? The most obvious and simplest though not the ideal standard is one based on the average weight of a sufficiently large sample of the general population. Weight varies somewhat systematically with age, even after the period of bodily growth is completed, and the standard must allow for this circumstance. Given these fundamentals, overweight may be defined and measured as the per cent of excess of any person over the average for his age and sex. This measure, if applied without further modification, suffers from the defect that a certain variation in body weight must be expected as a normal concomitant of body build. Accordingly some authors have made allowance for this, at least in first approximation, by segregating the people under observation into three broad classes, such as those commonly designated as the linear, the stocky or lateral, and an intermediate type. A few investigators have attempted a more precise gauge and have studied material classified according to such measures, as, for example, the quotient chest-girth/height.

Quite aside from "normal" variations in weight corresponding to variation in build there is a fundamental and unjustified assumption in using the *average* weight of a numerically adequate sample as standard of "normality." Much of the increase in weight with advancing age is not "physiologically" normal. Accordingly a table of "ideal" weights has been suggested which are recommended as the appropriate standard toward which personal hygiene may

advantageously be directed. (See, *Weight, Normal for Health*)

As to the influence of build aside from excess weight as such and variations in skeletal type, the figure appropriately described as "pot bellied" is most unfavorable. In a study of body build it was found that overweights whose abdominal girth was more than two inches greater than chest girth had an excess mortality of about 50 per cent over and above that associated with their particular degree of overweight. Generally speaking, solidly built, large-boned overweight is superior to the flabbier type.

Distribution of body weights in population. From a general point of view how much of a problem is overweight? What proportion of the population is overweight? What is the per cent distribution of men and women among underweights, "normals," and overweights?

Some figures can be quoted. In a study of physical defects based on nearly 17,000 male policyholders examined by the Life Extension Institute the following proportions were found at different age levels in persons 20 per cent or more overweight:

AGE	PER CENT
All ages	12.9
Under 25	4.9
25-34	8.1
35-44	14.4
45-54	18.9
55 and over	19.8

EXCESS MORTALITY OF OVERWEIGHTS

GENERAL MORTALITY FROM ALL CAUSES—After these preliminaries we now approach our central thesis: that material overweight tends to be accompanied by some excess mortality; this is evidenced beyond question by all competent studies. In round numbers, it can be said of men that "the penalty for overweight is from one fourth to three fourths excess mortality."

MORTALITY FROM SPECIFIC CAUSES—Since the broad fact of excess mortality among overweights is beyond reasonable doubt, an insistent question is: What are the specific causes of death to which overweights are particularly prone? The results of study of the experiences of Union Central Life Insurance Company are illuminating. Some of its principal finding are summarized in the following tables and chart.

The figures in the tables consistently indicate a definite excess mortality from most of the diseases exhibited. The excess is more marked in the higher age group and rises to the extreme of more than 1,000 per cent excess in the case of diabetes at ages forty-five and over. In addition it is immediately apparent from the tables that the diseases of later life —the so-called degenerative diseases— are the group particularly affected. Among causes not so specifically related to the aging process both accidents and suicide have a mortality somewhat above average among overweights. In the case of suicides this probably represents, at least in part, a personal reaction to ill health. However, among infectious diseases whose incidence spreads over the entire life period tuberculosis has a mortality that is actually less than average among overweights. This particular result is obviously influenced by the fact that underweights, especially young underweights, are, or have been in the past, predominantly susceptible to the disease.

EXCESS MORTALITY OF OVERWEIGHTS FOR SPECIFIED CAUSES OF DEATH (ALL AGES COMBINED)

CAUSES OF DEATH	RATIO OF MORTALITY OF OVERWEIGHTS TO THAT OF NORMALS
	Per Cent
All causes	132
Circulatory diseases	
Organic diseases of heart	151
Angina pectories	219
Diseases of the arteries	165
Acute endocarditis and pericarditis	163
Nephritis, acute and chronic	172
Cerebral hemorrhage and apoplexy	157
Cancer	111
Diabetes	257
Tuberculosis, all forms	47
Pulmonary tuberculosis	46
Respiratory diseases	
Pneumonia, lobar and unspecified	94
Diseases of the digestive system	
Appendicitis	118
Cirrhosis of the liver	167
External causes	
Accidents	112
Suicides	129

EXCESS MORTALITY AMONG OVERWEIGHT MEN FROM SELECTED CAUSES BY WEIGHT CLASSES AND BROAD AGE GROUPS

DISEASE, AGE

| | PER CENT OVERWEIGHT | | |
| | 5-15 | 15-25 | 25 and over |
	Per cent over average mortality		
Organic heart disease			
Under age 45	12	48	*
Over age 45	50	73	173
Angina pectoris			
Under age 45	133	*	*
Over age 45	88	139	148
Diseases of the arteries			
Under age 45	*	*	*
Over age 45	156	216	67
Nephritis, acute and chronic			
Under age 45	50	218	241
Over age 45	27	133	160
Cerebral hemorrhage, apoplexy, and paralysis			
Under age 45	6	35	*
Over age 45	51	70	135
Cancer, all forms			
Under age 45	*	5	*
Over age 45	8	24	30
Diabetes			
Under age 45	14	*	*
Over age 45	74	265	1,026

*An asterisk indicates that the deviation from "normal" was not significant for a sample of the size available.

MORTALITY AMONG OVERWEIGHT WOMEN—The study based on the experience of the Union Central Life Insurance Company was restricted to data on male lives. As this left a regrettable gap in the information and conclusions obtained, a later study was aimed specifically to secure data on female lives. The material analyzed was based on more than 300 000 standard policies (Regular Ordinary Branch) issued by the Metropolitan Life Insurance Company. The results of this investigation followed in the main those of the study of overweight males, but with apparently more moderate adverse influence of excess weight. This may, however, have been at least in part due to a factor in medical selection.

As to mortality from specific causes among overweight women, relatively high death rates were found for the cardiovascular-renal conditions, diabetes, gall bladder disease, cancer, and puerperal conditions. The excess mortality from accidents and suicide observed among overweight men was not appreciably noted among overweight women.

A supplementary study by the same company based on more than 120.000 substandard policies on female lives yielded results differing in some details from those observed in the standard experience. However, the conclusions followed essentially the same general lines, that excess mortality over average increases with degree of overweight above the average.

Conclusion—There is a wealth of evidence from a variety of sources that overweight, particularly in certain types of body build, is definitely associated with mortality and morbidity above average. Beyond this general conclusion the evidence points with equal clarity to certain causes as being those chiefly involved in this association, namely, the degenerative diseases characteristic of later adult life, especially diabetes and the cardiovascular-renal group.

MOSQUITO BITES   The mosquito is proof of Kipling's famous statement that "the female of the species is more deadly that the male." The male mosquito does not bite. The female mosquito is out for blood. The mosquito does not really bite but saws through the skin.

Investigators have found that mosquitoes prefer to bite some people rather than others. They have found, moreover, that some people react severely to mosquito bites whereas others do not react at all. The attractiveness of an individual for mosquitoes varies from time to time. Mosquitoes that bite prefer places

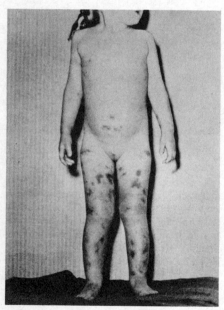

(A)

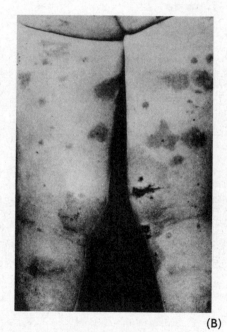

(B)

(A) Child exposed to multiple mosquito bites. The areas became black and blue and swollen, and the child had ill effects as a result of insect allergy.

(B) Close-up of back of thighs, showing mosquito bites and discoloration of the skin. Although mosquito bites are common, such allergic reactions are not.

with lots of people rather than those with just a few people or places that are empty. Mosquitoes are more attracted by numerous or unwashed sleepers than by a few people who are sleeping and who are well washed. Thorough cleansing with soap and water decreases the attractiveness of any individual for mosquitos. Mosquitos are attracted by warm objects, by lights at night, and by dark objects during the day.

Dark clothing is more attractive than light clothing for mosquitoes, and rough clothing is more attractive than smooth clothing. Mosquitoes prefer damp weather to dry weather, but in the cold seasons they prefer dry weather to damp weather. Mosquitoes prefer adults to children and men to women.

If you watch a mosquito as it alights on the skin you will find that it begins to move back and forth, causing the saw to penetrate the skin. If it feeds rapidly it swells up, and if you smack the mosquito a spot of blood will appear on the skin, indicating the amount of blood that has been taken. When the mosquito first inserts the proboscis into your skin it injects some saliva, which keeps the blood from clotting.

Mosquitoes carry malaria, yellow fever, and a number of other diseases. The mosquito can be eliminated by getting rid of pools of stagnant water in

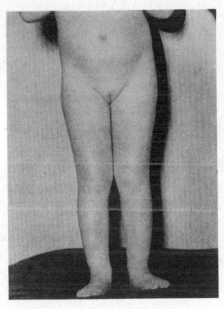

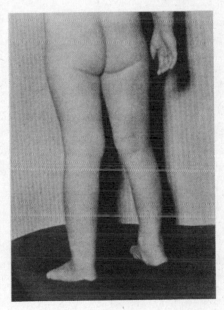

(C)   (D)

(C) Skin eruptions completely healed after hospitalization and treatment.

(D) Back view showing complete healing of the areas.

Postgraduate Medicine

the surroundings, by spraying surfaces of water with oil, by the widespread use of DDT, and by other well-established health engineering technics. The itching of the mosquito bite can be controlled by the use of one per cent menthol or phenol in calamine lotion or by the application of the ointments of antihistamines such as neohetramine, neoantergan, thephorin, pyrabenzamine, benadryl, diatrin, and others.

MOTION SICKNESS See *Seasickness.*

MOUTH, DISEASE OF See *Pyorrhea, Teeth, Tongue,* et cetera.

MOUTH, DISEASE OF—cancer: See article CANCER.

MULTIPLE SCLEROSIS Multiple sclerosis is probably third or fourth in frequency among all of the disorders that affect the nervous system. Usually this condition begins fairly early in life —between the ages of ten and forty. Then it gradually develops and becomes worse over a period of many years. Apparently the condition does not occur in families, nor does there seem to be any hereditary factor involved.

Occasionally the condition begins after childbirth or a surgical operation or some such incident, but apparently this may easily be coincidence and not have any direct relationship.

In multiple sclerosis the nervous system is involved with degenerative changes and secondary scarring as a result of which its functions are interfered with and disappear. This means that all kinds of combinations of symptoms can occur, including paralysis beginning with moderate weakness in the legs and symptoms like sudden jumping of the legs due to a spastic condition of the muscles. The arms are less frequently

involved than the legs and usually much later in the condition. Speech changes are somewhat characteristic, the speech becoming slow and monotonous, so that the person talks as if he were spelling out every word. There are tremors of the hands when some definite movement is attempted. Occasionally the head may develop a tremor.

The mental symptoms may include gradual deterioration with depression or instances in which there are serious disturbances of the emotions and the ability to think. Usually, however, patients with multiple sclerosis are optimistic and seem to feel well almost regardless of the extent of the disease.

Ultimately the important organs of the body involved in seeing, hearing, or taking care of the digestive functions become affected, which means that the patient will have to have nursing care.

The duration of these cases varies from a few years to many years, depending on the rapidity of progress of the disease.

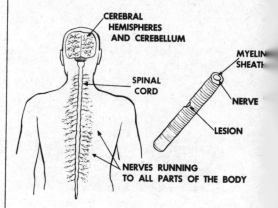

CEREBRAL HEMISPHERES AND CEREBELLUM

MYELIN SHEATH

SPINAL CORD

NERVE

LESION

NERVES RUNNING TO ALL PARTS OF THE BODY

Multiple sclerosis is a disease of the nervous system, where the white matter is destroyed. Drawing shows the areas affected by multiple sclerosis.

Medicine is still investigating to determine whether or not multiple sclerosis is due to an infection with a virus or an inflammatory disease produced by some toxin. So far a specific organism has not been identified as responsible for these cases.

Unfortunately specific methods of treatment that will definitely halt the disease or cure it are not known. Much comfort can be given by proper nursing and by attention to the individual symptoms as they develop. People with long chronic diseases die not so much from the disease as from the secondary complications.

Examination of the spinal cord shows that this disease affects chiefly the white matter of the nervous system. The portion affected is the sheaths of the nerves which change in their character to plaques, these interfering with the passage of nerve stimuli. Today the cause of multiple sclerosis is unknown and neither is there any specific treatment for the disease. Countless medications have been used and none of these has proved to be especially valuable.

This disease occurs most commonly in the damp cold climates of the temperate zones and patients who can manage to live where the climatic conditions are warmer and drier do better. Physicians have found that pregnancy often precipitates a relapse in a woman with multiple sclerosis and the condition sometimes comes on for the first time in a woman who is pregnant. Among other conditions which bring about exacerbations of multiple sclerosis are overexertion, physical fatigue, exposure to cold and dampness, emotional reactions and injuries of various kinds. Especially important have been the various procedures used in rehabilitation of handicapped which aid the patient with multiple sclerosis to make the best he can out of the body that has been injured.

In multiple sclerosis physicians have found that the blood serum shows a decrease in albumin and an increase in gamma globulin in the spinal fluid. These are simply facts which when put together may some day be valuable but for the present do not establish anything specific for diagnosis or treatment.

MUMPS When the glands in front of the ear begin to swell rapidly, associated with fever up to 101 degrees Fahrenheit, the condition is probably mumps. The swelling is generally below and in front of the ear but it may extend backward and may also involve other glands. Usually the swelling and the fever are about as bad as they are going to get by the second day, after which the temperature drops and the swelling goes down. Cases are known, however, in which the condition persists even for weeks.

The worst danger of mumps is the well-known complication, which occurs, however, in only 1 out of 100 cases. In serious epidemics as many as 10 per cent of cases have the complication of swelling of the sex glands—the testes in the male, the ovary in the female. This complication means more fever, more sickness, some pain, and in a good many instances destruction of the glands that are infected to the extent of depriving them of their function.

Mumps is caused by the smallest type of infectious agent—namely, the virus. This has been proved by transferring the infection from man to animals. The disease is quite contagious whenever there is close contact. It is not, however, as contagious as measles or chicken pox. The virus is found in the saliva during the disease and can be disseminated by droplets of the saliva or by contaminated hands.

Usually the disease affects children between the ages of five and fifteen. Rarely does it affect any child under ten months of age. Most cases of mumps occur in the early winter and in the spring. Usually a person has mumps only once because the first attack will give the body protective substances against subsequent attacks. Cases are known, however, in which the disease has occurred two or even three times.

Fortunately few people die of mumps and the treatment involves in most cases merely rest in bed as long as the fever and swelling persist, scrupulous cleanliness of the mouth, a diet with plenty of fluids. The doctor may prescribe drugs for the relief of pain if that is considered necessary.

When the complications occur, the physician will want to give the patient his special attention. This is necessary to relieve the pains and to make certain that the amount of damage to the tissues is kept at a minimum.

In time of war mumps becomes epidemic in camps. For instance in World War I one third of the men in one camp were infected during an epidemic of mumps. For that reason it is customary to isolate infected patients immediately when cases are discovered under such circumstances.

MUMPS—childhood disease: See CHILDHOOD DISEASES, article INFECTIOUS DISEASES OF CHILDHOOD.

MUMPS—contagious disease: See INFECTIOUS DISEASE, article THE PREVENTION AND TREATMENT OF INFECTIOUS DISEASE.

MUMPS—incidence: See INFECTIOUS DISEASE, article THE PREVENTION AND TREATMENT OF INFECTIOUS DISEASE.

MUMPS—incubation period: See CHILDHOOD DISEASES, article INFECTIOUS DISEASES OF CHILDHOOD.

MUMPS—sex glands may be scarred: See article ENDOCRINOLOGY.

MUSCLE CRAMPS Many people suffer with cramps in the muscles which come on during exercise or at night when they turn or stretch or sometimes when an arm or leg is held in an unusual position for a rather long time. The mechanism of the cramp is the occurrence of an involuntary contraction of the fibers imposed on a voluntary movement. The cause of the cramp is, therefore, this spasmodic contraction, which produces pain. Observations indicate that the cramps come on more frequently in the presence of fatigue, lack of sufficient blood supply, and inflammation of the muscle or nerve, a deficiency of thiamin, and a lack of sufficient calcium in the body.

Various technics have been developed for increasing the consumption of oxygen as a means of relieving the cramps, including, for instance, breathing into a paper sack which acts as a stimulus to the intake of oxygen. The suggestion has been made that the taking of extra calcium would be effective but an actual trial showed that it is ineffective. Certain drugs which seem to have the effect of stimulating the chemistry of muscles, among them quinine, have been used with some success. In the vast majority of cases, however, the cramps are hardly of sufficient significance to demand much beyond an encouragement to keep the tissues warm and to use enough exercise to encourage the circulation. If muscle cramps come with great frequency, a careful medical study needs to be made, particularly related to the efficiency of the circulation of the blood in the muscles.

MUSCLE DISEASES Muscles constitute a large portion of the body structure; involvement of the muscles by disease is likely to have a tremendous effect on the body as a whole. In most instances, however, diseases affecting the muscles result from damage to nerves by which the muscles are made to move or to be at rest. There are instances in which muscles are damaged by mechanical activities. There is, for example, tearing of a muscle fiber due to overstretching or a sudden jerk or blow Sometimes the biceps muscle in the arm is torn. Occasionally the large muscles which manipulate the thumb are pulled away. Many times the tendons or fibrous structures by which the muscles are attached to the bones are torn. Tearing of the muscles in the thighs and in the back of the foot occurs fairly frequently in running and in games like tennis and squash, where there are sudden turns of the foot and leg.

Usually the first sign of such an injury is a sudden severe pain at the point where the breaking of the tendon or muscle has occurred. Then there is weakness. Frequently there is a flow of blood between the fibers of the muscles. As long as clotted blood is present, there may be pain on motion.

When such an injury has occurred, the treatment naturally has to depend on the nature and severity of the injury, on the age of the person involved, and on the general condition. Sometimes it is necessary to repair serious tears of muscles and tendons by surgical operation as soon as the condition is discovered. Modern surgery has technics for sewing the torn parts under strictly sterile conditions and then, by the use of casts, holding them tightly until healing has occurred.

Following healing, it becomes neces-

There are over 600 muscles in the body, all attached to the 206 bones making up the skeleton. Many of these muscles are arranged in opposition to one another so as to make movement of the head, limbs, and other parts possible in several directions.
Cleveland Health Museum

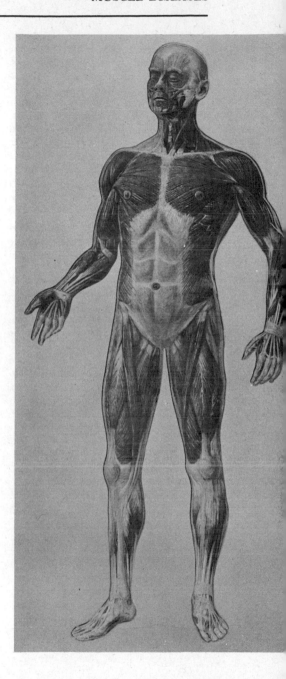

sary to use physical therapy in the form of heat, massage, and controlled movements to recover completely the function of the muscle. There are also conditions in which muscles become infected and inflamed due to invasion by germs. One inflammation which is localized in muscles is trichinosis, since this parasite localizes and grows in the muscle. There are instances, however, in which infectious germs also get inside muscles, producing pus and abscesses, with subsequent threat to life itself. Here again the diagnosis of the condition must be made by the doctor after careful study, and the treatment depends on what he finds as to the nature and extent of the inflammation.

There is also a group of diseases known as muscular dystrophies, in which the muscles waste away and lose their strength. The causes of these conditions vary. In many instances the causes are not known. In a typical case a child who seems to be normal at birth will begin at the age of four or five to be unable to use his legs properly and to tumble about. The back muscles become weak, so that the child cannot sit erect. Soon he finds difficulty in getting up when lying on the floor. In some cases there is complete wasting of the muscles, whereas in others there is continued progressive weakness without so much destruction of the tissues. As the muscles that are affected become weak, the stronger muscles pull, so that the body may become twisted and distorted.

MUSCULAR DYSTROPHY   A chronic crippling disease which mysteriously attacks the muscles. Unlike infantile paralysis, in which crippling effects stop at some point, muscular dystrophy progresses until all the muscles deteriorate. Although the presence of the muscle wasting is plain, the cause remains unknown.

The disease afflicts the proximal muscles first where a progressive wasting and weakness occurs. Eventually, this condition extends to practically all voluntary muscles of the body.

Postural changes that take place during the course of dystrophy include a waddling gait, lordosis and scoliosis (curvature of spinal column), and winged scapulae or shoulder-blades. In more advanced cases, contractures of the leg muscles force the person with muscular dystrophy to walk on his toes (pes equinus). Extreme weakness of the arms prevents the afflicted person from raising them above shoulder level. Eventually, all the voluntary muscles of the body are affected and the victim is bedridden. While Muscular Dystrophy itself is not fatal, the weakness it causes makes even a trifling intercurrent illness dangerous.

The four main types of Muscular Dystrophy are:

A — PSEUDOHYPERTROPHIC TYPE — the most prevalent form. It commences in childhood between the ages of three and ten; its course is more rapid than in any other type. It is hereditary in 35 percent of all cases. It affects three times as many males as it does females.

B — JUVENILE FORM — has its onset in childhood or adolescence. Its progression is slower, and patients may reach middle age. This form is hereditary. Males and females are equally affected.

C — FACIO-SCAPULO-HUMERAL FORM — Afflicts young adults and attacks the facial muscles, shoulders and upper arms.

D — MIXED TYPES — a group of conditions with onset between the ages of 30 and 50. Not inherited, they can strike anyone. The course of the disease is rapid, often causing death in from five to ten years.

A cure for Muscular Dystrophy has yet to be found. Research has indicated the cause of the disease may be allied with faulty metabolism of the muscles,

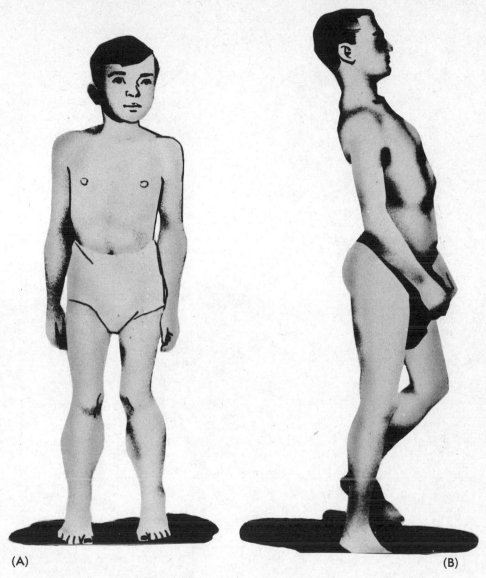

(A)

(B)

(A) The picture of the pseudohypertrophic form of muscular dystrophy is characteristic, especially the contrast between the thin
thighs and the enlarged calves. In pseudohypertrophic muscular
dystrophy there is wasting of some muscles and enlargement
of others.

(B) The rolling, waddling gait is typical—with curvature of the
spine and protuberance of the abdomen. Often the patient walks
on his toes with feet turned inward.

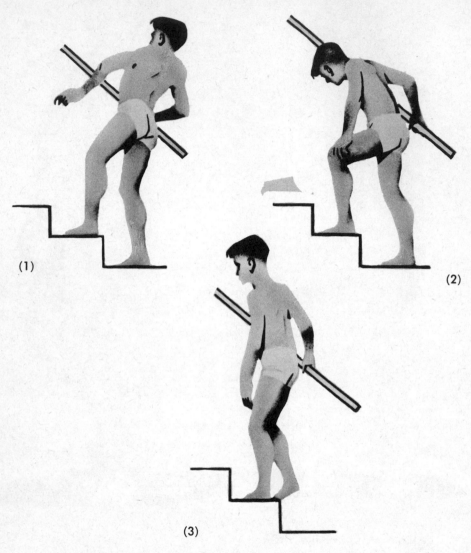

(1)

(2)

(3)

(C) Difficulty in climbing stairs may be one of the early symptoms of muscular dystrophy. (1) The railing is grasped for support and used to pull the body up. The leg is lifted by tilting the body, and using all possible muscles. (2) The leverage afforded by placing the hand on the knee assists in lifting the body and dragging up the other leg. (3) The ascent is made one step at a time, one foot does not pass the other.

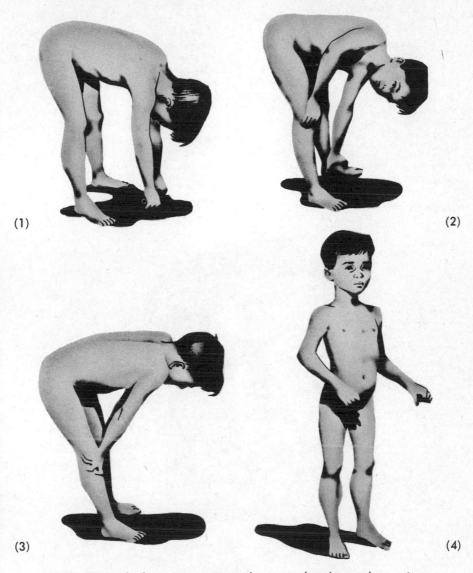

(1)

(2)

(3)

(4)

(D) (1) To reach the erect position the muscular dystrophy patient must extend the knees and gradually move the hands toward the feet. (2) Using the support of the floor as long as possible, the hands are brought to the lower extremities. (3) The hands are alternately moved up the thighs, erecting the body. (4) With the assistance of many accessory muscles the erect position is finally reached.

related to their inability to utilize vitamin E.

Since a specific treatment is not available for the cure of this disease, supporting treatment consists of physical therapy exercises, self-help and physical activity to be engaged in by the patient while he still has the use of his muscles, as inactivity hastens wasting.

The Muscular Dystrophy Associations of America, Inc., founded in 1950 devotes itself to research into the cause and cure of MD, and provides certain services for the estimated 200 000 victims of this disease in the United States.

In muscular dystrophy the muscles become progressively weak, the person affected becomes depressed and loses his appetite. Various attempts to control muscular dystrophy particularly with changes in diet to a one high in amino acids with extra folic acid and vitamin B_{12} have seemed to result in success but two recently controlled studies have established that this method was a complete failure. One trial on 42 patients and another on 33 failed to bring about any appreciable gain in strength, ability to work or to rise from a sitting or lying position.

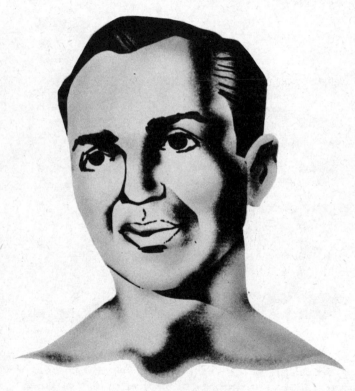

(E) The involvement of the facial muscles with prominence of the lips (tapir type). Weakness and asymmetry in smiling, and inability to whistle are characteristic of the facioscapulohumeral form of muscular dystrophy.

MUSTARD PLASTERS Mustard plasters are used as counterirritants with a view to drawing blood to the area where the mustard plaster is applied. They can be so strong that they will blister the skin. They should be milder for women and children than for men. Mustard plasters should not be left on for more than from fifteen to thirty minutes.

MUSTARD PLASTERS—dermatitis caused by: See SKIN, article THE SKIN.

MYASTHENIA GRAVIS Myas- thenia gravis is a condition in which there is progressive weakness. Previously it had been shown that neostigmine was specific in recovery from this condition. A new drug has been named Win-8077 and is called mysuram chloride. This is what is called an anticholinesterase preparation and is stronger than neo- stigmine. The drug can be taken by mouth. In certain instances the use of drugs in myasthenia results in further weakness and the doctor must detect the extent to which the drug is responsible beyond what is produced by the disease itself.

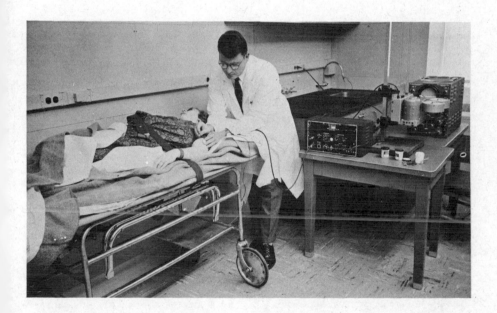

Myasthenia gravis is a weakness of the muscles, usually starting in the face and throat. The disease causes a breakdown of muscular coordination. Here, an investigator is conducting elec- tro-physiological studies to determine whether the site of the pathology lies in the nerve or the muscle.

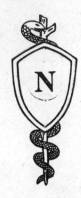

NARCOLEPSY Among the strange conditions that afflict human beings is narcolepsy, in which recurring attacks of sleep come on suddenly; in a number of cases sleep is continuous. Incidentally, there may be associated with this a condition in which the muscles of the body suddenly seem to lose their strength, so that the knees give way and the person falls to the ground without loss of consciousness. This is called tonelessness.

Cases of narcolepsy have been known to develop following serious injury to the head; some cases have been associated with tumors involving certain portions of the brain; some instances are known in which excessive sleepiness or ease of falling asleep was part of a purely mental condition.

Usually the person who has this condition is not what we would call dynamic—not one of those persons who simply overflows with energy. The person with narcolepsy has a sleepy look on his face and is disinclined to move around much. He will keep awake while working at something that interests him, but when left alone or when lying on a bed, he quickly falls asleep. Sometimes these people fall asleep while standing in a streetcar. One such person fell asleep while walking on the street and wakened only when he stepped off the curb. In most instances, however, the person is likely to fall asleep gradually while sitting. Sometimes these cases are associated also with a condition called bulimia, which means a morbid hunger.

The sudden weakness of the muscles that has been described is often associated with some emotion, such as amusement, laughter, anger, or fright. A woman, aged forty-four, had a tendency to fall asleep in church and at social gatherings but the condition became really serious when she fell asleep while standing at the cookstove.

Fortunately few people die of narcolepsy unless as a result of an accident.

It has been found that a remedy called ephedrine sulfate will help to prevent these attacks of sleep. More recently the product called amphetamine or benzedrine has also been found useful in controlling this condition. These remedies are powerful drugs and should never be used unless prescribed by a doctor, who will determine whether the product is to be used, the amount to be taken daily or nightly, and other controls to prevent harm.

NARCOTIC ADDICTION Twenty years ago a survey made by the United States Public Health Service indicated to the experts that there were between 110,000 and 150,000 people in the United States who were addicted to various forms of opium. It was estimated a few years ago that there were between 35,000 and 50,000 addicts in the United States. Obviously all such figures are estimates, since secrecy is the very life of the opium trade.

Women seemed to be much more likely to become addicted to the drug than men. Indeed it was rather well established before the new narcotic laws were passed that about two women were addicted for every one man. The figures now seem to indicate that four men are addicted for every one woman. It is believed that women became addicted in the earlier days because they led a more secluded and sedentary life and that they treated themselves with drug preparations containing dope or opium for all sorts of real or imaginary ills. Once, however, the use of such remedies was brought under control, it was not easily possible for women to obtain drugs; naturally women are much more law-abiding than men and are not as likely to get into bad environments as men.

Investigators of the United States Public Health Service point out that women were treated and cured in great numbers following the passing of the narcotic laws and that thereafter women avoided illegal contacts with opium. Men were still able to make such contacts and thus became addicted to the drugs.

The person who takes drugs and becomes addicted to them does so because he is emotionally unstable and is unable to adjust himself to his environment. He feels restless, discontented, and inferior. The taking of a drug which breaks down his mental processes gives him a sense of ease, contentment, and confidence. This, of course, gives him pleasure.

Some people still become narcotic addicts because they develop serious and painful chronic illnesses in which they obtain relief from pain only through the use of strong drugs. The addiction to narcotic drugs is harmful because it breaks down character.

When the Harrison Narcotic Act was passed, it became apparent that people who were addicted to drugs had to be cared for. In 1929 a law was passed creating two narcotic farms which are now located in Lexington, Kentucky, and Fort Worth, Texas. In these places physicians are investigating the nature of narcotic addiction and are undertaking work to rehabilitate narcotic addicts who are admitted to the farms. The narcotic addict who may be committed to one of these farms is, of course, not free to go as he will, but he is treated as a patient and not as a prisoner.

The method of treatment usually followed is to withdraw the drug rapidly from the patient, taking care of his physical health in the meantime so that he will not suffer unduly or seriously. This process requires from ten days to two weeks, after which measures are begun leading to the rehabilitation of the patient from both the mental and physical points of view.

It is recognized also that there are addictions to marihuana and cocaine, but these addictions are believed to be more of a police problem than addiction to opium.

The number of narcotic addicts in the United States is estimated to be between 50,000 and 60,000. Almost 80% of addicts are men and half of all of them are between 21-30 years of age. More than three-fourths of addicts in the United States use heroin. The solution of the drug problem, according to the Commissioner of Narcotics, lies in co-ordination of the efforts of narcotic enforcement agencies with provisions for medical care in hospitals especially equipped and staffed by psychiatric, occupational and recreational experts.

NASAL DISORDER (See also discussion under *Ozena* and *Vitamins*) Ozena (a nose disease associated with dryness, crusting, and a fetid discharge) and other similar nose conditions are sometimes greatly improved by large doses of vitamin A. Such conditions are associated with damage to the mucous membrane that lines the nose. In clinics in Denmark and Germany, 35 patients with such nose conditions were treated with massive doses of vitamin A. Although 5,000 units daily is the amount considered necessary to prevent a vitamin-A deficiency, these patients were given 300,000 units 2 days a week by injection into the muscles, and 150,000 to 300,000 units orally the other 5 days of the week. Although a few patients failed to respond well, in the majority the mucous membranes became more normal; the crusting and odor disappeared. None of the patients revealed symptoms of poisoning from excess vitamin A.

NAUSEA See *Vomiting.*

NAVEL, DISEASES OF The navel is the scar that is left when the umbilical cord, by which the body of the child is attached to that of its mother before birth, is cut. The scientific name for the navel is the umbilicus. After the cord is cut, there is a gradual shrinkage of the excess tissue. Once the scar has healed, the navel needs little attention unless it becomes involved in an infection or some other disturbance.

The care of the navel in a newborn child is important. The cord must be tied off satisfactorily at a sufficient distance from the body. It is covered with a sterile dressing and it is watched carefully until it is healed. Exceedingly dangerous would be a secondary hemorrhage from the cord or an infection.

Some years ago a distinguished surgeon wrote a two-volume work on diseases of the umbilicus. Most of the conditions which might concern this tissue represent failures to heal satisfactorily, leaving an opening or a fistula or a possible rupture, so that the tissues of the abdomen protrude through the opening. Such conditions demand surgical attention. The surgeon repairs the failure to close by sewing and reconstructing the area.

Because the navel contains creases and folds, it demands attention as far as its cleanliness is concerned. Removal of accumulations of tissue debris or of soap should be a part of the regular hygiene of daily life.

The tissues of the navel are like those of the skin. They become subject to any disease that affects the skin. When there is an ulcer in the umbilicus, the same attention should be given to it as to an ulcer anywhere else. This means removal of infectious material and the application of suitable drugs to control the germs that may be present. Instances have been described in which the tissue around the umbilicus developed a blue appearance. This has been due to an accumulation of blood inside the abdomen following rupture of one of the fallopian tubes of a woman or from a hemorrhage or any other cause.

NECK, BROKEN "Broken back" and "broken neck" once meant almost certain death or a lingering disability. With the discovery of the X ray and with the extension of its use, breaks in the bones of the spine are now found to be exceedingly frequent. Studies of 200 consecutive cases in New York showed that the break in the bone of the spine in 117 cases occurred when the person fell from a height; 69 were struck by moving objects, including 31 automobiles; 2 people were thrown; and in 12 instances the cause of the break in the bone of the spine was not determined. In 35 of these 200 cases death occurred, not, however, because of the break in the bone of the spine but because there was an associated serious injury to the head or a secondary pneumonia and in some instances severe shock.

Fractures of the spine may occur in the upper region, in the middle, or, as frequently happens, at the bottom. Most of the serious breaks occur in the region around the neck. A broken neck is much more serious than a break in the bones of the spine lower down. Sometimes the injury to the spine may be so forceful that the bones are twisted away from each other, making a much more serious condition than a mere breaking of one of the portions of one of the bones. The most serious results follow when there is a break directly into the center of the spinal column with the occurrence of hemorrhage around the spinal cord. Serious also are cases in which the material of the spinal cord itself is seriously damaged, or, as occurs in some cases, completely cut through.

When the patient loses all sensation below the level at which the injury occurred and loses complete control of the ordinary actions of the bowels and of the bladder, the symptoms may be taken as an indication that there has been serious damage.

The earliest possible attention of a physician who can do everything possible to remove pressure and to aid restoration of the tissues to their normal positions may save life. First aid, if correct, may save a life. People with an injury to the spine must be moved only when lying on a flat board and with the minimum amount of manipulation. If the injury is in the region of the neck, some technic should be found to hold the neck absolutely still. The shock is treated by the usual methods of application of warmth and the use of proper remedies. For this, of course, a physician is necessary.

As soon as the condition of the person who has been injured warrants, an X-ray picture is taken to show exactly how much damage has occurred. Then the surgeon or orthopedic surgeon arranges the proper supports and braces to hold the tissues in proper position and the physician makes certain that the functions of the body are cared for during the process of recovery.

When the patient recovers, careful study must be made by a specialist in nervous and mental diseases to determine the extent of the damage that has been done and the possibilities for further treatment to bring about complete recovery.

NEPHRITIS Whenever a man goes for a physical examination in relation to taking out life insurance, being inducted into the Army, or playing football with a high school or college team, the examination is likely to include some simple tests of the urine to determine whether or not the urine contains albumin. The presence of albumin in the urine is abnormal; that is to say, most healthy men are free from this condition. The presence of albumin may on occasion be due to a purely temporary condition (for instance, doctors recognize today what is called emotional albuminuria), but in most instances the presence of albumin means that there has been an inflammation of the kidneys sufficient to cause protein to leak through from the blood into the urine or perhaps sufficient to destroy enough tissue of the kidney itself to cause such waste material to appear in the urine.

The word "nephritis" means simply inflammation of the kidney. However, it includes a number of conditions which may be acute or chronic, all of which are characterized by the appearance of albumin in the urine and, in addition, occasionally by the appearance of blood and of portions of kidney tissue. Nephritis is usually listed as fourth in the list of the causes of death and each year in the United States is responsible for the death of something over 100,000 people, or about 7 per cent of all deaths.

An acute inflammation of the kidneys is so serious that no one is likely to neglect it long. Associated with the disturbance of excretion of urine, there are swellings of the tissues, waterlogging of the circulation, and even enough poisoning of the body in general to cause convulsions or unconsciousness. Chronic inflammation of the kidneys includes a number of different forms depending on the part of the kidney that is involved. Failure of the kidneys to do their work throws much more work on the heart.

For many years chronic inflammation of the kidneys has been known as Bright's disease. It was named after a famous London doctor, Richard Bright, who first demonstrated the association of swelling of the human body due to accumulation of water in the tissues and the presence in the urine of a substance which coagulated when the urine was boiled. These observations were presented to the medical profession in 1827, and Bright's name has been attached to this group of disorders since that time.

The kidneys—to make their nature clear—are two kidney-shaped masses which lie high up in the abdominal region behind the stomach, attached near the spine. Each of them includes millions of tiny grapelike masses of specialized blood vessels called glomeruli. Each little clump empties into a funnellike structure leading to a small coiled tube, and all of these tubes finally empty into a larger collecting space called the pelvis of the kidney. The urine is formed in these grapelike masses. It escapes from the clump of blood vessels through a small funnel that is only one seventh the size of the tube by which the blood entered the glomerulus. The action of the glomerulus is to squeeze out the fluid, like a wine press, so that the waste matter passes out of the body in the urine and the filtered liquid goes back into the blood. The amount of work done by this machinery can be realized from the fact that it handles about 150 quarts a day. Since there are something over 6 quarts of blood in the body, it will be realized that the blood goes round and round, being relieved on each passage through the kidney of the material to be passed out of the body.

Whenever there is an infection elsewhere in the body, the possibility exists that the poisons or germs may be carried into the kidney and set up some trouble in the kidney tissue. This would be called acute nephritis. The poisons that can set up an acute inflammation of the kidney are not always germ poisons, since it is known that poisonous metals and other toxic substances can produce this result. Whenever there is a suspicion that an inflammation of the kidney is present, an immediate examination of the urine should be made. When the urine is heated, the albumin, if present, will coagulate as a solid clot, much like the white part of a boiled egg. When strong acid is added to the urine, the albumin will coagulate. There are, of course, quantitative tests which will show about how much albumin is present in the urine.

The conditions which are likely to cause suspicion would include persistent headache, mental depression, and fatigue. The skin will develop a pale or pasty appearance. There may be puffiness and swelling under the eyes, on the backs of the hands, and around the feet. As the condition progresses, the blood pressure may be raised. The swellings due to accumulation of fluid may become enormous, so that even the abdomen and the space around the lungs and heart become filled and action of the organs impeded by the retained liquid. This may read like the text of some of the old almanacs which used to be freely circulated in selling somebody's kidney pills or kidney remedy. They usually showed a haggard individual, bent over, with his hand on the middle of his back. Usually the hand was not in a place anywhere near the place where the kidneys actually are. Most pain in the back is not due to disturbances of the kidneys. Enough people have symptoms like those that have been mentioned, however, to indicate that the presence of such symptoms should demand an immediate study of the urine.

When the urine of a person with inflammation of the kidneys is examined under the microscope, particularly after a fair amount of the urine has been caused to settle by the use of a centrifuge, the material will be found to contain not only some red blood cells but also molds which resemble casts of the tiny tubes of the kidney. Casts are of many different varieties, depending on the nature of the material that they contain. They are described variously as blood casts, hyaline casts, granular casts, and with other adjectives. In the presence of such kidney conditions the doctor can also learn a great deal by examination of the blood, since failure of the kidneys to function properly will produce chemical changes in the blood.

It used to be thought that acute Bright's disease was a fatal disorder. Now we know that this is far from the truth. It is the tendency of most cases to get well, given a reasonable opportunity. Indeed authorities say that about 90 per cent of all cases will recover completely if recognized early and if properly treated. In the remaining cases the disease tends to persist and eventually to pass over into what is called chronic nephritis. In the period between the acute inflammation of the kidney and the gradual change to the chronic form, there is an intermediary state that is sometimes called nephrosis. The urine in this form of kidney disease is usually decreased in amount, and the amount of albumin in the urine is considerable. The distinction between various stages of inflammation of the kidneys is difficult and depends largely on the experience of the doctor.

People with acute inflammation of the kidney are urged to go to bed and stay in bed until the kidneys function normally. They take a diet that is simple and nutritious, usually keeping the amount of salt and the amount of protein rather low in relation to the average diet. Indeed some physicians limit the patient with acute nephritis to milk and fruit juices for a few days. We know, however, that any fever or inflammation or infection tends to use up the protein of the body, and protein is required for repair of damaged tissue. Hence regulation of the protein in the diet is a delicate matter and one which is best left to the expert who is taking care of the patient. When there are signs of severe suppression of the flow of urine, many doctors choose to cause the patient to perspire freely so as to get some of the waste material out of the body.

There has been a popular belief that meat in any form is harmful to people with Bright's disease. If the blood shows a deficiency in protein, the amount of protein in the diet—and this means meat—may in most instances be increased.

Whenever there is swelling of the tissues due to accumulation of fluid, the intake and elimination of water from the body must be watched carefully. Such people are warned against taking excessive amounts of fluid, but some fluid is absolutely necessary for proper function of the tissues and particularly for the elimination of toxic waste materials. Among the most difficult conditions to overcome is accumulation of the fluid in the tissues. Sometimes the fluid around the eyes is so profuse that they may actually be swollen shut. Sometimes the legs swell so greatly as to make walking difficult if not impossible. If fluid collects in the brain in sufficient amounts, it will disturb thought and action. The diet and the elimination of the patient need to be watched particularly because many of these people will seem to be large, due to accumulation of fluid in the body, whereas actually they are undernourished and even emaciated. In the early stages the heart and blood vessels may not be affected, but later the damage to the heart and blood vessels may be so great that life is maintained with difficulty.

The competent doctor who is caring for a patient with inflammation of the kidneys will make studies of the blood, as has already been mentioned, and will frequently examine the urine and also test the functional ability of the kidney to determine whether or not it is doing its work satisfactorily. Repeated examinations will be made to determine whether or not the condition is getting better or worse. Any diet or fluids taken by the patient will be regulated by the results of the functional tests and in fact may serve to some extent themselves as a means of testing the ability of the kidney to work.

Nephritis is so variable as it occurs in different people that it is simply impossible to say in any given case what the rate of progress is likely to be. Since control of the disease depends on constant observation of its progress, everyone who has had albumin in the urine should have at least one annual survey, including study of the urine and the blood and functional tests of the various vital organs of the body.

BRIGHT'S DISEASE—See KIDNEY, article THE KIDNEY: ITS DISEASES AND DISTURBANCES.

BRIGHT'S DISEASE—defined: See KIDNEY, article THE KIDNEY: ITS DISEASES AND DISTURBANCES.

BRIGHT'S DISEASE—diarrhea caused by: See article DIGESTION AND DIGESTIVE DISEASES.

BRIGHT'S DISEASE—example of renal albuminuria: See KIDNEY, article THE KIDNEY: ITS DISEASES AND DISTURBANCES.

BRIGHT'S DISEASE—term 125 years old: See KIDNEY, article THE KIDNEY: ITS DISEASES AND DISTURBANCES.

NEPHRITIS—aims in treatment: See KIDNEY, article THE KIDNEY: ITS DISEASES AND DISTURBANCES.

NEPHRITIS—benign, postural, and other forms of functional albuminuria confused with: See KIDNEY, article THE KIDNEY: ITS DISEASES AND DISTURBANCES.

NEPHRITIS—calculosa: See entry CALCULI.

NEPHRITIS—causes: See KIDNEY, article THE KIDNEY: ITS DISEASES AND DISTURBANCES.

NEPHRITIS—death rate (fig.): See HEART, article DISEASES OF THE HEART AND CIRCULATION.

NEPHRITIS—formaldehyde vapors may cause: See article OCCUPATION AND HEALTH.

NEPHRITIS—gouty: See KIDNEY, article THE KIDNEY: ITS DISEASES AND DISTURBANCES.

NEPHRITIS—hypertension caused by: See article BLOOD PRESSURE.

NEPHRITIS—hypertension difficult to treat: See article BLOOD PRESSURE.

NEPHRITIS—meaning: See KIDNEY, article THE KIDNEY: ITS DISEASES AND DISTURBANCES.

NEPHRITIS—methyl alcohol may cause: See article OCCUPATION AND HEALTH.

NEPHRITIS—pregnancy: See BIRTH, article CARE OF MOTHERS BEFORE AND AFTER CHILDBIRTH.

NEPHRITIS—scarlatinal: See KIDNEY, article THE KIDNEY: ITS DISEASES AND DISTURBANCES.

NEPHRITIS—uremia: See KIDNEY, article THE KIDNEY: ITS DISEASES AND DISTURBANCES.

NEPHRITIS—urinary protein consists mostly of serum albumin and globulin: See KIDNEY, article THE KIDNEY: ITS DISEASES AND DISTURBANCES.

NERVE INJURY Injuries of nerves are also responding to new methods whereas formerly not much could be done. Nerve injuries may be caused by wounds, by cuts, by compression, by injections or by tearing or by various methods which stop the flow of blood to the nerve. Long periods of time may be required before the healing of injuries to the nerves. When nerves are injured, surgical operation may disclose a possibility of sewing together portions that have become separated. Important in treatment of nerve injuries is physical therapy including massage, passive movements and exercises, the use of splints to prevent the stretching of paralyzed muscles and stimulation of the nerves by electricity to help recover their action.

NERVOUS AND CONVULSIVE CHILDHOOD DISORDERS

NERVOUS AND CONVULSIVE CHILDHOOD DISORDERS (See also *Child Care, Chorea, Epilepsy*) Infants and young children seem to be more liable to convulsive disorders than are adults. Indeed the nervous system of the child reacts to infections and intoxications with an instability of the nervous system that is quite different from that seen in older people. The exact cause for this is not well understood. By actual tests the nervous system of the child is less sensitive than that of the adult. The response to irritation of the nervous system is least at the time of birth and increases until maturity.

Regardless of the cause of the convulsions or the mechanisms by which they are produced, parents confronted with twitching or spasms in a young child are likely to become greatly alarmed; certainly they cannot be blamed for it. The best advice is to report to the doctor the appearance of any convulsions, twitchings of the hands or feet or spasms or, in fact, anything that seems to be different from the ordinary behavior of the infant.

For many years people have been told that the best way to quiet a baby in spasm or convulsions is to put it in a hot bath. This is one of the most popular home remedies. However, doctors report any number of serious accidents from this self-treatment, principally because people confronted by convulsions in a child are likely to lose all sense of balance and judgment. They are anxious to get the water hot and to get the child into it so that children have been scarred or maimed out of someone's anxiety to stop a convulsion. Actually the convulsion itself is far less dangerous than the panic-stricken activities of those who are anxious to help.

The causes contributory to convulsions may include the irritations of the nervous system resulting from fever, from serious infections or from intoxications by waste products of the body. Sometimes even a mild inflammatory reaction in the bowels or the kidneys may be responsible for a convulsion. Convulsions have occurred in children with whooping cough simply because they were entirely out of breath from long-continued coughing and as a result were partially asphyxiated. In cases of inflammation of the kidney the waste products fail to be excreted from the body; their accumulation in the tissues may result in a convulsion.

We have learned from studies on people with diabetes that changes in the level of the sugar in the blood may be associated with convulsive reactions. Whenever the sugar in the blood passes a certain critical low level, convulsions occur exactly as they may occur in people who takes overdoses of insulin.

Another common superstition is the belief that teething and worms are the causes of convulsions in children. Actually, teething in itself is seldom sufficiently severe to arouse a convulsive disorder in a normal child. If, however, there has been a deficiency of calcium in the diet resulting in the condition called tetany, which is a spasmodic disorder of infants, any painful, continuous irritant may arouse a convulsion. As far as is known, worms are themselves not related to the cause of convulsions, but the severe diarrheas with loss of fluid from the body or the constant irritation in the bowel associated with the presence of worms may be a stimulus to a convulsion.

While it is true that convulsions may be preceded by restlessness and slight twitchings of the muscles of the face, hands, feet or eyelids, parents should not scan the child's face constantly for the presence of twitchings or be greatly disturbed by ordinary restlessness. In the true convulsion the twitching is definite, and sometimes the entire body shakes as in a severe chill. The muscles of the face may contract, the head be thrown back, the hands clenched with the thumbs buried in the palms. The child may lose consciousness for from one to three minutes, and breathing may be shallow. Since asphyxia is a frequent associate of a convulsion, the face may appear blue, especially around the lips. Because of the inability to control the tissues of the body, rattling sounds may be heard in the throat. Parents should remember, however, that convulsions terminating fatally are rare. A convulsion itself seldom is a cause of death. True, there have been instances in which the asphyxia or loss of oxygen from the body in long continued convulsions has resulted fatally, but these are exceedingly unusual.

WHAT TO DO BEFORE THE DOCTOR COMES—Since the convulsions rarely lasts longer than two or three minutes, it is usually over by the time someone has filled a tub with hot water, made sure of the temperature, removed the clothing from the child and transported the child to the bathroom. Modern physicians, therefore, deprecate the idea of controlling convulsions by putting the child in a tub of hot water. Until the doctor arrives, the child may be placed in a warm bed, and if the child has a fever, an ice cap may be applied to the head. Parents should not try to quiet the convulsion by giving the child drugs of any kind because these may interfere with the study of the condition that the doctor will want to make.

The doctor should be called immediately so that he can see the child as soon as possible after the convulsion and determine, if possible, its cause and then decide the method of treatment. If the cause of the convulsions is seriously in doubt, the physician will want to make studies of the blood or want to take a specimen of the spinal fluid for examination; he will measure the blood pressure and study the condition of the tissues back of the eye. He will want a specimen of the child's urine so as to determine the presence of albumin—an indication of inflammation of the kidneys—or of blood or of pus. As has been stated, he may wish to determine the level of sugar in the blood. In exceedingly difficult cases he will wish perhaps to have an X ray picture made of the spine and of the skull and perhaps also a tracing of the areas of excitation in the brain such as can be secured with the electro-encephalograph.

In many instances a child who has had a convulsion at the beginning of an infectious disease or in association with whooping cough may never have another similar attack. If, however, convulsions are prolonged and if they occur again and again, the condition demands the most careful study so that the proper procedures may be applied.

CHOREA One of the disorders seen in children in which there may be twitching of the muscles of the body is called chorea and is better known as St. Vitus' dance. Nowadays this condition is believed to be due to infection by a germ of the streptococcus type. Girls have St. Vitus' dance about two and one-half times as often as do boys and more than 80 per cent of all of the cases occur during early childhood. A person who has St. Vitus' dance makes involuntary muscular jerks and twitches, and when the twitching affects the muscles of the face, it is of course more noticeable.

The child with chorea needs to be studied particularly with relation to the nature of the infection because chorea may be associated with rheumatic conditions and even with the serious condition affecting the heart called rheumatic fever.

TETANY—Tetany should not be confused with the word *tetanus,* which is lockjaw. Tetanus is caused by a germ. Tetany, on the other hand, is usually associated with a lack of calcium in the body and hence is frequently associated with rickets. Most parents now know that every child ought to have adequate amounts of calcium and vitamins A and D in order to prevent the bowing of the legs, the beading of the ribs and the pot belly and deficient growth of the bones that are characteristic of rickets.

We now know that the nervous system can be excessively irritable if there is a lack of calcium taken in and absorbed by the body. The characteristic symptom in tetany is spasm, with which there may be pain. Since the spasm may even affect the tissues of the throat, there may be associated asphyxia with blueness and secondary convulsions. Indeed convulsions are exceedingly common in the presence of tetany. Because of the irritability of the nervous system any stimulus, even a mild one, may bring on the convulsions.

The doctor can determine the presence of the condition by a careful examination, and proper treatment controls it. The symptoms of tetany can be prevented by the proper giving of calcium to the child. Nowadays the people have been so well educated about the necessity of preventing rickets by the use of adequate amounts of calcium and cod liver oil that tetany is seen much less often than it used to be observed by the doctors.

EPILEPSY—Epilepsy in all of its forms is a fairly common disease. Probably as many people in the United States have epilepsy as have diabetes or active tuberculosis. The word *epilepsy* comes from a Greek word that means seizure.

In the typical epileptic attack there is a temporary loss of consciousness, accompanied by muscular movements, which may include anything from the slight twitching of the eyelids to a violent shaking of the entire body. We do not know the exact cause of epilepsy. Apparently there is a tendency to development of a constitution of the body and the brain that is excessively irritable and particularly responding to certain stimuli. The response is an attack of a convulsive type such as has been mentioned.

A device called the electro-encephalograph is capable of measuring the irritability of the brain. The use of this device shows one person in every ten has some irregularity of the brain-wave pattern and about one in every 200 has seizures of the type of epilepsy. These seizures come when the irritation factor reaches a certain threshold. Mothers need not be unduly alarmed, therefore, if a young child has several convulsions. Seventy out of a thousand children have one or more convulsions during their first five years of life. That is because the nervous system of the infant and young child is much more irritable than that of the adult. Many people tend to acquire lessened irritability as they grow older so that only five out of every thousand grown-ups have convulsive symptoms.

Doctors recognize several varieties of epilepsy, from the very serious type known as grand mal to the minor seizures, which are called petit mal. Frequently these may involve only rhythmical twitchings of the eyelids, a sudden, slight loss of consciousness or the presence of temporary confusion. In the majority of cases these symptoms tend to disappear or to be relatively insignificant as the child grows older.

Parents should realize, however, that first aid for a person with epilepsy requires calmness and judgment. The ordinary mild petit mal attack does not require special attention. In the case of a severe convulsion of the grand mal type, the person who wants to help must make certain, first of all, that the epileptic does not injure himself during the attack. He should be allowed to lie on the floor and away from contact with furniture or machinery of any kind. A folded handkerchief placed between the back teeth on one side of the mouth will prevent the person in a convulsion from biting his tongue or breaking his front teeth. Above all, the parents or those who are taking care of a child in a convulsion should be calm because panic, tension or fear in an adult is readily transmitted to the sick child. Be sure to prevent the earnest doers of good from throwing buckets of water on a person in a convulsive attack, from pouring whiskey down the throat or from rushing the child to a hospital. Remember again that nothing is to be gained by plunging the child into a tub of hot water.

Fortunately modern medicine has developed a variety of useful drugs for lowering the threshold of irritation of the person who is subject to a convulsive disorder. We have learned that diets which are small in amount and properly chosen help to diminish the threshold of irritation and lessen the number of convulsive attacks. New drugs include not only a variety of barbituric acid derivatives but also dilantin and tridione, which have been described as capable of eliminating convulsions entirely in many cases of petit mal.

NERVOUS BREAKDOWN Nervous breakdown includes a wide range of mental disorders.

With the public interest in mental disturbances a whole new vocabulary of terms has come into common use. Some of these terms have vague meanings. The term "breaking point," which really has a physical meaning, has now been applied to the human mind. Other terms now applied to mental factors are stress, tension, pressure, weight, force, and impact. Even the specialist in disorders of the mind finds it difficult to define exactly what is meant by "nervous breakdown."

Often the person who has what is called a nervous breakdown has begun with emotional instability. Out of his lack of tolerance of a situation in which he finds himself, he begins to develop changes in the secretions of the stomach that may lead eventually to ulcers, difficulties in vision that may finally be called eye strain, or pains in different portions of the body that receive the classification of neuralgia.

What we call morale in a human being appears to be emotional stability. Many men who might break down when left to themselves are able to sustain their morale when they are in a large group through the influence of leadership. They break down when this protective influence is removed.

Not all men have a mental breakdown under severe stress. Some men seem to be able to stand almost any trial or disturbance. But even these men may eventually develop physical changes or organic diseases which alter their mental stability.

Nervous breakdown in children may result in refusal to go to school and similar infractions. These children are different from those who are simply truant and refuse to go to school out of what might be called "meanness." They are neurotic children, and their symptoms may involve the whole family.

Frequently they are depressed and often overly preoccupied with sex questions. The children refuse to obey orders; they become aggressive, which contrasts with their formerly timid behavior. The child who formerly went easily to school now clings to his home and may refuse to leave his mother. Usually if the child is allowed to remain at home the acute symptoms tend to lessen, but they appear again if attempts are made to force the child back to school. In several cases reported this impasse continued for months. Obviously a mother confronted with a problem of this kind in the home becomes anxious and depressed and soon is entirely unable to handle the child.

Truant children may steal and lie, but the neurotic child is of an entirely different character. The latter represents a case of mental difficulty and must be treated from that point of view. The neurotic child is in most instances above average intelligence but is also timid, sensitive, and dependent. Often he is the only child and has been spoiled by parents who have yielded to the child and favored him in every way. These children are finicky about their food. Usually their emotional disturbances are related to the mother.

Attempts to treat these cases have indicated that treatment is difficult and must often be carried on for a long time in order to secure satisfactory results. The complete co-operation of the parents is required. Sometimes the best first step is to remove the child from contact with the parents to a suitable hospital or home where study may be made and proper treatment administered. Thus the child is saved a great deal of anxiety and misery. Moreover, the treatment is much easier if the child is removed from the emotionally highcharged atmosphere of the home. When the child is away from home, he can go to school each day from the hospital and gradually become relieved of the causes of the excessive emotional reactions.

NERVOUS DISEASES (See also discussion under *Amnesia, Brain, Brain Concussion, Brain Hemorrhage, Brain*

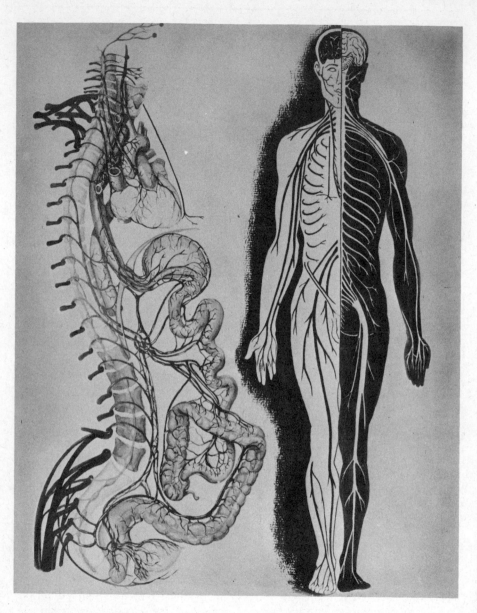

The nervous system is the body-coordinating system. Shown here are the nerves making up the peripheral system leading to the muscles, internal organs, and other parts of the body outside the brain and central nerve cord.

Tumor, Epilepsy, Meningitis, Nerve Injury, Paralysis Agitans, Shingles, Sympathetic Nervous System) In recent years, several conditions affecting the spinal cord and the nerves of the body which were formerly considered hopeless of benefit or treatment have yielded to medical science. Because of new approaches to the nervous system, these conditions have become controllable. The central nervous system is located in the cavity of the skull and in the spinal column. Thus the nervous tissues are protected by bony cases but the disadvantage lies in the fact that any disturbance is hard to get at because space is limited. Any growth, blood clot or abscess is constricted and the tissue damages are great whereas tissues of the abdomen for instance would not be damaged under similar circumstances because of the space available. The discovery of new devices like the electroencephalograph, contrast media which when used with the X ray make the tissues of the nervous system visible, radioactive isotopes which tend to localize in certain areas and new tests devised for use in the laboratory by the doctor directly on the patient have all tended to bring to light conditions affecting the nervous system which were formerly more difficult to understand. With these new improvements in diagnosis have come a number of drugs which have effects directly on portions of the nervous system and which are of the greatest significance in relieving diseases. Most conspicuous among symptoms brought about by damage to the nervous system are convulsions, inability to walk, changes in function of the limbs, the tongue, the eye and the special senses and particularly of speech.

Among the peculiar phenomenon related to speech may be the fact that a person is unable to name practically any object. Sometimes he can name the object as a whole but will have lost the ability to name parts of the object. People may develop an inability to read or an inability to write. They suddenly find that they are unable to add, subtract or multiply. In the course of his examination, the doctor discovers whether or not the patient can coordinate his movements, whether or not he has lost the strength from the muscles and, above all, whether or not some of the standard reflexes like the knee jerk or the bending of the big toe or similar responses to stimuli have become disordered. By such tests the doctor locates the area of the nerve or the portion of the spinal column that may have been involved.

Next come chemical tests of the spinal fluid and visualization of the contents of the spinal canal by introducing a substance like pantopaque which is a synthetic iodized oil that makes visible the spinal cord. Similarly examinations may be made with the X ray of portions of the brain.

The various X ray techniques are also valuable in distinguishing the presence in the spinal column and cord of displaced discs. The cartilages between the bones of the spine may be shoved out of position. By pressure on nerves, they produce severe symptoms and pain. Surgical operations can remove the disc and thus fully relieve all the symptoms.

NEURALGIA Pain in a nerve is called neuralgia. Neuralgia may, therefore, be facial neuralgia or sciatic neuralgia or dental neuralgia, depending on the nerve that is involved. In facial neuralgia there is a characteristic pain, stabbing and knifelike, which follows the course of one of the chief nerves which is known as the fifth or trigeminal nerve. This nerve spreads over the face, coming from a spot over the ear. In facial neuralgia the nerve may be so sensitive that even a cold current blowing on the face, or the light touch of a finger or feather to the face, may cause this stabbing pain to pass through the nerve.

Dental neuralgia usually begins with the decay of a tooth or an inflammation of the pulp cavity. At first the tooth is painful but soon the pain will spread from the tooth along the upper or lower jaw but not across the mid-line to the other side.

The typical pain of neuralgia of the facial nerve is called tic douloureux or trifacial neuralgia. This condition occurs usually in people around middle life and most often in those above fifty. Women are more frequently affected than men.

The exact cause of neuralgia has never been determined. Occasionally the condition may be controlled by using inhalations of a drug called trichlorethylene. However, the relief obtained by this method tends to wear off. Alcohol has been injected directly into the nerve area, and this technic gives relief for a certain length of time. It has been suggested that in certain instances the administration of large doses of thiamin has been helpful, these being given by injection, but again it has not been established with certainty that this produces long-continued relief or will prevent the condition.

In the very severe cases of neuralgia it is customary to do a surgical operation which destroys the nerve roots along which the sensation of pain is carried.

Whenever neuralgia affects any nerve, it is customary for the physician first to determine the nerve area involved and then to see what can be done to prevent the passing of the sensation of pain along that nerve. For this purpose sedative drugs are used, local anesthetic substances are injected into the nerve area, alcohol has been injected with a view to destroying the nerve, and X rays have been used, as well as similar technics.

There are instances, of course, in which the sensations of pain limited to certain nerve areas are more mental than physical. That makes such neuralgias a special problem in diagnosis for the doctor.

NEURALGIA—herpes zoster causes: See SKIN, article THE SKIN.

NEURALGIA—pain relievers: See MEDICINE CHEST, article THE FAMILY MEDICINE CHEST.

NEURITIS Any inflammation of the nerves is called a neuritis. The condition appears with pain and tenderness over an area supplied by the nerve. Sometimes there is loss of feeling or disturbances of sensation; sometimes paralysis, so that it is impossible to move a part supplied by the nerve. There are many different causes of neuritis, including alcohol, infections with germs like the diphtheria germ, or infections by malaria, which would supply the diagnosis of alcoholic, diphtheric, or malarial neuritis. When neuritis occurs in diabetes or rheumatism, the condition is known as diabetic or rheumatic neuritis. If more than one nerve is affected, it might be called multiple neuritis. Obviously the treatment of the condition depends on determining the cause and directing the treatment toward the cause. For relief sedative drugs may be used, fixation of the tissues to prevent movement, the application of heat, and other specific measures which the doctor prescribes.

PERIPHERAL NEURITIS—Peripheral neuritis is a condition in which there is inflammation of the nerves that extend from the spine toward the surface of the body. Sometimes peripheral neuritis follows a deficiency of vitamin B_0 or pyridoxine.

NEURITIS—diabetes: See article DIABETES.

NEURITIS—pain relievers: See MEDI-CINE CHEST, article THE FAMILY MEDI-CINE CHEST.

NEURITIS—pregnancy: See BIRTH, article CARE OF MOTHERS BEFORE AND AFTER CHILDBIRTH.

NEUROSIS Any functional disorder of the nervous system is known as a neurosis in contrast to a neuritis, which is an actual inflammation of the tissues. Because a neurosis is more likely to be mental than physical, it is sometimes called a psychoneurosis. A neurosis is sometimes related to certain tissues of the body, so that it can be called a cardiac neurosis as related to the heart, a gastric neurosis as related to the stomach, or a sexual neurosis when it involves the sex functions. Sometimes the neurosis is described in terms of the mental side, such as an anxiety neurosis, in which there are abnormal fears, or a compulsion neurosis, in which the person feels absolutely compelled to say or do certain things. A neurosis may be related to the occupation or profession, in which it is called a professional or occupational neurosis, or to a condition that causes anxiety, such as a war. This gives us the term "war neurosis."

Recent experiments have shown that people in a state of anxiety characteristically excrete in their urine excess amounts of hippuric acid. This suggests that neurotic persons, and those who suffer excessively from anxiety, can be distinguished from other persons by determining whether they have excessive excretion of hippuric acid at a time when there is no objective reason for anxiety. The presence of excess hippuric acid in the urine may also help identify persons who have a tendency to become neurotic.

NEUROSIS— See also entries EMOTIONS AND MENTAL DISEASE.

NEUROSIS—digestive troubles mistaken for: See article DIGESTION AND DIGESTIVE DISEASES.

NICOTINIC ACID DEFICIENCY (See also, *Vitamins*) The chief symptoms of pellagra, which is associated with a deficiency of niacin or nicotinic acid, include a red inflammation of the skin, a burning red tongue and mouth, diarrhea, and in late stages some mental disturbance. Many people in backward areas of the United States live on diets consisting largely of corn meal, fat meat and molasses. The meat is usually salt pork or side meat. The chief deficiency in such diets is the lack of animal protein such as milk, cheese, lean meat, and eggs, and the failure of the diet in leafy green vegetables. Apparently exposure to sunlight of a person who is deficient in niacin brings out the symptoms.

Almost 7000 people died of pellagra in the United States in 1928. By 1946 the educational campaign on proper nutrition had been so effective that only 804 deaths were reported.

While few cases of the complete development of pellagra are seen nowadays, there may be many instances of beginning symptoms or what doctors call a subacute condition. First come such symptoms as fatigue and loss of appetite. Then following exposure to the sun, the burning and stinging of the skin appears and next the soreness of the mouth and tongue. With these symptoms the patient is nervous, irritable, and finds difficulty in sleeping.

Since the condition is a deficiency disease, the treatment is primarily the taking of adequate amounts of niacin which is now available in several forms. If the condition is severe the doctor will inject the niacin rather than give it by mouth. The diet can be provided with the important niacin containing foods. The doctor will look after the patient's skin condition and make sure that he

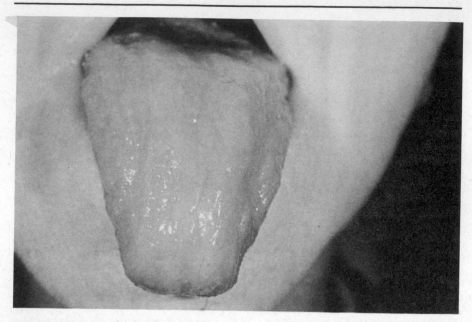

Acute glossitis with atrophy of lingual papillae associated with nicotinic acid deficiency. The gingivae, cheeks, lips, and tongue are fiery red in color, and a great deal of pain may be present. Ulcerations develop along the lateral margins of the tongue where it comes in contact with the teeth.

Chas. Pfizer & Co. Inc.

gets proper nursing care during the severe symptoms of the disease. Some physicians give large doses of liver extract. With proper treatment patients improve rapidly.

NIGHT CRAMPS (See also discussion under *Calcium, Muscle Cramps, Varicose Veins*) Seventy percent of people over 50 years old have occasional cramps of the legs at night. The pain is usually associated with a sudden contraction and hardening of the muscles of the calf of the leg. Stretching the leg, rubbing the calf or pressing the foot against the floor seems to bring relief. In any event, the severe pain leaves in about a minute, leaving some tenderness or soreness. The symptom may occur in people without evidence of any disease although it may be associated with hardening of the arteries, varicose veins or diabetes and occasionally with insufficient salt in the diet. In prevention and treatment of this condition quinine has been found valuable. A new drug that produces relaxation of muscles is Mephenesin. People with varicose veins benefit by keeping the legs elevated on a pillow or by raising the foot of the bed eight or nine inches. Another report says that calcium when prescribed prevented the cramps.

NIGHT EATING SYNDROME (See also discussion under *Appetite, Emotions, Hygiene, Personal, Obesity, Overeating, Weight, Over- and Under-*)

Psychosomatic studies on 25 obese women in the New York Hospital and Cornell Medical Center gave rise to defining a new type of case of exceedingly fat people which the authors describe as "the night eating syndrome." These people eat large amounts of food during the evening and night, whereas the food intake of people who are not too fat is negligible during the evening and night. With this comes insomnia and a loss of appetite in the morning with a small food intake at breakfast. The physicians feel that this type of obesity is not a result of overeating but rather represents response to stress of a type peculiar to certain obese patients and that it is intimately related to the overeating that leads to their obesity. They conclude that people with obesity due to emotional disturbances should not be put on rigid diets because it will be difficult for them to lose weight and they may attempt weight reduction only at a risk far outweighing the benefits to be derived.

NIGHT TERRORS If it were not for adults, babies would never be afraid, because they would not know the difference between what is dangerous and what is not dangerous. Babies become frightened because older people frighten them. They tell the baby about the "boogeyman" and teach babies to fear the policeman and the doctor and most of the other people on whom they must really depend for protection and health.

Apparently a baby may be born with a fear of a loud, sudden noise and a fear of falling. Those things we call instinctive. The baby learns to be afraid, however, of many things by seeing his parents suddenly draw back in fright. Babies learn from their parents to be afraid of thunder and lightning. A baby can be made afraid of his nursing bottle or his mother's breast if something that burns or tastes bitter happens to come to the baby in that connection.

Certain fears are so completely abnormal that they are reflected in the child's dreams and sleep. These are recognized in medicine under the name of night terror or by the Latin words *pavor nocturnis,* which means the same thing. These night terrors are usually a remnant of something that has happened during the day. The parents are likely to attribute them to something that the baby ate that he should not have eaten or to overstimulation by the radio or moving picture. Scientific investigation by child mental specialists, however, reveals that in most instances these night terrors occur in children whose parents are overanxious and excessively affectionate and also in those who are constantly being threatened with damage or mutilation by parents or nursemaids who know no other way in which to discipline a child.

A common source of the development of night terrors is the threat that the child's hands or his organs will be cut off because the parent or nursemaid is displeased with something the child was doing. Sudden attacks at night in which a child awakens screaming are occasionally associated with nervous disorders, which in turn are precipitated by similar unfortunate experiences.

From time to time the conditions have been blamed on adenoids, worms, or various infectious diseases. Occasionally the child screams at night because he is having a dream that he is being threatened or pursued. In some cases children who have sick headaches are likely to waken screaming at night. Since these headaches have been shown to be due occasionally to sensitivity to various protein substances, that type of investigation should be made so that that kind of stimulus can be avoided if it can be determined. Obviously, however, prevention by education of parents as to the proper attitudes toward the child and by the control of such physical defects as can be found is the ideal way to get rid of night terrors in children.

NOISE Unnecessary noise is a health hazard. The nervous reaction that follows exposure to noise is called echeosis.

Certain sounds are painfully loud and are therefore harmful to the ear or the brain or both. Rhythmical sound has the effect of preventing or postponing fatigue, as for example in soldiers who are marching. Sounds that are not rhythmical may startle, disturb, or irritate.

While the healthy man can stand the ordinary noises of the streets, including even unexpected blowing of motor horns, a hypersensitive man will suffer greatly from such disturbances. In cases of pneumonia infection, heart disease accompanied by insomnia, and in the case of people who are weakened after surgical operations, noise may be a serious menace. For this reason most cities provide for zones of quiet around hospitals and sanitariums.

Experiments have been conducted to determine the results of constant impinging of sound on the nerves. The investigators report that the noise raises the blood pressure and that a degree of noise sufficient to awaken a sleeping person will cause the muscles to contract and remain tense for as long as thirty minutes before they relax.

It has been shown that hardness of hearing, dizziness, and headaches may develop in persons who earn their living in noisy places. It is said that it requires 19 per cent more energy to perform a duty in noisy surroundings than to perform the same duty in a quiet environment. A healthy person can adapt himself to all sorts of peculiar disturbances but invariably adaptation

brings about some wear and tear on the nervous system.

Fortunately various methods have been developed for diminishing noise, and modern society recognizes noise as an unnecessary nuisance. For those who are especially sensitive to noise, rubber ear stoppers or defenders serve to reduce the noise or to shut it out. Much better, however, is the prevention of unnecessary noises by careful study to determine the causes and by the elimination of every source of noise that can be eliminated.

Noise Tolerance—See article Occupation and Health.

NOSE The nose is composed of small bones and cartilages and soft tissues which surround two cavities. Also directly related to the nose are the nasal sinuses.

Most important in the nose from the point of view of health and disease is its mucous membrane, or lining. The mucous membrane of the nose is one of the most sensitive tissues in the body. When it is bruised or hurt in any way, when it becomes infected, the response is prompt and the effect on the general health of the body may be serious.

Minor infections occur particularly in the hair follicles or in the roots of the hairs in the nose. The purpose of these hairs is to filter out dust or infectious material which comes into the nose with the air. Such germs as the streptococcus, the virus of influenza, and similar organisms are widespread. Many germs float in the air. When they get into a tissue which has in any way been damaged or of which the resistance has been lessened, they may set up an infection which eventually may spread throughout the body. The pernicious habit of pulling hairs out of the nose, squeezing pimples, or picking crusts is often the first step in injury leading to secondary infection.

An infection in the lining of the nose manifests itself by redness, swelling, discomfort, and pain, which increases steadily. If the swelling is sufficiently great, the outer aspect of the nose becomes swollen, and the swelling may extend even up to the eyelids. Whenever there is a swelling in the nose, a physician should inspect the area to determine the presence or absence of infection and to provide for a release of infected material so as to obviate the danger of a generalized infection.

The right way to take care of the nose is to remove carefully, by proper use of the handkerchief, such materials as can be reached easily. Those which cannot be reached may be washed out by the use of a mild spray without pressure. There are now generally available all sorts of sprays and materials which can be sprayed into the nose safely. Under no circumstances should materials be put in the nose under high pressure. This applies particularly to oils of various kinds, since it has been found that such oils may get into the lungs, and on occasion pneumonia has resulted from such procedures.

NOSEBLEED When serious hemorrhage occurs from the nose, the patient should be put flat on the back. Cold may be applied. If the bleeding persists, sterile gauze packs may be used to make pressure.

FOREIGN BODIES IN THE NOSE—Children, particularly infants, are likely to put into their mouths almost anything they happen to pick up. Occasionally also they push things into the nose. A substance of fairly small size taken into the mouth is not likely to be harmful, providing it is clean, even after it is swallowed. The digestive passages are big enough in most instances to let it pass through. Usually after eighteen to twenty-four hours the foreign materials will have disappeared from the body.

The breathing passages are much smaller than the digestive tube. Moreover, the breathing passages are curved and their walls are rigid. A substance forced into the nose is likely to remain there and serve as an obstacle which blocks the passage of air. Even more serious, however, is the fact that it will block the outflow of secretions.

Buttons, beans, pieces of chalk, or erasers that have from time to time been pushed into the nose get lodged there. Occasionally they are inhaled and get into the windpipe. Then an exceedingly serious condition develops.

The continuous presence of a foreign substance in the nose results eventually in the damming back of secretions and in the development of secondary infection. Soon there is a bad odor, a secondary swelling, and danger to life itself.

A doctor can utilize some of the special instruments that he has available and get a foreign substance out of the nose without very much trouble. The great danger of trying to get out a hard object like a button or piece of chalk is the damage to the tissues that results from manipulation. In many cases it is necessary to give the child an anesthetic to prevent jerking and moving of the head or interference by the hands and arms.

When a foreign substance is inhaled into the tube that leads to the lungs or into the lung itself, it is an immediate menace to life. Under such circumstances there must be no delay. An X-ray picture is taken as soon as possible, which aids the doctor in localizing the foreign substance. Special instruments have been developed which permit the placing of a tube down into the lung, and forceps and similar devices have been developed by which a foreign

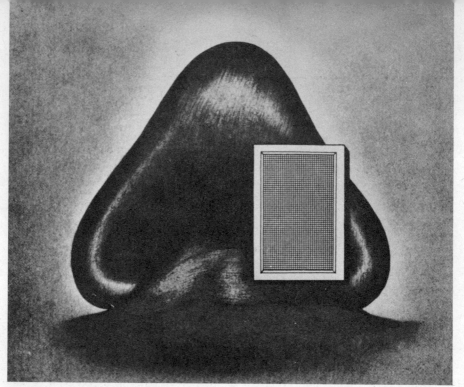

(A)

(A) One of the functions of the nose is the removal from the air that is breathed; of dust, pollens, insects, germs which flow on fluid, or other impurities. Within the nostrils are found hairs which help this screening process. These hairs also carry away the mucus which keeps the inner portions of the nose moist. In the picture, the screen is a symbol of this function of the nose.

(B) A second function of the nose in breathing is the warming of the air to bring it to the temperature of the body, which is 98.6° F. This is accomplished by the circulation of the blood through the lining of the nose which contains a considerable number of small blood vessels.

(C) The blood vessels, which are profuse in the membrane that lines the nose, also supply the liquid that is necessary for moistening air that is drawn into the body. With each breath about a pint of air is taken into the lungs; the total in a single day is 12,000 quarts of air which passes in or through the nose.

Winthrop

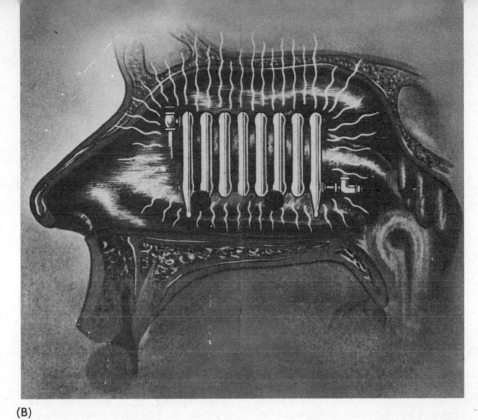

(B)

(C)

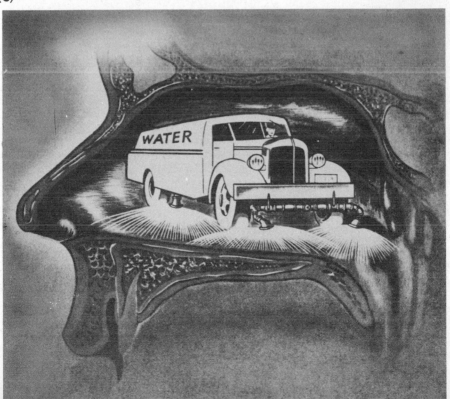

substance can be grasped and removed from the body.

PLASTIC SURGERY—When for any reason the nose is lost entirely, the facial expression naturally suffers. When the bridge of the nose disappears, as sometimes occurs in certain infections, the resulting appearance is anything but beautiful.

Automobile accidents which bring about sudden contact of the nose with the windshield often leave an expression on the face which, while not one of continual surprise, is nevertheless one that arrests attention. Falls, industrial accidents, railroad wrecks, and gunshot wounds pick the nose as a special target. Finally, the results of boxing are a constant source of income to specialists in nasal reconstruction.

As if the nose itself were not sufficiently prominent with most people, nature helps the situation by bestowing upon it a hump, a knob at the tip, or a deviation to one side or the other. Forms of the nose have been described as long and short, upturned and downturned, humped, flat, wide, pointed, narrow, and saddle-shaped.

Modern surgery has developed many different technics for changing the shape and appearance of the nose. These operations are done under conditions which insure reasonable success in most cases. Operations are done from inside the nose so that the scars do not appear on the surface. Unfortunately most of the people who want nasal reconstruction have a mental condition, so that the new nose still lacks something of perfection to them. As one expert in plastic surgery said, "They study themselves in the mirror until the mirror itself gets tired of looking at them."

If the loss or destruction of tissue in the nose resulting from an accident is such as to injure the health of the person concerned, surgical attention is desirable. There are many ways of building up a broken-down or absent bridge. Some surgeons transplant bone or cartilage or similar materials. Humps are removed by dissection and scraping or cutting away the excess material. During World War II many a man had been provided with an almost completely new nose by the transplantation from other parts of the body of large amounts of tissue.

Obviously a field of this kind can be made exceedingly lucrative through exploitation of the patient. Hence people who are going to invest in plastic surgery on the nose should make certain that the surgeon who is doing the work is one of recognized skill and established honesty. They will do well also to make certain that the work is to be done in a hospital that is known for proper scientific control over its surgery. They will do well also to have a clear understanding as to the approximate cost of the procedure, the amount of time likely to be lost from work, and their ability to meet the necessary requirements.

NOSE—See EAR, article THE EAR, TONGUE, NOSE, AND THROAT.

NOSE—blowing: See RESPIRATORY DISEASES, article THE RESPIRATORY DISEASES.

NOSE—changes during stress: See article STRESS AND DISEASE.

NOSE—drops: See article ALLERGY.

NOSE—foreign bodies: See article FIRST AID; EAR, article THE EAR, TONGUE, NOSE, AND THROAT.

NOSE—hygiene: See SKIN, article THE SKIN.

NOSE—infections: See entry COLDS.

NOSE—measles: See CHILDHOOD DISEASES, article INFECTIOUS DISEASES OF CHILDHOOD.

NOSE—plastic surgery: See EAR, article THE EAR, TONGUE, NOSE, AND THROAT.

NOSE—polyps: See EAR, article THE

EAR, TONGUE, NOSE, AND THROAT.

NOSE—sprays: See RESPIRATORY DISEASES, article THE RESPIRATORY DISEASES; EAR, article THE EAR, TONGUE, NOSE, AND THROAT.

NOSE—tumors: See EAR, article THE EAR, TONGUE, NOSE, AND THROAT.

NOSE—worms: See EAR, article THE EAR, TONGUE, NOSE, AND THROAT.

NOSEBLEED—See EAR, article THE

EAR, TONGUE, NOSE, AND THROAT.

NOSEBLEED—first aid: See article FIRST AID.

NOSEBLEED—menstrual period: See WOMEN, article HYGIENE OF WOMEN.

NOSEBLEED—typhoid fever: See article TRANSMISSIBLE DISEASES.

NUTRITION See *Weight, Over-* and *Under-*.

NUTRIENT YARDSTICK
DAILY REQUIREMENTS

	MAN	WOMAN	BOY 13-17 YRS.	CHILD 4-6 YRS.
CALORIES	3000	2500	3200	1600
PROTEIN GRAMS	70	60	85	50
CALCIUM GRAMS	.8	.8	1.4	1.0
IRON MILLIGRAMS	12	12	15	8
VITAMIN A INT. UNITS	5000	5000	5000	2500
VITAMIN B₁ MILLIGRAMS	1.8	1.5	1.6	8
VITAMIN B₂ MILLIGRAMS	2.7	2.2	2.4	1.2
NIACIN MILLIGRAMS	18	15	16	8
VITAMIN C MILLIGRAMS	75	70	90	50

The minimum daily requirement of certain foods and nutrients is determined in part by age and sex. Deficiency results in disease and, in children, malformation or poor growth. On the other hand, overeating results in obesity which causes general body weakness and a shortened life span. Cleveland Health Museum

Investigations in the Nutritional Research Laboratory of St. Luke's Hospital in New York and in St. Luke's Convalescent Hospital in Greenwich, Conn., have shown that infants' need for lysine, one of the essential amino acids, is about twice that of adults. Amino acids aid body growth and repair. A preparation containing lysine, thiamine, pyridoxine and vitamin B_{12} stimulated the appetite and rate of growth of infants. Underweight old people with poor appetites were also benefited. The mixture called "Incremin" was prepared as a liquid of which 10 to 20 drops are added to food each morning.

NUTRITION, EDUCATION IN

The average man in the United States today, obtains enough food to prevent serious deficiency diseases. This does not mean, however, that he is obtaining enough food of the right kind to give him optimal health. Neither does it mean that his children have the proper food for optimal growth, for developing resistance to disease, for preventing chronic disease, for overcoming unusual stress on the human body which may be associated with infection or serious illness, or to give them sufficient extra energy to enable them to keep pace with current drives.

The answer to the problem of improving nutrition is probably to be found in better education in the field of nutrition. A survey made by General Mills, Inc. covering 60,000 children in 38 states indicates that children's diets become poorer as the children grow older, that boys' diets are notably deficient in fruits and vegetables, that diets are related closely to the occupation and economic status of the parents, and that adolescent girls drink far too little milk in the belief that milk is especially fattening. Particularly significant in the field of diet is the choice of foods for pregnant women and industrial workers and for the aging population. No doubt nutritional science can do about as much for meeting the problems of the aged as any other form of scientific control.

NUTRITIONAL DISORDERS

Great numbers of people believe that most diseases come from wrong food. As a result innumerable dietary fads and fancies attract them. Really the body is a chemical plant which manufactures some of the substances it absolutely must have to survive. Fundamental mineral substances cannot be manufactured by the body. Vitamins cannot be manufactured by the body and must be taken in food or otherwise since the body depends on them for health and growth.

Dietary deficiencies naturally occur most often among people who get insufficient food but also among those who get the wrong foods. The most common dietary disorder is overweight or obesity.

At present the vitamins which human beings must have for health include Vitamin A and carotene, which is its precursor; thiamin and riboflavin and niacin which are parts of the Vitamin B complex; also Vitamin C and Vitamin D, Vitamin K, folic acid and Vitamin B_{12}.

The Food and Nutrition Board of the National Research Council has prepared a table of recommended daily dietary allowances for persons of both sexes, various ages, during pregnancy and nursing, for sedentary, physically active persons, and for heavy workers. Calorie intake various from 2000 daily for sedentary women to 4500 daily for male heavy workers. Women's needs increase during pregnancy and nursing of their babies. Children's needs vary with their ages, sex and activity also.

The lists of substances to be assured in the diet include good proteins, calcium, iron, the vitamins. Also needs must be met for water, salt, iodine, phosphorus, copper, Vitamin K and folic acid. Simple tables can be secured from the United States Public Health Service and other governmental agencies.

UNDERNUTRITION—Throughout the world, elsewhere much more than in the United States, people suffer from getting inadequate nourishment. These inadequacies may involve the total intake, the proteins and amino acids, the vitamins, and the minerals.

Loss of weight is not necessarily an indication of undernutrition nor is maintenance of weight assurance that the intake is proper. Troubles of salt and water balance such as occur in a variety of conditions affecting the heart, kidneys, liver and glandular organs may greatly affect the body weight. Starvation due to loss of appetite or profound neuropychiatric disturbances produces nutritional disorders. While the human body can build up reserves of some substances others are used up daily and must be regularly replenished. The effects of undernutrition may be aggravated by excessive action of the thyroid, by heat and by cold.

The regulatory mechanism of the body provides for using up fat to provide energy before drawing on the vital protein. A gram of fat provides 9 calories. A gram of protein or carbohydrate yields 4 calories. The body conserves its protein and for that reason a fat person can stand starvation much better than a thin one. The carbohydrate is stored in the liver as glycogen, and this is used up in a day or two by starvation.

Carbohydrate and fat conserve protein. The protein consists of amino acids of which ten are essential. Twelve other amino acids are classified as nonessential. People on a high carbohydrate diet can develop protein deficiency because they have not had enough protein

or because they have not had the essential amino acids in their protein. Eggs, meat, and milk best supply the essential amino acids. Growing children and pregnant women and nursing mothers need excess protein.

OVERWEIGHT—The social historian who looks back on 1956 will be interested in political movements and wars, but if he judges by our newspapers and magazines he may characterize the period as the one in which people became especially conscious of the relation of overweight to life and health. Articles on weight reduction are featured everywhere. Weird diets and reduction fads have their day or month and disappear. Even the old Hollywood 18-day-diet is being revived. Formerly just the women were interested, but now whole series of articles deal with the weight of men and boys.

Obesity is a disorder of the body's functioning which results in deposits of excess fat throughout the tissues. Doctors take special note of obesity because of the relationship between overweight and disorders of the heart, high blood pressure, diabetes, and joint disturbances.

Most experts are now agreed that by far the most frequent cause of obesity is the taking of too much food in proportion to the amount of energy that the person uses. Most people eat without too much attention to the weight problem, and yet the body can adjust itself reasonably well to getting rid of what is not used.

Some families consistently overeat and therefore the children imitating their parents, become overweight. Occasionally executives find that a snack enables them to carry on at their desks beyond the onset of fatigue; eating becomes a substitute for needed rest. As we get older we tend to walk and climb and move about less than previously. Unless we reduce the food intake overweight appears. Occasionally an illness stops physical activity and obesity may result.

OBESITY—The person who habitually overeats is always looking for an alibi. He points to someone else who eats a great deal and doesn't get fat; then he argues that his own body is different and that he absorbs where the other does not. I have seen a fat woman eating one chocolate cream after another while complaining sadly: "Everything I eat turns to fat." People do differ as to the extent to which their bodies will take up fat stores, and people also differ in their basal metabolic rates. Rarely however is overweight due to glandular deficiencies. The glands are more concerned with the areas of the body in which the fat is deposited—for instance, female hips, breasts and buttocks —the male jowls and paunch—than with overweight as a whole. Certain diseases with degeneration of important glands may be accompanied by weight increase. However, Dr. George Thorn says: "Many endocrine disturbances result from rather than cause obesity."

Everybody knows the obvious difficulties of the body associated with overweight. Fat people get out of breath, get tired easily and have pain in the joints of the knees, hips, and lower back. Fat people can't stand hot weather, they get more headaches, irritations of the skin and digestive disturbances. Fat women have more trouble with gall-bladder difficulties, diabetes, blood pressure and disturbances of their periodic functions than do the thin women. The gall bladder patient is frequently the fat woman who is fair, over forty, and who has had four pregnancies.

All authorities are now agreed that the proper way to reduce weight is to lessen the intake of food below the amount needed for the individual's energy. However, any person must still get the essential protein, vitamin and mineral substances necessary to maintain health.

WEIGHT REDUCTION—Anyone who is much overweight and who is serious about reducing should begin with a thorough examination by the doctor which will cover heart, lungs, glands, height, weight, blood pressure, condition of the blood and similar factors. A careful study of the urine should be made for presence of albumin and sugar to rule out nephritis or diabetes. The doctor will want to get at the patient's emotional condition and any psychologic conditions that may be responsible for the overeating. Dr. Edward Rynearson says a "will-power-pill" is needed by which he means to emphasize the necessity that the person really wants to reduce. By wise counsel the doctor can support the patient's motivation.

At first cutting down the calories results in some loss of energy and drive but this is less noticeable as the program continues. The loss of weight is most noticeable during the first few weeks when the basal metabolic rate of the patient readjusts itself to the lessened food intake and when there may be quite a reduction in water that is held in the body. Because of the depression and fatigue first noticed, some physicians recommend that the patient on a dietary reduction regime have some benzedrine not only to help his spirits but also because such drugs tend to diminish appetite.

Reduction in the intake of salt results in a prompt loss of water from the body and therefore rapid loss of weight, but this is not significant as far as fat is concerned. Actually the body gets rid of water beyond that needed for its proper functioning and the patient on weight reduction should not unduly restrict his intake of water.

Young people can reduce more easily than older ones. Because patients may be depressed by failure to observe large reductions, some physicians recommend that the patient be weighed only once each week.

NYSTAGMUS Nystagmus is an involuntary, rapid movement of the eyeball. It is especially associated with disturbances of, the nervous and brain tissues involved in control of eye movements. Sometimes it appears in certain occupations, as in the case of miners.

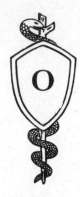

OBESITY (See also *Weight, Over-* and *Under-*) Of all of the annoyances that affect human beings, overweight is the one likely to receive least sympathy.

There are probably many different causes for overweight, but the main cause is taking in more food than is used up by the work of the body. Therefore the matter of stabilizing the weight at a proper level is simply a matter of physiologic bookkeeping.

The experts say that the "extraordinary thing is that more people do net really become fat." The reason more people do not become overweight without regulating the amount of food they eat is adjustment by the appetite to meet the ordinary needs of the body. In time, however, this adjustment may lose its delicacy, and people will begin to eat for a variety of reasons which have nothing whatever to do with appetite. They may eat purely as a habit. They may eat to overcome states of fear or social maladjustments. Sometimes they eat just to spite other people.

In a few instances overweight is due to some disturbance of the pituitary or thyroid glands, which fail to develop their secretions properly and in sufficient amounts. These are, however, the minor rather than the major number of cases.

The basal metabolic rate of the human being has a great deal to do with the speed and efficiency with which he uses up food for the production of energy. However, two people with the same basal metabolic rate may differ—one gaining weight readily and the other not. This is due to the fact that

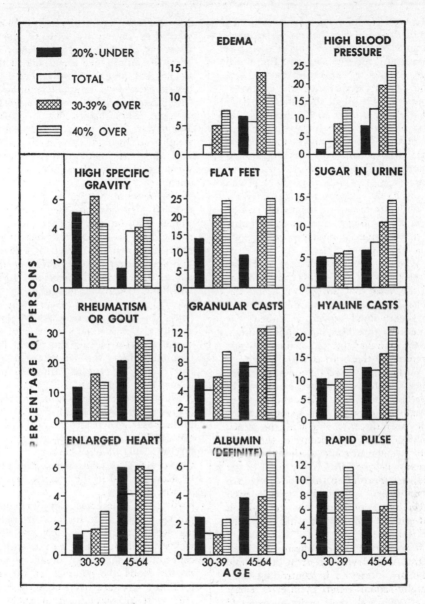

Chart showing rate of physical impairment among persons under or over standard weight. Impairment increases as weight increases. Note the graph on high blood pressure in the upper right corner. There is a definite rate of increase in high blood pressure associated with an increase in weight.

the total metabolism may be different from the basal metabolism. Extra muscular work and the taking of food will accelerate the metabolism. Emotional disturbances will speed up the metabolism. Total metabolism is the basal metabolism plus all of the other activities of the type mentioned. Probably for this reason people who are placid and calm tend to gain weight more rapidly than those who are excitable and "nervous." The placid person reacts less intensively to stimuli than the one who is excitable. People who gain weight readily are usually phlegmatic, worry less, sleep longer and more soundly, and relax more completely than people who are thin.

When overweight first begins, the fat tends to be deposited in certain portions of the body that are known as fat depots. These are the area of the breasts, the abdominal covering called the omentum, the hips, and similar areas. Later, however, fat can actually invade organs like the heart and the liver.

Ordinary overweight does not produce symptoms. However, excess weight can be associated with shortness of breath on exertion, an increased tendency to fatigue, trouble with the joints, increased danger of failure of the heart, and damage to some of the other vital organs. People with obesity seem to get diabetes more often than those who are of ordinary weight. Fat people with high blood pressure tend to have a lowering of the pressure when they take off weight.

The prevention of obesity is much better than trying to treat it. People who are interested in controlling their weight should weigh themselves every day and watch their waist measure. If the weight is steadily increasing and the waist measure likewise, it is best to begin to restrict the total consumption of food. The will power of the fat person is the fundamental factor in relief.

No one can be satisfactorily reduced who does not really wish to reduce. Most fat people, though they may not admit it, simply love to eat, and if they do not eat much at meals, they begin taking extra food in small amounts all through the day and before going to bed at night. These habits must be broken. Women are more likely to reduce their weight successfully than men because with them the desire to have a handsome appearance plays a considerable part.

The rate at which weight can be reduced depends on the amount of weight and on the manner in which the reduction is accomplished. Ordinarily two pounds a week is sufficient. For very heavy people, three or four pounds a week may be necessary. At the beginning the rapid loss of weight is due chiefly to loss of water from the body. In most severe cases of overweight the best results have been accomplished by putting the person in a hospital, where the exact amount of food taken in can be controlled over a long period of time.

Most recent in the control of obesity is the use of certain drugs which control the appetite. These drugs are, however, exceedingly stimulating and have a tendency to produce insomnia. They should never be taken unless prescribed by a doctor and in the amount that the doctor prescribes.

All sorts of special diets have been proposed from time to time for reducing weight. The best diets are those which cut down largely on fats and the concentrated sugars, on bread, and on starchy foods like potatoes. In the diet for those who are overweight the protein must be maintained at about 60 grams of protein per day. A reduction in protein below that amount tends to weaken the patient by using up the protein of the body. Fruits and vegetables which are low in carbohydrates

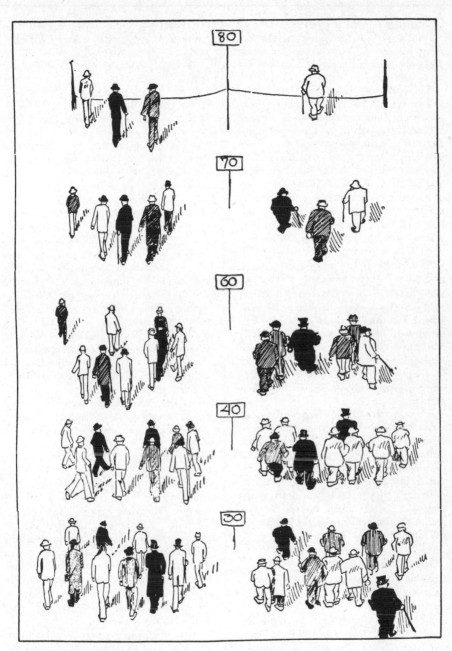

How 10 fat and 10 lean men fare as they walk through life.
Obese persons have less chance of living a long life.

(so-called 5 and 10 per cent vegetables) are invaluable in reducing weight because by their bulk they reduce hunger. They also supply necessary mineral salts and vitamins.

There is no single diet that is desirable for all patients who are reducing weight. The doctor can plan the diet to meet the requirements of the individual patient. For very severe cases of overweight, doctors put patients in hospitals and reduce the diet as low as 300 calories a day. For the average, diets of 600 to 800 calories a day can be prescribed which will take off weight rapidly. All such diets are best supplemented with the necessary vitamins and mineral salts, since it is exceedingly difficult, on diets as low as 600 calories, to get all of these essential substances. Diets have also been developed of about 1200 calories a day which can be continued for long periods of time combined with vitamins and mineral salts and thus hold the weight stable.

Coupled with these diets there should be a program of prolonged gentle exercises which, however, must be taken regularly.

Thyroid extract has frequently been taken by people to speed up the metabolism. Thyroid should never be taken unless prescribed by the doctor and in the amounts that he prescribes. Amphetamine, benzedrine, or dexedrine are prescribed by the doctor to destroy appetite. A sweet taken one half hour before a meal will also allay hunger or kill appetite.

OBESITY—basal metabolism rarely responsible: See article ENDOCRINOLOGY.

OBESITY—diabetes: See article DIABETES.

OBESITY—dinitrobenzene as reducing agent: See article OCCUPATION AND HEALTH.

OBESITY—hypertension favored by: See article BLOOD PRESSURE.

OBESITY—ovarian hormones will not prevent or cure: See article ENDOCRINOLOGY.

OBESITY—skin stretched: See SKIN, article THE SKIN.

OBESITY IN CHILDHOOD, CAUSES OF

(See also, *Overweight Children; Overweight Children, Treatment of.*) Fat children are fat because they eat too much. This simple sentence summarizes the results of numerous studies. Obvious as this statement appears to be, it may be considered a new discovery. People used to attribute obesity to glandular or endocrine disturbances. Plain overeating seemed too simple a cause to explain the unnatural distortions of size and bodily proportions in obese children. The statement, "fat children are fat because they eat too much," is simple only if read as referring solely to the physical aspects, the "how" of getting fat. The situation becomes a complicated psychological problem if the question of "why" is raised.

Before considering the food habits of fat children a few words need to be said about the glandular theories of obesity. Even parents who do not know much about the body and its function may inquire whether there isn't a "bad gland" that makes their children so fat. Once parents have accepted this belief it is difficult to convince them that their children do *not* suffer a glandular disease. They may quote some person in authority, a teacher, nurse, or even a physician who has told them that the "glands" were out of order. In a way parents are quite eager to believe this. "Bad" or "lazy" glands seem to explain all the peculiarities and shortcomings of the children. It sounds "scientific" and is therefore concinving.

It is difficult to say why this belief that "glands" are the cause of obesity has ever become so widespread. There are no objective studies that support such a diagnosis. True, in rare cases obesity may develop in a child who suffers from a true endocrine disorder or who is mentally defective. Such children are entirely different from the ordinary overweight child who, fortunately, is essentially normal in his physical make-up.

The relation of the endocrine glands to growth and development has been known for many years. A child will not grow properly if the thyroid or pituitary glands are underactive. These two glands are blamed most frequently as causing obesity by underactivity. Obese children, however, are not short; on the contrary, they are definitely *taller* than other children of the same age. Some are veritable giants. An obese child of six may be as big as an average child of ten years or more. The large size may lead to difficulties for the child. Often such children are judged according to their size and not their age, and too much is expected of them. They may be called mentally dull and backward if they do not measure up to their physical appearance. Yet it is not true that obese children are mentally retarded. Most of them have excellent minds and rate high on intelligence tests.

Accelerated physical development and good intelligence are sufficient to exclude the existence of thyroid disorder. Many other observations speak in the same direction. The maturation of the bones can be studied by X-ray examination. In obese children the bone development is more or less accelerated. In cases of glandular deficiency it is generally delayed. Of greatest practical importance is the fact that puberty occurs at a normal or frequently at an early age in obese children. It is a mistake to think that obesity in a child, particularly in a boy, is a sign that he will not develop sexually. Much misery and unhappiness have been caused through this false belief.

There is one laboratory examination for which every obese patient will either ask or will quote a former examination as a proof that the glands are wrong I am referring to the so-called basal metabolism test. Many people think that this test could be used to learn something about the cause of obesity and that a "low" test indicates glandular disorder. I cannot explain here in detail how many errors are made in the interpretation of these tests. The source of error has something to do with the state of obesity itself. Sufficient to say that the true observation is that obese children produce more, not less, calories than normal children.

The absence of specific endocrine disturbances does not exclude the possibility of some inherent tendencies in obese children which facilitate their growing fat. Such inherent qualities, which cannot be described more definitely, are often referred to as "constitutional" or "inherited," which is merely labeling them as existent. They do not explain the development of obesity or do away with the necessity of investigating and ameliorating, if possible, the factors and circumstances under which obesity becomes manifest. There are probably many more children who could become obese if they were exposed to similar environmental conditions, just as there are other children who develop entirely different symptoms seemingly under the same circumstances.

The chief cause of obesity is overeating. One reason why this obvious fact has not found due consideration in the past is that fat people, particularly the parents of fat children, are not inclined to give accurate information about their food intake. The question itself is sometimes reacted to as an insult or lack of tact. The replies are frequently evasive and deny the existence of a problem. Most mothers will say, "not much" or "just normal" or even "very little," and they will describe the composition of the food in a similar way: "All I give him," or "The same as other children eat." If one gives a mother the chance to express herself freely about the child and her feelings and problems in relation to him, she will frequently revise her statement within the same interview and give a vivid description of what the food intake really is like, how much the child demands, or what she expects that he should eat.

It may happen that the mother of a fat child seriously complains about his poor appetite, and it is not uncommon that a fat child is brought for examination not because he is overweight, but because he no longer overeats. So long as he is a large eater the obesity does not concern the parents; they consider it to be natural. They become alarmed when a child stops overeating but remains fat. There seems to be the expectation that the fat would then disappear at once. A large appetite is so commonly considered an expression of good health that it is not mentioned as a complaint.

It is difficult to say exactly how much obese children overeat, since even the normal requirements show wide individual variations. One may ask older children to keep diaries of their daily intake before any instruction has been given. Although one may be sure that the diary itself serves as a check, it helps in gaining a picture of eating habits of fat children. The most striking factor beside the large amounts is the one-sided preference for starchy food such as bread and spaghetti and for sweets. National and family customs sometimes are determining factors for the food on which the child overeats, although the craving for sweets and ice cream and their use by mothers for reward or punishment is found with great uniformity.

Mothers often resent being asked details about such intimate personal subjects as eating. Some seem to be aware of the faulty upbringing which it implies, and they are therefore defensive about being exposed. One mother was particularly embittered about her previous physician, whom she had consulted about the boy's "glands." She did not like it at all that he had found nothing wrong, and she planned to see some "really big specialist." She could hardly control her anger while recounting her experience. "What does he mean, calling him a beast? He is not beastly." Explanation of the word "obese" did little to appease her. The baby was a boy of seven weighing more than 100 pounds. "Do I have to go there to have him tell me I force too much food on him? I never force him. He eats what he wants. He is a small eater." It is, of course, impossible to obtain accurate information from such a mother. One may infer that the "baby" got fat on nothing by listening longer to her. "I don't buy him candy, not very much. He is so demanding. If I don't give it to him he torments me. My nerves are not very strong. It seems that everything I do is wrong."

The fattest boy in my group came for treatment at the age of eleven and one half with a weight of 265 pounds. The school record indicated that he had more than doubled his weight during the last three years. He had gained himself the nickname "Jumbo." He certainly did not deny that he ate too much. On the contrary, it was his biggest asset and had made him an important person in his neighborhood. He would be called in to finish whatever leftovers there were, and his schoolmates also took an active interest. They were all his friends, and each boy would bring an extra sandwich for Jumbo's lunch at school. One can just see them gleefully watching him munch his daily dozen—or more—and gradually spread in dimension. In addition he had his regular meals at home with about one pound of spaghetti at each meal and two loaves of bread per day.

There are many stories about this boy, all of them illustrations of the characteristic attitude of obese children toward food. Typical was one episode while he was losing weight, also at an amazing rate. He came faithfully to the office for weekly checkups and always had lost. Then one day he had gained. He looked very sullen and guilty. I asked him, "What is the matter?" and he said, "I gained." I asked him to tell me some more about it, and he said, "I ate chocolate." I asked, "Why?" and he explained, "My mind told me to." By means of such a monosyllabic conversation it came out that he had made a bet with his friends that he could get his weight below 200, and he had won. When he collected his winnings he invested them in chocolate.

In giving the information the fat children themselves sometimes repeat their mothers' assurance of getting fat on practically no food. Generally, however, the very change in alertness when asked about their favorite dishes or the general subject of food reveals their exaggerated interest in and enjoyment of food. Quite often the family has recognized this, and descriptions like "food is all he speaks and thinks of" or "her heart goes out for food" are not uncommon.

The statement that the fat child eats "too much" contains an implicit reference to his needs. Eating of large amounts of food would not lead to obesity if the body needed as much. The amounts which rapidly growing and physically active adolescents can consume without getting fat are proverbial. Appetite increases normally with increased energy output. In the obese this normal balance is disturbed, and one finds the combination of very large food intake and little or no exercise. One might say that eating is the only activity the fat child really indulges in and enjoys.

Information about inactivity is usually given much more freely and with less falsification than that on eating habits. Depending on the parent's emotional attitude, it is mentioned in praise of the child that he is a nice quiet boy who has nothing to do with the rough fellows in the neighborhood or that she is a sweet girl who plays house with other nice quiet little girls. Reversely, it will be quoted in a derogatory way as evidence of a child's undesirable qualities that he cannot do any of the things in which other boys excel or "that even the girls chase him away."

It is rare indeed to see a fat child on an athletic field or tennis court. Even hiking, swimming, and bicycle riding are avoided by most. The occasional fat youngster who participates in the activities of his age group may avoid the strenuous side. There was a twelve-year-old boy who took part in everything his friends did, but his nickname was "the politician." His mother explained, "He lets the other fellow do the work. If he goes down to play baseball, he keeps score, and if he works on the newspaper he takes the part of the editor and lets the others run about as reporters."

There is another much less conspicuous aspect to the inactivity of fat children, namely, their lack of independence, the failure to do things for themselves. This may extend to every detail of daily life and bodily function. There are children ten years of age or more who never had a bowel movement without being coaxed, or even accompanied, to the bathroom. Enuresis persists in about 40 per cent of such children above six years of age. Some of eight years or more continue to be spoon-fed. Persistence of bottle feeding and unwillingness to chew are not unusual up to five years.

Sometimes young obese children express a desire to do things for themselves. Without encouragement and opportunity they fail to develop motor skill according to their age and gradually lose interest in becoming independent. If demands are made upon them later on, they are so slow and incompetent that they become discouraged and soon give up, especially when nagged and driven to greater hurry. In many cases the saving of energy by avoiding the ordinary activities of daily life is of equal, if not of greater, importance than the saving due to avoidance of sports and games.

There is nothing noteworthy about the fact that a child who persistently overeats and is at the same time underactive grows fat. The question is *why* the normal regulation between eating and energy requirements is disturbed. This question becomes answerable if we turn from physiological to psychological considerations. The description of food habits and underactivity has already indicated the strong emotional meaning of these symptoms. Food has an exaggerated positive value for the obese child. It stands for love, security, and satisfaction. Muscular activity and social contacts, on the other hand, are associated with the concept of danger, threat, and insecurity. The simultaneous occurrence of love of food and avoidance of activity thus becomes comprehensible.

Eating and activity acquire this peculiar emotional significance in a family setting which, though not specific, is characteristic for obesity. The typical obese family is of small size. Quite often it is the youngest or an only child who becomes obese. Fathers usually play a subordinate role in the emotional life of the obese family. The mothers are dominant in their influence and have a particularly close hold on the potentially obese child. Many mothers live out their own problems and frustrations in these children. They cannot give their children respect as individuals nor permit them independence and the dignity of personal achievement. These mothers try to realize in their children their own dreams of a life of luxury and idleness of which they themselves may have felt deprived. Their expression of affection is over-feeding the child and sparing him the necessary tasks of doing things for himself. The mother's attitude toward the obese child is like that toward an inanimate and prized possession, one to which they give the very best of care in order to retain it. A characteristic aspect of this possessive attitude is the frequently expressed wish for a daughter instead of a son, because these mothers feel that a daughter represents a more permanent possession than a son. In bringing up their sons they give them the role of a daughter in their emotional life. The "feminine" characteristics of obese boys seem to be related to this attitude of the mother. There certainly is no evidence that it is an expression of abnormal or delayed sexual maturation.

Mixed with the expression of affection, which overprotectiveness and overfeeding represent, is an underlying hostility which many mothers feel in relation to the fat child. Far-reaching protective measures are devised to spare the mother the anguish of her own anxiety for the safety of the child, even though these measures interfere with the child's normal psychological growth and social adjustment. At the same time the mother is irritated by the demands which this excessive care makes upon her. She nags and criticizes the child and often resorts to beating him in order to find relief from her own exasperation. Yet in her heart she wants to retain his affection and loyalty, and food is a constant bribe with which she keeps him close and dependent. As long as the child is young there is prestige for her in having a well-fed child. As the child grows older and the obesity becomes a handicap the mother will be unrelenting in nagging and belittling him for his awkward appearance and in berating him for his greediness.

The family frame of obese children thus reveals influences which lead to inactivity and overeating and distort their personality maturation. The most serious aspect in this mal-development is the interference with the development of an adequate sense of security, competence, and worth-whileness. The obese child grows up with fundamentally low self-esteem and with the conviction of his helplessness in a world which has been represented to him as a dangerous place in which he is lost without a protecting mother. Such an attitude toward life makes an individual a constant victim of uncertainty and anxiety. His only defense against this anxiety is to turn back to mother, and, since the mother is a person who is unable to give of herself but has appeased all his needs with the offering of food, food becomes his weapon against anxiety and source of comfort in periods of emotional distress. For many obese people eating is the only known source of comfort and satisfaction. Other sources of satisfaction, comfortable relations to people, and the realization of inherent creative and constructive abilities have remained seriously crippled under the unfavorable influences of their upbringing.

OCCIPITAL NEURALGIA (See also, *Neuralgia*) Pain at the back of the neck, called occipital neuralgia, brings on severe tenderness, and the skin may be so sensitive to touch that it is impossible even to brush the hair. Since there are other causes of pain at this portion of the body, the doctor has to make a most careful investigation to determine that it is the involvement of two nerves coming from the spine to this area that is responsible.

Obviously, any inflammation, new growth, poisoning, or other irritant factor that can reach a nerve can cause severe pain that persists and that demands medical attention. Pain involving the shoulder and arm may occur from arthritis, from inflammation of a bursa, from a job involving constant arm use, such as telegraphy. Whenever the pain is diffuse and involves the muscles and joints it is unlikely to be neuralgia and more likely to be some of the other conditions that have been mentioned.

Occupation and Health

BY

CAREY P. McCORD, M.D.

Consultant, Institute of Industrial Health, University of Michigan, Ann Arbor.

INTRODUCTION: OCCUPATIONAL DISEASES

EVERY JOB ON WHICH *anyone works brings with it some degree of exposure to risk from contact with chemical substances, with electric power, with conditions of temperature, humidity or similar changes in the environment that may cause illness. The occupations are now recognized as of first importance as a factor in causing disability.*

The human body has in it certain factors for controlling its own temperature, but sometimes outside conditions become so severe that the body's own thermostatic function will not control. Cold constricts the blood vessels in the skin; heat expands them. Sudden changes of temperature, particularly from extreme heat to cold, result in discomfort and are believed to be associated with pains in the limbs and with catching cold. Excessive heat for long periods of time can produce changes in the body leading to unconsciousness and even to death.

In the article which follows, Dr. Carey P. McCord considers first the general conditions associated with occupational diseases and then classifies them ac-

cording to the chief factor involved in bringing about the illness. For example, if anyone is exposed to extreme dry heat he can develop heat stroke. This is associated with fever, a rapid pulse, flushing of the skin, profuse sweating, and a fall in the blood pressure. Eventually, of course, exposure to extreme heat may so affect the organs and tissues of the body that anemia, inflammations of the skin, disturbances of the kidney, and breakdown of many of the other organs of the body may follow. There are innumerable occupations in which heat is a factor, particularly such occupations as those of blast-furnace and boiler-room workers, of workers in the chemical and cement industries, of cooks, laundry workers, tinners, and similar occupations.

Sudden changes in the temperature are particularly likely to occur to men in the ice industry, to butchers, to candy makers, cooks, drivers, electrotypers, fishermen, florists, miners, packing-house employees, soap makers, and similar occupations.

INDUSTRIAL SKIN DISEASES

Occupational skin diseases comprise about 75% of all occupational diseases. The number of substances used in various industries which may affect the worker is legion. Among florists there may be sensitivities to plants, as described under allergic diseases, or irritations of the skin from water, or poisoning from such substances as nicotine and arsenic used to destroy insect pests. Furriers may be poisoned by paraphenylendiamine, as described under diseases of the skin. Workers with chromium in electro-plating develop chrome ulcers. There are also inflammations of the skin from acids, alkalis, soaps, dyes, and drugs. The physician will usually inquire as to the occupation of his patient and as to any unusual substances used in that occupation.

Incidentally, all workers except those in a few especially hazardous trades are more likely to suffer from ailments unrelated to work than from occupational diseases that result directly from conditions in which the worker toils. Modern departments of industrial health in state and municipal health departments do much to control conditions of work.

DAMPNESS

Occasionally workers are employed in places which are exceedingly damp. This happens particularly in such occupations as those of the fisherman, leather preparers in the glove industry, laundry workers, packing-house employees, workers in the paper industry, pottery workers, sewer workers, and farmers. Most occupations in which dampness occurs are also associated with high and low temperatures and with high humidity.

There are, however, some conditions in which the wetness alone is the serious factor. Exposure to dampness is usually associated as a contributing factor with coughs and colds, in rheumatic disease, and in changes in the skin. Of course, the human being is not adapted to living in exceedingly damp areas; hence he should endeavor to avoid the dampness by wearing waterproof clothing, rubber boots, and similar protective coverings. Moreover, accumulation of water can frequently be prevented by digging channels or ditches to carry away the excess.

DUST AS A HAZARD

The most serious hazard today in many industries is dust. The dusts not only block the tissues, but in some cases act as an irritant, so that there are inflammation, swelling, and even destruction. Moreover, the dusts sometimes carry germs with them into the tissues, and once in the body the germs may set up inflammations.

Among the most dangerous of the dusts which affect mankind is silica. This produces a condition known as silicosis. X-ray pictures show the lungs full of nodules following the lodgment of the silica in the lymphatics. When the disease is well advanced, the lungs do not expand, and breathing is difficult, and there may be continuous coughing.

The dust from asbestos produces the same type of inflammation that silica produces, although apparently milder. In order to prevent silicosis, workers in any industry in which silica is much used should avoid inhalation, and the head of the industry can aid the worker with certain simple procedures. Water or oil may be used to wet the dust, thus preventing it from rising and filling the air. Exhaust systems can be applied to remove the dust at the point where it develops. Sometimes the work can be done in an enclosed chamber with the worker outside. Finally, where dust is exceedingly excessive, helmets may be worn by the workers to cover the head and neck, and they can get their air by breathing through pipes from a non-dusty area.

Workers in such an industry should have their lungs X-rayed regularly, and there should be a physician in the plant who is familiar with the changes that take place in the lungs under exposure. Whenever a worker in a dusty trade has a cough, a dryness of the nose and throat, pain on breathing and hoarseness, whenever he coughs or expectorates blood, and develops colds which simply refuse to clear up, he should begin to wonder whether or not the dust is affecting him unfavorably. There are hundreds of industries in which dust is a serious factor. In all of them it is a hazard, but when it is silica or asbestos dust, it is a menace to health and life.

INFECTIONS OF INDUSTRY

Certain industries are associated with the likelihood of special infections of the body. For example: workers with hides and animal hair are constantly exposed to infection with anthrax. This begins as a malignant pustule, an inflamed pimple or a boil, which becomes hard, has a purple center and a deep red zone around it. Gradually this breaks down and discharges a thick, bloody material, and eventually may even become gangrenous. The lymph glands in the neighborhood swell, and the veins become inflamed. Associated with this there may be a general weakness, including chilliness, loss of appetite, vomiting, and a high fever.

Anthrax is a dangerous disease, and workers with hides must do everything possible to prevent infection. Foreign skins or hair should never be carried on the unprotected shoulder. All hides and animal hair should be thoroughly sterilized. The workers should wash their hands frequently in antiseptic solutions, and those who sort hair should wear breathing devices to prevent inhalation.

As is pointed out elsewhere, the body may become infected from the tissue of infected rabbit with tularemia, from infected straw with actinomycosis, from a contaminated nail with tetanus, from infected milk with undulant fever, and so on, from various substances. Workers in mines and on farms who walk about barefooted may develop hook-worm infection.

Every cut, scratch, or abrasion sustained in any industry should be treated at once with suitable antiseptics, such as iodine, to prevent infection. Industries in which infections of the skin, such as boils, carbuncles, and abscesses, are most likely to develop are those of the butcher, the canner, feather workers, fertilizer makers, garbage workers, glue makers, hair workers, dairy workers, silk workers, soap makers, and veterinarians.

RADIANT ENERGY DISEASES

Among the most serious of the occupational diseases recently developed are those associated with the use of radium, the X-ray, and various radioactive substances. Exposure to X-rays and to the emanations from radium may produce serious burns and irritations of the skin which result in cancer. They also affect the blood and the blood-forming organs seriously, so that deficiencies of both the red and the white blood cells are exceedingly common.

Employees in watch factories who prepare the luminous dials have sustained generalized radium poisoning with disastrous results. Workers must learn to protect themselves against these hazards, first of all, by suitable screening against the rays through the wearing of aprons and gloves infiltrated with lead. Brushes for radium painting should never be pointed with the mouth or lips.

Another type of radiant energy which may produce damage to the human body is that associated with ultraviolet and infra-red rays. These are occupational hazards particularly in welding and cutting. The ultraviolet rays are invisible. They cause intense irritation of the eyes and a burning of the skin. Sunblindness and desert-blindness represent the type of injury that can be caused to the eye by ultraviolet rays. The infra-red rays are essentially heat rays and can cause all the damage that heat of intensity applied to the human body can cause in other ways.

Workers around ultraviolet or infra-red rays may protect themselves against these rays by wearing goggles, helmets, shields, and masks equipped with colored lenses especially designed to exclude dangerous rays. The rays cannot penetrate ordinary clothing, so that covering of the body with a sufficient thickness of clothing will prevent injury and damage to the skin.

Among the industries in which exposure to ultraviolet and infra-red rays are most common are blacksmiths, cutters who use oxyacetylene gas, furnace workers, glass blowers, iron and steel mill workers, and everyone working in the motion-picture industry. The welders who use the arc for cutting and welding steel are also constantly exposed to dangerous rays.

In the following article, Dr. Carey P. McCord has presented some of the general considerations associated with occupational diseases, and he presents a consideration of the one hundred and fifty most common hazards likely to be found in industry. Any worker associated with any of the poisons here listed should take steps to protect himself against exposure by inhalation, by contamination of the skin, and by other sources.

M. F.

OCCUPATION AND HEALTH

The outstanding characteristic of Americans is their zest for work. This willingness to work, along with great technical, economic, and social advances in our industrial world, have procured luxuries for all of us far beyond the dreams of kings of old—automobiles, good food, television sets, family-owned homes —to name but a few. The health to enjoy these good things has been enhanced by advances in medicine generally—the care of infants and the care of the aged; the new wonder drugs; new surgical techniques, including surgery of the heart; new procedures for diagnosis, and the improved organization of preventive medical programs in government and industry. Since nearly all adult men and many women spend forty or more hours per week at their jobs, occupational medicine has played no little part in this scheme of positive health promotion.

The industrial physician or medical department is the public health department for the worker at work. Safety programs to prevent accidents work effectively in industry. Carriers of workmen's compensation have found that excellent surgical care and the liberal use of specialists for sick workers is good for themselves as well. All large industries and most moderate-sized concerns have well-developed medical departments. There is also a rapidly increasing trend for small plants to procure good part-time medical consultation so that they, too, can participate in the positive benefit programs. Care for injured workers is by no means the only function of these medical departments and medical consultants. The pre-employment examinations prevailing in industry today are used not to prevent people from working, but rather to advise management of the type of work that a prospective employee can do without harm to himself or his fellow workers. For instance, a person with some disease of the heart might well do light work, whereas the work of a stevedore would soon disable him completely. Occupational medicine enables such men to work and earn, at the same time protecting health. Likewise by the pre-employment examination many people are for the first time made aware of some curable defect and encouraged to seek help from the personal physician of their own choice. However, people with communicable diseases may be prevented from exposing fellow employees until such time as they may safely mingle with them.

Nonetheless, the detection of disease or defects and personal health education do not complete the job of those charged with maintaining the health of the men and women who work. In the work environment there is sometimes encountered toxic vapor, fume, gas or dust, harmful radiation, undue alterations of temperature, excesses of humidity, noise or vibration, any of which may cause an occupational disease. An occupational disease is any abnormal state of the body or mind resulting from work. It differs from an accident in that some time must pass between the first exposure to the causative agent and the development of symptoms. A painter may be exposed over a period of days to the action of a paint solvent. This slowly irritates the skin, so that in the course of a week a rash appears on his hands or forearms. An employee in a battery-manufacturing plant where there is inadequate medical and engineering protection from exposure to lead may inhale lead dust for months and only gradually develop loss of appetite and weight, increasing constipation, and abdominal cramps. A miner may work for twenty or thirty years breathing silica dust before there is any evidence of silicosis as seen in X-ray films. These are occupational diseases.

Monumental research has been done by our universities, our government agencies, and above all by industry itself on the pathologic changes produced by exposure to these substances and on methods to control them in order to maintain healthful surroundings in which to work. The efficacy of these advancements in occupational medicine is attested by the rarity of occupational disease. In California in 1950 there were only 12,245 cases of occupational disease reported to the State Bureau of Adult Health. At the same time there were 136,814 lost-time industrial accidents.

Purely from an interest point of view, and to give some idea generally of the types of occupational disease which may occur, the reported cases are herewith broken down as to the organ affected and the principal groups of causative agents:

Infectious and parasitic disease		205
Diseases of the eye		1,726
Flash burns (from welding rays)	1,672	
Other	54	
Diseases of the ear		38
Diseases of the respiratory system		331
Diseases of the skin		6,615
Poison Oak	3,302	
Other	3,313	
Diseases of the bones and organs of movement		1,703
Strains & inflammation of the tendons	1,469	
Other	207	
Systemic poisonings by industrial chemicals		339
Poisoning by other substances, including venom (insect bites) & pharmaceuticals		620
Weather		273
Heat	246	
Other	27	
Burns (repeated exposure to chemicals)		234
Other specific causes		156
Not specified		5
Total		12,245

Much effort has been exerted to ascertain the effects of noise on people and to devise standards of noise tolerance. Also, with the advent of the atom bomb and the numerous radioactive substances that have been placed in common usage as a result of knowledge of nuclear physics, the increased control of radiant energy has become one of the greatest problems in the technical aspects of industrial medicine.

NOISE

Sound is that form of vibrational energy which produces the sensation of hearing. It is usually transmitted to the ear by air but may also travel through bone. Sound is propagated by vibratory disturbances. Whereas musical sound or tone is due to regularly recurring vibrations, a noise results when the impulses are irregular or confused. Both the loudness or intensity of the sound waves and their frequency play a part in the effect of a given noise on the ear. To be audible, vibrations must have a rate of at least 12 to 15 per second, and shrill, high-pitched tones may be heard with a rate of vibration of approximately 20,000 per second. High frequency sounds are more annoying and damaging than sounds of low frequency. The decibel is the usual unit of measure for sound. Some idea of the value of the decibel can be obtained from the following comparisons:

The tick of a watch at 3 feet may be measured as 10 to 30 decibels on the sound intensity or loudness scale; ordinary conversation as 40 to 60 decibels, and a pneumatic drill at 10 feet as 70 to 90 decibels. The threshold of feeling noise (in contrast to hearing it) occurs at 100 to 120 decibels, depending on the frequency. Since the bel, and accordingly the decibel, is determined on a base 10 logarithmic scale, 10 decibels is 10 times as loud, 20 decibels is 100 times as loud, and 30 decibels is 1,000 times as loud as 1 decibel.

Noise may produce effects ranging through mental inefficiency, nervousness, fatigue, indigestion, temporary deafness, and permanent injury to the ear. Deafness resulting from industrial noise may usually be distinguished from other types of deafness because occupational deafness occurs in certain frequency ranges peaking at 4,096 vibrations per second. Although there is no doubt that industrial deafness occurs, as illustrated by the old-time boiler maker, considerable duration of time, even with exposure to high noise levels, is necessary to produce permanent deafness. Opinion as to the exact levels at which noise may produce lasting detriment to the ear varies, but the majority of data indicates that some harmful effect may result from prolonged exposure to noise of intensities from 85 to 110 decibels. The incompleteness of data upon which to base standards of noise tolerance has been one of the deterrents to efforts aimed at controlling noise in industry.

Personal protection against noise and vibration is available. Airborne noise can be reduced by the insertion in the external ear of pliable materials such as wax, or foam rubber. Commercially produced ear plugs of various designs are available. Protection against bone-conducted noise and vibration requires the use of soft-soled shoes, felt or rubber mats, and chairs or platforms mounted on springs. However, these methods are employed only in situations where it is impracticable to control noise at its source.

The trend toward reducing industrial noise is apparent in the recent design of modern office machines such as the "noiseless typewriter." However, the same trend has developed in the field of manufacturing and processing equipment, and in many instances this has included alteration of production methods. Noise is reduced when welding replaces riveting, when hydraulic presses displace the old trip hammers, when V-belts replace growling gears, and when advanced foundry practice reduces or eliminates chipping and grinding of castings. The shock and noise created by metallic impact generally characteristic of metal fabrication may often be reduced at its source by damping materials such as rubber or the "hydro-pneumatic metal" of Chamberlain. The latter can be used as inserts in hammers, punches, dies, and as durable shock-absorbing mounts for heavy machinery. It was used successfully in World War II to prevent shock to delicate equipment on battleships and as shoe inserts to prevent fractured ankles when large bombs exploded under water in proximity to battleships.

Thus there are means of measuring noise, of determining its effect on organisms, and, to a certain extent, of reducing such harmful effects.

RADIANT ENERGY

The tremendous power of atomic energy for benefit or destruction was far from the minds of the German, William Roentgen, and the Frenchman, Antoine Becquerel, some fifty years ago when they respectively discovered the X-ray and what we call radioactivity. Becquerel found that uranium salts had developed a photographic film in the dark, and his pupils, Pierre and Marie Curie, went on to discover radium, the first known radioactive element always present in uranium.

Radioactivity, the giving off of charged particles, results from the breakdown of the element itself. As radium dissipates its energy it eventually turns into lead. Although this radiation from the atom is extremely harmful to human flesh and bone, no appreciable heat is felt and there is no way of immediately recognizing by the physical senses the dire effect of its penetration into the tissues, so that early there was no thought of the tremendous energy involved. What is this atom of which we speak so glibly? Everything is made up of invisibly small particles called atoms. However, small as they are, atoms are made up of even smaller particles known as electrons, protons, and neutrons. An atom consists of a nucleus (positively charged particles, the protons; and neutrons, without any charge) about which revolve the negatively charged electrons. The electrons are attracted to the nucleus, but their terrific speed of rotation exerts a centrifugal force that prevents their moving closer to it. It is the difference in the proportion of protons that makes one element different from another. Most elements are stable unless by bombarding with particles like those given off by radium or by slowed neutrons, a portion of the nucleus can be knocked off, producing a different element and giving off energy. This is the principle employed in the atom bomb.

The radiations produced in this manner consist primarily of three types of moving particles: alpha rays, beta rays, and gamma rays, which differ in their response to electric forces. Protons and neutrons may also be given off as energized particles. Similar to these are X-rays produced when a moving electrically charged particle strikes against a hard target. Such radiant energy produces undesirable effects in the human body whenever it is absorbed in excess of certain amounts to which the human organism has been accustomed in its natural surroundings. Injury results only when the radiation releases ions (electrically charged particles) within the cell structure, and the injury is proportional to the ionization produced. So far as the effect on the cell is concerned, it does not matter greatly whether these ions are produced indirectly by secondary emanations from X-rays or gamma rays or directly by the impact of primary particles such as beta and alpha rays.

The X-rays and gamma rays are penetrating radiations which, in contrast to other types of radiant energy, can pass entirely through any part of the body with only moderate diminution of their intensity. X-rays are used in the doctor's office to photograph bones and other parts of the body. In this instance the radiations are carefully controlled so that a single dose does not exceed the safe level.

Alpha particles have a very low penetrating power, and when originating outside the body produce no appreciable biologic effect. They are stopped by a few inches of air. Beta rays from radium and from many artificially produced radioactive substances have a much greater penetrating power and are able to traverse a fraction of an inch of animal tissue. Overexposure to beta rays will produce burns, most frequently of the hands.

Neutrons are known as slow or fast. They are without electric charge and do not cause ionization of tissue, but the fast neutron may collide with hydrogen atoms, imparting some of their energy to them and producing rapidly moving charged particles capable of harm.

Radiant energy may produce burns of the skin and cancer. Generalized radiation by penetrating rays causes nausea, vomiting, diarrhea, and anemia. Leukemia may result Radium, if absorbed, is stored in the bones and affects both the blood-forming marrow and the bone itself. It is important to iterate that these symptoms are not immediately present. The senses give no warning of impending harm. Injury is only apparent after a latent period of several hours to one or two weeks or more. It may take many years for the results of repeated small exposures to radiant energy to become apparent. If the cells concerned in reproduction are injured, there is also the possibility of mutations (abnormalities) developing in subsequent generations.

Radiant energy may be encountered in an atomic explosion, in industrial X-ray processes to detect flaws in metal, in the work of medical technicians, in radium dial painting, and in the handling of radioactive isotopes, which are coming into more general usage.

Protection against the effect of radiation is twofold—medical and engineering. Pre-employment medical examinations are necessary to prevent exposure of persons already anemic. Periodic examinations of the blood to detect early changes, examination of the exhaled air for its radioactivity, and the wearing by workers of detecting devices or photographic film, are essential to protection. Shielding of processes by sufficient distance (remote control), adequate amounts of lead or other materials—in the case of fast neutrons, hydrogen barriers are used—and removal of contaminated air, are essential engineering controls.

In spite of the tremendous hazard from exposure to radiant energy with the development and application of atomic physics—once the problem was known—industrial medicine has done and continues to do an amazingly fine job in minimizing the harmful effects of radiation.

TOXIC SUBSTANCES THAT MAY BE ENCOUNTERED IN INDUSTRY

Acetanilid, which is well known as a dangerous drug in the treatment of headache, is extensively used in the manufacture of many chemicals, such as paranitranilin. It is commonly taken into the body under industrial conditions in the form of dusts. The action of acetanilid simulates that of aniline oil. An outstanding manifestation is a blue discoloration of the skin, notably of the lips, finger tips, and ears, which is due to the formation of methemoglobin in the blood.

Acetone (dimethyl ketone) is a much used industrial solvent, especially in the manufacture of munitions. It is representative of a long series of ketones, all of which possess about the same order of toxicity. While inhaled vapors may lead to some damage to the respiratory tract and other portions of the body, this takes place only when vapor concentrations are comparatively high. Acetone is much less toxic than such other agents as benzene or carbon tetrachloride. In contact with the skin, acetone is a defatting agent and thus favors the appearance of dermatitis.

Acetylene gas is in itself probably nontoxic, except that it may act as a simple asphyxiant; that is, it may displace oxygen in the air to an extent that life may not be supported. However, the use of acetylene as in torch welding may be associated with a number of other exposures. If acetylene welding be done on galvanized metal, zinc chills may arise from that metal used in the galvanizing. The same is true in torch work in brazing brass. Chemical rays from acetylene torch work may lead to injury to the eyes, producing such conditions as conjunctivitis or retinitis.

Ammonia gas causes profound local action on the skin, eyes, and respiratory tract. Four hundred parts of this substance per million of air constitute the threshold for immediate irritation of the throat. Prolonged exposure to one fourth of that amount is the maximum tolerable for prolonged periods. Although ammonia accidents may be severe and fatal, it is unlikely that ammonia as such enters the body.

Coatings, such as lacquers and varnishes, may contain *amyl alcohol* or related amyl compounds. Toxicity is not great, but it may lead to low-grade irritation of the eyes, nose, and throat.

Aniline oil is a much used chemical in a variety of industries, especially in the manufacture of chemicals. A large number of compounds derived from aniline exert a harmful action similar to that of aniline itself. Aniline is definitely toxic, producing both acute and chronic poisoning. It readily enters the body through the unbroken skin, leading to poisoning. Also poisoning may take place through inhalation or ingestion of the oil or its dusts or vapors. In severe acute poisoning there may be observed sudden prostration with blue coloration of lips, nose, and fingers, and unconsciousness with or without convulsions.

Both *arsenic* and its compounds are highly toxic. Arsenic is widely used in industry, and in addition is present in many industrial substances as impurities unknown to industrial workers. Unsuspected poisonings arise in scores of industries making no direct uses of this substance. It may enter the body in the form of gases, vapors, fluids, or dusts. Local action may be produced on exposed parts. In constitutional disease the principal systems or organs involved are: gastrointestinal tract, the kidneys, the liver, the nervous system, and the respiratory tract. The loss of hair and of nails, together with bronzing of the skin, are common features.

Asbestos, which is a complex calcium magnesium silicate, may from the breathing of its dust give rise to a lung disease known as asbestosis. This disease resembles silicosis, but in fact is not silicosis, which is only produced by silicon dioxide. Many years of dust exposure may be required to establish the disease. Once established, it is permanent. The X-ray picture of the lungs is fairly characteristic.

Asphalt is not a chemical entity but a tarry substance of inconstant make-up, found in nature or resulting from petroleum or coal distillation. Asphalt contains many toxic agents, notably skin irritants. Operations involving hot asphalt constitute greater practical dangers than the handling in cold form. Possible skin cancer may be caused by contact with asphalt.

Bakelite is the trade name for a synthetic resin produced from the interaction of phenol and formaldehyde. Several other trade names are associated with this product. In the manufacture of bakelite some exposures may be found in phenol, formaldehyde, various resin solvents, and "hex" (hexamethylenetetramine). The latter is a frequent source of dermatitis.

Benzene (benzol) differs from benzine. The former chiefly originates in coal-tar distillation but it is known that benzene or substances chemically closely akin to benzene may be obtained from some petroleums. Benzene is highly toxic. Concentrations above one hundred parts per million of air are to be regarded as harmful. Vapors enter the body along with respired air. High concentrations may lead to immediate action, characterized by convulsions, unconsciousness, and prompt death; but the greater number of cases are chronic and center about the results of destruction of several forms of blood elements. Some persons are far more susceptible to the action of benzene than others. Chronic poisoning is characterized by damage to blood-forming organs, kidneys, liver, nervous system, and by increased susceptibility to ordinary infections. Hemorrhage into the skin, from the nose, mouth, and stomach, rectum, lungs, and genitalia, are prime manifestations. Benzene in contact with the skin may be absorbed and produce systemic poisoning, or local skin action may take place leading to a dermatitis.

Benzine is a nontechnical term applied to various derivatives of petroleum distillation, such as gasoline, naphtha, etc. The action of this chemical may be local on the skin, or systemic after the inhalation of vapors. This substance is more toxic than commonly believed, and may give rise either to "naphtha jags" (which is an acute disease resembling alcoholic intoxication), associated with respiratory tract irritation, or rarely to chronic forms characterized by profound changes in the nervous system, liver, and kidneys. Chronic benzine poisoning may simulate multiple paralysis.

Beryllium. There are many industrial processes in which beryllium may exist. It forms an alloy with several metals, most outstanding of which is beryllium copper, used in making springs and diaphragms for altimeters. Beryllium glass is used to filter out strong or reflected electrons in X-ray streams. Formerly the element was used extensively in the manufacture of fluorescent lamps and this was the chief source of poisoning. Although ulcers and nodules may be produced on the skin, the reaction in the lungs is of paramount importance. Beryllium causes weakness, shortness of breath, cough, nervousness, and loss of weight. Distinct changes in the lung, not unlike those found in tuberculosis, are produced.

Bichromates are extensively used in lithography, photography, blueprint work, the dye industry, etc. Their action is similar to that of chromates and chromic acid. Local action may be extensive and intractable. It may produce a dermatitis of unbroken skin, deep burrowing ulcers ("chrome holes"), perforation of the nasal septum, inflammation of the respiratory tract, and a condition akin to sensitization may be instituted by chromium, in which trivial exposures produce profound inflammation of large areas of the skin not in contact with the irritant. Damage from chromium is always slow in healing. Not all compounds of chromium are injurious. This depends upon differences in valency.

Bisulphide of carbon is much used in artificial silk manufacture and in the rubber industry. Its action is primarily exerted on the central nervous system, causing conditions resembling insanity. It may lead to blindness, paralyses of various groups of muscles, and in addition damage to the kidneys and the gastro-intestinal tract takes place. A rapid heart is the rule.

The manipulation of *brass* in cold form is not known to produce characteristic damage. Brass dust may induce a mechanical dermatitis, and the skin and hair may become green from the copper content of the brass. When, however, brass is in molten state, metal fume fever may arise, which primarily depends on the action of zinc rather than the copper or the brass. The disease produced is variously termed "zinc chills," "brass ague," "foundrymen's chills," etc. In addition, workers about molten brass may acquire lead or arsenic poisoning as the result of these metals being present as impurities in the brass.

Much stated in respect to the hazards of brass work applies to *bronze* workers. Especially, lead may appear in bronze, and lead poisoning is not a rarity.

Bronze powders is a term extensively applied to the divers metallic powders used in printing and decorating. All such bronze powders are capable of producing inflammation of the skin. Low-grade respiratory tract irritation is common. Some so-called bronze powders actually are colored aluminum powders. Fine aluminum powders are inflammable and explosions have occurred.

Butyl alcohol is a widely used ingredient in solvents. Its toxicity is believed to begin at about one hundred parts of the vapors per million of air. In addition to being a respiratory tract irritant, butyl alcohol may lead to damage to the kidneys, liver, lungs, and to the causation of anemia.

Various compounds of *cadmium* may enter the body through the lungs in the form of dusts or fumes, and to a lesser extent dusts may enter the stomach. Edema of the lungs may be produced, with or without pneumonia and related injuries. Some scar tissue may be produced. Cadmium likewise injures the liver, kidneys, and intestinal tract. Vomiting may take place, together with diarrhea. On a comparative basis, cadmium is more toxic than lead.

Wherever used, *carbolic acid* (phenol) is a potential source of severe injury.

Harm may be either local, beginning with a slight burn and culminating in gangrene, or may be systemic, following skin absorption, inhalation, or accidental swallowing. Deleterious action is swift, and death may be produced within a few hours. Any portion of the body may be affected. Commonly the respiratory and intestinal tracts, the liver, the kidneys, and blood-forming elements are damaged.

Carbon dioxide is not toxic except as it displaces oxygen necessary in respired air. It is a simple asphyxiant. Deaths in industry from exposure to undue amounts of carbon dioxide are fairly frequent and commonly may be construed as accidents rather than occupational diseases. The presence of low quantities of carbon dioxide in the air constitutes no index of air vitiation. Instead, some carbon dioxide is essential as a stimulant to normal breathing.

Carbon monoxide is one of the most widespread and insidious hazards of industry. Carbon monoxide easily combines with the hemoglobin of the blood and inhibits the oxygen-carrying power of the blood. The commoner features of acute poisoning are headache, nausea, dizziness, visual disturbances, abdominal pain, discoloration of the skin, which may be pink, greenish or yellowish-red, followed by unconsciousness and convulsions in severer cases. This form of poisoning either in or apart from industry may be regarded as an accident rather than a disease. After severe poisoning with prolonged unconsciousness, various serious after-effects may arise of prolonged duration. Chronic carbon monoxide poisoning is at this time disputed. Prompt artificial respiration after removal from exposure is highly desirable when respiration has ceased.

The action of *carbon tetrachloride* is characteristic of a group of chlorinated hydrocarbons, including ethylene dichloride, trichlorethylene, and chloroform. The threshold of danger begins at about one hundred parts of the vapors per million of air. Poisoning may be acute, delayed, and possibly chronic. In acute poisoning the essential manifestations are headache, vomiting, diarrhea, abnormal pain, sense of moving masses in the abdomen, and irritation of the kidneys. The delayed poisoning may arise twenty-four to forty-eight hours after exposure. Delayed poisoning largely centers about destruction of liver tissues and damage from the subsequently produced guanidine. The damage from acute poisoning is believed to be readily repaired without significant after-effects, but some physicians recognize the possibility of a chronic form of the disease. Exposure through inhalation is the usual mode of entry, but skin absorption is possible and local skin action has been observed. This material is widely used in industry such as in dry cleaning, metal degreasing, in fire extinguishers, etc.

In the manufacture and industrial use of *chloride of lime,* dusts and gases may lead to asthma, inflammation of the eyes, injury to the respiratory tract, and skin diseases. Harmful action is probably subsequent to liberated chlorine, although impurities may account for some damage.

Chlorine is an irrespirable gas, hazardous in small quantities, leading to prompt swelling (edema) of the lungs and air passages. The chronic form of intoxication, due to the intake of minute quantities over long periods of time, is characterized by severe bronchitis, persistent coughing, and pain in the chest.

Many of the widely used household *insecticides* consist of ground-up chrysanthemum buds used, as such, as a powder, or are extracted by such agents as ethylene dichloride, kerosene, etc. Both in the manufacture of these insecticides and in their use, extensive skin damage may be occasioned. In the powder form the offending agent may be pyrethrotoxic acid; in liquid forms, this combined with the solvent constitute damaging agents. In industry the disease state is more prevalent in summer months, due to the additional extracting action of perspiration. Allergic diseases from pyrethrum are more often in households than in industry.

Any toxicity connected with the industrial uses of *copper* is questionable, other than dermatitis and metal fume fever. Green perspiration and discoloration of hair may lead to an unwarranted degree of apprehension. The copper ion is no less toxic, if, in fact, it enters the body under any circumstance in quantities other than traces.

Creosote is an indefinite term covering various tarry substances from wood, coal, or petroleum. It contains many irritant constituents to the skin, eyes, and respiratory tract.

In the shaping of metal objects with lathes and similar machinery, coolants, cutting compounds and other *anti-friction agents* are in wide use. These agents may be oils or solutions of irritant salts, such as soda ash in emulsions. Irritation to the skin may be produced mechanically by the plugging up of the openings of the skin, sealing in effete materials, or by the direct action of the cutting compounds or their decomposition products. In addition, some harm may be created by bacteria from spitting into containers of these compounds.

Cyanides are extensively used in highly different industries, such as metal plating, case hardening, and insecticidal work. Action may be local, in the production of extensive ulceration, or systemic. The action is that of or is related to that of hydrocyanic acid. Cyanides are highly toxic industrial agents. Cyanides apart from causing skin disease act as internal asyhyxiants.

Dichloro-difluoromethane, used chiefly as a refrigerant, is a substance of low toxicity, acting solely or foremostly only as a simple asphyxiant, thus being dangerous only as it replaces oxygen in the respired air.

Dinitrobenzene is an intermediate in the manufacture of many chemicals, including dyes. It causes systemic disease, characterized by chocolate-colored blood, jaundice, marked loss of weight, labored breathing, mental sluggishness, impaired vision, and other changes. Its use by the obese to reduce weight is dangerous.

Ethyl benzene is a solvent for paraffins, resins, and lacquers. It causes dizziness, unsteady gait, trembling of extremities, slow, labored breathing, together with local irritation.

Ethylene dichloride is one of a series of chlorinated hydrocarbons with action similar to carbon tetrachloride. Its use is increasing in dry-cleaning plants, in the making of insecticides, in the disinfestation of grain elevators, etc.

Ethyl nitrate is a by-product in the manufacture of mercury fulminate. The latter is employed as detonator in gun cartridges. Exposure to fumes leads to low blood pressure, flushing of the skin, rapid heart, rapid respiration, excruciating headache, and abnormal temperature.

Formaldehyde is a gas, and when this gas is combined with water, formalin is produced. The liquid formalin exerts a destructive action on the skin. Formaldehyde vapors leave the solution. Systemic action is cumulative, leading to the degeneration of the liver and to nephritis. Severe damage may be done to the respiratory tract through irritation and subsequent edema.

Grain itch is a disease of the skin having many names, such as "prairie itch," "threshers' itch," "Texas mange," and "Ohio scratches." This disease is common around threshing operations and hay baling but may appear as a non-occupational disease in bunkhouses where straw mattresses are utilized. This disease is due to an animal parasite, an itch mite technically termed *pediculoides ventricosus.*

Granite is a form of siliceous rock with a high content of free silica. It is a common source of silicosis, to which disease reference should be made.

Heat, or the absence of heat, is the source of a number of specific occupational conditions, such as thermic fever, sunstroke, heat exhaustion, chilblains, etc. Heat is not the source of characteristic occupational diseases, but of ill-defined systemic impairments productive of degenerative diseases and fatigue. The specified conditions, with the exception of chilblains, may, with propriety, be regarded as accidental injuries.

*"Hex"—hexamethylenetetramine—*is known in medicine as urotropin; it was formerly used in the curing of rubber. It is now used in molding plastic objects, such as in bakelite molding. It is a source of severe dermatitis, which occurs more frequently in summer.

Hydrogen is an explosive gas with a low degree of toxicity. It is a simple asphyxiant, causing the displacement of oxygen. It is also a slight irritant to the eyes and is found about plating vats, battery charging, etc.

Hydrogen sulphide, a highly toxic gas widely distributed in industries, such as tanneries, artificial silk mills, and oil fields, is a source of ulcerated eyes. The upper limit of tolerance for this gas is only 20 ppm of air. Its odor is characteristic and any general concentration that imparts odor may be regarded as dangerous.

Some complex compounds of *hydroquinone* eliminate all skin pigmentation after extended contact. The skin of the Negro may become albino-like white. No injury is known, the damage being cosmetic and usually temporary.

The manufacture of many *insecticidal* agents designed for use in households and elsewhere involves hazardous exposure. Among others, potentially dangerous agents are chrysanthemum buds, formalin, ethylene dichloride, hydrocyanic acid, etc.

Kerosene is a petroleum distillate with a higher boiling point than benzine. The toxic properties are the same as those for benzine, only less dangerous because of a higher boiling point.

Lead constitutes a foremost occupational disease danger, with potential exposure in no less than two hundred different industries. Practically all forms of lead are poisonous, although the less soluble compounds constitute less dangerous hazards. This substance may enter the body through inhalation of dust, ingestion of dust, or paste (such as lead in oil), the drinking of fluid, such as lead-bearing drinking water; some organic lead compounds are absorbed through the skin. Minute traces, such as 1.5 mg. daily, may produce lead poisoning as a result of cumulative properties. Some persons are far less susceptible than others to lead. The principal lesions are found in the neuro-muscular system, circulatory system, gastro-intestinal tract, and brain.

Lime, chemically known as calcium oxide, may produce local burns of every degree of severity. These burns are deep, leading to tenacious eschars, which delay healing. Lime may contain impurities, including arsenic, that give rise to poisoning characteristic of these impurities.

Litharge is a form of lead oxide, much used in storage battery manufacture. The poison that may result from this substance is similar to that caused by other forms of lead.

Manganese is a metal associated in the ore form with zinc, lead, etc. Manganese enters the body primarily as a dust through inhalation and ingestion. After several months of exposure those who become affected gradually develop a deterioration of the central nervous system leading to permanent, irreparable paralysis. Patients develop masklike faces, become clumsy in all motions of the body, are unable to stop while in motion, and are permanently disabled. Manganese dust has been described as the cause of chemical pneumonia. This may be true in Europe, but is little known in the United States.

Meerschaum is a complex magnesium silicate. Mining and the shaping of articles from meerschaum lead to dusts that create a fibrosis of the lung tissues, similar to that from talc and possibly ashes too.

Mercury poisoning is one of the oldest occupational diseases, which has been well described by Ramazzini (1700), although he was not the first writer to discuss this subject. Both mercury and its compounds are the source of the poisoning. These intoxicants may enter the body through the skin, by inhalation, or by ingestion. No less than two hundred occupations provide exposure to mercury or its compounds or both. Outstanding manifestations are salivation, gastro-intestinal inflammation, urinary changes, skin ulceration, neuromuscular lesions, particularly tremors, and mental depression.

Mesothorium is a disintegration product of thorium, between thorium and radiothorium. This term, however, is applied to extensive series of similar bodies, such as thorium X, thoron, etc. Activity of commercial mesothorium is due to the presence of radium mesothorium I and its transformation products, alpha, beta, and gamma emanations.

Methyl alcohol, also designated by such terms as methanol, wood alcohol, Columbian spirits, wood naphtha, and wood spirits, may be made synthetically from the combination of carbon monoxide (or carbon dioxide) and hydrogen, under conditions of high pressure and temperature. The natural product is derived from wood distillation. Both the natural and the synthetic products are highly toxic. The threshold of toxicity is near the concentration of five hundred parts of vapor per million parts of air. Methyl alcohol may enter the body through the skin, by inhalation, and by ingestion. Characteristic lesions are optic atrophy, nephritis, toxic degeneration of the liver, gastro-intestinal, and pulmonary tract inflammation.

Methyl chloride is employed as a refrigerant and as such has been responsible for a number of cases of poisoning. Due to the fact that methyl chloride appears to decompose into wood alcohol in the body, the clinical manifestations are the same as those of methyl alcohol poisoning. Gross exposure leads to a primary intoxication, with death from narcosis. Known industrial accidents in hotels, apartment houses, etc., have been of the acute narcotic form. Death by methyl chloride from refrigerator leaks is well established.

Methyl violet is an aniline dye used in making indelible pencils. There is considerable variation in constituency of dyes termed methyl violet. This agent is especially toxic to the tissues of the eye. Necrosis of the cornea of the eye may readily be produced by flakes of indelible pencil lead material entering the eye. Puncture wounds from indelible pencils are healed with difficulty.

Mica is the name given various siliceous minerals, and dusts therefrom in any of its forms are siliceous. Silicatosis may be induced if the exposure to concentrated dust is prolonged. Mechanical injury of the skin from mica particles has long been recognized. Among other industrial uses, mica is employed in electrical insulation factories and in stove foundries.

Narcissus bulbs, which so closely resemble onions, contain a deadly alkaloid named narcissin. The eating of narcissus bulbs has caused deaths from the action of narcissin. Industrially, the only harm known to arise is a skin disease, which also is attributed to the narcissin.

The toxicity of *nickel* is often mentioned but rarely proved. Workers in nickel-plating departments truly develop divers intoxications, but in many instances these may be attributed to the adjuvants in plating departments rather than to nickel itself. The so-called nickel rash is a term covering practically all forms of dermatitis from whatever source arises around nickel-plating works. Nickel spectacle frames may cause a dermatitis on the wearer.

Nickel carbonyl is a clear, pale straw-colored liquid which boils at a temperature of 43° C. This salt is quite volatile and possesses toxic properties. In the milder forms of poisoning workers suffer from headache, giddiness, unsteady gait, nausea, and at times dyspnœa, which symptoms quickly disappear upon removal to fresh air. Severe poisoning is manifested by dyspnœa, which after a lapse of 12 to 36 hours is increased, accompanied by cyanosis, a rise in temperature with coughing, and with more or less bloodstained expectoration. The action of the heart is increased but otherwise normal. Delirium of varying types is generally present. Fatal termination of a case takes place usually from the fourth to the eleventh day of illness.

Nitrobenzene (oil of mirbane), an intermediate in the formation of aniline, may produce local skin burns, systemic disease from skin absorption, and intoxication by inhalation. Manifestations are weakness, loss of appetite, burning sensation of skin, abnormal sensation, anxiety state, reeling gait, stammering speech, abnormal reflexes, and convulsions. Later these may be followed by paralyses, amblyopia, brown-colored blood, methemoglobin, and in chronic cases yellow skin. Still later degeneration of red corpuscles and condition of hematoporphyrin are manifested. It is frequently fatal.

Nitrocellulose in its many forms is believed to be relatively harmless. Danger may arise from the many chemicals employed in its manufacture. It is possible that the coatings applied to nitrocellulose for special purposes, such as waterproofing, may be harmful.

Nitrogen oxides represent a series including the nitric, the dioxide, the tetroxide, etc. High concentrations such as 100 ppm may cause pulmonary edema. These oxides may be produced in connection with arc welding and less so in torch welding. Nitrous oxide is the well known laughing gas anesthetic.

Nitroglycerin is responsible for "dynamite head," a condition well known to blasters. The characteristic picture of nitroglycerin action is an intolerable headache associated with a rapid pulse. The keeping of a small portion of dynamite, or other explosive, about the person, perpetuates the tolerance, which apparently is readily established. Enough nitroglycerin may adhere to the clothes of explosive workers to bring about nitroglycerin harm to other persons in their homes. When nitroglycerin explodes, toxicity from the resulting gas is not due to nitroglycerin but to products of combustion.

Nitrous chloride is a highly irritating and asphyxiating gas, possessing insidious delayed action leading to pulmonary edema and respiratory tract inflammation. This gas is highly explosive, notwithstanding which fact it is somewhat extensively used in industry.

Nitrous gases or oxides are frequently encountered in industry such as in arc or torch welding. Of the series, nitric oxide is probably the most toxic, but as such is seldom found. Nitrogen dioxide is the more stable form, but even this in the presence of moisture is changed over into nitrous and nitric acid. The threshold of danger begins at about 100 ppm, but many published standards are at lower levels, such as 40 or even 10 ppm.

Phosgene or carbonylchloride is used as a chemical warfare agent as well as in industry. Its harmful action is apparently limited to the lungs, respiratory tract, and the blood stream, with secondary cardiac impairment. Violent lung inflammation develops with edema, later followed by necrosis of the lung tissue. Death frequently occurs. Lesser exposure may lead to minor degrees of impairment, as mentioned above, which eventuate in emphysema, bronchitis, bronchiectasis, and dysfunction of the heart.

Phosphorus, because of its toxicity, is not employed to any great extent in the United States at the present time. It is utilized, however, in the manufacture of fireworks, in the making of phospho-bronze, and in the chemical industry. White or yellow phosphorus is severely toxic. Susceptibility to poisoning varies. Red phosphorus is essentially free from toxicity. Phosphorus primarily acts upon the bones, leading to necrosis and periostitis. The common site of this bone affection is the jaw, entry of the phosphorus being made by way of carious teeth. Soft tissues in the region of the bone become involved as a secondary process. Phosphorus necrosis is a continuous process and may result in deformity or death.

Extensive exposure to *phosphureted hydrogen* leads to prompt death without .symptoms indicative of phosphorus poisoning. Symptoms are shortness of breath, marked gastro-intestinal irritation with vomiting and diarrhea, prostration, tremors, and finally active convulsions and death from respiratory failure. Long continued lesser exposure may lead to bone changes, nephritis, etc. Phosphureted hydrogen constitutes an insidious hazard in the manipulation of ferrosilicon, etc.

Recent advances in the field of insect control include the use of *organic phosphates,* examples of which are hexaethyl-tetraphosphate (HETP), tetraethyl-pyrophosphate (TEPP), which is the active toxic ingredient in HETP, and parathion, also known as Thiophos and Vapophos. These products are rapidly absorbed through the intact skin or by inhalation of their vapor or dust. Symptoms of poisoning are headache, nausea,· vomiting, dizziness, abdominal cramps, and constriction of the pupils of the eye. Manifestations of severe poisoning are a feeling of tightness in the chest, diarrhea, difficulty in breathing, twitching of the muscles, convulsions, or loss of consciousness. Poisoning can be prevented by proper attention to safe methods of handling. Contacts of bare skin must be avoided, and natural rubber gloves must be worn. Material that gets on the skin should be quickly removed with large amounts of soap and water. Cleanliness of clothing and skin is necessary and repellent garments where drenching of the clothing is possible. Adequately designed respirators may be necessary.

Picric acid or trinitrophenol enters the body through skin absorption, by inhalation, and by ingestion of dusts. The commonest lesion is a dermatitis (picric itch). This may be brought about by use of picric acid and picrates. In addition to the dermatitis, there may be yellow pigmentation of the skin suggesting jaundice, gastro-intestinal disturbance with pain, degeneration of the blood, nephritis, and degeneration of the liver.

Putty commonly contains ground whiting and linseed oil, but rarely lead compounds. Colored putties may contain skin-irritating dyes.

Pyrene is a trade name for one brand of carbon tetrachloride. When decomposed by heating, pyrene may give rise to phosgene vapors.

Quinine compounds have been the cause of a dermatitis among pharmaceutical workers; also of edema of eyelids with conjunctivitis and itching. It is a low-grade respiratory irritant.

In the manufacture of rayon and other artificial silks, many harmful agents may be utilized as intermediates and adjuvants. The outstanding objectionable agent is *carbon bisulphide.*

Rotogravure ink has been associated with dermatitis. Paranitraniline red or a similar substance is probably the active agent leading to that type of dermatitis. Readers of freshly printed rotogravure newspapers may become affected.

Sandstone is a silica-bearing rock with a high free silica content. It is known as a source of silicosis.

Sealing wax of various brands may differ in composition. It may contain resinous materials from coal tar or petroleum or from vegetable matter. At times it is colored with arsenic. Turpentine and other harmful solvents have been employed.

Sewer gas may contain hydrogen sulphide, carbon monoxide, carbon dioxide, any of which may lead to disasters.

Shellac itself, which is an Indian resin, is probably nontoxic, but may be a skin sensitizer. The substances in which it is dissolved may be poisonous, and in the past have caused many scores of poisonings and some deaths. As a solvent, wood alcohol has been the source of blindness and death.

Free silica, in any of its many forms, when taken into the body through the respiratory tract, in sufficient quantity, slowly leads to a dusty lung disease known as silicosis. Silicosis is probably the result of chemical action of the siliceous materials. Cases may be produced within less than one year of exposure, but the usual case requires several years to develop. Patients may complain of difficulty in breathing, of pain in the chest, of coughing, but often the disease is symptomless until far advanced. No treatment is efficacious. Tuberculosis is a common concomitant. This disease is encountered among workers in granite and sandstone quarrying, in stone dressing, in mining, and in foundries among many other industries.

Silver, or its salts, as used in industry, significantly is harmful from just one standpoint, and that is that it produces black deposits within the skin, a condition known as argyrosis.

Sulphur dioxide is the commonest household refrigerant, with the exception of ice. It is also used extensively in a variety of industries or is the product of other materials. Twenty parts per million of air will produce some irritation; fifty parts per million is dangerous. Injury chiefly is limited to the respiratory tract and to reflex actions. Contrary to common belief, tolerance for sulphur-dioxide action is not established. Chronic bronchitis and other persistent manifestations are well known. It may also produce acidosis.

Talc is magnesium silicate. As such, it is capable of producing fibrosis of the lungs.

Tannic acid may attack the unbroken skin and may partially tan the skin. A dermatitis is universally present among hide handlers in the tanning yard using the tannic acid process. When the skin is broken, deep undermining ulcers may arise. In low percentages tannic acid solutions constitute a valuable medicament for the treatment of skin burns.

Tar is a general term applied to a variety of substances derived from wood, coal, or petroleum. Tar cancer is a rare affection among persons exposed. Skin diseases and irritation of the respiratory tract are common.

Tetraethyl lead is an organic lead compound utilized as an antiknock substance in motor vehicles. The opportunities for intoxication are largely limited to the manipulation of this substance in its manufacture. It is one of the few forms of lead entering the body through the skin. Apparently this form of lead has a special predilection for brain tissues, leading to encephalitis.

Thallium, a toxic metal, forms salts which are useful in the making of rat poisons, in the preparation of depilatories and other pharmaceuticals, in disinfectants, in dye manufacture, and in lead alloys. When taken into the body it causes loss of hair, optic atrophy, distorted color vision, lymphocytosis, etc. On skin contact, hair is destroyed and possibly through skin absorption the other actions mentioned may arise.

The *tin* industry is attended by some exposures in mining, smelting, and refining, but these are probably due to impurities, heat, etc., rather than to any toxic properties of tin itself under industrial conditions. At the present time scant proof of the toxicity of tin exists, but some compounds of tin may be injurious.

The *tobacco* industry affords a number of opportunities for injury. Tobacco workers may acquire nicotine poisoning, but rarely do due to the development of a tolerance for this substance as does the tobacco smoker. Tuberculosis and other respiratory disease rates are reported as high in this industry, but a direct causative connection is not established. Arsenic is a potential danger from its use as an insecticide during the growing period. In the curing of tobacco, carbon dioxide is given off which may lead to asphyxiation. Cyanides are sometimes used for tobacco disinfection. High temperatures and humidities characterize certain departments.

Toluene (toluol) is closely related to benzene. It is advocated as a substitute for benzol, owing to lesser capacity for intoxication. It is more active as a narcotic agent than benzene, but less frequently produces chronic intoxication. When poisoning occurs, the clinical picture is similar to that of benzene poisoning.

Trichlorethylene is a chlorinated hydrocarbon akin in action to carbon tetrachloride.

Pure gum spirits of *turpentine* is less dangerous than other types, such as wood or steam distilled or naphtha extracted turpentine. It may, however, produce irritation of the skin and mucous membranes, gastritis, salivation, genito-urinary manifestations, etc.

Vanadium is a metal of restricted industrial use. Its salts find use in photography and in the manufacture of steels. Toxicity has been attributed especially to the trioxid. The outstanding manifestations are marked irritation of the respiratory tract, eventuating in hemorrhage, rapid loss of weight, nephritis, optic atrophy, and general condition simulating nervous breakdown. This condition is so rare as to be open to question as to its existence.

White damp is a term used by miners for carbon monoxide in mines. Black damp is ordinarily carbon dioxide. Stink damp is usually hydrogen sulphide.

Xylene (xylol) is chemically related to benzene (benzol). It is more toxic than benzene in producing acute narcosis, and is less toxic in the production of chronic conditions. The clinical disease produced, although rarely, is similar to that of benzene poisoning.

Industrial *zinc* is probably nontoxic. Recently produced zinc oxide, as in the manufacture of brass or in galvanizing, may lead to zinc chills, also termed brass chills, brass workers' ague, etc. The condition is characterized by great thirst, marked chilling with or without elevated temperature, eventuating in deep sleep with profound physical depression. Zinc is not involved in any chronic form of poisoning.

Zinc chloride is much used in wood preservation as a fire repellent and fungicide. It is associated with the production of dermatitis. Zinc sulphate produces marked alimentary tract inflammation, culminating, in severe cases, in ulceration of the stomach or duodenum.

All of the above items are but examples of industry's injurious work materials. Several hundred additional items might have been listed.

OCCUPATIONAL THERAPY Occupational therapy is recognized as a significant part of medical practice. Actually occupational therapy is employed in all sorts of diseases such as chronic arthritis, tuberculosis, chronic heart disease, and recovery from all forms of paralysis. Indeed occupational therapy is needed whenever a person is confined to bed for a fairly long period of time. Occupational therapy varies, moreover, from the kind of work that can be carried on when the patient is flat on his or her back in bed to the therapy that is carried on by patients who move about and use all kinds of machinery. It may begin with such light work as basketry, weaving, braiding and drawing and move on to the building of looms, ornaments and furniture or power apparatus.

Now let us see how occupational therapy can be helpful to an injured workman. Here is a man whose hand was badly cut. The wound may be healed but the fingers are still stiff and the tendons which move the fingers may be bound down as a result of infection and lack of use. This man is obviously not fit to return to work. It would be quite possible for a masseur to give him hours of treatment every day and thus to bring about suitable motion in the hand, but the man himself might not thus be encouraged to make such use of the hand as would be required for complete recovery. He might get a great deal of benefit from weaving, using a small hand loom and shuttle of a proper size to fit his grip.

Incidentally some of these patients who are using occupational therapy get so interested in the work that they begin using the well hand instead of the damaged one. Every patient must be studied, however, to pick out for him a job that is suitable to his particular disability.

Here is a man with an injury of the ankle who has lost strength because of the injury and whose tissues are stiff because of the swelling and lack of use. He can be put to work on a foot power scroll-saw with pedals like those of a bicycle. The pedals can be adjusted so that only a slight motion of the ankle is required and then can be gradually changed so that increased motion occurs. At first he will work on a thin, soft piece of wood which requires little foot power. Then as his strength increases, hard wood and thicker wood will be supplied so as to give him opportunity for the greatest improvement. It is also possible to adjust these pedals so that the greatest pressure will come on the front of the foot or on the heel so as to give the best result for this patient.

As you go through the school, you will find some patients working at benches doing carpentry and using planes, screwdrivers, saws and hammers. You will find other patients doing metal work. Some will be weaving. Some will be making toys. Others will be learning book binding, printing, pottery, wrought iron, willow or cement work. And not all of it is work! Frequently games like pool or billiards will accomplish the same motions that may be accomplished by work, but there is something about the accomplishments associated with work by the production of a finished object that is more stimulating even than winning a game of pool or billiards.

The person who learns to do occupational therapy must be not only a teacher of motions but a psychologist. It is necessary to keep in mind the former occupation of the patient and to select a type of work with which he is familiar. If, however, the tissues have been damaged so that there is no opportunity for the patient to return to his former occupation, it will become necessary to direct the training to employment in a different field.

Occupational therapy is scientific.

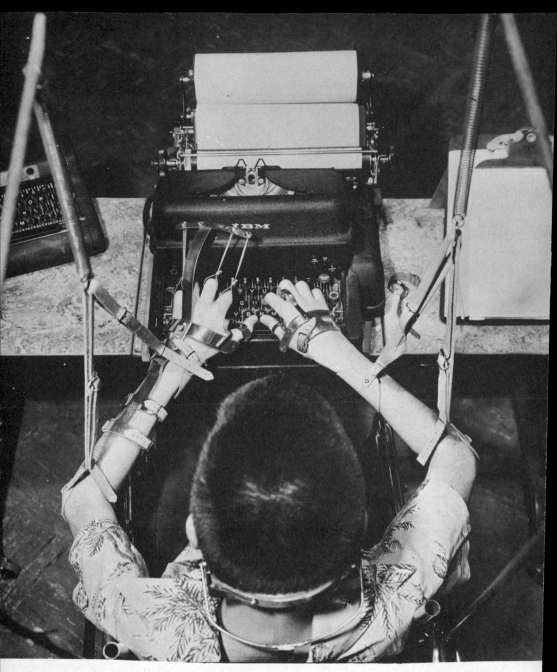

With the use of special appliances handicapped persons are able to engage in various handicrafts and pursuits of interest under the guidance and encouragement of the occupational therapist. In one of the photographs a patient is seen "re-learning" to feed himself during occupation therapy. The young lady who is painting is developing a latent talent.

National Foundation For Infantile Paralysis

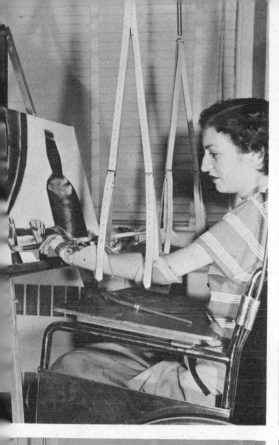
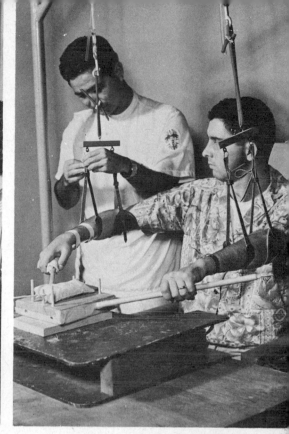
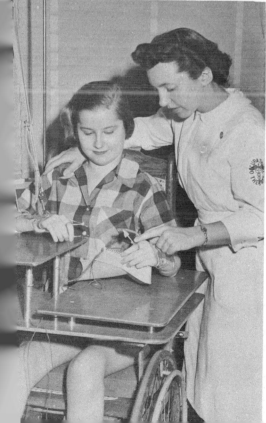
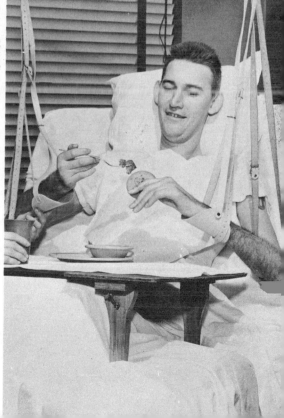

Records are kept of the work from day to day so that the therapists will know exactly how much improvement is occuring and thus be able to determine whether or not the methods used are successful. A person who is left-handed must be taught left-handed work, but if the left hand is so injured that it seems impossible to continue with the left hand, the right hand must be taught to function. Moreover, always the occupational therapist must keep in mind the fact that he or she is working not with well people but with sick people. All of the work must be definitely related to the sickness of the patient and the conditions that are desired to be reached—also those which obtain at the moment.

ODORS Among human beings the ability to smell varies greatly. Few, if any, human beings have the power to detect odors and to identify those odors in relation to certain hazards that attaches to many of the lower animals. Moreover, the ability to detect odors by the use of the olfactory nerves and the portion of the brain associated with them may be seriously damaged by such ordinary conditions as the common cold or allergy.

Several devices have been invented for measuring the ability to detect odors, one of them inelegantly named the "stinkometer." This apparatus consists simply of a lot of bottles with chemical solutions which respond to certain chemical substances that are associated with vaporized materials. One stinkometer is used to evaluate the freshness of foods by measuring the odors.

Doctors recognize a condition called anosmia, which means a complete loss of the capacity to smell. This may be permanent or temporary, depending on whether or not it involves damage of the nervous structures or their complete destruction. If a person loses the sense of smell on only one side, it is called hemianosmia. Such defects in smelling may be due to dryness of the mucous membranes in the nose, infection, injuries, the actions of drugs or deterioration of the tissues. The term hyposmia means a partial loss of the ability to detect odors, whereas hyperosmia means that there is an excessive response to odors. This may be associated with hysteria or may result from excessive irritability of the tissues involved in smelling.

Sometimes people think they are smelling something when the reaction is purely mental. Some people complain of constantly smelling fish; others of smelling roses—which is certainly more pleasant. The sensation of smelling an odor that does not exist may be the result of a hallucination.

If the doctor can find something positive in the tissues to account for disturbances of the olfactory sense, the patient is fortunate. Such conditions are frequently correctable. Most difficult of all are the cases in which the disturbances related to odors are mental.

The ordinary healthy person is not subject to offensive odors, provided he keeps himself clean. Some people who work in sewers, stockyards, and chemical works, as well as students in dissecting rooms, carry odors around with them to which they have become quite accustomed but which are immediately detectable by other people. One of the chief advantages of air conditioning in modern industry is the help it gives in getting rid of disturbing smells, some of which may be of human origin.

In many instances people have unpleasant odors on the surface of the body which cannot be controlled by bathing or changing garments. Everyone knows that garlic can produce a smell about the body, which is frequently associated with nationalities that have a great deal of garlic in their diets.

Young people are usually less odorous than older people. Sometimes odors attach to people who suffer with disease conditions such as diabetes or cancer. These represent in most instances disintegration of tissues. The odor frequently associated with feet is due to maceration of the skin between the toes.

Certain drugs are known which can diminish the output of perspiration and thus control unpleasant odors. Furthermore the use of the X ray, which must be done only by experts because of the danger, can destroy sweat glands and thus diminish odors.

ODORS—associations: See EAR, article THE EAR, TONGUE, NOSE, AND THROAT.

OLD AGE   See *Senescence.*

Old Age

BY

MORRIS FISHBEIN, M.D.

Former Editor, *Journal American Medical Association;* Chicago; Editor, *Excerpta Medica, Bulletin World Medical Assn.; Post-graduate Medicine.*

ALTHOUGH ONE HUNDRED YEARS of life is possible to human beings, only 30 people in 3,000,000 reach that age. And more than two thirds of the persons who do reach that age are women. The reason for this latter fact is that women are usually less exposed to accident and infection and, what is more important, are more apt to lead temperate lives.

Census figures from Great Britain show that the average number of persons more than 100 in the British Isles is about 110, and that 80 of this number are women.

These figures are not absolutely accurate, since most old people are proud of their age and tend to exaggerate. For example, in nearly every census, more people who give their ages as over 91 are found than people who give their ages as between 85 and 90. British health authorities assume that many jump from 85 to 91 in a year or two.

THE SPAN OF LIFE

However, the span of life is gradually increasing. And in time we may expect to have more and more people above 90. The chief reason for this remains the rapid decline in death rates for infants. Thus, a man born in 1854 had a life expectancy of 40 years. Now he may reasonably expect to live to be 68. Having reached the age of 60, a man's expectancy of life is now 14½ years, and a woman's 16 years.

Since heredity seems to play a large part in longevity, it is conceivable that encouragement of intermarriage between families that tend to live long would produce stock that tended to live long. However, such experiments among humans are almost impossible, and this theory must remain largely a matter of conjecture.

One of the real problems we have to face is to make the lives of the aged happier and healthier. They must realize their own shortcomings in regard to strength and ability to throw off disease, while those around them should always take into consideration the changes which come with advanced age. If older persons observe the simple rules of health, there is no reason why their declining years should not be happy.

CHANGES IN OLD AGE

One of the things which every person over sixty must realize is that his organs are functioning more slowly than in his youth and that allowances must be made for this change. The glands tend to function less in old age, so that the skin becomes dry. Even the gastric juice carries a lower percentage of hydrochloric acid, and for this reason there is difficulty with digestion. Moreover, the mucus in the intestines becomes less, so that there is a tendency to dryness of the intestinal contents and therefore to constipation.

One of the significant changes in old age is the blunting of sensibility to pain. This is very important, because the breaking down of the tissues leads to sensations that are uncomfortable. For the same reason disease in old age comes insidiously.

Whereas pneumonia, heart disease, stones in the kidney or gall bladder may cause agonizing pain to a young person, they come on so insidiously in older ones they may be unrecognized until they have reached the point where help is difficult. Even cancer comes on insidiously in the aged.

The sensations of taste and smell also become weaker, so that food is not so appetizing. Everyone knows also that sight and hearing are greatly depreciated in the elderly.

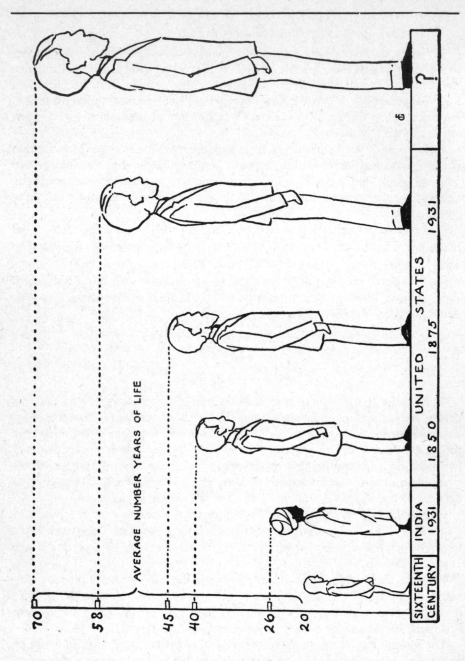

AVERAGE NUMBER YEARS OF LIFE

70 58 45 40 26 20

SIXTEENTH CENTURY | INDIA 1931 | 1850 | 1875 | UNITED STATES | 1931 | ?

Life expectancy.

One of the most interesting aspects of old age is the change in the mind and ability to sleep. Because the aged sleep less continuously, they frequently estimate the amount of sleep at much less than it really is. However, it is quite certain the aged are able to use much less sleep than vigorous, active people, and it is not desirable to get them into the habit of taking sedative drugs. It is likely, according to Sir Humphry Rolleston, that excessive sleep is more harmful to them than too little.

The mind becomes much more easily fatigued in old age than in middle age. Gradually the power of affection wanes in the old, perhaps because they have become habituated to the loss of relatives and friends. Possibly they are more self-centered; time passes slowly, and their minds are occupied with their own feelings.

THE BODY IN OLD AGE

In Great Britain a foundation was established to study the problem of aging and the care of old people. They point out that old age is actually a quality of mind and body and that the time of onset of old age varies from person to person. For a number of reasons old age has been taken to begin at 60 for women and 65 for men, and these figures are taken as standard in pension acts.

People in advanced years require more medical attention than do those of younger ages. Nevertheless, one fourth of all the old people studied had gone for three years or more without seeking medical aid and in many instances had virtually never required any. More than 12 per cent of the people had gone so long since seeing a doctor that they could not remember when the last time was, and more than 7 per cent were certain that they had 20 years or .more of good health.

They found relatively little undernourishment among the old people; in fact, only 3 per cent were classed as undernourished. The chief nutritional disturbance was a lack of iron, which affected about 5 per cent of the women.

It was found also that men tend to remain normal in body build as they grow old, whereas women show much growth variation in the direction of either leanness or stoutness. Twenty-five per cent of women over 85 years of age were undeniably obese.

As people grow old, they find more or less difficulty in getting around as well as they used to. Only 2½ per cent of the people over 60 years of age were confined to bed, and it was thought that the figure was low because old people who live at home have in most instances to help in looking after themselves. For that reason, if the aged find it necessary to be continuously in bed, they are transferred to institutions.

Almost one-fourth of the old people were capable of only limited getting about in their immediate districts. After 70 years of age the specific symptoms of old age are likely to become emphasized. These include weakness, dizziness, difficulty with traffic, inflammation of the back and lack of confidence.

Caring for old people at home puts a severe burden on the younger generation, many of whom carry this strain for years and years without relief.

Stairs are a particular problem when old people are concerned and when they are in poor health. At least one-third of old people have trouble getting up and down stairs or both ways. Stairs are especially a hazard when they are steep and when they lack a rail. Whenever old people are compelled to use stairs, there should be a rail to help them. Over 6 per cent of old people were unable to use stairs at all. The trouble with stairs was especially hard on old women because of their desire to participate in housework. Old people themselves recognize the special problem that is presented by stairs, and a large majority think that bungalows are the ideal type of home.

Among the medical conditions that affect old people most are rheumatism or arthritis, the effects of falls or accidents, and bronchitis.

Almost half of all old people are troubled with coughs, and men more than women. Rheumatic conditions of one kind or another affect more than half, and they vary from just twinges of pain to crippling incapacity from involvement of the joints. Women are more frequently affected than men, and this is particularly hard on them because of the nature of their work in the household.

Men have a liability to gout nearly ten times that of the women. Pain in the feet affects nearly 40 per cent of the old people and women twice as often as men. Another symptom that causes much distress is frequency and urgency of emptying the bladder. This affects one-third of all the old people. It is commoner in women than in men, and it makes shopping difficult.

Difficulties in hearing affect men more than women. Some dizziness is experienced by at least 75 per cent of the women over 85 years of age, and difficulty in getting about in the dark is a symptom for more than 90 per cent of women over 85. However, in general, old people are extremely unsteady in walking, some of it due to dizziness, some to failure to lift the feet properly.

DISEASES OF OLD AGE

Even premature senility may occur in youth. Heart disease, atrophy of the brain, and hardening of the arteries may also occur in comparatively young people. However, most of the diseases that occur in the aged are the result of gradual breaking down of the tissues. These include hardening of the arteries, heart failure, hardening of the liver, enlargement of the prostate, cancer, obesity, and indigestion. However, old age does modify any disease, so that it is different from the same condition in youth.

Measles, scarlet fever, typhoid, and diphtheria occur very rarely in old people, probably because they have been infected in youth and thereby developed immunity from these diseases. The form of sick headache called migraine usually becomes less troublesome as age advances and may disappear with increasing years. A recent conception of this disease indicates that it may be the result of sensitivity to some protein food substance, and perhaps the repeated attacks eventually bring about desensitization.

Even when an aged person is in good health, he must keep a close watch for the diseases to which his age makes him particularly susceptible. Happiness for all elderly persons is principally a matter of health, and so health must be guarded more and more closely as time goes on.

The changes that occur in the skin of the aged are due to gradual loss of activity on the part of the glands and of the tissues responsible for immunity. Because the aged are likely to be a little less scrupulous in the care of the skin, slight infections occur repeatedly. There are also bed sores. Itching is a stimulus to severe scratching and secondary infections take place in the scratches.

The blood vessels may lose their contractile power, and there are occasionally tiny hemorrhages under the skin. One of the most severe conditions that affects the aged is the reaction called herpes zoster. It is a form of shingles which develops along the course of a nerve and which in the aged may be exceedingly painful. Moreover, once the attack has passed, the pains may continue and return at intervals without the eruption. These conditions must be watched closely and treated immediately.

Of course, the aged suffer frequently with dizziness due to many possible causes. Sometimes it is due to accumulated hard wax in the ear, sometimes to changes that have taken place in the internal ear; frequently it is associated with high blood pressure, hardening of the arteries, and changes in the circulation of the blood in the brain. Sometimes the result is a difficulty of coördination between the eye, the ear, and the sense of balance, so that the aged may stagger or fall when the eyes are raised suddenly or under some similar stimulus.

One of the diseases more likely to occur in the aged than in the young is paralysis agitans, or the shaking palsy. Although this disease may occur in youth, the vast majority of cases occur in people between fifty and seventy years of age. The disease occurs twice as often in men as in women. It is marked by tremor of the hands, with a pill-rolling movement, and it tends to progress, running a complete course in from ten to fifteen years.

The aged should be especially careful to consult a good physician when any of the symptoms described in this article occur. While they may be simple results of old age, without more serious implication, they should be checked at frequent intervals by the family doctor.

EXERCISE AND HYGIENE

Old people have particular difficulty in walking, for many reasons. First, there may be weakening in the circulation; sometimes pain in the muscles results from imperfect circulation. Often older persons walk with short steps, because in this way they are better able to control their sense of balance.

While the aged may have high blood pressure, it is not so serious as in youth.

Of course, old people suffer with disturbances of digestion because of the changes that have taken place in their secretions, and also because they have difficulty in keeping infection away from their teeth and because they do not chew the food properly. The constipation of old age is now largely controlled by the taking of mineral oil which serves the purpose of softening the intestinal mass and making elimination easy. This remedy is practically harmless and adds years of health to many older persons. Hemorrhoids are frequent in the aged and are, of course, associated with constipation.

There was a time when the teeth of the human being gradually fell out as he grew older so that he found himself, by the time he reached old age, able to take only liquid food or food that was soft. Modern dentistry has made it possible for the aged to chew steaks or vegetables of considerable fibrous content. It is for this reason that the aged must frequently resort to laxatives or to mineral oil in order to aid the weakened intestinal muscles in handling the waste material.

The aged are likely to suffer particularly with accumulations of mucous material in the lungs; with diminished power of the lungs to repair themselves, small areas of degenerated tissue break down, and the material accumulates and has to be coughed out of the lung. The continued inhalation and coughing results in disturbances such as bronchopneumonia or similar complaints.

The elderly are particularly prone to varicose veins, to inflammations of the joints, and to fixed joints which follow inflammation.

CANCER IN OLD AGE

Cancer has always been recognized by the medical profession as a disease of old age. More recently it has seemed to occur fairly frequently among younger people, and there are many explanations advanced for this fact. It is recognized that heredity plays a large part in cancer, and that inbreeding may bear some responsibility. The British statistician, Karl Pearson, found that the maximum incidence of cancer occurs at the age of forty-six in women, and of fifty-six in men. The chief cancer period is from forty-six to sixty-four years.

It is well established that cancer is associated with long continued irritation of susceptible spots in the tissue. Obviously aged people are more subject to long continued irritation than are the young. Men suffer, of course, much more frequently than do women with cancer of the lips and tongue, perhaps because of their smoking habits. Even though women have begun to smoke cigarettes regularly, it is unlikely that they will suffer as much with cancer of the lips and tongue as do men, because women are much more careful about the state of their mouths and teeth. Men suffer with cancer of the prostate; women with cancer of the organs particularly concerned with childbearing.

There have been many attempts to explain cancer in old age, but all of them are theoretical. In old age the degenerative process in the cells leads to the formation of new tissue, and the repeated demands made on the cells in this way may result in the sudden rapid growth that is called cancer. Warthin, eminent pathologist, considered cancer to be merely a sudden rapid aging of a group of cells.

Whatever the cause may be, older persons should be especially careful to treat all slight infections and to visit a physician if these irritations do not respond readily to treatment.

The chapter on cancer in this book gives the most recent and reliable information available.

THE CRITICAL AGE FOR MEN

Pediatricians say that the first year of life is the most critical. Others insist that the first 10 years are the hardest. Some call adolescence with the transition from childhood to adult life the most critical period.

The great control that is now asserted over infant mortality and the elimination of many of the diseases that used to affect youth make the majority of doctors today think that the most serious age is the period of transition from maturity to old age. Men enter the most critical period of their lives at 50.

This is the time when they begin to need glasses to read the print in the telephone book. Now they begin to get tired a little earlier in the afternoon.

Occasionally, the onset of these conditions induces resentment. Many a physical culture expert or the proprietor of a health institute or a gymnasium has earned an excellent livelihood from the fact that these men take up exercise and try to prove to themselves that they are better than they really are. The wise man will realize that aging is a natural process and that the conditions that come with advancing years must be treated with respect. If the thyroid gland, the sex glands and the pituitary are less efficient, the deficiency will be reflected in the body generally. A doctor can prescribe glandular substances to overcome such deficiencies in part.

Hardening of the arteries and high blood pressure are two of the most important symptoms. Many years ago a wise physician said that a man is as old as his arteries. Incidentally, men are more frequently affected with hardening of the arteries than are women.

Arthritis is another condition that occurs many times to people after the age of 40 and which cripples and disables a good many older people.

Medicine can do a great deal for these disturbances if they are brought soon enough to medical attention. But man is not immortal and the wise man will recognize the aging process and conduct himself accordingly.

THE OLD MAN AND THE JOB

Women in the home keep on at their job of running the household and taking care of the family as long as they are able. Many of them find work ready to handle even up to seventy-five or eighty years of age. By contrast the man retired at anywhere from sixty to seventy years of age may find himself full of the desire to work and produce and to contribute to the public good and yet be shut out of his opportunity to do the work that he can do best.

The professional man who can serve as a doctor, a lawyer, a clergyman, an artist or a writer can keep on without too much difficulty. The worker in industry finds the situation much more difficult, regardless of his physical or mental age. As a man gets older he loses speed and those who operate machines find that they cannot keep up. Furthermore, the conditions of industry do not provide for continued work at a lesser wage but insist that the full wage be paid regardless of advancing years. Insufficient study has been given to the kinds of work that are especially suited to the older worker, aside from employment as a timekeeper or foreman or administrator. If the old men are kept on too long the younger men complain that there is no opportunity to rise in the establishment. Power and increased income are likely to go with promotion and few old men wish to go back to positions of less influence or income.

Many men anticipate with the greatest of pleasure the day when they are to retire from work. These are the men who dislike the job to begin with, and who have an avocation which gives pleasure and to which they can devote themselves after retirement.

Physicians are convinced that a busy rather than an aimless life is the ideal prescription for old age. For too many instances are known of fairly young men who retired only to die within a few years from what seemed simply to be the ultimate effects of boredom and self-neglect.

A survey in Britain showed that the care of the aged for the most part rests on the family, and then the neighbors where there is real community life and spirit. In one community 57% of the burden rested on one daughter and there was little indication that multiple daughters shared the responsibility. Usually it was the youngest daughter that carried the burden, and the older ones reserved the right of criticism.

EMOTIONAL PROBLEMS OF OLDER PEOPLE

An editorial in the American Journal of Public Health calls attention to recent scientific studies of the special emotional hazards that are characteristic of advancing years.

As people grow older they develop limitations on vision and hearing and a reduction of physical activity and of endurance. They also begin to have difficulties in remembering and in coördination. Fortunately the specialists in sight and hearing are now able to give great aid toward supplementing weaknesses in sight and hearing. We are also learning much about rehabilitation and measures for helping people who are failing physically.

Older people often begin to find incomes steadily reducing with expenses steadily increasing. True social security aims to help in meeting the situation but other trends incline toward putting older workers completely on the shelf.

Many older people having given up their steady occupations have failed to develop any hobbies or outside interests to which they can turn their attention. Their lives assume continuous boredom and ultimate depression.

As a husband or wife is lost the friends of the family incline to fall away from the remaining member and social contacts diminish leading to loneliness and introversion.

In ancient societies the aged were viewed with respect and came to be the Nestors, advisers and counsellors. Our modern civilization drifts to an opposite extreme where all the emphasis is placed on youth.

The American Journal of Public Health says "we would do well to recognize the assets as well as the liabilities of senescence; to train ourselves in middle age for ripe and fruitful later years; to provide the medical and psychiatric and rehabilitative aids needed for healthy aging; and to regard the elderly not as outcasts but as essential and potentially valuable elements in the life of the family, the neighborhood and the nation."

Useful (youthful) old age. From left to right, starting at the top: Luther Burbank (1849-1928), American naturalist, author, and plant originator. Had more than 3000 experiments under way at age 77. Benjamin Franklin (1706-1790), American statesman and philosopher. Attended Constitutional Convention at age 75; president of Pennsylvania at age 73. Thomas Alva Edison (1847-1931), American electrician and inventor. In last years was still conducting extensive experiments and improving existing inventions. George Washington Carver (1864-1942), agricultural researcher. Developed over 300 products from the peanut alone. Robert Latou Dickinson (1861-19), gynecologist and author. Created birth series models at age 78 for Chicago World's Fair. Susan B. Anthony (1820-1906), American suffragist and reformer. Delegate to International Council of Women at London at age 79. Clara Barton (1821-1912), American philanthropist who founded the Red Cross. Was active in relief work in Cuba at age 77. George W. Crile (1864-1943), internationally known Cleveland surgeon. Founder of Cleveland Clinic and a medical researcher. George Bernard Shaw (1856-1950), Irish dramatist and critic who led a full and active life.   Cleveland Health Museum

OLDER PEOPLE (See also discussion under *Death Rate, Fall in, Degenerative Changes, Senescence*) Life expectancy at birth now approximates the Biblical three score years and ten for men but women live longer. The aged used to be 3% of the population. Now people over 65 constitute almost 10%. The specialty which does research on problems of the aged and takes care of old people is geriatrics.

An Ohio state psychologist surveyed accomplishments of several thousand outstanding older people. Advancing years bring certain strengths, knowledge, and judgment which are impossible for people in their early youth and maturity. An elderly physician continued to serve his long-standing patients, his practice becoming largely geriatric and his competence enhanced by his long acquaintance with his patients. A law-

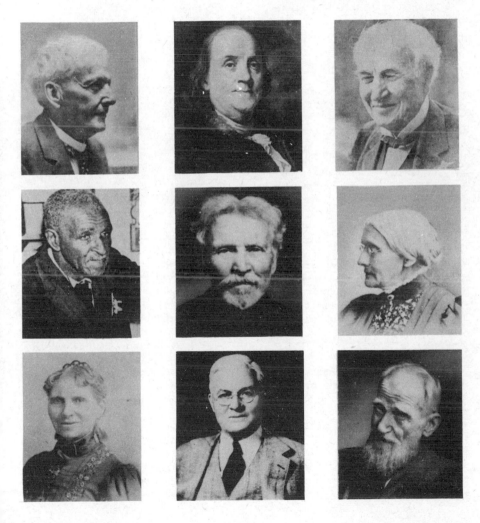

yer well up in years became a specialist in local property problems in a city where he had spent most of his life. A 97-year-old entomologist wrote a history of his field. A 92-year-old former newspaper man served his community as justice of peace. No longer able to continue his highly skilled work, a 72-year-old mechanic in a small manufacturing firm continued his employment there where he was put in charge of the tool cage.

A group was organized in St. Louis in 1954 to make the accumulated experience of its members available, without charge, to social, civic, and business enterprises. Queried on the compensations of old age, most of the members listed more advantages than handicaps. Prominent among the advantages listed were those which result from leisure and lessened business pressure—"more time to do the things that one has always wished to do," and "more time and relaxations." "Better understanding of life's problems," and "freedom from false and unimportant desires," were also listed as advantages of age.

OLFACTORY The sense of smell is known as the olfactory sense. This may be disturbed in a variety of conditions. Frequently in examining for disturbances of the brain, tests are made of the ability to smell various odors.

OMENTUM The omentum is a large membrane which is a part of the peritoneum, or lining of the abdominal cavity. It covers various organs of the abdomen and portions of the omentum extend from the stomach to adjacent organs. Like other tissues of the body, it may become inflamed and subject to various infections or tumors requiring surgical procedures.

OMENTUM—See article DIGESTION AND DIGESTIVE DISEASES.

OPEN HEART SURGERY (See also discussion under *Surgery of the Heart*) Open heart surgery has been found to be *corrective* surgery for congenital defects which would otherwise lead to increasing disability. Since 1952, Dr. C. Walton Lillehei of the University of Minnesota stated 160 cases have been operated in this way. He feels that in a few years, most operations on the heart will be done by the open heart technique or by hypothermia. The latter, however, is more successful with lesions higher in the heart such as atrial septal defects because of the cooling effects to conduction mechanism. The lower chambers with interventricular septal defects are better dealt with by the cross circulation technique. Earlier work on these defects utilized the arterial reservoir method and the canine lung preparation to oxygenate the blood during open heart surgery.

In the cross circulation donor technique, the oxygenation of the patient's blood takes place in the pulmonary circulation of the donor, through transference tubing and pumps.

The artificial oxygenator has been in use since March 1955. In this system, plastic tubing is utilized along with a pump mechanism to provide external artificial oxygenation. With this system, there have been 47 patients operated on, with a survival of 33 patients.

This open heart technique has been particularly helpful, and life saving, in the repair of ventricular septal defects; as 50% of these patients usually die before the age of one year.

Seventy-five cases of this type have been done with a survival risk of 75% It is felt that the risk of operation is greater when the pulmonary artery pressure is greater than 70% of the aortic pressure. The ideal candidate for this procedure was found when the patient was older than two years, had no associated heart lesions, and the pulmonary artery pressure was between 60/40 and 80/50. There have been no deaths in the group of patients in this category.

OPHTHALMIA An inflammation of the eye is called ophthalmia. The term "ophthalmus" refers to the eye and there are a wide variety of conditions with the prefix "ophthal-." Thus ophthalmoplegia is a paralysis of the eye; ophthalmitis, an inflammation of the eye; ophthalmoscope, an instrument for looking into the eye; ophthalmology, the study of diseases of the eye, and a specialist in diseases affecting the eye is known as an ophthalmologist.

OPHTHALMIA, SYMPATHETIC—See EYE, article THE EYE.

OPHTHALMOSCOPE—See PHYSICIAN, article THE CHOICE OF A PHYSICIAN; EYE, article THE EYE.

ORCHITIS Orchitis is an inflammation of the testicle. The prefix "orchid-" has nothing to do with the flower of the same name but in medicine is used to refer to any condition affecting the testicle. When there is inflammation of the testicles, the symptoms include pain, swelling, and a feeling of weight. Such an inflammation may be due to the organism of gonorrhea or to any other germ such as that of tuberculosis or syphilis. Treatment depends altogether on determining the nature of the disturbance. Sometimes surgery is required.

ORTHO- The prefix "ortho-" in medicine means straight. Thus orthopedics has to do with the correction of deformities of the joints and spine; orthodontia with the straightening of the teeth; orthopsychiatry with the straightening out of behavior and personality.

OSTEOARTHRITIS (See also discussion under *Arthritis*) Few real advances have been made in the attack on this disease. The cortisone drugs when they are administered properly will sometimes afford partial relief of the pain and stiffness but experts now feel that in the majority of patients the disability is not sufficient to warrant the possible side effects of these drugs. Many studies have been made of the relationship of the hormones to degenerative joint diseases and the entire matter is still under study.

In attempting to arrive at the nature of osteoarthritis the electron microscope has been used. These studies have shown that with advancing years there is a gradual and irregular disappearance of the fluid mucoid material that is responsible for holding water in the cartilages. Much of the tissue's elastic property seems to depend on the presence of a chemical called chondroitin sulfate which is a portion of the cartilage. This substance is gradually lost in osteoarthritis. The loss of chondroitin probably accounts for the decreased resilience and increased susceptibility to wear and tear that comes with aging and with osteoarthritis. As these changes occur in the cartilages, particularly of the spine, new formation of bone and projecting tissues develop which in turn affect the nerves; the nerves are injured by the shortening of the spine that occurs due to degeneration of the cartilagenous discs between the vertebra; sharp angulation of the nerve roots may result and with this comes irritation and degeneration of nerve fibers.

The use of the X ray shows that some osteoarthritis is found in all elderly persons ·but symptoms that require medical care develop in only about 10%. Even the abnormal stresses that develop from overweight and occupational strain are not however sufficient to explain all of the phenomena of this disease. Hence both heredity and altered glandular functions are taken into account as exerting some influence. In studying cases of osteoarthritis, doctors found that degenerative changes of the terminal joints of the fingers with the formation of the little lumps that are called Heberden's nodes have a striking familial tendency. They appear predominantly in women to the extent to about ten to one and they are most likely to begin during the menopause.

OSTEOMYELITIS   Osteomyelitis is an infection of the bones of the body. Most of these cases are due to the pusforming organisms like the staphylococcus and the streptococcus but instances are known in which the pneumococcus and the typhoid germ caused osteomyelitis.

In most cases the germs get into the bones by way of the blood stream. Occasionally, however, infections in the tissues near the bones work through into the bony area. This happens particularly when a bone is infected from a joint.

The long bones of the body, like the bones of the legs and arms, are most frequently affected but any bone may be involved. It is known that infections of the jawbone are much more serious than a similar infection in a long bone.

The first sign of osteomyelitis is pain in the infected bone. This comes on suddenly and is associated with fever and rapid pulse and all of the usual signs of infection. Frequently also there are swelling, redness, and the other signs of disturbance at the spot that is infected.

When the doctor makes an examination of the blood, he will find that there has been a great increase in the white blood cells. The child with an infection of the bone will probably refuse to have the arm or leg examined and will be apprehensive about having it touched.

Because the bones are associated with the production of blood for the body and because the blood may carry the infection from a bone throughout the body, osteomyelitis is always a serious condition. When just one bone is involved, the difficulty is, of course, much less than in the case of multiple osteomyelitis because cases are known in which the infection has attacked one bone after another, and in the past, cases have been seen in which twelve or thirteen different bone abscesses have developed in the same person.

Nowadays with the use of the X ray and modern methods of diagnosis, osteomyelitis is discovered and treated much sooner than used to be the practice thirty or forty years ago. Before the discovery of the sulfonamide drugs and of penicillin, there were few remedies which were able to get at a deep-seated infection in the bone. These newer remedies, however, which have a specific effect on the streptococcus, the staphylococcus, and the pneumococcus, are able to do much more in controlling osteomyelitis. Nevertheless, good medical practice still demands surgical treatment so that the bone is opened, the damaged and infected tissue removed, and the infected area treated directly with applications of penicillin as well as by injection of penicillin into the muscles or into the blood.

In a previous generation osteomyelitis affecting the jawbone was considered to be an almost invariably fatal disease. The astounding recovery of several such cases treated with penicillin was the most impressive observation early in the use of this amazing drug.

Indeed the publication of the reports of these cases focused the attention of all the medical world on the great value of penicillin for the control of infections by the pus-forming germs.

OSTEOPATHY Osteopathy is a system of treatment of disease in which there is manipulation of the bones, joints, and other tissues of the body with a view to restoring what is conceived to be a deranged mechanism. The osteopaths themselves define osteopathy as "that system of the healing art which places the chief emphasis on the structural integrity of the body mechanism, as being the most important single factor to maintain the well-being of the organism in health and disease." In many states osteopaths are limited wholly to such manipulations. The osteopathic course of instruction now includes some college education and four years of osteopathic education in which osteopaths are taught something about germs and drugs. Thus in some states osteopaths are also permitted to prescribe certain drugs and to undertake surgical procedures.

OTITIS MEDIA, OR MIDDLE EAR INFECTION (See also, *Ear Infection* of the interior of the ear after a sore throat is not nearly so frequent as such infections used to be. The specific action against staphylococci, pneumococci, streptococci, and other germs that infect noses and throats wrought by the antibiotic drugs and the sulfonamides has enormously reduced such complications. However, neglect of a sore throat or a virulent infection may be occasionally followed by spread of the germs to the middle ear. One or both ears may be infected. The condition usually begins with a pain in the ear and a high fever. The pain is continuous but may be irregular and is usually worse at night. When the doctor looks at the eardrum it is seen to be bulging. If the drum is not opened the pressure may cause it to burst. Then a thin watery discharge will come out, often changing to thick creamy pus. When the eardrum is cut or bursts the pain stops immediately and usually the temperature falls. The discharge may persist for a long time.

OTOSCLEROSIS (See also *Deafness*) One of the most common causes of progressive deafness is a change in the internal ear in which spongy bone appears and in which the small bones of the internal ear fail to function. The experts in ear disease prefer to call the condition otospongiosis because of the changes that take place.

The exact cause of otosclerosis is not known. Innumerable studies have been made to determine whether or not it was hereditary or due to some vitamin deficiency or some failure of the glands to function, but unfortunately it has not been shown that any one of these factors is primarily responsible. Most authorities consider this to be a chronic inflammatory disease with the destruction of formation of new bone in the internal ear.

The condition seems to occur more often in women than in men and often the first complaint is an annoying and distracting ringing in the ears. Associated with this there is a gradual loss of hearing which goes on progressively. Although the condition may begin on only one side, eventually both ears become affected.

Sufficient hearing will remain in some cases to permit the person to follow ordinary conversation but in other cases the progress is so great that it becomes necessary for the affected person to learn lip reading or to avail himself of other technics in order to be able to hear the spoken voice. It has been found that the pitch of the raised voice is heard more easily in otosclerosis, so that some of these people hear better in noisy surroundings because the people who speak to them raise the pitch of the voice.

Whenever there is a gradual loss of hearing going on for months or even years, the suspicion is warranted that otosclerosis may be present. Indeed doctors have a saying to the effect that "otosclerosis is a disease in which the doctor sees nothing and the patient hears nothing."

Specialists in diseases of the ear have a good many different tests which they apply to such cases in order to make certain that the condition is actually otosclerosis and not any other disturbance of the mechanism of the internal ear which might develop similar symptoms.

As has already been said, all sorts of treatments have been applied to these cases but unfortunately the methods thus far developed, outside of certain surgical procedures, the use of lip reading and of hearing aids, have not been of special benefit. The doctor will, of course, make certain that all of the accessory factors involved in hearing are properly functioning. This includes cleansing of the Eustachian tubes by the technic which the doctor uses for blowing through the tubes. It includes also the administration of a suitable diet, the control of the dosage of vitamins, and the application of proper glandular materials when any glandular failure of function is found. Sometimes the ringing in the ears needs to be controlled by various sedative drugs. The operation for the making of a window from the outside into the internal ear, known as the Lempert operation, is still the subject of investigation but a good many cases have already been reported in which this operative procedure has been of definite benefit.

OTOSCLEROSIS, SURGERY FOR (See also discussion under *Deafness* and *Otosclerosis*) Otosclerosis is a disease that involves the formation of spongy bone in the tissues of the ear. It usually begins between ages 16 and 30 and leads to progressive deafness. The condition is much more common in women than in men; its cause is unknown. An investigator believes otosclerosis results from damage to the blood supply of the tissues involved. Tests for otosclerosis include listening to a low voice from a 20-foot distance, listening to a tuning fork or watch ticks, or being tested with an electric audiometer. People with the deafness that results from otosclerosis hear conversation better in noisy than in quiet surroundings.

A new method of treatment is the fenestration (or window) operation, in which an opening (or window) is made behind the ear to permit sound waves to reach the internal ear by a different route than the eardrum. The operation is most successful when done early in the development of the deafness, for in earlier cases the operation has a 75% chance of success, in later cases it has only a 30% chance.

Another new operation is designed to loosen the fibers that keep the little bones behind the eardrum—called the hammer, anvil, and stirrup—from moving easily.

OVARY The ovary is the name given to the sex gland of women. There are two of these in a normal woman— one on each side in the lower portion of the abdomen.

It is the function of the ovary to provide the female egg cell which passes once each month down the fallopian tubes to the uterus. The ovary also develops various glandular secretions which are important in maintaining the female body structure and the functions which are peculiar to women.

In case the ovary becomes infected and it becomes necessary to remove it by surgery, the lack of these secretions brings about changes in the body. Hence one of the greatest discoveries in modern medicine is the determination of the nature of these secretions and the development of extracts or artificial substances which can be injected into the body and which serve to take the place of the secretions that are missing.

Since the ovary is supported in the abdomen by a tissue which holds it to the abdominal wall, it becomes possible for various symptoms to be associated with a stretching or twisting of these tissues, which are called ovarian ligaments. Twisting or stretching of these tissues may also affect the blood supply of the gland. Therefore symptoms of pain, swelling, or failure of functions in the ovaries which are associated with abnormal twisting or stretching of the ligaments may also require a surgical operation.

Occasionally also the ovary is subject to the formation of cysts, which are large collections of fluid in the form of glandular material or degenerated material of the gland itself. Cysts also occur when there is a hemorrhage into the gland. A cyst may remain small and not cause much disturbance. In other instances, however, the amount of fluid material develops tremendously, so that cysts may become exceedingly large and thus require surgical removal.

The ovary also becomes infected occasionally by the passing of infection along the tubes which carry the cells to the uterus. Infections like gonorrhea, tuberculosis, or streptococcic infections are accountable for more than 90 per cent of all infections of the ovary. When there is pus or infected material in the fallopian tubes—so-called pus tubes—it passes along by pressure to the ovary and thus carries the infection. In the presence of the pain, the swelling, and the fever which occur under such circumstances, the immediate treatment is the application of heat or of an ice bag. It is quite possible under modern circumstances to treat such infections with the sulfonamide drugs or with penicillin, and the physician must make the decision as to how long such treatment is to be carried on before surgical operation becomes necessary for the removal of the tube or the ovary.

Finally, tumors of all sorts may affect the ovary, including cancer. The doctor cannot determine from any examination that he can carry on from the outside of the body the exact nature of such a tumor. It is, therefore, generally believed that the treatment of all tumors of the ovary is the performing of an immediate operation, at which time the doctor decides the nature of the tumor and exactly what is to be done.

OVARIES—See articles SEX HYGIENE; ENDOCRINOLOGY; BLOOD PRESSURE.

OVARIES—cancer controlled by removal: See article CANCER.

OVARIES—development during adolescence: See article ENDOCRINOLOGY.

OVARIES—function in menstruation: See WOMEN, article HYGIENE OF WOMEN.

OVARIES—hormones made artificially: See article ENDOCRINOLOGY.

OVARIES—hormones used for complaints associated with menopause: See article ENDOCRINOLOGY.

OVARIES—location (fig.): See article ENDOCRINOLOGY.

OVARIES—old at forty-five: See article SEX HYGIENE.

OVARIES—pituitary stimulates: See article ENDOCRINOLOGY.

OVARIES—purpose: See article SEX HYGIENE.

OVARIES—skin affected by: See SKIN, article THE SKIN.

OVARIES—women with one not less capable of reproduction than those with

two: See BIRTH, article CARE OF MOTH-
ERS BEFORE AND AFTER CHILDBIRTH.

OVEREATING (See also discussion
under *Appetite, Emotions, Hygiene,
Personal, Night Eating Syndrome,
Obesity, Weight, Over- and Under-*)
Overeating and the obesity that results
from overeating are often associated
with an emotional problem; they can
be controlled through the removal of
anxiety and hostility. Insecurity, sensi-
tiveness, neurotic fears, and guilt all
create anxiety. A person who overeats
resorts to food in an attempt to allay
anxiety, for food, especially high-carbo-
hydrate food, unconsciously represents
either emotional or financial security,
according to psychoanalysts. An obese
person may also seek gratification from
food during moments of unhappiness
and self-pity. Food, particularly sweets,
becomes the one thing in life he knows
will invariably afford him pleasure. He
may also use food as a reward and treat
himself to an extra-special meal or a
sweet delicacy as a reward for what
he considers a personal noteworthy
achievement.

Probably the most important cause
for overeating is repressed hostility. A
fat person represses his hostility because
he fears retaliation and disapproval;
thus he gives an appearance of passivity
and submissiveness. His inability to
assert himself or express hostility is a
result of conditioning in early childhood; usually at least one of his parents
was a cruel and strict disciplinarian
who would not tolerate the expression
of hostility or rebellion.

Psychotherapy is an important tool
in treating overeating and resultant
obesity. Group therapy has recently become prominent as an approach to this
problem, and in several respects has
been found to be superior to individual
psychotherapy; patients benefit by working together and sharing a mutual
problem.

OVERWEIGHT CHILDREN (See
also, *Obesity in Children, Causes of;
Overweight Children, Treatment of*)
Overweight children, like all other
children, grow up in families. As with
all other children, the parents' ways in
bringing them up are of profound importance for their physical and psychologic development. Here we are concerned not only with the problems of
the overweight children themselves, but
also with the role which the families
play in the development and treatment
of obesity in childhood.

The old saying that there are three
stages of obesity known respectively as
the enviable, the comical, and the piti-
able aptly describes the different attitudes to overweight children and adolescents. It applies not only to the degrees
emotional reactions toward obese chil-
of overweight, but also to the changing
dren at different ages.

Every mother enjoys and takes pride
in a healthy bouncing baby. Years later
a mother, desperate about the outsized
proportions of her adolescent daughter,
may still sparkle with pride when she
recalls how all her neighbors envied her
because she had such a big and well-fed
child, how the little girl was held up as
a shining example for other puny, poorly
eating children.

In the normal course of events children outgrow their baby fat. Some, however, do not. For a while they are looked
upon with kindly eyes, and their chub-
biness is considered cute. They will appear in this light much longer to their
mothers than to the more objective and
critical eyes of the outside world. Many
a mother comes to a doctor's office to
find an ally against a teacher or relative
who tells her that her child is too fat.
Such a mother is quite honest when
she says, "She doesn't look that way to

me." She may even offer a belligerent statement: "The family thinks the bigger he is the better he is."

Even the most bindly devoted mother will wake up someday to the realization that there is something wrong with her child: that he is *too fat*. What admonitions of relatives, teachers, and physicians have failed to do will be accomplished by comparison with other children. As we shall see later, fat children often spend the early part of their lives isolated from other children and in the exclusive company of their mothers, who themselves have no interest outside the narrow events of their immediate families. Quite often we learn that these children have been kept away from nursery school or kindergarten. School is their first experience outside their own home, and it is a social event for which they are entirely unprepared.

The lot of fat children is sad. They move awkwardly like clumsy giants among the lively, graceful, and slender children. They grow ashamed of their misshapen bodies and ungainly appearance. Some would want to take part in active games and have fun like other children. "I can run a race, but I never win. I have to carry all this fat around," complained an eleven-year old fat boy. Another one, only nine years old, had already resigned himself to his fate. "I have nothing to run for," was his reply when asked about his interest in games.

The social and psychologic problems which obesity creates for a child become increasingly more serious as the child grows older. To be different comes to mean to be not so good as the rest. This applies to all kinds of handicaps and infirmities, and a child will do anything to keep his peculiarities a secret. Fat children have no way of hiding their problem. They are conspicious and attract attention by their very size. Obesity is often not taken seriously, not even by adults. Quite often it is considered

"funny." Fat children usually become the butt and laughingstock of their schoolmates. They are called "fatso," "fat stuff," or some other derisive names. Although they look big, they are not good fighters. Usually they are fearful and not capable of defending themselves against their tormentors. They may assume an attitude of "I don't mind." This is only a feeble defense against the insults which hit a fat child day by day and make him miserable and often drive him into seclusion.

This is the picture that confronts the mother of a fat child when she begins to look on her child as part of his social group. She is apt to become exclusively concerned with his obesity as if her child were just a "fat body." All his other qualities and interests in which she formerly took pride are overlooked and are considered of no value in comparison with the shame of her child being an object of ridicule. All her anxious efforts will now be bent on making him thin. She may upbraid him for being greedy and urge him to more activity after having overprotected him all his life and kept him away from it as "too dangerous." At this point many fat children are brought to the doctor. Quite often an open struggle over the need for reducing has been going on in the family.

This turning point in a family's attitude toward a fat child may occur at widely different ages. The more isolated a family is the later this will occur, sometimes not until adolescence is well advanced. There is also a great variation in the degree of obesity which prompts a family to seek help. An eleven-year-old boy was brought for treatment because he could no longer bend down and tie his own shoes. His weight at that time was 265 pounds. Up until then his fatness had been looked on in the light of a joke.

Some mothers never recognize that

their child is too fat. Immigrant mothers may remember how they had suffered from hunger in their own childhood and cannot understand why they should deny food to their children when there is plenty. In the "old country" only the rich could afford well-fed children. To them it is part of the new life and freedom to have a fat child.

From what has been said thus far it should be apparent that there is no clear line of demarcation between what one might call in a child a state of blooming nutrition and an abnormal degree of obesity. Obesity becomes a problem that needs medical and often psychiatric attention when the fatness interferes with the happiness of living and stands in the way of sound social and psychologic development.

OVERWEIGHT CHILDREN, TREATMENT OF (See also, *Overweight Children; Obesity in Children, Cause of*) Awareness of the psychological factors makes it understandable why treatment of obesity has always been such a baffling problem, although from a nutrition point of view it is a very simple task to calculate a reducing diet. Since overeating has made him fat, all one has to do is to tell an obese child how to reduce his food intake. The very low-caloric diets which have been recommended for adults are not suitable for children. The main task is to educate a fat child and his family to eat well-balanced meals of moderate caloric value. Adequate protein, mineral, and vitamin intake must be assured. A diet composed of milk, meat and fish, eggs, cheese, fruits and vegetables, and moderate amounts of whole-wheat bread will fulfill this requirement. Sometimes it is advisable to add vitamins, particularly the fat-soluble ones, the intake of which may be inadequate if the fat content of the diet is restricted. We have found

that diets of from 1200-1800 calories result in adequate weight loss.

In prescribing a diet a number of factors have to be taken into account: the degree of obesity, that is, the amount of excess weight; the rate at which the child has gained during the preceding period; the daily routine and special activities; the child's preference for, and dislike of, certain food. Sometimes in a rapidly growing child who is only moderately overweight it will not be necessary to plan for weight reduction. All one has to do is to help him to keep his weight constant so that he can "grow into his weight." It is this "outgrowing" for which the family always hopes and which rarely takes place unless the eating habits are changed.

The child whose weight is so high that it exceeds that of a normal adult or in whom the obesity is so severe that it interferes with his physical health and social adjustment should be placed on a restricted diet which leads to a loss of weight. In most instances this should be accomplished gradually. The main fact to be kept in mind is that this should not be just a reducing diet, which has to be adhered to religiously for a short time, but that an eating program should be planned which can be followed indefinitely, one which is sufficiently flexible to permit adjustment to the changing needs of the child.

If a child follows such a diet he will invariably lose weight, particularly if he follows also the advice of being more active. In those rare instances where simple ignorance of food values is the outstanding cause for the faulty food habits or where external circumstances have enforced idleness (for instance, confining illness or accidents) the child will be able to follow the prescribed regime with satisfactory results.

Yet anybody familiar with the treatment of obese children knows only too well how poorly they co-operate. They just do not eat the perfect, well-balanced, and adequate diets which the doctor prescribes. The situation is paradoxical: fat people really suffer from their condition and ask anxiously for advice, but they will not, or cannot, adhere to it. The word "adequate" to them means something quite different from what it means to the average person or to the physician. A diet which appears to be perfectly adequate may inflict real hardship on a fat child and even more on his parents. They may either flatly refuse to try it, like the father of a fat child who indignantly said, "I brought her to a clinic to lose weight, not to get a diet." Or there may be a brief period of adherence and corresponding loss in weight, and then the child begins to gain weight in spite of the beautiful diet which we calculated.

Under controlled conditions and strict supervision of a hospital or in the fashionable "success schools" of the beauty salons such unco-coperative and reluctant children and adolescents may lose weight, sometimes at an astonishing rate. The "successes," however, are often short-lived, as expected from a purely symptomatic treatment. The best that this mechanical reducing can achieve is to produce "thin fat children." By this expression I mean that if the fundamental attitude and the life habits of a child and the disturbed relationships in the family remain unchanged, the child or adolescent will regain the lost weight, if not at once, then as soon as he is faced with difficult life situations or problems that challenge his low capacity for independent decisions and achievement.

These strict reducing periods have one positive value: they demonstrate to the child and the family that weight reduction is possible. Quite often they had been convinced that the child could not respond to a diet. This prejudice is a serious obstacle in a rational treatment program.

The basis of effective treatment of obese children is an understanding of the underlying emotional problems. The first question is whether or not a child should reduce at all. Sometimes a mother brings a young child for examination only because the school or some relations urge her to do so. She herself considers the child to be in the best of health. There is very little one can do except leave the door open for later contact when the mother is more ready to see the obesity as a real handicap to the child. In mother situations the psychological problems are so grave and the emotional balance is so precarious that one should not interfere with the overeating lest one block the only way in which a child can fight overwhelming anxiety and find some feeling of comfort. There are even situations in which a more permissive attitude toward eating is indicated, namely when the continuous fight about reducing has aggravated the existing emotional problems to such an extent that the child is in danger of becoming mentally ill. Such children require intensive psychiatric treatment.

Such grave situations are rare. They should serve as a warning that dieting for a child is not a simple matter of calculating calories. An evaluation of the emotional climate is necessary in all cases in order to prevent a deadlock in treatment.

In prescribing a diet for fat children it has to be kept in mind that these children are unhappy and poorly adjusted in their whole way of living. Depriving them of food will only add to their unhappiness. It is necessary to help them to find new sources of satisfaction and, even more important, more self-respect.

One can help many fat children toward a better adjustment by showing true interest in their problems and a friendly and respectful attitude. Frequent contacts, if possible, at weekly intervals are necessary. Asking a fat child to eat less places a very hard task before him. He has had little chance to develop self-reliance, and a doctor's continuous interest has to supply him with a confidence which he himself does not feel. This means also that one should not assume a punitive or disgusted attitude if a child does not adhere to the diet. It is more helpful to find out what made the effort so difficult during that particular week. Thus one learns about the daily problems of a child, his joys, and his sorrows. In this way one may be of help to a fat child in developing independence and finding a more constructive outlet for his energy. In many cases psychiatric help may be needed to disentangle the close emotional ties to the mother.

If in order to insure regular visits to the office some prescription is given, this will not interfere with a rational psychological approach as long as the drug is not presented as a magic pill that will do the job. There is, however, strong psychological objection against the use of endocrine products for treatment of so-called sexual maldevelopment in obese boys. Cases in which there is true indication for such treatment are so exceedingly rare that they can be neglected in this general discussion. In a very large number of obese preadolescent boys who are made the object of such therapuetic zeal there is no medical justification whatsoever for exposing the family to unnecessary expense and the young patient to the emotional trauma of being branded as suffering from an essential physiological deficiency. Such young people are already handicapped by grave adjustment problems due to the difficulties of their background and the embarrassment of being fat. The additional psychological injury of such unwarranted diagnosis and treatment further aggravates the situation, since it seems to confirm their worst fears about being inadequate for life. Treatment for an obese adolescent means help with his personal difficulties so that he can give up the pleasure of overeating and find new satisfactions. Whether or not treatment of an obese child or adolescent will be successful will depend to a large extent on whether or not he develops self-reliance and independence and learns to make constructive use of his good physical and mental endowment so that he can give more meaningful expression to his creative drives than the static form of physical largeness.

OXYGEN Oxygen once was just an emergency remedy rushed in when patients were at the point of death.

Today it is well established as a useful remedy in many forms of disease, and it is recognized that early use of oxygen may be far more beneficial than any attempt to delay its application, in certain types of cases, until an emergency exists.

New oxygen devices include incubators which keep premature infants in a high oxygen atmosphere. For grownups there are oxygen tents, oxygen rooms, and special devices for breathing oxygen on a more limited scale.

In use of the oxygen tent, the oxygen in the air is kept down at about a 50 per cent level in contrast with the normal level. About one standard tank of oxygen a day is required.

If an oxygen tent is not available, a temporary emergency type of apparatus can be made, consisting of an anesthetic mask with a rebreathing bag. It is also possible to introduce the oxygen through a tube in the nose. In setting up such a system, the oxygen must be passed through water to prevent too much drying of membranes of nose and throat.

Oxygen should be used in all cases in which breathing is difficult and in which the patient suffers from an actual shortage of air. This occurs in all types of asphyxia, such as carbon monoxide poisoning or pneumonia.

The shortage of air which occurs with diseases of the heart is seldom greatly benefited by treatment with oxygen, since this type of shortage is largely due to a slowing of circulation of the blood.

On the other hand, oxygen may help cases of angina pectoris, because in these cases there may be a deficient amount of oxygen in the heart muscle.

Persons whose attacks of angina pectoris are readily controlled by rest or by treatment with the usual drugs do not need oxygen, but those who have frequent and severe attacks of angina, which come on with the slightest amount of physical effort, may find themselves greatly benefited by this treatment.

All that is to be known about the value of oxygen in various forms of disease has not yet begun to be established, but investigations are being carried out in many hospitals and laboratories and increasing use is found for this substance.

Since there is danger of fire and of violent explosion of oxygen under wrong conditions, it is never to be used except under direction of an experienced attendant.

OXYGEN—asthma: See article AL-LERGY.

OXYGEN—blood takes on fresh supply in right ventricle: See HEART, article DISEASES OF THE HEART AND CIRCULA-TION.

OXYGEN—hemoglobin transports: See BLOOD, article THE BLOOD AND ITS DISEASES.

OXYGEN—how furnished to tissues by circulation: See HEART, article DISEASES OF THE HEART AND CIRCULATION.

OXYGEN—measured by basal metabolism test: See article ENDOCRINOLOGY.

OXYGEN—needed to burn fuel in blood: See HEART, article DISEASES OF THE HEART AND CIRCULATION.

OXYGEN—pneumonia: See RESPIRATORY DISEASES, article THE RESPIRATORY DISEASES.

OXYGEN IN THE BODY The tissues of the body have to have oxygen to live. When the supply of oxygen is inadequate the condition is called anoxia. The shortage of oxygen may be apparent in the circulating blood. The red cells of the blood may be inadequate in amount or in the red coloring matter necessary to carry oxygen. Anything that blocks the circulation will also block the oxygen supply. Sometimes the cells of the body are unable, because of changes, to take up the oxygen that reaches them.

Since all parts of the body must have oxygen a shortage will affect all of them. However, some tissues of the body are much more dependent on oxygen than are others. Most sensitive of all are the tissues of the nervous system. Sudden lack of oxygen to the nervous system results in impairment of judgment, lack of co-ordination of movements, and a condition which, in general, resembles that of a person who is drunk. After the lack of oxygen has persisted the person becomes fatigued, drowsy, inattentive, and unable to respond to ordinary stimuli.

If lack of oxygen to the brain persists death will result from inability to breathe.

A failure of sufficient oxygen to reach the liver and the muscles where foods are broken down to their ultimate condition for use by the body, results in acidosis and is therefore also incompatible with life. The body tries to meet the threat of anoxia by increasing the breathing rate, by increasing the number of red blood cells, and the amount of red coloring matter. The heart and the kidneys are likewise affected unfavorably if oxygen is not supplied to their cells. The increase in red blood cells and hemoglobin in response to anoxia may begin gradually and continue for weeks. At high altitudes the total increase may reach 40 per cent above the usual.

CYANOSIS AND ARGYRIA—The word "cyanosis" means blueness, but in medicine it is restricted to the kind of blueness that follows a reduction in the amount of hemoglobin or red coloring matter in the blood. A condition called "argyria" which is due to deposit of silver in the skin gives a silvery blue appearance. Blueness due to lack of oxygen in the blood is best seen in the lips, the white of the eye, the fingernail beds, the ears and the area over the cheek bones.

Certain poisonous substances including drugs may lead to cyanosis by changing the nature of the hemoglobin or red coloring matter of the blood. Among these drugs are the nitrates which are sometimes used to dilate blood vessels and lower blood pressure. Also hydrogen sulfide and acetanilide may have this effect. When people are poisoned by carbon monoxide gas the blood develops a cherry red color rather than blue. Occasionally people who take sulfonamide drugs get bluish blood due to a chemical change.

When there is any interference with the flow of blood through the skin the color may seem blue or a pale bluish-gray. Such difficulty may come from a weak heart, an obstruction of the flow of blood or simple exposure of the skin to severe cold. Some people suffer constantly with cold and bluish hands and feet because of poor circulation in the extremities.

Obviously the determination as to just which mechanism is responsible for the blue appearance of the body is highly important in relationship to what will be done about it. The doctor must determine whether the difficulty is due to the heart, or the lungs or some trouble in the blood itself. By special signs such as clubbing of the fingers, the duration of the condition in relationship to employment, examinations of the heart and lungs, and chemical and physical studies of the blood, he can make the distinction.

TOO MANY RED CELLS—POLYCYTHEMIA—Doctors put together names of diseases frequently out of portions of words. "Poly" means multiple or too many; "cyth" refers to cells; "emia" means the blood. An alarming increase in the number of red blood cells might also be called an erythrocytosis which merely means a condition of the red blood cells. An excess number of the cells may develop as a result of an insufficient oxygen supply such as occurs at high altitudes, or as a result of an excess manufacture producing a disease the cause of which is not known. This true polycythemia is also called Osler's disease and Vaquez's disease after physicians who first noticed it.

Polycythemia comes on gradually and persists for ten or twenty years. The person with this condition has constantly a deep red flush which may have a bluish appearance. Usually the spleen and the liver are enlarged. The blood clots easily. Hemorrhages in various parts of the body are not uncommon. Whereas the blood count ordinarily is around five to six million the count rises in this condition to nine to twelve million cells in each cubic millimeter of blood.

Among unusual causes of secondary polycythemia in addition to residence at high altitude are disturbances, such as silicosis, which interfere with receipt of oxygen by the lungs, abnormalities of circulation of the blood through the lungs; cases which occur in infants that have been unable to get a good oxygen supply before birth; and even certain tumors of the brain and failure of the adrenal glands. Among methods of treatment now used to control excess production of the cells are X-ray of the bone marrow, giving of radioactive phosphorus and use of the nitrogen mustards.

OZENA An extraordinary and unfortunate disease which affects the mucous membranes of the nose is called ozena, a word which comes from a Greek word meaning stench. The doctors have apparently never been very sensitive about describing the disease because the French word for this disease is *pue-nez,* which means stinking nose, and the Germans with their characteristic bluntness simply call it *Stinknase.*

In this disease there is a gradual degeneration of the membrane that lines the nose. Then a mucous or mucopurulent discharge collects and dries, so that there are large foul-smelling crusts. All sorts of investigations have been made to find out the cause of ozena and whether or not any special germs are present to produce the characteristic bad odor. The most recent point of view is that continued infection of the nose in infancy gradually produces atrophy and death of the nasal mucous membrane, so that the nasal opening becomes too wide and thus permits the collection of crusts and the secondary infection. Certainly this should be a warning to parents never to neglect infection of the nose in children but to see to it that infection is controlled as soon as possible.

Strangely also, from Great Britain comes the report that this disease occurs chiefly among young girls, mostly of the servant class, and that it is seen most often in public dispensaries and rarely in private practice.

Incidentally this disease, which was quite frequent in a previous generation, has now almost disappeared, as is the case of another disease in young women called chlorosis. This gradual disappearance of ozena is believed to be due to the improved diet, the outdoor life and exercise, and the increasing medical attention to infections occurring in childhood.

Formerly it was the custom to treat ozena by copious washing of the nose with alkaline lotions and antiseptic lotions. It was customary to keep the nose filled with gauze containing antiseptic materials. Modern treatment includes particularly proper attention to the diet and a glandular study so as to bring the patient into the best state of health possible. Attempts are made to stimulate the mucous membrane of the nose to restore, if possible, its lost function. Attempts have even been made by surgical procedures to transplant mucous membrane but fortunately the gradual disappearance of the condition by prevention and by the changes that have taken place in the general hygiene of the body are more important than surgical cure.

Unfortunately the large majority of people do not apply for treatment to infections of the nose until the damage has become well advanced. The occurrence of even a few cases of ozena should be a warning to secure prompt treatment in all such cases.

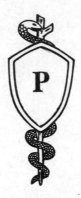

PAIN Pain is one of four elementary sensations, the others being touch, heat, and cold. Studies by the physiologists show that there are in the skin little points or nerve endings specialized to detect pain, touch, heat, and cold. The ability to feel pain is a protective mechanism for the human being, since it warns us of danger.

When for any reason an area has lost sensation, pain is the first sensation to be recovered. Moreover, there are more pain spots in the skin than heat or cold, although the touch spots are just about as frequent. In other words, you can feel that something is touching you at just about the same time you feel pain, if the sensation is painful.

As with other sensations, the detection of pain varies in different people. Some people are much more sensitive to pain than others.

The scientists have been making special studies of the pain sensation in recent years, particularly with a view to measuring the effects of various drugs that are used to diminish the sensation of pain. One technic includes the use of heat to the point of feeling of pain; another, the use of cold or freezing to the point at which it becomes painful. It has been found that morphine raises the threshold at which pain is felt to twice its normal level; codeine raises it only 50 per cent; alcohol, 45 per cent; and aspirin, 33 per cent. Beyond a certain dose extra quantities of any drug do not have any extra effect. Two drugs in combination do not raise the pain threshold any higher than one effective drug by itself. The only reason for using two drugs is that one has a more prompt effect and the other has a longer effect.

Studies also show that the speed at

which a sensation moves along a nerve varies.

With our new knowledge of pain, it has become possible to diminish the pain during surgical operations by blocking the nerves, by cutting the nerves, and by the use of pain-relieving drugs.

The scientists also distinguish between pain on the surface, pain in the bones, in the blood vessels, or in the organs of the body. Pain is first felt in the little terminal points of the nerves which then carry the sensation, with a small change in electric potential, to the spinal column and up the spinal column to the area in the brain. From this point the feeling is reflected back to the point of origin, so that one feels the pain in the finger, the toe, or some specific spot. Because of the pathways by which the sensation is carried to the brain, there are instances in which pain is felt in a tissue that has been removed, as, for instance, pain that is felt in a leg that has been removed, because of irritation of the nerves along which that sensation would ordinarily pass.

Scientists also recognize what is called psychogenic pain, which is wholly mental. Such pain does not possess the qualities of pain that are associated with pain that is physical. The psychogenic pains are vague, they are irregular in their ap-

pearance, they are likely to be exaggerated in description, and they are usually accompanied by signs of excellent health otherwise. Pains that are more psychogenic than physical are likely to clear up

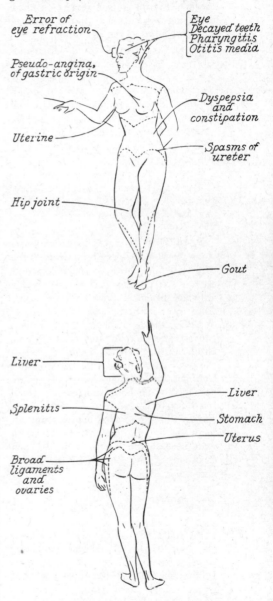

These drawings show some areas where pains referred from other tissues are felt. Pain may develop in a part of the body but the cause of that pain may be situated in another area. A well-known example of referred pain is the pain which arises in the heart and is referred to the neck and the left arm (angina pectoris).

when the mental reason for the pain disappears. Doctors refer, for instance, to the kind of pain that is felt by a person following an accident on a railroad or in a motorcar which promptly disappears when the person receives a check from the railroad or insurance company as compensation for his injury.

PAIN THRESHOLD—A modern superstitition that American Indians are less sensitive to pain than white people led to a comparison of the pain threshold among Indian, Eskimo, and white subjects. The research showed that age, sex, race, or national origin has no effect on the pain threshold of the human skin.

PAIN RELIEVERS—in medicine chest: See MEDICINE CHEST, article THE FAMILY MEDICINE CHEST.

PALENESS (See also discussion under *Anemia, Blood Conditions, Child Care, Sleep*) Pale children make mothers anxious. Frequently pallor is associated with persistent fatigue which results from emotional strain, lack of sleep, or overstimulation. Among the common causes of anemia in infants and young children are deficient iron in the diet of the prospective mother, failure to absorb iron because of digestive disturbances, damage to the bone marrow in which red blood cells are formed (such damage resulting most frequently from infection), and failure of the liver to store needed iron for the body. In such cases prescription of iron by the doctor had a beneficial effect.

PALSY See *Paralysis Agitans.*

PANCREAS The pancreas is a large gland situated in the abdominal cavity near the stomach, liver, and gall bladder. Its functions include the development of secretions which are important in re-

lation to the use of sugar by the body and to the digestion of proteins in the intestines.

The common association of inflammations of the gall bladder with inflammations of the pancreas has led doctors to believe that inflammations of the gall bladder are particularly dangerous because of the possibility of extension to the pancreas. Sometimes this glandular organ becomes infected directly with germs brought by the blood when people happen to have boils, mumps, influenza, pneumonia, or similar infections. Occasionally the pancreas is infected directly from an ulcer of the stomach. Men past middle age are much more frequently affected by inflammations of the pancreas than are women.

When this gland is infected, there are frequently attacks of dyspepsia and pains like those that occur with disease of the gall bladder. Often pains come on immediately after a heavy meal. There may be distention of the abdomen, vomiting, and localized pain and swelling. Usually also the doctor finds, when he examines the blood, that the white blood cells are greatly increased, which is usual when there is infection inside the abdomen. In a serious case of this kind the only definite life-saving measure is an immediate surgical operation to check the progress of the infection. In other instances the infection in the pancreas may not be sudden and severe but possibly in a milder manner over a long period of time. This is called chronic pancreatitis, or chronic inflammation of the pancreas. Associated with such infection, there are loss of appetite and weight, nausea and vomiting, a feeling of fullness, and occasionally much disturbance of digestion accompanied with diarrhea and the passing of a good deal of undigested material.

The pancreas may also be involved by the formation of cysts, stones, and tumors. Under such circumstances there may be excessive secretion of the glandular materials, so that the symptoms are related to this fact. An excess amount of insulin in the blood, with an insufficient amount of sugar in the blood, gives the same symptoms as are associated with an overdose of insulin. This includes giddiness, unconsciousness—perhaps with convulsions—periodical attacks of intense fatigue, and shortness of breath. Indeed cases are known in which people who have been suffering with an excess amount of insulin in the blood have been diagnosed as intoxicated by alcohol. In one instance a man was arrested for murder with a motorcar due to driving while intoxicated, and it was shown later that he was suffering with an excess amount of insulin in his blood.

The pancreas is one of the vital organs of the human body, equal in its importance to the liver and the thyroid gland. Too few people really have any knowledge that there is such an organ.

PANTOTHENIC ACID DEFICIENCY (See also discussion under

Vitamins) A recent report from the State University of Iowa on induced pantothenic acid deficiency in humans is significant. After a twelve-day control period, a pantothenic-acid-deficient diet was administered to four healthy young men. In addition, they received a new vitamin antagonist (omega-methyl pantothenic acid).

During the second week of this regimen, low blood pressure when standing, rapid heart beat after exertion, and fatigability developed. The third week brought complaints of gastric distress, anorexia, and constipation. Emotional changes were noted in the fourth week—irascibility, discontent, and quarrelsomeness. These were associated with numbness and tingling of the hands and feet, hyperactive reflexes, impaired sense of balance, and weakness of certain finger muscles. An increased susceptibility to infection was also observed.

Metabolic alterations that occurred during the period of pantothenic acid deficiency caused progressive weight loss in spite of a 3,000-calorie diet which included 100 grams of protein daily. There was a decline in blood cholesterol; also, changes revealed by eosinophil tests and urinary hormone excretion were indicative of diminished function of the adrenal cortices.

Some of these manifestations of the deficiency improved when pantothenic acid was added to the experimental diet-plus-antagonist. Other signs and symptoms, however, progressed; and because the investigators became alarmed at the resemblance of the syndrome to adrenal cortical insufficiency, cortisone and parenteral fluids were administered. These measures, in addition to a full diet and oral and parenteral vitamin B complex (with pantothenic acid supplementation), led to a prompt recovery.

Thus it appears that pantothenic acid (or its metabolic derivative, coenzyme A) is essential in man. That a spontaneous deficiency from inadequate intake is unlikely can readily be understood since this vitamin is widely distributed in foods and is resistant to chemical or thermal destruction.

PARALYSIS See also discussion of paralysis due to brain hemorrhage under *Apoplexy*.

PARALYSIS—agitans: See article OLD AGE.

PARALYSIS—benzine poisoning may stimulate: See article OCCUPATION AND HEALTH.

PARALYSIS—encephalitis: See article TRANSMISSIBLE DISEASES.

PARALYSIS—hardening of brain arteries: See article BLOOD PRESSURE.

PARALYSIS—infantile paralysis: See entry INFANTILE PARALYSIS.

PARALYSIS AGITANS In 1817 a London doctor named James Parkinson described a disease in which there was involuntary tremulous motion with lessened muscular power in parts of the body not in action and even when supported. He called attention also to a propensity to bend the trunk forward and to pass from a walking to a running pace. These are characteristic symptoms of what is now called Parkinson's disease or the shaking palsy, known scientifically as paralysis agitans.

The condition comes on most often in the sixth or seventh decade of life, but in rare instances a similar condition occurs in young people following epidemic infections of the brain.

Unfortunately nothing certain is known about the cause of paralysis agitans, although changes in the blood vessels of the brain and changes in the tissues of the nervous system and brain have been found. The disease is not especially associated with high blood pressure or brain hemorrhage.

In the very early stages of paralysis agitans a cessation of the ordinary swing of one arm may be the first visible sign. Another sign is a gradual appearance of fixity in the facial expression and slowness with which the ordinary movements of expression come and go. The condition tends to appear first in one limb and then to spread to the other limb on the same side and finally to the opposite limbs. The usual order of involvement is arm, leg, opposite arm, and opposite leg. After rigidity invades the muscles of the trunk of the body, the person with paralysis agitans tends to take a stooping attitude and to take shorter steps when he walks. Then he tends to take increasingly rapid steps, so that he breaks into a shuffling trot when he walks. Gradually all movements become slower and more limited in range.

The rate of progress of paralysis agitans varies. In many instances the condition may be confined to one limb for months or even a year before any other portion of the body is affected, and similar periods may pass before the condition spreads to other parts of the body. The general health of such a patient may remain remarkably good for many years.

Palliative treatment tends to postpone the arrival of complete disability and to give the patient relief from some of the disturbing symptoms. The drugs that influence rigidity are drugs of the belladonna type, and several technics have been developed for giving these drugs so as to bring about ease and apparent improvement. A new surgical approach involves stopping the flow of blood in certain blood vessels of the brain.

A specialist has observed that some strong emotional stimulus may suddenly bring about temporary amelioration of the disability. Sudden fright or danger may do this, but soon after there is a relapse into the previous condition.

Everything possible should be done

for these patients to improve their general health and strength. Massage and suitable baths tone the skin and muscles. Sedative drugs tend to reduce the restlessness and the tremors.

SHAKING PALSY—See article OLD AGE.
SHAKING PALSY—encephalitis symptoms similar: See article TRANSMISSIBLE DISEASES.

PARANOIA When human beings develop a mental disorder which is characterized by extraordinary ambitions and suspicions about persecution and grandeur expressed in logical form, the condition is called paranoia. There are many different types of paranoia.

PARANOIA—See MENTAL, article NERVOUS AND MENTAL DISORDERS.

PARATHYROID GLANDS The parathyroid glands are the smallest known organs of internal secretion. Usually there are four parathyroid glands —two on each side. They lie in the throat behind the thyroid gland. They are small, so that the entire four glands weigh only a tiny fraction of a pound.

Apparently the effect of the secretion put out by the parathyroid glands is to influence calcium and phosphorus as used in the human body, raising the total amount of calcium in the blood and lowering the total amount of phosphorus. When it is necessary to increase the amount of calcium in the blood, the material is obtained either from the bones or from extra calcium taken into the body. The great importance of calcium in the human body has often been emphasized, since it is the material which makes up the bones and teeth and since it is also involved in stabilizing nervous reactions. Thus in certain convulsive disorders, such as tetany, there may be too small an amount of calcium in the blood. The condition called tetany, which is

a sign of insufficient activity on the part of the parathyroid glands, is characterized by a tendency of the muscles to go into a condition of painful, prolonged spasm. This involves the muscles of the forearms and hands and the throat but may involve almost any muscles of the body. Associated with the spasms there may be tingling sensations, a feeling of weight on the chest, and general numbness. Occasionally twitchings occur in various muscles. People with tetany due to insufficiency of calcium may also be nervous, self-centered, emotional, or depressed.

Once it was exceedingly difficult for doctors to treat such patients successfully, but nowadays there are many ways in which calcium may be put into the body promptly. In many instances, however, the symptoms of tetany are produced by other conditions which are not related to a deficiency of action of the parathyroid glands. Thus the condition called rickets, or osteomalacia associated with characteristic changes in the bones may produce similar symptoms. In all such conditions the calcium in the blood is low due to defective absorption of calcium from the food. In many instances symptoms like those of tetany are due to excessive alkali in the body.

The first step for the doctor in all such cases is to find out exactly what is the state of the blood and the cause of the symptoms. Sometimes the condition is controllable by providing a diet with a low amount of phosphates, supplemented by the giving of large amounts of calcium salts. A diet low in phosphates would eliminate meat, yolk of egg, and also cut down the amount of milk.

The opposite condition is excessive action of the parathyroid glands, likely to be characterized by serious changes in the bones. This produces a condition called fibrous inflammation of the bones, or osteitis fibrosa. In this condition the bones are soft and can be cut with a knife due to the elimination of calcium from the bones. The bones actually become porous, producing a state that is also characterized by the name osteoporosis. Because of the excessive mobilization of calcium in the blood derived from the bones, stones are often found in the various organs of the body. Softness of the bones and the failure of the calcium to be used properly in their development may produce strange deformities in the body. To the twisting and disturbance of the bones the name "osteomalacia" is given. Sometimes the excessive action of the parathyroid glands is due to a tumor growth in these glands. In such cases surgical removal of the gland is the only help.

PARATHYROID GLANDS—See article ENDOCRINOLOGY.

PARATHYROID GLANDS—location (fig.): See article ENDOCRINOLOGY.

PARATHYROID GLANDS—skin affected by: See SKIN, article THE SKIN.

PARENTAL ANXIETY (See also discussion under *Child Care, Demand Feeding, Emotions, Feeding Schedule*) A review of current theories on child rearing, made by a leading pediatrician at New York University, concludes that the effects of current psychiatric teaching have been to increase parental anxiety, shake parents' faith in their own ability to rear children, and undermine parental authority. This results, the review claims, from unsubstantiated ideas that frustration is invariably harmful, and that every infantile and childhood experience will have a permanent effect on a child's future emotional life. Concentration on the importance of parental affection has led parents to fear that discipline may jeopardize a good parent-child relationship. While parents have learned that a strict schedule for feeding, sleeping, and similar activities is not absolutely necessary, this changing attitude has re-sulted in an over-all breaking down of the confidence of parents in their ability to rear a child. Experience shows that in general children thrive best in a home atmosphere where they believe their parents love them, and where they are given a reasonable amount of discipline, have a good example set by the parents and adequate reward for proper behavior.

PARESIS About 3 per cent of people who became infected with syphilis in the past developed late in life a condition called variously general paralysis, general paresis, general paralysis of the insane, or, by the doctors, dementia paralytica. In this condition the syphilis is found to have infected the brain and the coverings of the brain with damage to the tissues sufficient to result in paralysis and mental disturbance. Strangely, this form of syphilis occurs three to five times as often in men as in women.

Customarily the person who has had syphilis and who is developing paresis first shows the condition by slight changes in manner, including irritability, carelessness about the clothes and the body generally, lack of judgment, absent-mindedness, inability to concentrate, slowness of comprehension, and similar irregularities. Since all of these symptoms may occur as the result of a variety of other conditions, their appearance in a person should not necessarily be considered the sign of beginning paresis. It is the assemblage of the symptoms and their characteristic development and continuance that permit the expert to make the diagnosis.

Associated with the mental symptoms affecting the nervous system there are others of a motor character, such as disturbances of dexterity, tremors of the hands, inability to make co-ordinated movements, even changes in the facial expression and often speech defects, so that the patient cannot say such trick phrases as "she sells sea shells," "third riding artillery brigade," and similar phrases.

One of the signs long known to be associated with paresis is the change in the pupil of the eye, so that when the doctor makes the test the pupil of the eye does not react to light but does react to accommodation; that is to say, the pupil will not grow smaller with light and larger without light but will adjust itself to looking at objects close up or at a distance.

As paresis develops, there comes one of the symptoms which is most dramatic, namely, a condition called euphoria, an extraordinary sense of well-being in which these people are grandiose, elated with delusions of wealth and great power, and in which they feel better than ever before. This appears in around 15 to 20 per cent of the cases. These delusions take strange actions. One man of ordinary income went into a department store and ordered a thousand dollars' worth of silk underwear. A baker doing an ordinary business ordered twenty-seven delivery trucks to take care of an increase in business which he thought was going to occur.

In other cases there are depression, anxiety, fear of danger, and self-accusation. In still others there are loss of memory, difficulty in calculation and writing, and difficulties in judgment.

Eventually the damage becomes so great that the patient with paresis has to be put to bed, and a general paralysis of all of the muscles of the body ensues.

Once paresis was considered to be an invariably fatal disease. If a man or woman developed this condition, which was often called softening of the brain around 1900, the outlook was bad. There was the possibility of death, the likelihood of years of confinement in an institution for the insane. Today the out-

look for such a person is far from hopeless.

The improvement in outlook has resulted from the gradual development of a number of important discoveries in medical science related directly to an understanding of this disease. The famous Japanese investigator Noguchi was the first to prove that general paresis is caused by syphilis. Another investigator found that the injection of such patients with the germ that causes malaria resulted in a fever which tended to stop the progress of the paretic condition. Next came treatment by the use of heat, which is developed either through passing an electric current through the body or by putting the patient in a body-baking device. Then came various drugs of the arsenic type, such as salvarsan or 606, scientifically called arsphenamine, and another more specific arsenic drug called tryparsamide. All of these methods are difficult to administer and are used only in a hospital.

Most recent in the treatment of paresis and of other forms of syphilis of the nervous system is the use of penicillin. It is now rather well established that penicillin is effective in the treatment of early syphilis, often bringing about recovery, as nearly as can be determined by modern methods, within weeks or months. In many instances excellent results are secured by combining the treatment of syphilis with penicillin and one of the arsenic preparations.

A joint investigation conducted by experts in various parts of the country under the direction of the National Research Council has shown that 80 per cent of 30 cases treated with penicillin improved to some degree, nearly half improved 50 per cent or more, 8 improved 75 per cent and 1 was restored to normal. Even in long-continued paresis in which deterioration had occurred, 2 out of 10 improved 75 per cent, 1 out of 10 improved 50 per cent, but in 7 the deterioration had been so great that improvement was not possible.

Apparently there is new hope for the person with paresis.

PARESIS—age at onset: See MENTAL, article NERVOUS AND MENTAL DISORDERS.

PARESIS—syphilis micro-organism causes: See MENTAL, article NERVOUS AND MENTAL DISORDERS.

PARKINSON'S DISEASE, SURGERY IN (See also *Paralysis Agitans*) As an example of a surgical approach to a condition formerly considered wholly medical, one may cite attempts to control paralysis agitans better known as Parkinson's disease or the shaking palsy by surgical procedures. Attempts have been made by removal of portions of the cortex of the brain to stop the tremors. The operation itself is so severe and the end results so doubtful that this operation proposed in the late 1930s has been virtually abandoned. Next came attempts to section certain nerves within the brain with a view to stopping tremor. This method also bore great risk and doubtful success. Most recent is an attempt to halt the muscular tremor and the fixation of the muscles in the face by tying off an artery called the anterior carotid artery which supplies with blood those sections of the brain responsible for the tremor. The operation performed by I. S. Cooper is believed to be of value in persons less than 60 years old and without any sign of hardening of the arteries. Cooper reported that in 9 out of 11 cases so treated in which Parkinson's disease followed previous inflammation of the brain a definite benefit was obtained. Tying off of an artery is not a serious surgical procedure and the end results do not carry the hazard to life that was associated with some previously mentioned surgical procedures.

PARTURITION (See discussions under *Pregnancy* and *Prenatal Care*) Parturition is the process of giving birth to a child.

PATCH TEST The patch test is a technic in which a small patch of adhesive, containing a substance to which a person may be sensitive, is applied to the skin. The appearance of redness and inflammation is considered to be a positive test.

PATCH TEST—See article ALLERGY.

PEDIATRICIAN A pediatrician is a specialist in the treatment of children's diseases. This specialty is called pediatrics.

PELLAGRA Certain diseases are called deficiency diseases, which means they result from failure of the body to receive something that it needs for growth, repair, and development. One of the most serious of the deficiency diseases is called pellagra, which for many years has caused great harm and suffering to mankind. At one time many thousands of cases of this disease occurred throughout the United States. Today it is seen only in certain areas where the diets of people are greatly limited because of economic, social, or agricultural conditions. In 1917–18 at least 200,000 people in the United States suffered from this disease. In 1915 it was reported that 10,000 people had died of pellagra.

Today we know that the condition occurs largely because of the absence of certain necessary vitamins and proteins from the diet. Most important is nicotinic acid, also known as niacin. This substance, which is a part of the vitamin B complex, is absolutely necessary for the health and growth of the human body. When it is absent from the diet, there occur changes in the skin with redness and irritation and secondary cracking and ulceration. Soreness of the mouth and a violent red appearance of the tongue are other serious manifestations. We know from postmortem examinations that this redness and irritation may extend along the entire intestinal tract. Superimposed on these conditions there may be irritability, anxiety, delirium, and burning sensations in the nerves. The soreness of the mouth and of the intestinal tract prevent people with pellagra from eating as they should. Hence the condition develops into what is called a vicious circle.

Experiments have shown that feeding of people who have pellagra with yeast, liver extract, fresh milk, eggs, and lean meat brings about prompt recovery. Also the necessary vitamins may be either injected into the body or provided in other ways. Whenever a single vitamin is absent, it is likely that other vitamins also will be missing from the diet. This means that the diets of all of those with pellagra have to be investigated. Often it is found that these people have been living on pork fat, corn bread, soda biscuits, and corn syrup. Their diets need to be supplemented not only with the foods

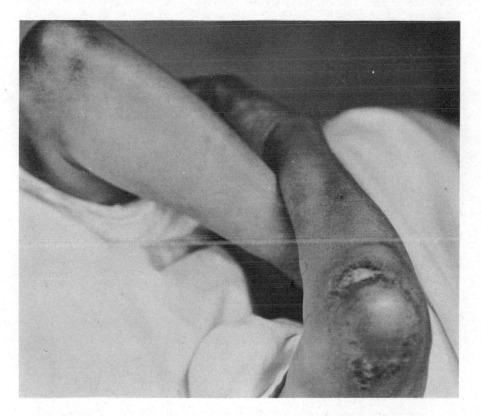

Pellagrous lesions on the elbows. Lesions usually appear on areas exposed to sunlight and subjected to frequent friction or trauma.
Chas. Pfizer & Co., Inc.

1567

that have been mentioned but also with tomatoes, green peas, other green and yellow vegetables, and similar foods.

An interesting sidelight on pellagra is the suggestion that Job, when he complained about his boils and when he was stricken with a terrible skin disease that involved his entire body from the soles of his feet to the crown of his head, was actually suffering from pellagra. The condition appears wherever poverty exists. It will be remembered that Job had lost his money and had become a pauper.

PELLAGRA—See article DEFICIENCY DISEASES.

PELLAGRA—diarrhea caused by: See article DIGESTION AND DIGESTIVE DISEASES.

PELLAGRA—niacin: See article DEFICIENCY DISEASES.

PELLAGRA—pyridoxine: See article DEFICIENCY DISEASES.

PELLAGRA—result of shortage of niacin: See INFANCY, article CARE AND FEEDING OF THE CHILD.

PELLAGRA—skin changes: See SKIN, article THE SKIN.

PELLAGRA—United States: See article DEFICIENCY DISEASES.

PELVIMETRY The obstetrician before childbirth measures the dimensions and capacity of the pelvis of the woman who is going to have a child. The pelvis is the basin-shaped ring of bones at the bottom of the trunk. It joins the legs below and the spine above.

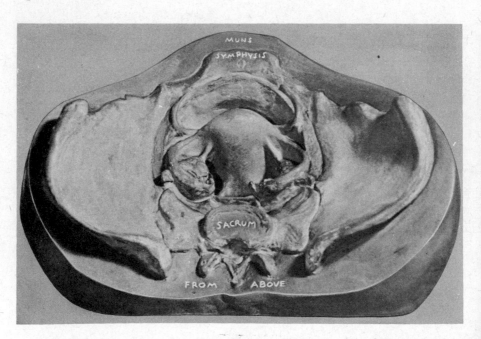

Model of the female pelvis. Before childbirth the obstetrician measures the diameters of the pelvis with an instrument shaped like calipers.

Cleveland Health Museum

PELVIC ORGANS—female (fig.): See WOMEN, article HYGIENE OF WOMEN.

PELVIS—girl's broader than boy's: See article SEX HYGIENE.

PEMPHIGUS A disease of the skin in which there are large blisters which break and leave pigmented spots is called pemphigus. Frequently itching and burning appear in connection with the development of the blisters. There are many different forms of skin disease in which such blisters appear and there are many different varieties of pemphigus.

PEMPHIGUS—See SKIN, article THE SKIN.

PENICILLIN A mold known as *Penicillium notatum,* when grown in a suitable mixture, gives off a secretion that can be dried and extracted as a powder. This material is called penicillin. It has been found to be immensely effective in the treatment of all sorts of infections by germs of many different varieties.

PENICILLIN—allergy to: See article ALLERGY.

PENICILLIN—allergy treated by: See SKIN, article THE SKIN.

PENICILLIN—chicken pox: See CHILDHOOD DISEASES, article INFECTIOUS DISEASES OF CHILDHOOD.

PENICILLIN—diabetic gangrene: See article DIABETES.

PENICILLIN—diphtheria: See CHILDHOOD DISEASES, article INFECTIOUS DISEASES OF CHILDHOOD.

PENICILLIN—erysipelas: See article TRANSMISSIBLE DISEASES.

PENICILLIN—German measles: See CHILDHOOD DISEASES, article INFECTIOUS DISEASES OF CHILDHOOD.

PENICILLIN—gonorrhea: See VENE-REAL DISEASES, article THE VENEREAL DISEASES.

PENICILLIN—hemolytic streptococcic infection: See HEART, article DISEASES OF THE HEART AND CIRCULATION.

PENICILLIN—hives may be caused by: See SKIN, article THE SKIN.

PENICILLIN—impetigo: See SKIN, article THE SKIN.

PENICILLIN—infectious diseases: See INFECTIOUS DISEASE, article THE PREVENTION AND TREATMENT OF INFECTIOUS DISEASE.

PENICILLIN—pneumonia: See RESPIRATORY DISEASES, article THE RESPIRATORY DISEASES.

PENICILLIN—pus-producing skin infections: See SKIN, article THE SKIN.

PENICILLIN—rat-bite fever: See article TRANSMISSIBLE DISEASES.

PENICILLIN—rheumatic fever: See HEART, article DISEASES OF THE HEART AND CIRCULATION.

PENICILLIN—scalp infections: See HAIR, article THE HAIR.

PENICILLIN—scarlet fever: See CHILDHOOD DISEASES, article INFECTIOUS DISEASES OF CHILDHOOD.

PENICILLIN—seborrheic dermatitis: See HAIR, article THE HAIR.

PENICILLIN—sinuses: See EAR, article THE EAR, TONGUE, NOSE, AND THROAT.

PENICILLIN—skin antiseptic: See SKIN, article THE SKIN.

PENICILLIN—skin eruptions caused by: See SKIN, article THE SKIN.

PENICILLIN—syphilis: See BLOOD, article THE BLOOD AND ITS DISEASES; SKIN, article THE SKIN; VENEREAL DISEASES, article THE VENEREAL DISEASES.

PENICILLIN—tetanus: See article TRANSMISSIBLE DISEASES.

PENICILLIN—throat lozenges: See EAR, article THE EAR, TONGUE, NOSE, AND THROAT.

PENICILLIN—Vincent's angina: See article TRANSMISSIBLE DISEASES.

PENICILLIN—wens: See SKIN, article THE SKIN.

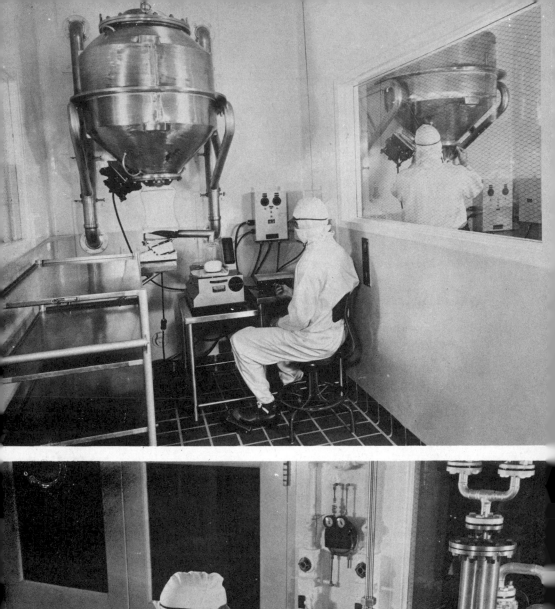
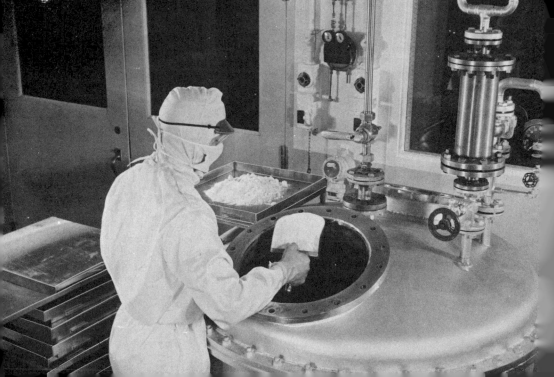

PENIS The penis is the male sex organ used in sexual intercourse. Various disorders as well as infections may affect the organ. Surgical procedures have been developed for correcting structural disorders, particularly when there is an abnormal opening of the tube called the urethra which carries the urine from the bladder to the outside. One of these disorders is called hypospadia, in which there is a splitting of portions of the penis so that the opening comes on the inner side instead of at the front.

PENIS—cleaning child's: See INFANCY, article CARE AND FEEDING OF THE CHILD.

PENIS—gonorrhea: See VENEREAL DISEASES, article THE VENEREAL DISEASES.

PENIS—function: See article SEX HYGIENE.

PENIS—how to get rid of a chordee: See VENEREAL DISEASES, article THE VENEREAL DISEASES.

PENIS—washing: See article SEX HYGIENE.

PEPTIC ULCERS IN CHILDREN (See also, *Ulcers*) It is now known that children have peptic ulcers. If a child complains of pain in the upper abdomen, X rays should be taken and the necessary studies made to determine whether an ulcer of the stomach or duodenum is present. A report from Texas tells of 6 cases of ulcers in children who ranged from 7 to 12 years of age. Two of the children were nervous, irritable girls who had personality problems and difficulties in family adjustment. Treatment was given to relieve the ulcers, but the doctors also advised psychiatric study for the girls. Another doctor says his observations lead him to believe that from 0.1 to 0.2 per cent of children between the ages of 1 and 6 may have peptic ulcers and that emotional factors have played a prominent role in causing them. He defines the typical candidate for a childhood peptic ulcer as a tense, bright, nervous youngster; such a child tends to keep his emotions repressed. Treatment of childhood ulcers usually includes a bland diet and drinking of milk between meals and before going to bed at night, plus the medical treatment for ulcers in adults.

PERICARDITIS The heart lies in a sac which is called the pericardium. This sac may become infected and inflamed, in which case there is pain over the heart, a rapid pulse, and often severe coughing. Since the infection tends to roughen the lining and to produce fibrinous material, the doctor can hear a sound of the rubbing of the roughened portions when he uses the stethoscope in cases of pericarditis. There are many different varieties of pericarditis, depending on the nature of the germ that produces the infection and on the extent of the symptoms.

PERICARDITIS—See HEART, article DISEASES OF THE HEART AND CIRCULATION.

PERICARDITIS—uremia: See KIDNEY,

Penicillin is an antibiotic used to combat infectious diseases. It is very valuable as a prophylactic agent used to prevent infections during surgery and dental extractions. The photographs show two steps in the manufacture of pencillin. Operator removes penicillin from the tank in which final purification has been accomplished. After drying and milling, penicillin of uniform particle size is filled and weighed into glass jars for transfer to sterile packaging area.

Chas. Pfizer & Co., Inc.

article THE KIDNEY: ITS DISEASES AND DISTURBANCES.

PERINEUM The space between the genital organs and the anus or lower opening of the bowel is called the perineum. Women frequently have disturbances in this area associated with tearing and pressure because of childbirth. The area may also become infected by the ringworm that attacks the groins, in which case there is severe itching and sometimes blistering in this area.

PERITONITIS The peritoneum is the name given to the membrane that lines the abdominal cavity just as the lining of the chest cavity is called the pleura. This tissue is subject to such conditions as affect linings elsewhere in the body. Thus it may rupture through the wall of the abdomen in the case of a hernia, or rupture. There may be cysts of the folds of the peritoneum that go down to the organs. This part of the peritoneum is called mesentery and the cysts are called mesenteric cysts.

The most serious condition that affects the peritoneum is peritonitis, which means inflammation of the peritoneum. When this tissue becomes inflamed, the results are always serious. Sometimes inflammation of the peritoneum develops after injury to the abdomen but in most instances the peritoneum is infected by germs which come by way of the blood or by secondary infections by the organs that lie within the abdomen, like the appendix. If, for instance, the appendix becomes infected and ruptures, the most dangerous complication is secondary peritonitis. Sometimes the peritoneum becomes infected by the rupture of an ulcer of the abdomen or the stomach. Pain begins almost immediately with infection and is felt at the point where the infection originated. As the inflammation progresses, the patient becomes seriously ill because of the absorption of the poisonous materials. There is fever, rigidity of the abdominal wall, and tenderness when the wall is touched. Thus whenever there is severe abdominal pain accompanied by tenderness of the abdominal wall, by vomiting and fever, the doctor suspects peritonitis. Unless acute peritonitis is promptly treated, it may be fatal. The time between the occurrence of the peritonitis and death may be only a matter of a few hours to a few days, depending on the severity of the infection. Obviously, therefore, the prompt diagnosis of peritonitis is of the utmost importance in saving life.

In most instances treatment of this condition is surgical. The doctor opens the abdomen and removes the infectious material, sometimes applying drug treatments directly to the peritoneal cavity.

Since the germs which affect the peritoneum are in most instances of the types that yield to sulfa drugs and to penicillin, physicians anticipate great improvement in the records of deaths from peritonitis in the forthcoming years. It is doubted that the condition will be considered as seriously fatal in the future as it has been in the past. However, even the sulfa drugs and penicillin cannot be considered helpful in cases of this type unless the diagnosis is made promptly and treatment given at once.

See article DIGESTION AND DIGESTIVE DISEASES.

PERITONITIS—mistaken for acute indigestion: See article DIGESTION AND DIGESTIVE DISEASES.

PERITONITIS—perforation: See article DIGESTION AND DIGESTIVE DISEASES.

PERITONITIS—tonsillitis may cause: See EAR, article THE EAR, TONGUE, NOSE, AND THROAT.

PERITONITIS—uremia: See KIDNEY, article THE KIDNEY: ITS DISEASES AND DISTURBANCES.

PERSPIRATION In hot weather human beings get especially interested in perspiration, the chief use of which is to regulate the heat of the body and keep it normal. The sweat glands are the chief paths by which water reaches the surface of the skin; a good deal of water passes through the skin by what is known as insensible perspiration. Perspiration is about 98 to 99 per cent water.

Tests have been made in the hot desert to determine how much fluid may be lost from the body by way of sweat. People vary as to the speed with which they begin to perspire and as to the amount of salts and water that they lose from the body during perspiration. People vary also as to the amount of perspiration from various portions of the body. One investigator found that the perspiration from the palms and soles is five to ten times as much as from other parts of the body. Incidentally, people who do not perspire fairly easily should not live in tropical countries.

The odor of the sweat varies according to the part of the body from which it is secreted. Ordinarily it is acid, but after profuse perspiration it tends to be neutral or alkaline.

There is a division of work between the skin and the kidneys in excreting water. For that reason the urine is light-colored in winter when perspiration is slight and darker in summer when the skin is secreting a great deal of water.

Perspiration is increased by heat, by the drinking of warm drinks, by psychic causes such as fright and anxiety, and by a number of the drugs which are known to increase the flow of water from the skin. Perspiration is decreased by external cold and by various drugs which have been proved capable of decreasing perspiration.

A number of special diseases affect the sweat glands. One of them, which describes excessive sweating, is called hyperhidrosis, in which the hands are continually moist, clammy, or dripping with fluid. This perspiration is usually cold. Serious states of this kind should be treated by specialists in diseases of the skin who have special remedies that can be prescribed.

Excessive perspiration may be the symptom of a serious general condition. Often perspiration is affected by the emotional state. People who perspire freely should wear underwear that does not retain moisture—a mixture of silk and wool, light in weight, for winter, and cotton and silk in summer. More important, however, than the type of underwear is the amount of clothing. Care should be taken not to wear too much clothing, particularly by those who perspire excessively. Many people now find it advantageous to wear the same weight of underwear all year round. Medicine has developed several different substances which are useful in limiting the amount of perspiration. These drugs, however, are in most instances sufficiently potent so that they should be used over large sections of the body only when specifically prescribed by the doctor. Many different dusting powders useful in excessive perspiration are also available.

There is another condition in which sweat fails to be secreted by the body. This is exceedingly rare.

In a third type of case there is an

offensive odor to the sweat. This is known as bromidrosis.

In another condition the sweat is colored, and this condition is called chromidrosis. The appearance of colored perspiration is believed to be due to infections with various kinds of germs.

The odor of the perspiration under the arms was found to be due to decomposition of germs and their action on the secretions of the sweat glands. It was established that fresh sweat does not have any odor but assumes the odor only after standing for several hours. In an experiment carried out by W. B. Shelley a flask of fluid from the glands under the arms did not develop any odor after standing for 14 days. When the areas under the arms are washed with a solution of hexachlorophene this helps to eliminate the germs. Shaving the hair gives better opportunity for the antiseptic to act. Aluminum chloride such as is found in various underarm preparations was also effective but not through preventing the secretion of perspiration. Rather it came about by the antibacterial action. This investigation lends scientific support for the practice of fastidious persons of shaving the hairs, washing frequently under the arms, using a mild aluminum preparation and changing to freshly washed clothing frequently.

PERSPIRATION—acid at times: See KIDNEY, article THE KIDNEY: ITS DISEASES AND DISTURBANCES.

PERSPIRATION—alum in sponge bath to prevent: See RESPIRATORY DISEASES, article THE RESPIRATORY DISEASES.

PERSPIRATION—amount: See article STRESS AND DISEASE; KIDNEY, article THE KIDNEY: ITS DISEASES AND DISTURBANCES.

PERSPIRATION—antiperspirant preparations: See article ALLERGY; SKIN, article THE SKIN.

PERSPIRATION—constipation may be in-

duced: See article DIGESTION AND DIGESTIVE DISEASES.

PERSPIRATION—detergents and deodorants: See article ALLERGY.

PERSPIRATION—excessive: See SKIN, article THE SKIN.

PERSPIRATION—feet: See FOOT, article THE FOOT.

PERSPIRATION—glands: See BIRTH, article CARE OF MOTHERS BEFORE AND AFTER CHILDBIRTH; article ENDOCRINOLOGY; SKIN, article THE SKIN.

PERSPIRATION—infantile paralysis: See CHILDHOOD DISEASES, article INFECTIOUS DISEASES OF CHILDHOOD.

PERSPIRATION—infants with rickets: See INFANCY, article CARE AND FEEDING OF THE CHILD.

PERSPIRATION—response to germs: See INFECTIOUS DISEASE, article THE PREVENTION AND TREATMENT OF INFECTIOUS DISEASE.

PERSPIRATION—salt loss: See DIET, article ADVICE ON THE DIET.

PERSPIRATION—scalp: See HAIR, article THE HAIR.

PERSPIRATION—skin function: See SKIN, article THE SKIN.

PERSPIRATION—water eliminated daily: See article STRESS AND DISEASE; KIDNEY, article THE KIDNEY: ITS DISEASES AND DISTURBANCES.

PERTUSSIS See *Whooping Cough.*

PHARYNX In the throat, between the mouth and the opening of the esophagus which leads into the stomach, is an area that is commonly called the pharynx. In the pharynx are found the tonsils and a good deal of lymphoid tissue. It is customary to divide the pharynx into parts, including the nasal pharynx, which is the part that goes up toward the nose, and the laryngeal part, which goes down toward the larynx and trachea.

Whenever anyone catches a severe cold or gets a sore throat or acute tonsillitis, the pharynx is likely to be inflamed at the same time. When the infection is caused by a streptococcus, usually known as the hemolytic streptococcus, the condition known as septic sore throat develops. In this condition the mucous membrane becomes swollen, purple, and glazed. The uvula, which is the little piece of tissue which hangs down into the throat from above, may become swollen and the tonsils may become seriously infected. Sometimes this swelling is so severe that the patient finds it difficult to breathe.

With a septic sore throat the patient is gravely ill, the breath develops a foul odor; it is difficult for the patient to eat. Moreover, the infection is rapidly absorbed from the throat, so that the patient may become generally ill and secondary infections may be set up in other parts of the body.

Fortunately the streptococcus of septic sore throat is susceptible to treatment with the sulfa drugs and penicillin, so that this condition has been largely brought under control by modern technics.

Most important when an epidemic of septic sore throat strikes a community is to find out exactly where the epidemic originated and how it spreads. In the past, before strict control of milk supplies was the rule, epidemics were usually due to infection from the udder of the cow, often from a milker who was himself infected with septic sore throat, and often from a milker with severe infections of the fingers. Septic mastitis in the cow, which merely means streptococcus infection of the udder, is associated with epidemics of septic sore throat in the communities that use the milk.

Another condition that affects the pharynx is Vincent's angina, a form of infection of the throat caused by germs. This condition also requires special treatment since the organisms of Vincent's angina are known to be susceptible to treatment with several specific remedies. Most important, however, in such cases is for the doctor to make certain of the diagnosis of the condition so that specific remedies may be applied.

PHARYNX—location (fig.): See EAR, article THE EAR, TONGUE, NOSE, AND THROAT.

PHENOL POISONING (See also, *Poisoning*) Once phenol, known as carbolic acid, and related material like the cresols were common causes of poisoning. Now other antiseptics have been developed and have replaced phenol as a commonly used germ destroying material. Phenol is a dangerous caustic substance which damages tissue with which it comes in contact. Moreover, it is absorbed and then injures the body generally. When absorbed it affects the centers in the brain responsible for breathing and for the circulation of blood.

Contamination of the skin or clothing with phenol demands immediate attention. The clothing should be removed and the skin washed as soon as possible with warm water or 50 per cent alcohol. Artificial respiration may be necessary and also rest and warmth.

PHENOLPHTHALEIN Phenolphthalein is a neutral drug that acts on the large bowel as a purgative. Some people are allergic to it and break out with skin eruptions. In general, however, it is among the least toxic of the usual laxatives. It is a constituent of a good many patent laxative drugs.

PHENOLPHTHALEIN—cathartic: See MEDICINE CHEST, article THE FAMILY MEDICINE CHEST.

PHENOLPHTHALEIN—laxative during pregnancy: See BIRTH, article CARE OF MOTHERS BEFORE AND AFTER CHILDBIRTH.

PHLEBITIS The human being walks upright so that the veins in his legs have to carry the burden of a column of blood returning to the heart. These veins have valves which may remain capable of holding up the column of blood throughout life. In many instances, however, the valves break down, and the result is the appearance of varicose veins.

If infections occur, the linings of the blood vessels become inflamed. Clots may be formed which are then carried off from the veins to appear elsewhere in the body. The blood may accumulate in the tissues of the legs, causing swelling and pain. Any illness which slows the circulation of the blood and during which there is a long period of lying in bed may induce the formation of clots in the blood vessels. If you happen to be walking when a clot forms, there is lameness in the leg, and the foot may swell and become blue.

In such cases relief is had by elevating the foot of the bed moderately or sleeping with the legs elevated. After about ten days of cautious exercise and the wearing of a semielastic bandage recovery will usually occur.

Inflammation of the blood vessels with the formation of such clots is known as thrombophlebitis, which comes from the words "thrombo," meaning clots, and "phlebitis," meaning inflammation of the veins.

After about 1 per cent of cases of childbirth and after about 2 per cent of severe operations in the abdominal cavity, thrombophlebitis occurs as a secondary complication. Sometimes if the infection is severe, there will be fever with chills. The chief danger from thrombophlebitis is the possibility that a portion of a clot may break away and get into the blood stream, eventually blocking an important blood vessel in the lungs, heart, or brain. Fortunately this complication is not exceedingly frequent. More frequent is the possibility that a clot may get into some other part of the body and set up a secondary infection or abscess.

A vein with thrombophlebitis is frequently painful. The doctor may prescribe many soothing remedies to overcome the pain and also to bring about relief. Since the pain may be due to a spasm of the blood vessels or of the muscles, remedies used to overcome spasm are helpful. Carefulness in keeping the legs elevated and taking pressure off the veins whenever possible often brings about complete relief in these cases.

PHOSPHATE Phosphates are essential for all life and have a multitude of functions in the body. The most obvious use of phosphates is in the formation of bone and teeth. Bones and teeth consist mostly of calcium triphosphate. Because phosphate forms this insoluble compound with calcium, the amount of phosphate present determines the amount of calcium in solution in the blood. The whole mechanism of calcium and phosphate deposition in bone and solution in blood is regulated by the parathyroid endocrine glands. Phosphate is required for the absorption, breakdown and storage of glucose (dextrose or grape sugar). Phosphate is contained in many enzymes, including those used in the breakdown of fat and glucose. Among its many other uses in the body, phosphate functions in energy balance. There are certain relatively unstable compounds, called active-phosphates, which have a high potential energy content. When these active phosphates break down, their energy is released, and it is this energy that is used in muscle contraction. Almost all energy that is obtained from food is either released as heat or stored as active phosphate.

PHOSPHORUS

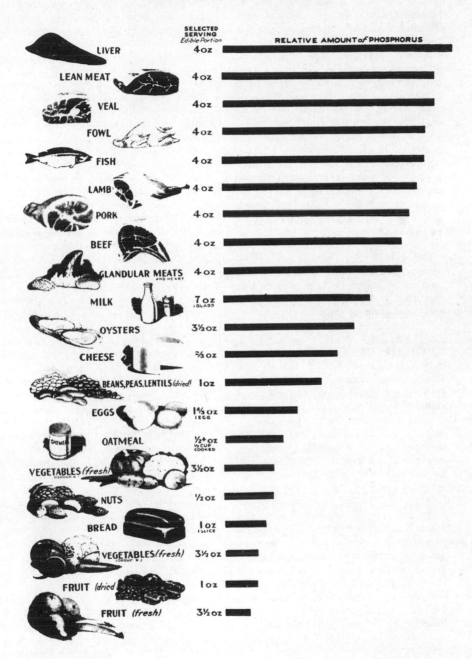

	SELECTED SERVING Edible Portion	RELATIVE AMOUNT of PHOSPHORUS
LIVER	4 oz	
LEAN MEAT	4 oz	
VEAL	4 oz	
FOWL	4 oz	
FISH	4 oz	
LAMB	4 oz	
PORK	4 oz	
BEEF	4 oz	
GLANDULAR MEATS AND HEART	4 oz	
MILK	7 oz (1 GLASS)	
OYSTERS	3½ oz	
CHEESE	⅔ oz	
BEANS, PEAS, LENTILS (dried)	1 oz	
EGGS	1⅘ oz (1 EGG)	
OATMEAL	½+ oz (½ CUP COOKED)	
VEGETABLES (fresh) (GROUP A)	3½ oz	
NUTS	½ oz	
BREAD	1 oz (1 SLICE)	
VEGETABLES (fresh) (GROUP B)	3½ oz	
FRUIT (dried)	1 oz	
FRUIT (fresh)	3½ oz	

1577

PHOSPHORUS Phosphorus is poisonous and is used extensively in preparations which kill roaches and rats. The heads of matches contain phosphorus, and these may be a source of accidental poisoning. The symptoms of phosphorus poisoning do not appear until several days after ingestion. Degeneration of the liver, kidneys and other organs are the immediate causes of the many, varied symptoms. While phosphorus as such is not normally found in the body, compounds containing phosphorus are needed. These compounds have an electrically charged unit (radical) containing a phosphorus atom in combination with four oxygen atoms and are called phosphates. (*See phosphates.*)

PHTHISIS (See *Tuberculosis*) Pulmonary consumption, or tuberculosis, used to be called phthisis because this condition produced progressive wasting and emaciation of the body.

PHYSICAL AND MENTAL GROWTH OF CHILD (See also, *Adjustment Problems of School Age Child*) The younger a child is, the faster it grows old. Children grow more rapidly during the early years of life than they do later. By carefully observing the growth of the child and its development the doctor can determine whether or not there are any deficiencies in its hygiene of living and correct any errors in the baby's care.

A routine physical examination of the baby includes its weight, height and other dimensions, a study of the bones to determine whether or not they are growing satisfactorily and coming together as they should, examination of the teeth and an estimate of the mental development of the child, including the use of its eyes, ears and other senses. An experienced doctor, just from looking at a child, can tell whether or not it is properly nourished, but the weight of the baby is an accurate measure of its nutrition. However, weight may be misleading, as for instance when fluid is accumulating in the body.

Babies should be weighed at least once every week during the first six months, every two weeks for the rest of the year, and every month during the second year. From that time on weights should be taken at fairly frequent intervals to determine the child's growth.

There is no normal weight for a baby at the time of birth. Children vary in their weight according to their heredity, the stock from which they come, the nutritional state of their parents and similar factors. During the early months of life there should be a gain of weight of from five to six ounces a week. During the second half year the average weekly gain should be from two and one-half to three ounces a week. The rate at which the child gains after two years of age is one-tenth that of early infancy.

Measurement of the height of a child is important because the child may be well nourished and may be gaining regularly in weight but may still be suffering from some of the conditions that cause dwarfing. As the child grows, there is a relative decrease in the size of the head and a relative increase in the rate of growth of the arms and legs as compared with the trunk. The size of the baby's head is usually followed with care during infancy because an undue increase in its size may be associated with such disturbances as accumulation of water in the brain, whereas a very small head may be associated with defective development. Fortunately, both these conditions are rather rare.

Parents are likely to worry a great deal about the speed of development of muscular activity by the child. If it seems at all slow in learning to walk, they become greatly disturbed. From the time the average baby is nine to 18 months of age it begins to creep, then to pull itself up by a chair, and then to walk. A child 15 months old can get upstairs by holding onto the banister or walking on all fours. It usually will come downstairs by sitting on the top step and then gradually sliding down one step at a time. However, some babies prefer to back downstairs. Either conduct is quite within the range of the normal. Usually a child 18 months old can go upstairs standing upright by holding onto the railing. There are records of children that have walked at nine months of age and even some that have walked at seven months. However, 40 per cent of children walk when they are a year old, and 67 per cent walk by the time they are 14 months old. A few children who may be otherwise quite normal may not walk before they are 18 to 20 months old. This may be due to lack of practice or perhaps in some cases to weakness.

Children must learn to walk. This activity requires coordination and strength of the muscles. When a child does begin to walk, parents must recognize the accomplishment and praise the child suitably. If the child cries too easily or becomes too much afraid of falls and bumps, it will learn to walk slowly. Fears created thus early in life may modify life thereafter. Among other factors that delay the acquirement of walking by children are overweight, rickets and bad nutrition generally. The child does not trust the strength of its muscles. Overweight should be controlled by suitable feeding, about which the doctor can advise; this applies equally to undernutrition. Rickets is a serious disease with bowing of the legs and muscular weakness, usually associated with lack of sufficient amounts of vitamins A and D, calcium and phosphorus. The doctor can with the X ray

study the development of the bones and the muscles and can prescribe suitably for a child with the insidious beginnings of rickets.

Some children learn to walk slowly because they are kept too long in play pens and not allowed freedom of movement. In some homes the floors are too slippery or too dirty or too drafty to practice walking. Some mothers, misguided as to their responsibility, will keep little children a long time in dresses that are too long and in shoes that are too soft.

Again any coordinated physical activity of the body is largely dependent on the mental state. If there is any doubt as to the child's development, the physician should be consulted promptly.

By the time a normal baby is 18 months old, it can get itself up into a child's chair and can climb into an adult's chair. Many times the baby will fall. However, normal babies pay little attention to such falls unless they are actually accompanied by injury.

Dr. Arnold Gesell of Yale University has made extensive studies of the rate of development of babies, taking motion pictures of babies of all ages doing various tasks. A one year old child can hold a cube in one hand and reach for another. Such a baby may occasionally get one cube on top of another but will never build a tower. By the time the baby is 18 months old it can build a tower with cubes, can throw a ball and can even try to turn the pages of a book, although a baby of this age is likely to turn three or four pages at one time.

A one year old baby will wave bye-bye as a sort of nursery trick. An 18 months old baby will bye-bye and mean it. It knows that "bye-bye" means the end of the visit. I have seen an 18 months old baby indicate to its parents that it was ready to leave by saying "bye-bye" to everyone in the vicinity. Such development means that the child has a brain with the ability to perceive and reason.

A one year old child has a sort of fragmentary sense that it is somebody. An 18 month old child can distinguish between itself and other people and will occasionally insist on owning certain toys and other belongings. A reasonably well developed 18 months old child will participate in family life by fetching and carrying on request and imitate the actions of older people.

Babies must learn certain things that are necessary for comfortable living. They must learn to tell the difference between people and things and between their own people and strangers.

Very young babies will stare at brilliant objects. Older babies will follow moving objects with their eyes. Young babies will grasp anything put into the hand. At the end of the third month the baby will begin to wave such objects about and to scratch them or pound them on the floor or on the table. By the fourth or fifth month hand and eye movements begin to be associated. By the sixth month the baby will look on the floor for something that it drops and will endeavor to pull toward itself any object that it cannot reach. Another test of mind and muscle is the ability to draw. Still more important is the kind of stories that interest children and willingness to listen to stories and to acquire information that they receive.

A two year old child can fold paper, use simple sentences and phrases, name familiar objects such as keys, pennies and watches, listen to stories, look at pictures, and even attempt to describe its own experiences. A child of three, when asked, will indicate its mouth, nose and eyes, repeat two numbers that are not consecutive and pick out a boy, a dog, a tree or a car in a picture.

TALKING—Speech is fundamental in differentiating human beings from other animals. The progress of speech, therefore, is one of the best tests of the men-

tal advancement of children. About the most exciting time in an average family is the moment when the baby begins to talk. In the first few months of life babies make sounds with little significance. However, these sounds must be a source of satisfaction to the baby or it would not spend so much time working at them. The first sounds that a baby makes are variations of the sounds of the vowels a and u. Then the consonants m, p and b are added to the vowels. These are the sounds that can be made with the lips closed. After the baby is three months old it will combine these sounds, so that sounds like umm, da, ma and goo are formed. If the baby puts two da's together, the father is flattered. If it puts two wah's together, the mother will insist that the baby wants a drink of water.

Soon the normal baby will see that there is value in the sounds that it makes. People bring things. Then the baby will imitate adult sounds, and soon it will learn to speak. As soon as the baby makes noises that sound like words and people begin praising and encouraging the baby, it will try to imitate itself and become proud of its ability. Such encouragement is a great help in teaching the baby to speak.

A baby can probably understand many words before he can say any of them. A bright baby will speak his first word about the time he is eight or nine months old. Almost any baby can be expected to say something by the time he reaches the tenth or twelfth month. The ability to combine words into phrases and sentences comes usually between the time the baby is one and one-half and two years old. From that time on the vocabulary will grow almost daily. By the time a child is seven years old he is probably familiar with almost 3,000 words. However, the number of words that a child can use varies with its intelligence. In general, smart children talk earlier and dull children talk later than the average. The development of speech is one of the methods that experts use for measuring intelligence. The extent to which parents work and live with their children may have a great deal to do with the ability of the child to acquire speech.

Remember that the child learns most of its speech through imitation. Parents should not use baby talk to the child because the child will imitate the kind of talk that it hears. Parents should not scream at their children without expecting the children to scream back. Talking in a well modulated voice with proper emphasis may be developed by training into a habit of which the child will be proud. Here are some good rules to follow in developing good speech habits in your children:

1. Do not correct the child's pronunciation or enunciation. Applaud that which is right. Do not stress that which is wrong.

2. Do not imitate the child's baby talk. When you say "dravy" for gravy and "wed" for red, simply because the baby talks that way, you confirm him in his difficulty. But do not correct him too severely. If you keep on talking English, he will talk it as soon as he can.

3. Never talk down to babies and little children.

4. Do not nag, coax or raise your voice in an effort to get the baby to talk. Speech will come naturally.

5. If the baby's uncle and aunt stammer, or if you stammer yourself, give the baby a chance to learn how to talk from someone else. Children will imitate.

6. Give the child a chance to talk and listen to him when he talks. This will encourage him.

7. Tell the child to listen. Do not ignore him but include him whenever possible in the conversation.

Finally, the inability to speak well often results from inability to hear well. Children who have severe colds and infected ears during childhood frequently lose enough of their hearing to interfere with the proper development of speech.

Statistics show that about 10 per cent of our people have some type of speech defect. Perhaps 1,500 000 children stutter and stammer; perhaps another million require help for other bad habits of speech. Any disorder of speech is so significant in the future life of a child that parents will do well to consult competent advice in this regard at the earliest possible moment. The child that stammers and stutters may be so seriously concerned by its disability as to become melancholic and unable to make the social contacts that are necessary for normal living.

The Choice of a Physician

BY

MORRIS FISHBEIN, M.D.

Former Editor, *Journal American Medical Association,* Chicago; Editor, *Excerpta Medica, Bulletin World Medical Assn.; Post-graduate Medicine.*

THE FAMILY DOCTOR

Of ALL THE PROBLEMS that may concern the average family, there is probably not one in which the decision is of more ultimate importance for the health and happiness of the family than the choice of the family physician. The family doctor of an earlier day was mostly learned in the school of experience. In many instances he had studied with a preceptor and perhaps had a course of lectures in some medical school lasting six months and devoted but slightly to the practical side of medicine. Such knowledge he obtained by studying cases with his preceptor. He did, however, develop an intimate personal relationship with those whom he served, which is recognized today as the basic feature of the best type of medical practice.

In the old days the family loved, indeed almost worshiped, the family doctor. He was their guide in health as well as in sickness. He alone, of all the community, knew the family secrets, and he could be depended on to keep the faith. True, his remedies were occasionally harsh and his diagnosis largely guesswork, but his record of cures is surprising. He was especially known for his ability to practise the art of scientific observation, using to the utmost his five senses. The physician of today has available innumerable scientific devices for aiding, prolonging, and extending these senses, but unless brains are carefully mixed with the application of the devices the end result may be confusion rather than scientific diagnosis, and the cost far beyond the necessary cost for first-class medical practice.

GRADUATION FROM A MEDICAL COLLEGE

In choosing a physician be sure you know the answers to the following questions: First, is he a graduate of a recognized medical school that requires at least four years of thorough training? There was a time when there were more medical schools in the United States than in all the rest of the world. We had almost 200 medical schools in this country around 1900. Today there are more than 80 medical colleges in the United States. Now all of these are rated as Class A by the Council on Medical Education and Hospitals of the American Medical Association. A Class A college is one with a certain definite number of full-time teachers and with a well-established graded curriculum. At least two years of college education are required previous to studying medicine, four years of medical education of approximately nine months each, and around one year or two years of internship after graduation before the prospective physician can get his diploma.

LICENSE BY THE STATE

Is the doctor licensed to practice medicine in the state in which he has his office? The majority of the states conduct regular examinations for a license to practise, these examinations being given by a group of physicians known as the State Medical Board of Registration and Licensure. In some states the doctor is required to renew his license every year. Before he can get a license he must usually show evidence of his graduation and also undergo a written and practical examination in the basic medical subjects. He must also present certificates of good moral character from at least two physicians who know him.

THE DOCTOR'S INTERNSHIP

Has the doctor had actual training as an intern in a hospital? Or has he been associated with a practising physician long enough to obtain practical education in medicine? Has he at the time of consultation a direct connection with a good hospital? There are in the United States almost 7,000 hospitals acceptable to the joint rating board of the American Hospital Association, the American Medical Association, the American College of Physicians and the American College of Surgeons. Of the 220,000 physicians in the United States more than 130,000 are directly affiliated with these hospitals as members of the staff.

The appointment of a physician to the staff of a good hospital indicates that he has been passed upon according to his qualifications by the medical staff of the hospital and frequently also by the board of directors of the institution.

MEMBERSHIP IN THE COUNTY MEDICAL SOCIETY

Is the doctor a member of his county medical society, of his state medical society, of the American Medical Association, or of any other recognized, organized body of physicians? The American Medical Association is organized like the United States government. It has county societies which pass carefully on physicians who wish to join. Before a man can belong to his state medical society he must belong to his county medical society. Before he can belong to the American Medical Association he must belong to both county and state medical societies. Before he can belong to any of the recognized special societies, such as those in surgery, diseases of the eye, ear, nose and throat, skin, and other specialties, he must belong to the American Medical Association or to his state and county medical societies.

While membership in a medical society is not an absolute guarantee of honesty or of good faith, the physician who belongs to such a society is subject to the criticism of his colleagues and subject also to being called before special committees to explain actions that are not considered ethical or satisfactory. A patient is much better off with a doctor who belongs to a recognized medical society than in the hands of one who is utterly independent of such organizational control. There are, of course, numerous medical organizations which are not recognized or established or scientific. There is even an organization composed of innumerable quacks who practise all sorts of strange medical cults and promote many unestablished notions.

CHARACTERISTICS OF AN ETHICAL DOCTOR

An ethical physician may be differentiated from a quack by certain well-established characteristics. An ethical physician does not advertise his methods or cures in a newspaper. He does not give out circulars concerning his work or his fees. He does not indiscriminately distribute his picture. He does not put large signboards on his windows or outside his office, advertising his extraordinary merits, or otherwise promoting his wares. A competent ethical physician seldom finds it necessary to travel from town to town to secure patients. He usually has an established place of residence and of work to which patients come when they require his services or to which they send, requesting his attendance when they themselves are unable to travel. The traveling doctor who moves from town to town is not to be consulted or to be considered a safe family physician.

There has been for years a tradition in medicine that new discoveries are freely published to the profession in the various medical periodicals and are not held as secrets by certain men which only they can apply. The public may therefore well beware of any doctor or group of doctors who advertise or publish broadcast the fact that they have discovered a new cure or method of treatment that other doctors do not know about, or who claim they can cure such serious conditions as cancer, tuberculosis, the venereal diseases, or rheumatic disease in a short time by some secret manipulation or by some unestablished method.

THE SCIENTIFIC ADVANCEMENT OF MEDICINE

The advancement of medicine has been associated with the introduction of innumerable complicated devices used not only in the diagnosis of disease but also in treatment. The sense of vision is aided by the microscope which enlarges invisible objects so that they may be seen. There are other instruments such as the cystoscope, the otoscope, the laryngoscope, and the ophthalmoscope which enable the physician competent in their use to look directly into various body cavities. By means of the X-ray, opaque tissues are brought into the field of vision, and by the use of various dye substances combined with the X-ray most of the organs and tissues of the body can now be seen during life.

The development of physics, of chemistry, of bacteriology, and of many sciences on which medicine rests has made it possible for physicians to determine to the thousandth of a gram the content of the blood and of various secretions and excretions of the body, determining thus the presence of sugar, of protein, of various salts, and of other substances related to the functions of the body in health and in disease. In surgery new devices have been developed for cutting tissues without hemorrhage, for keeping the patient quiet or anesthetized during operation, and for keeping conditions so clean that there is no danger of infection.

New methods have been discovered which aid the specialist in diseases of the nose and throat in looking into the sinuses, in determining their contours, in examining the ear externally and internally, and in peering into the very depths not only of the larynx but even of the lungs.

DEVELOPMENT OF SPECIALISTS

The employment of the special devices used in medical practice requires hours of study and practice for the development of proper technic. As a result of the tremendous expansion of medical knowledge specialization entered the field, so that today not only is medicine practised by general practitioners who, it has been determined, can easily take care of 85 per cent of the conditions for

TEST	PURPOSE OF TEST	HOW TEST IS MADE
Schick	To determine if person tested is susceptible to diphtheria.	Minute amount (1/10 cc.) of diluted diphtheria toxin is injected into skin on front surface of forearm with hypodermic syringe and needle.
Dick	To determine if person tested is immune to scarlet fever.	By injecting 1/10 cc. of diluted scarlet-fever toxin into skin on front surface of forearm with hypodermic syringe and needle.
Widal	To determine if person tested has typhoid or paratyphoid fever.	The finger is pricked, and about 1 cc. of blood is collected. Several dilutions of the blood serum are made with salt solution; it is then added to cultures of typhoid bacilli and paratyphoid bacilli. These mixtures are placed in an incubator at about 98° F. for an hour, then are examined to determine if the germs have been clumped by the serum.
Tuberculin	To aid in determining presence of tuberculosis infection.	Diluted solution of tuberculin is injected into the skin, usually on front surface of forearm. Tuberculin is prepared from culture of tubercle bacilli. Test is examined after forty-eight hours.
Sedimentation	To aid in diagnosing tuberculosis and acute infections such as rheumatic fever.	Five to 10 cc. of blood are drawn from patient's vein and mixed with one drop of a potassium-oxalate solution. Special tube is then used to determine amount of settling of red blood cells. Speed of settling is called sedimentation rate.
Complement Fixation	To aid in diagnosing syphilis. (Also called Wassermann, Kahn test, etc.)	To blood serum or spinal fluid from patient are added various extracts and serums.
Aschheim-Zondek	To determine if pregnancy has occurred.	Specimen of urine from the patient is made slightly acid, filtered, and then injected into number of young, normal mice. (In Friedman modification, rabbits are used.)
Basal Metabolism	To aid in diagnosing thyroid and other glandular disturbances.	Patient breathes into and out of container of oxygen. His heat-production rate is determined by his rate of oxygen consumption. Percentage of variation from normal heat-production rate is called his basal-metabolic rate.
Hemoglobin Determination	To determine amount of hemoglobin in blood.	Patient's fingertip or ear lobe is punctured, and a measured amount of blood is drawn into a pipette. Prior to further laboratory test, blood is placed in tube containing hydrochloric acid.
Red Blood Cell Determination	To determine presence of anemia or polycythemia.	A drop of patient's blood is diluted in a special pipette, and after proper preparation, the red blood cells are counted.
White Blood Cell Determination	To aid in determining presence of infections or leukemia.	Blood from patient is diluted with a special fluid that destroys the red blood cells but does not injure the white cells. After proper preparation, the white cells are counted.
Urine	To determine presence of kidney disease or diabetes.	Urine specimen is examined for presence of albumin, red and white blood cells, and sugar.
Clotting Time	To test clotting ability of blood.	Skin is punctured and time estimated before bleeding stops.
Prothrombin Time	To determine vitamin-K deficiency.	Test to determine adequacy of a substance in blood necessary for clotting.
Blood Pressure	To detect high or low blood pressure.	Measured with mercury column or spring instrument by putting cuff around patient's arm and getting record at contraction (systolic) and relaxation (diastolic) of heart.

INTERPRETATION OF TEST	REMARKS
Positive reaction shown by red area at point where toxin was injected. Negative reaction indicates person is immune to diphtheria.	Schick testing of children about every two or three years is advised by many physicians; also testing of adults before inoculation during epidemics.
Positive reaction consists of red area one centimeter or more in diameter, occurring eighteen to twenty-four hours after injection. No reaction indicates immunity to scarlet fever.	Some physicians do not consider the Dick-test results comparable in dependability with those of the Schick test.
Clumping of germs brought about by this serum indicates that patient has typhoid fever.	Test is of no value if person has had typhoid fever previously, or if he has been vaccinated against the disease.
Positive reaction is a red area about the point of injection after forty-eight hours.	Tuberculin test should always be considered in conjunction with other examinations.
Speeded-up sedimentation rate is evidence of the presence of some infection.	Many factors influence sedimentation rate, such as room temperature, concentration of red blood cells, length of sedimentation tube.
Reactions are judged by degree to which destruction of red blood cells is prevented.	Some doctors now deem it advisable to report the complement-fixation reactions only as positive, doubtful, or negative.
If the mice's ovaries are enlarged, test is positive for pregnancy.	Test stated to be reliable after tenth day following first missed menstrual period. Test remains positive until seven days after the birth of a full-term baby. Other new tests involve use of frogs, rabbits, etc.
Ten percent or more above or below normal—between plus or minus seven—indicates an abnormal condition. Above is a sign of hyperthyroidism.	Useful only in conjunction with physical examination and study of patient's symptoms. For accurate results in test, patient must be completely relaxed. Test is made after patient has fasted for twelve hours and has rested thirty minutes just before test.
Decrease in hemoglobin means anemia.	Sahli's method is briefly described here. There are other methods, but none is absolutely accurate.
Decrease of red blood cells below 4,500,000 to 6,000,000 per cubic millimeter indicates anemia.	When normal care is taken in this test, results are invariably reliable.
Above normal usually indicates infection.	Same as above.
Albumin may indicate acute or chronic kidney inflammation or infection of kidney. Red blood cells may be present in acute nephritis and in tumors or stones of the kidney. Large numbers of white blood cells indicate a bladder infection or infection of the kidney pelvis. Sugar usually means diabetes.	Color and odor of urine, presence of sediment, its reaction—that is, whether alkaline or acid—its specific gravity, are all important in diagnosing kidney and related disorders.
Usual time is one to three minutes.	Used in purpura and hemophilia.
Test shows insufficient amount of substance necessary for clotting blood.	Technique used before gall-bladder operations and in liver inflammation.
Normal rate is approximately 120 plus years, over twenty to thirty.	Routine in life-insurance examination.

which patients consult physicians, but it is practised in some eighteen to twenty specialties of various types, such as those which concern themselves wholly with internal medicine and diagnosis; surgery, which is divided into orthopedic surgery, genito-urinary surgery, brain surgery, abdominal surgery, and similar branches. There are also specialists in diseases of the skin, in diseases of women, in diseases of children, in obstetrics, in nervous and mental diseases, in diseases of the stomach and intestines, in industrial medicine, in preventive medicine, in anesthesia, and in several other more confined branches.

There is not as yet any legal method for determining who shall be considered competent to practise a specialty in medicine and who shall not. It therefore becomes possible for any physician who wishes to do so to set himself up as a specialist in any medical field. The rewards of specialization are usually beyond those of general practice in the form of shorter hours of work, more time for research, higher pay for work accomplished and, no doubt, much more interest in the work. Various means have been developed by the medical profession itself for limiting, if possible, entrance of unworthy men into various specialties. Some of the specialistic societies will not admit any man until he has had at least five years of experience in a specialty and until he has done sufficient research work and published enough scientific papers to prove his competence.

Moreover, the medical profession has itself established examining and certifying boards which now undertake, after a young man has been at least five years in practice, to give him both a written and a practical examination and, provided he is qualified, to issue to him a certificate of competence.

CONSULT THE FAMILY DOCTOR FIRST

In the vast majority of cases people who wish to consult a specialist will do well to go first to their family doctor or general practitioner so that he may, after a study of the case, select for the patient such specialists as may be necessary for consultation as to diagnosis or for specialistic treatment. In this way the patient may save himself a great deal of time and money. Numerous instances are recorded in which a patient with a pain in some portion of the body went directly to a specialist, only to find out that the pain which concerned him was not due to an organ within the field of that specialist but perhaps to some entirely different cause.

For instance, such a condition as ordinary dizziness may be due to causes arising in the digestive tract, in the heart and circulation, in the internal ear, or in the brain. Only a careful study of the history of the case, the nature of the symptoms, and similar factors, will enable a physician to see which one of these organs or systems may be concerned. Similarly, bleeding from the throat may be due to conditions in the throat, in which case a general practitioner or a specialist in diseases of the throat might be consulted. On the other hand, it might be due to tuberculosis of the lungs, to a tumor of the esophagus or to hemorrhage taking place in the stomach, in which case a specialist concerned with those organs might be needed. Hence, for the vast majority of complaints the patient should first of all consult a family physician, preferably one to whom he has gone for some time. He may confidently be guided by his advice.

PICKING A FAMILY DOCTOR

When coming into a community you may select your physician in various ways. If you will call the secretary of the county medical society the secretary will probably be willing to give you a list of general practitioners in his vicinity. You may then determine by meeting these men and by inquiry into their qualifications whether or not you care to commit the illnesses of yourself and of your family to their care. If you are a member of any well-established fraternal organization or church, association of commerce, business organization, or similar group, you may on inquiry among your associates in these groups find out who are the competent physicians in the community, and then, by making your own inquiries as to competence along the lines of the questions that have been suggested earlier in this chapter, determine which of those that have been recommended is suitable to your needs.

Once a physician has been selected and has been found competent to give not only the type of scientific advice needed for ordinary cases, but also to give the personal intimate attention that is the distinguishing characteristic of the best type of family doctor, you will do well to cling to that family physician and to recognize in him a friend and a counselor. Remember also that the servant is worthy of his hire. Far too often physicians' bills are the last to be paid because the very nature of the profession has in the past made the physician willing to wait until the bills for food, for clothing, for shelter, for fuel, and the other necessities of life have been taken care of. The physician must himself provide these things for his family. A physician who receives from his patient conscientious and responsible treatment is likely to return to that patient even more conscientious and responsible attention than he himself has received.

PICA Children frequently crave unnatural articles of food, eating dirt, sticks, plaster, or all sorts of similar materials. The condition is known as pica.

PICA—See BIRTH, article CARE OF MOTHERS BEFORE AND AFTER CHILDBIRTH.

PILES See *Hemorrhoids.*

PILONIDAL CYSTS At the very bottom of the human spine there is occasionally a glandular organ that does not close completely at the time of birth or that perhaps continues to secrete material which does not find an easy outlet, so that the end result is a cyst, a collection of fluid in a gland without any outlet. The point where the cyst appears is at the very end of the spine, where the tail would be if human beings had tails.

These cysts apparently cause greatest disturbance in men between the ages of twenty and forty-five, and they were a real problem for the surgeons of the United States Army and Navy during the war.

Ancient people gave the pilonidal cyst its name, since the words "pilus" and "nidus" simply mean a place where there is hair or a nest of hair. If the little opening becomes infected, there is inflammation with pain on sitting or motion. Sometimes attempts are made to treat this by the use of hot sitz baths, the application of hot-water bottles, minor incisions merely to let out the fluid that is under pressure, and similar temporary procedures. When, however, the openings get blocked with hair, with dirt or with body secretions, competent surgical action is needed.

With soldiers in jeeps, fliers who sit for long periods of time and come down with a bump, or truck drivers, the cyst frequently becomes inflamed. If the blocking is sufficient to cause large accumulations of material, the cyst may grow to the size of an egg.

A proper surgical operation for pilonidal cyst includes the cutting out of the abnormal tissue and sufficient time in the hospital to permit complete healing. Since this may involve the removal of a large amount of tissue, some reparative or plastic surgery procedures may ultimately be necessary to bring about completely satisfactory results.

Attempts have been made by experimentation to find ways to inject the area with caustic substances and to obliterate it as one obliterates varicose veins. However, these methods are still considered in the experimental stage.

PINEAL GLAND The pineal gland is another gland whose activities seem to cease at the time of maturity. This gland lies within the skull at the lower portion of the brain. As yet we do not know with certainty what its functions in the human body actually are. The gland is tiny—about the size of a pea when it is flattened out. When, however, it becomes enlarged from any cause, it tends to close up the canal by which the cerebrospinal fluid circulates from the brain into the spinal cord. If this canal is closed, the fluid in the brain develops a high pressure with symptoms so serious that they may lead to death.

We learn about the functions of the glands in various ways. One of the methods is to destroy the gland completely in an animal or to remove it from the animal's body and then observe the animal to see what happens. Another method is to make an extract of the gland and feed it to animals in excess to see what an excess of this glandular material will do to the animal.

Various effects have been observed following the injection of extracts of the pineal into animals. It is supposed to have some effect in stopping over-action by the sex glands and also to inhibit too rapid growth. These effects are doubtful. No method has yet been found for making an extract of the pineal gland which with certainty has definite activity. Generally animals fed with this material grow larger and stronger muscularly, although there may be trouble with the development of the genital organs. In guinea pigs, if the gland is destroyed, the sex organs grow more rapidly and become larger than those of animals which do not have their pineal gland destroyed.

Here is a gland in the internal system which is obviously of some importance in the life of the human being but which needs to be studied far more extensively before we can say exactly what its functions are.

PINEAL GLAND—See article ENDOCRINOLOGY.

PINEAL GLAND—location (fig.): See article ENDOCRINOLOGY.

PITUITARY GLAND The pituitary gland is a veritable storehouse of hormones or important glandular principles. At least five of these are already well recognized. One is known as the growth hormone, another as the sex hormone, the third as the thyroid-stimulating hormone, the fourth as the milk-stimulating hormone, and the fifth as the adrenal-gland-stimulating hormone.

Any trouble with the growth hormone is promptly reflected in the size of the animal or child concerned. If the hypophysis, as this gland is sometimes called, is removed from a young animal, its growth is stopped. In a few weeks its long bones will discontinue increasing in length. Moreover, the body weight as a whole remains low.

The pituitary gland secretes a substance which is definitely related to the activities of the sex glands. Unless this portion of the gland is functioning adequately, the sex organs and the glands do not grow satisfactorily, and the person does not mature.

When a woman becomes pregnant, the substance secreted by the gland which maintains her periodic functions is no longer needed by the body and is found in the urine. This fact is the basis of the tests which have been developed for determining whether or not a woman is pregnant. In these tests, known as the Aschheim-Zondek test, the urine of the patient is injected into immature mice or rabbits. Within a few days, if the hormone is present in the urine, these animals become mature. Urine from a woman who is not pregnant will not produce maturity in the animals. This test is known to be effective in from 98 to 99 per cent of cases and constitutes one of the greatest advances of medical science in recent years.

Since the hormone is known to exist in the urine of pregnant animals, it has become possible to isolate it and to use it as a medicine in the treatment of various conditions. These conditions are practically all of the type involved in action of the sex glands. The determination as to whether or not the pituitary principle is to be used must rest with the physician after a most thorough study of the condition in the individual patient.

In the same way it is recognized that there lies in the pituitary gland a substance which is important in relation to the secretion of milk and other substances which are definitely related to the flow of the urine. There is, moreover, a portion of the gland which seems to be primarily concerned with the action of the thyroid gland.

These glandular substances are used in the treatment of a variety of conditions. Some are still in an exceedingly early experimental stage. But more and more is being learned as to how the human body may be influenced through this interlocking directorate of glands.

The posterior portion of the pituitary gland has a definite effect on the unstriped muscle mechanism in the human body, serving to stimulate it when it is not active. It is, therefore, used to aid the action of the organs in childbirth, to stimulate motion of the bowels when they seem to be paralyzed under various circumstances, and, finally, to have some effect in stimulating the development of the blood sugar.

In general, when the pituitary gland is inactive, the patient is slow and sluggish, both mentally and physically. Fat increases in various portions of the body, and the patient falls asleep readily. If the condition occurs before the child i. grown, mental development is retarded. the sex glands remain small, and maturity is delayed.

When there is overactivity of the gland as a whole, there may be all sorts of symptoms due to the enlargement of the gland in addition to the overgrowth and overdevelopment already mentioned.

In addition to the functions of the pituitary gland that have already been mentioned, it has a definitely established place as a controlling gland over some of the other glands in the system. For instance there is one substance from the pituitary which is called the diabetogenic substance, because it is known that the pituitary can definitely influence the use of both carbohydrates and fats in the body.

The investigators are convinced that the pituitary has some definite relationship with the islands of Langerhans of the pancreas, important in the control of sugar. When these islands are deficient, diabetes develops. For instance it is known that removal of the pancreas will result in the appearance of sugar in the blood and the urine of the animal, after which removal of the pituitary will considerably ameliorate these symptoms. The death of an animal with the pancreas removed is considerably postponed if the pituitary gland is removed at the same time.

Moreover, the removal of the pituitary gland from an animal in which the pancreas is intact will result in a lessened amount of sugar in the blood and in the urine. At the same time the amount of sugar stored in the muscles and in the liver as glycogen is lessened.

Next the pituitary gland secretes a substance which helps to control the thyroid gland. Whenever there is a deficient action of the thyroid gland, the pituitary increases in size. Patients who have a deficient action of the pituitary gland tend to have a basal metabolism that is lower than normal. Administration of the substance from the pituitary which is known to control the thyroid will result in enlargement of the thyroid.

Another principle of the pituitary controls the adrenal glands. Removal of the pituitary is followed promptly by a breakdown of the adrenal glands. Thus it is thought to be possible that the substance in the pituitary gland may set up the first steps of the disease which follows complete destruction of the adrenal glands. This disease, which is called Addison's disease, may be treated by the administration of the cortex of the adrenal glands. Formerly patients who had a breakdown of the adrenals invariably died. Now by the use of this extract, which is called cortin, their lives may be lengthened. It is conceivable that the giving of the pituitary adrenal principle would also help in such cases.

Finally, there is a definite effect of the pituitary on the parathyroid glands, which are largely concerned with the handling of calcium by the body and with the growth of bones.

The substance in the pituitary that controls the adrenal cortex is ACTH or corticotropin. Investigators also believe a substance in the pituitary that controls growth may have some relation to various forms of cancer. Experimental removal of the pituitary in one case stopped a cancer of the prostate gland.

PITUITARY EXTRACT—diabetes insipidus: See article ENDOCRINOLOGY.

PITUITARY EXTRACT—diabetes mellitus: See article DIABETES.

PITUITARY EXTRACT—menstrual irregularity corrected by: See article ENDOCRINOLOGY.

PITUITARY EXTRACT—underactive testes or ovaries supplemented by: See article ENDOCRINOLOGY.

PITUITARY GLAND—See article ENDOCRINOLOGY.

PITUITARY GLAND—age affects: See article OLD AGE.

PITUITARY GLAND—associated with peculiar changes in body structure: See article ENDOCRINOLOGY.

PITUITARY GLAND—diabetes insipidus: See KIDNEY, article THE KIDNEY: ITS DISEASES AND DISTURBANCES.

PITUITARY GLAND—hair growth: See HAIR, article THE HAIR.

PITUITARY GLAND—hormones used for arthritis, gout, and rheumatism: See article ARTHRITIS, RHEUMATISM, AND GOUT.

PITUITARY GLAND hypertension influenced by: See article BLOOD PRESSURE.

PITUITARY GLAND—location (fig.): See article ENDOCRINOLOGY.

PITUITARY GLAND—menstruation: See WOMEN, article HYGIENE OF WOMEN.

PITUITARY GLAND—secretion of Langerhans islands influenced by: See article DIABETES.

PITUITARY GLAND—skin affected by: See SKIN, article THE SKIN.

PITUITARY GLAND—testes stimulated to grow and secrete: See article ENDOCRINOLOGY.

PLAGUE In the Middle Ages plagues of various kinds used to devastate mankind. Now we have learned that these plagues were due to the spread of certain germs which are known as the germs of plague or pestilence. The two most common forms of plague are bubonic and pneumonic plague, depending on whether the germs infect the lungs or are associated with the appearance of a swollen abscess in the groin, commonly called a bubo. Modern medicine has developed methods of vaccination against plague and technics of control which prevent the spread of the disease so that it is exceedingly rare in civilized countries. There have been only a few cases of pneumonic or bubonic plague in the past fifty years.

PLAGUE—cause determined: See INFECTIOUS DISEASE, article THE PREVENTION AND TREATMENT OF INFECTIOUS DISEASE.

PLAGUE—fleas: See INFECTIOUS DISEASE, article THE PREVENTION AND TREATMENT OF INFECTIOUS DISEASE.

PLAGUE—occurrence: See INFECTIOUS DISEASE, article THE PREVENTION AND TREATMENT OF INFECTIOUS DISEASE.

PLANTAR WARTS (See also, *Feet, Warts*) Among the most painful of all warts are those that occur on the sole of the foot, commonly called plantar warts. These are probably caused by infection of the rubbed skin with a specific virus. A wart on the sole of the foot soon becomes so painful as to interfere with walking.

Plantar warts are treated in a variety of ways. The hard skin on the bottom of the foot must be softened, and the wart removed. The damaged tissue is protected by proper bandages and antiseptics during the process of healing. Such warts may be removed by surgery, by electrocoagulation, sometimes by radium or X-ray.

PLEURISY The lining of the cavity of the chest is called the pleura. Any inflammation or infection of this lining leads to symptoms which are grouped together under the name "pleurisy."

The pleura covers the inside of the chest wall, the top of the diaphragm, and the outer side of the lungs. When the pleura becomes inflamed, it tends to give off a good deal of fluid. The accumulation of this fluid in the chest cavity develops a condition that is called pleurisy with effusion. If the fluid given off becomes secondarily infected with pus-forming germs, there is a purulent pleurisy or an empyema. If the condition heals, there may be thickening of the wall. Inflammation and the accumulation of fluid also limit the breathing, displace the heart and other organs, and cause a good deal of pain.

Usually pleurisy is secondary to disease in some other part of the body, so that the infection of the pleura follows a disease of the lung or the carrying of germs from an abscess elsewhere in the body to the pleura. Occasionally pleurisy follows damage to the chest wall.

Pleurisy may begin with a sudden, severe stitch or pain in the side. Difficulty in breathing brings on a cough. There is expectoration. If there is a severe infection, there may also be chills and fever.

Pleurisy is a painful condition, and the patient who has it will show evidence of his distress. He will try to lie so that the pain is relieved. When the doctor listens to the chest, he can hear a rubbing that is characteristic of the roughened lining membranes when they touch each other.

The control of pleurisy, when there is not any outpouring of fluid into the chest cavity, involves rest in bed and treatment of the disease so as to eliminate the infection. The pain is relieved with heat. Often it becomes necessary, however, to strap the chest tightly with adhesive tape so as to reduce its motion.

Once fluid has developed in the chest cavity, it is necessary to determine its presence by the usual methods which the doctor follows and also by use of the X ray. The doctor can put a needle into the chest wall and remove the fluid, which brings about prompt relief. In case of serious infection with the production of empyema, surgical operation may be necessary. However, the development of the sulfonamide drugs and of penicillin now makes it possible in many instances to produce cures by draining the cavity and by putting in solutions of these remedies which act directly on the infecting germs.

PLEURISY—symptom of rheumatic fever: See HEART, article DISEASES OF THE HEART AND CIRCULATION.

PNEUMONIA In the vast majority of cases of pneumonia the cause is a germ known as the pneumococcus. There are at least thirty-four different types of this germ, and they may be identified by the physician through laboratory tests of the sputum. Many cases of pneumonia are caused by germs other than the pneumococcus. In some instances the streptococcus produces pneumonia that is even more serious than that caused by the pneumococcus. Recently there have been many cases of pneumonia associated with infection with specific viruses. In most instances pneumonia comes on after a severe cold or in association with some other infectious disease.

Until recent discoveries, such as the sulfonamides and penicillin, pneumonia was among the most feared of all diseases. That fear has not entirely disappeared. Any condition that attacks a vital organ of the body is serious. Diseases that strike the heart, lungs, and brain are more feared than those that affect the digestion or the muscles of the body. Some diseases cause death in a short time; human beings fear most those diseases that produce death rapidly.

Doctors combated pneumonia twenty-five years ago chiefly by good nursing, by the use of drugs to support the heart and the circulation, and by controlling excessive fever and intoxication of the body. Nowadays the mainstays in the treatment of pneumonia are the sulfonamide drugs, penicillin, and the use of oxygen. With these new methods of treatment the number of deaths from pneumonia has been cut more than two thirds. The death rates for pneumonia in the Army are the lowest that have ever been recorded. Whereas 17 per cent of the men in our Army who were infected with pneumonia died of the disease in World War I, less than 1 per cent of those infected with pneumonia died in World War II.

In a typical case of pneumonia the person who has had a light cold or some infectious disease is taken suddenly with a shaking chill and a sharp, stabbing pain in the side. This pain is made worse by breathing. Then comes a cough with bloody or brownish expectoration and fever. Frequently headache and nausea disturb the patient, and occasionally there is vomiting. Sleep is difficult because of the general misery and the pain. Among the worst of the symptoms are prostration and weakness. However, in some instances, weak as the patient may be, he has delirium and sudden urges which may cause him to attempt to leave the bed.

As the infection develops, the outpouring of blood and serum into the lung causes it to solidify, so there is insufficient breathing space and great difficulty in causing the blood, which comes back to the heart through the veins, to go through the lungs in order to receive new oxygen. As a result, the fingernails and the skin turn blue, and there is great shortness of breath. The breathing is shallow and grunting.

As the disease continues to become worse, the abdomen becomes distended, there is delirium and occasionally even jaundice. The fever becomes higher and the illness profound.

As the patient recovers, the temperature and the pulse return to normal, but the patient will remain weak for weeks or months and only gradually regains strength. Sometimes the recovery is delayed by complications, such as secondary infection in the chest, producing the condition called empyema. Such collections of pus cause the temperature to be high in the evening and low in the morning, and surgery may be necessary to let the pus out of the chest. However, the use of the sulfonamide drugs and penicillin has greatly lessened this complication.

The care of a patient with pneumonia taxes to the utmost the skill of the doctor and the nurses. Pneumonia patients must be kept at rest and should remain in bed for at least a week after the temperature, the pulse, and the breathing rates have returned to normal. The diet of the patient with pneumonia is usually ample, with plenty of salt and enough fluids to maintain the fluid content of the body. If there has been purging or elimination of great amounts of fluid by vomiting or by the bowel, this fluid must be restored.

Relief from pain and discomfort can be had by the prescription of suitable drugs. Especially valuable also for the relief of the pain in pneumonia is strapping of the chest to prevent excessive stretching of the ribs. The application of poultices, jackets of various kinds, and electric applications may afford comfort but certainly do not have any direct action on the pneumonia, and they sometimes interfere with the breathing of exhausted patients.

The greatest danger to life in pneumonia is in the extremes—that is, in the very young and in the very old. The disease is usually more dangerous to women than to men. It occurs more frequently to those who suffer from exposure to bad weather by their occupations, who are weakened through undernourishment, or who have indulged excessively in alcohol.

For a long time physicians depended in the treatment of pneumonia on a variety of serums which had been developed and which were specific to a certain extent against the individual types of infection. Today the sulfonamides and penicillin have been found so efficient in this condition that the use of serums is likely to disappear except in occasional cases when the physician may consider it necessary.

Particularly valuable against pneumonia is that form of the sulfonamides known as sulfadiazine. Combinations of sulfadiazine with other sulfonamide drugs are also useful in pneumococcus infections.

The shortness of breath in pneumonia is one of the most serious of the symptoms and used to be treated by making sure that the windows were kept wide open and that there was plenty of fresh air in the room. More recently the value of oxygen has been established, so that the shortness of breath and the blueness associated with insufficient oxygen are overcome by the use of oxygen chambers or oxygen tents for those seriously ill with pneumonia. Sometimes also the patient who is short of breath is helped by a semisitting position rather than being permitted to lie flat on the back.

It used to be said that recovery from pneumonia depended on the heart, and drugs to stimulate and aid the heart were frequently given. Nowadays so much benefit is derived from overcoming the infection itself and the intoxication caused by the infection and by the use of oxygen that remedies directed to enforcing the action of the heart are less often used. However, the constant attention of the physician in a case of pneumonia is exceedingly important, since he can detect difficulties related to the heart at the earliest possible moment and give the relief that is indicated when symptoms affecting the heart appear.

Especially important in all cases of pneumonia is the period of recovery. The greatest danger lies in the endeavor to get the patient up and back to work too soon.

In most cases the fever persists from five to ten days, although occasionally even longer. Then the condition improves by a crisis, which is one of the most striking features of the disease, or by a gradual improvement. When a crisis occurs in pneumonia, the patient seems to be on the verge of collapse; suddenly he begins to perspire freely, there is a rapid drop in the temperature to normal or subnormal, a slowing of the breathing and pulse rates, and in a few hours the person looks and feels better and drops off into a quiet sleep. There is no truth to the statement that the crisis always occurs on an odd day, like the fifth, seventh, or ninth.

Unlike other acute infectious diseases, pneumonia may occur more than once in the same person. Indeed there is a belief that recurrence of pneumonia appears more often than that of any other infectious disease. There does not seem to be any truth in the belief that a person who has had one attack of pneumonia is likely to have others of the same type; rather we now know that there are several different kinds of pneumonia and the person who has had one kind of pneumonia may get one of the other types.

BRONCHOPNEUMONIA—old people: See article OLD AGE.

BRONCHOPNEUMONIA—vitamin A deficiency: See article DEFICIENCY DISEASES.

PNEUMONIA—See RESPIRATORY DISEASES, article THE RESPIRATORY DISEASES.

PNEUMONIA—albuminuria may result: See KIDNEY, article THE KIDNEY: ITS DISEASES AND DISTURBANCES.

PNEUMONIA—arthritis can result: See article ARTHRITIS, RHEUMATISM, AND GOUT.

PNEUMONIA—atypical virus: See RESPIRATORY DISEASES, article THE RESPIRATORY DISEASES.

PNEUMONIA—bronchial asthma mistakenly diagnosed: See article ALLERGY.

PNEUMONIA—cause determined: See INFECTIOUS DISEASE, article THE PREVENTION AND TREATMENT OF INFECTIOUS DISEASE.

PNEUMONIA—chemical: See article OCCUPATION AND HEALTH.

PNEUMONIA—cold may introduce: See RESPIRATORY DISEASES, article THE RESPIRATORY DISEASES.

PNEUMONIA—convulsions in infants at onset: See INFANCY, article CARE AND FEEDING OF THE CHILD.

PNEUMONIA—danger in infantile paralysis: See CHILDHOOD DISEASES, article INFECTIOUS DISEASES OF CHILDHOOD.

PNEUMONIA—death rate: See article DIABETES; HEART, article DISEASES OF THE HEART AND CIRCULATION.

PNEUMONIA—diabetes: See article DIABETES.

PNEUMONIA—diabetes mortality lower: See article DIABETES.

PNEUMONIA—endocarditis may occur: See HEART, article DISEASES OF THE HEART AND CIRCULATION.

PNEUMONIA—febrile nephroses may result: See KIDNEY, article THE KIDNEY: ITS DISEASES AND DISTURBANCES.

PNEUMONIA—gall bladder may be affected: See article DIGESTION AND DIGESTIVE DISEASES.

PNEUMONIA—glanders symptoms similar: See article TRANSMISSIBLE DISEASES.

PNEUMONIA—herpes associated with: See SKIN, article THE SKIN.

PNEUMONIA—infants: See INFANCY, article CARE AND FEEDING OF THE CHILD.

PNEUMONIA—inflammation of colon: See article DIGESTION AND DIGESTIVE DISEASES.

PNEUMONIA—lungs: See INFECTIOUS DISEASE, article THE PREVENTION AND TREATMENT OF INFECTIOUS DISEASE.

PNEUMONIA—pneumococcus causes: See INFECTIOUS DISEASE, article THE PREVENTION AND TREATMENT OF INFECTIOUS DISEASE; RESPIRATORY DISEASES, article THE RESPIRATORY DISEASES.

PNEUMONIA—pneumococcus in lungs: See INFECTIOUS DISEASE, article THE PREVENTION AND TREATMENT OF INFECTIOUS DISEASE.

PNEUMONIA—primary: See INFANCY, article CARE AND FEEDING OF THE CHILD.

PNEUMONIA—psittacosis resembles: See article TRANSMISSIBLE DISEASES.

PNEUMONIA—resistance reduced by chronic disorders: See INFECTIOUS DISEASE, article THE PREVENTION AND TREATMENT OF INFECTIOUS DISEASE.

PNEUMONIA—respiratory disease: See RESPIRATORY DISEASES, article THE RESPIRATORY DISEASES.

PNEUMONIA—rheumatic fever sometimes accompanied by: See HEART, article DISEASES OF THE HEART AND CIRCULATION.

PNEUMONIA—rheumatism can result: See article ARTHRITIS, RHEUMATISM, AND GOUT.

PNEUMONIA—Rocky Mountain spotted fever may introduce: See article TRANSMISSIBLE DISEASES.

PNEUMONIA—secondary: See INFANCY, article CARE AND FEEDING OF THE CHILD.

PNEUMONIA—sinus infection may cause: See EAR, article THE EAR, TONGUE, NOSE, AND THROAT.

PNEUMONIA—virus, frequently attacks

patients with lung cancer: See article CANCER.

PNEUMONIA—whooping cough frequently precedes: See CHILDHOOD DISEASES, article INFECTIOUS DISEASES OF CHILDHOOD.

PNEUMONIC PLAGUE See discussion under *Plague*.

POISONING Hardly a substance exists in nature but is capable of producing unsalutary effects on the human body if taken in sufficient amounts or under the wrong circumstances or in relationship to certain tissues. Any substance capable of producing such deleterious effects is known as a poison. For every substance there is a safe dose and a poisonous dose.

When a physician is confronted with a case of suspected poisoning, he must provide first aid, which is designed to remove the dangerous substance from the body and overcome the dangerous symptoms. First try to ascertain the nature of the poison taken. An empty bottle in the vicinity, the presence of some of the substance in a cup or utensil, or the presence of some of the substance on the tablecloth, the floor, or the clothing may be a valuable sign. By examining the breath or the mouth of the patient one may sometimes determine the possibility of poisoning. If the person has taken the poison accidentally, he may be willing to tell the doctor, provided, of course, that the patient is still conscious.

If poisoning is suspected, the doctor should be called immediately. Before the doctor arrives, it is well to give whites of eggs, milk, or strong tea, which are antagonistic to many poisons.

In order to get the poison out of the body as rapidly as possible, one may provoke vomiting. This may be done by tickling the back of the throat or by giving a cup of warm water with salt or by using a stomach tube, provided a stomach tube is handy and one knows how to use it. Perhaps the simplest procedure is to put a heaping teaspoonful of salt in a cup of lukewarm water, stir until the salt is dissolved, and have the patient drink the mixture, repeating every three or four minutes until vomiting is provoked. Usually vomiting will occur promptly and will serve to wash out the stomach. Thereafter the case must be treated as any other case of dizziness, faintness, or shock.

The symptoms must be treated according to the severity of the poisoning. If the patient is greatly weakened or prostrated, he must be kept reasonably warm, recumbent, and his general strength must be sustained.

In poisoning with narcotic drugs it is customary to provoke vomiting and then to give strong black coffee, at the same time doing everything possible to keep the patient awake. Sometimes it is necessary to walk the patient about forcefully. As long as the person is awake, he will continue to breathe; if he is permitted to sleep, breathing may stop.

For many common poisons there are special antidotes. Few people have time to consult tables of antidotes; few people remember where an antidote is to be found.

In considering the care of cases of poisoning for purposes of first aid, it is preferable to consider them in groups according to the nature of the poison. More deaths are due to carbon monoxide gas than to any other poison. Many of these deaths are suicidal; others are accidental; and in a few instances carbon monoxide gas has been used for homicide. The person who has been poisoned with carbon monoxide gas has a purple appearance, the blood is fluid and cherry-red in color. All of the organs are congested and cherry-red in color. The most important sources of carbon monoxide gas are coal and coke in charcoal stoves, various industrial and chemical industries, the exhaust gas from motorcars, the exhaust gas from internal-combustion engines, mine explosions, blasting operations, factory furnaces, blast furnaces, and tunnels in which carbon monoxide gas accumulates.

As soon as a person has been removed from the gas, the cherry-red coloration may be considerably reduced. After recovery from carbon monoxide poisoning, depending on the severity of the poisoning, there may be headaches, inflammations of the nerves, and in some instances mental disturbances.

In warfare many gases capable of poisoning the human body were once used. These include blister gases, mustard gases, and lewisite, which gives burns like those of mustard gas. The blister fluid from lewisite contains arsenic.

There are also lung-irritant gases which are sometimes found in industry. These include chlorine, phosgene, and chloropicrin. Their effects are primarily on the lungs.

Other gases are tear gases which cause the eyes to fill with tears and make vision difficult if not impossible. Such gases as methylchloride, sulfur dioxide, and ammonia, used in various types of refrigeration apparatus, have also the possibility of poisoning the human body when the person is exposed to a considerable dose.

In connection with war defense, technics of detection and protection against all these gases have been developed.

The corrosive acids include hydrochloric acid, nitric acid, and sulfuric acid; the alkalis include potassium, sodium compounds, and ammonia. The taking of these substances in fairly large amounts will so damage the tissues that death ensues, often in a few minutes.

Following the taking of such substances, there is immediate burning, pain from the mouth to the stomach, with destruction of the mucous membranes of the mouth. Then come shock and collapse, with a rapid feeble pulse, coldness of the extremities, clammy sweating, thirst, and depression.

The treatment of acid poisoning involves the giving of alkalis, but the carbonates and bicarbonates are usually avoided because they create carbon dioxide gas. The substances best given are solutions of lime water and, in an emergency, soap solutions may be used. Substances like milk, oil, or barley water also help to control the damage.

In acid poisoning or alkali poisoning the damage is usually so severe that hospitalization and the constant care of a physician may be required.

When a person is poisoned with an alkaline substance, it is customary to give him a dilute acid like vinegar or lemon juice. If a carbonate has been taken, it is customary to give potassium salts, which means magnesium sulfate. The whites of egg, barley water, or oily solutions may help to overcome the damage. The great danger of poisoning with such substances is the scarring that occurs with complete closure of the throat or the esophagus, so that long-continued treatment, or even surgery, may be necessary to make it possible for the patient to live.

There are innumerable drugs which can poison the human being. (Each of these is discussed under the appropriate alphabetical designation.) Reports have been made of unnecessary deaths due to bichloride of mercury, kerosene, and gasoline. Commonly used in households for cleaning purposes are substances like benzene and carbon disulfide, which also have poisoning possibilities.

More rare are cases of poisoning by substances like arsenic, zinc, and thallium. In connection with poisoning by substances of this kind, it is well to remember that we are confronted with the possibility of chronic poisoning through the taking of small amounts over a long period of time as well as with the acute cases which follow the taking of a large dose.

Children have died from strychnine poisoning because they ate large amounts of sugar-coated cathartic pills which contained strychnine. There are numerous reports of people who have taken overdoses of medicines for sleeping or for relieving pain. These substances are not poisonous in ordinary amounts but become poisonous when too much is taken.

People have been poisoned by nicotine sprays used on plants.

Once great numbers of people suffered from lead poisoning. Babies have suffered from such poisoning due to chewing paint on cribs, baby carriages, play pens, or toys. Lead pipes occasionally are used in plumbing and enough lead has been known to get into water or beer or wines conveyed in pipes to produce cases of poisoning. An unusual instance of lead poisoning was brought about by the burning of discarded storage-battery casings as fuel. Altogether, however, the danger of lead poisoning is much less than it used to be because scientific controls have been developed in industry following the detection of this hazard. For years people have joked about the possibility of dying from lead poisoning due to bullets. Finally, however, a scientific report has appeared which proves definitely that lead could be discharged from bullets in the body and produce damage.

ACETANILID POISONING — Acetanilid and phenacetin, as well as pyramidon, are frequent constituents of headache remedies which in sufficiently large doses will bring about death. In addition to the measures usually tried in poisoning, it may be necessary in severe cases to use artificial respiration in order to force the breathing to continue.

ARSENIC POISONING—No matter how arsenic gets into the body, it is eventually passed into the intestines from the blood, although small amounts are eliminated in the hair and considerable of it may be carried to the skin to produce pigmentation.

If small doses of arsenic are taken into the body over long periods of time, irritation of the nerve endings is produced.

Years ago arsenic was found to contaminate beer made under bad conditions in England, and there was an epidemic of such irritation of the nerves among persistent beer drinkers.

Workers in arsenic may have the skin of the hands so severely affected that there will be ulceration down to the bone.

BARBITURATE POISONING—Stories continue to appear about people who die either purposely or by accident from large doses of "sleeping pills." The most common ingredient of sleeping pills is barbituric acid in the form of salts called barbiturates. Among the most commonly known of those are luminal, seconal, phenobarbital, pentobarbital, amytal, dial, ipral, neonal, and ovipal. Every drug manufacturer deals in products of this kind.

Most states have laws that require prescription of the tablets by a physician; some states require a new prescription before an old prescription can be filled. All these drugs can put people to sleep. They differ in the speed of their action, the duration of their effect, and the extent to which the body can get rid of the drugs. With excessive doses people find themselves unsteady in their walking. At the same time the drug slows the breathing, increases the heart rate, causes a fall in the blood pressure and the temperature. Some people become used to the drugs and think they are able to take larger and larger doses without hazard. Eventually many pass the margin of safety and are found unconscious or dead.

The doctor when called to see such patients must find first the cause of the unconsciousness. Cases are known in which people have taken from five to ten times enough to produce sleep and have still recovered. Once the average dose is exceeded the risk begins. The doctor must make sure that the throat is clear of mucus and that the patient will get enough air. If there is blueness, oxygen is given at once. The oxygen will cause the blueness to disappear if the patient is able to use the lungs. If, however, the breathing is feeble it may be necessary to supply artificial respiration with one of the machines available for this purpose. A suggestion has been made to put a small amount of a drug that can cause vomiting in each pill. If too many pills are taken the patient vomits and thus gets rid of the poisonous sedative.

Several drugs are antidotes for this condition, the most important of these being picrotoxin. This is given promptly, particularly when the blood pressure is falling or when the respiration is seriously depressed despite the giving of oxygen.

BENZENE POISONING—Benzene, also called benzol, has many uses in trade and commerce. It is used as a motor fuel; as a solvent in the manufacture of rubber goods of one type or another; sometimes also in the manufacture of spray paints, floor cleansers, floor waxes, varnish removers, and indeed as a solvent for all sorts of materials. Benzene is a clear fluid known as a coal tar product.

Ordinarily the vapors are heavier than air, which is important in relationship to poisoning, as is also the fact that the heating of benzene will cause it to become lighter, to rise, and to spread throughout the air.

A person who has been poisoned by benzene acts much like a man who has become intoxicated by too much alcohol; either he will become unconscious or appear to be dazed. He will stagger when walking or, if sufficiently affected, become drowsy and gradually unconscious, so that finally he dies.

In milder cases there is depression, nausea, vomiting, and a tendency to sleep. Moreover, there are likely to be changes in the blood which are revealed by other symptoms, such as bloody spots appearing suddenly over the body.

A person subjected to repeated inhalations of benzene shows loss of vigor and fatigue. Of course the most important point in making a diagnosis of this condition is to determine that the person concerned has been in contact with benzene.

If a man who has been cleaning a still or a tank, or one who has been painting the inside of a tank with a paint containing benzene, suddenly develops these symptoms, it may be taken for granted that he probably has benzene poisoning. If anyone engaged in spray painting or removal of various paints or varnishes develops such symptoms, the paint or material used should be investigated at once as to its benzene content.

It is, of course, of first importance for the person concerned to be removed as soon as possible from the situation in which he is exposed to the benzene.

The physician sees to it that he is put immediately at rest, that he gets sufficient sleep, that his heart is properly supported by the right kind of remedies, that there is plenty of fresh air, and that his nutrition is adequate. If the blood damage has been great, it is, of course, important to pay special attention to building it up.

BORIC ACID POISONING—Boric acid in ordinary quantities is not a dangerous poison but infants have been seriously poisoned by drinking boric acid solutions instead of water. Thirty grams of borax also have been reported as being fatal to adults. For this type of poisoning it is necessary to clean out the stomach and bowels as soon as possible, to give coffee for stimulating, and to protect the kidneys by giving fairly large doses of alkaline drinks.

COAL OIL POISONING—Occasionally children drink kerosene or coal oil by mistake and as a result may develop poisoning.

Dr. Julian P. Price has reported four cases of children who drank kerosene, one without any serious effects; one with immediate collapse from which he recovered; one who developed fever, difficulty in breathing, and later recovered; and one who died. The patient who died was a white boy, eleven months old, who while crawling around the floor picked up a container holding coal oil and started to drink.

Immediately he began to cough and attracted the attention of the nurse, who rushed him to the office of the family doctor. The family doctor gave him some sweet cream, followed by a drug, which caused the child to throw up the mixture in the stomach. Everything possible was done to keep the child stimulated and to restore his circulation and breathing, but the next day he died from terminal pneumonia.

When coal oil is first taken into the stomach, there is a burning feeling in the mouth, throat, and stomach, colic in the abdomen, vomiting, and thirst. If the poisons of the coal oil are absorbed, the patient develops drowsiness, shallow breathing, feeble pulse, and turns blue, then becomes unconscious and not infrequently dies.

In grown-up persons who take a small amount of coal oil or who work for a long time in an atmosphere where they inhale a great deal of coal oil, symptoms develop like those of a mild jag which is called a "naphtha jag."

The first symptoms are a sense of excitement and lack of self-control; later, however, there is depression, headache, nausea, roaring in the ears, irritation in the throat, and a trembling in the hands and arms.

If a sufficient amount of the fluid is absorbed, signs of shallow breathing, weak heart, convulsions, and death follow.

Thus far medicine knows no specific antidote for coal oil poisoning. Therefore under such circumstances the first thing to do is to wash out the stomach and give a mild laxative.

Then stimulants are used in order to sustain life and the patient is watched constantly so as to lend him such support as can be given by medicine for the organs that need it.

CYANIDE POISONING—For years the writers of detective stories have depended on cyanide poisoning as a technic for quickly getting rid of someone in a novel. Cyanide poison is commonly believed to be invariably fatal. Since the product is used in the silver industry and also for the destruction of insect pests, it is fairly well known. Of course every pharmacist is exceedingly careful to make certain that purchasers of cyanide are properly registered. Every year in the United States anywhere from 80 to 245 people die as a result of cyanide poisoning. The medical records show that 22 people who had taken such poison have recovered.

Usually it is difficult to find out how much cyanide the person took and this makes difficult the determination of its exact poisonous character. Treatment of cases of cyanide poisoning has usually been unsatisfactory because the drug is actually rapidly fatal. Many studies have been made on the use of a variety of substances which might act as anti-dotes to cyanide poison. One of these was methylene blue. Another substance frequently used is glucose, which is given by injection. More recently pharmacologists have tried the effects of amyl nitrite, sodium nitrite, and sodium thiosulfate, which have been found more effective than methylene blue alone in protecting animals from the effects of such intoxication.

LYE POISONING—Household lye is a menace to little children. The substance is commonly used as a cleansing agent. Lye is a caustic alkali. Such substances are found also in washing powder, drainpipe cleaner, and paint removers.

When lye gets into the throat of a child, burns of the throat, the larynx, or voice box and of the esophagus or swallowing tube occur. These result in secondary scarring which may block the passages and even lead to death. Immediately following the swallowing of lye the lips and the tongue and the throat become swollen and ulcerated.

First try to neutralize the alkali with a weak acid such as diluted vinegar, lemon juice, or orange juice. Nothing is gained by trying to pump the stomach to get the substance out because it has already produced its maximum damage. The substance is never taken in sufficiently large amounts to offer any possibility of recovery of any of it.

The visible burns have to be treated by application of oils like olive oil. Usually sedatives have to be given to control the pain.

Once the first wounds have healed, doctors have a technic for reopening the passages so that the child may breathe and swallow. This is accomplished by causing the child to swallow a piece of string. Then bulbs which are gradually increased in size are forced down the string to dilate the passage.

Caustic substances should always be labeled "poison." Following the passage of laws regulating labeling, there has been a decrease in the number of such accidents. Nevertheless, enough cases still occur to indicate that carelessness in leaving caustic substances such as lye around the house continues to result in serious damage to great numbers of children.

MERCURY POISONING—Bichloride of mercury is one of the most dangerous poisons. A doctor should be called at the earliest possible moment because this drug acts on the tissues of the body and, if not removed soon enough from the tissues, the effects of bichloride of mercury are usually fatal. In severe cases a person who has been poisoned with bichloride of mercury suffers from pains in the abdomen, vomiting, and a good deal of purging. In bichloride of mercury poisoning it is customary to give egg white as soon as possible and also some milk. Every case of bichloride of mercury poisoning is so serious that the attention of a most competent physician should be secured immediately.

MUSHROOM POISONING—Two couples went out into a near-by woods and picked a large quantity of mushrooms. Into the pan in which these fungi were cooked a quarter was dropped, in the belief that any poisonous mushrooms would be revealed if the silver coin became tarnished.

The quarter did not tarnish, so that night the four sat down and had a hearty meal of the delicacies.

At two in the morning one of the women awoke with a severe abdominal pain, associated with nausea, vomiting, dizziness, and prostration. At four, her husband suspected that the mushrooms might have been poisonous, so he took a large dose of salts.

A doctor was called at six to treat the woman. Later the other couple felt the same symptoms. For thirty-six hours all four were exceedingly sick, developing severe jaundice. Finally two died.

When their bodies were examined, the livers and the kidneys were found to be badly damaged. Even the nervous systems and the brains showed signs of severe damage.

This incident should bring home to you two important lessons:

1. To be sure that mushrooms are not poisonous, buy them from an experienced dealer who can take the responsibility.

2. If you do happen to feel any symptoms of mushroom poisoning, as I have described above, call a doctor immediately, because prompt action means the difference between life and death.

Mushrooms have been eaten by human beings as far back as history can record. The ancient Babylonians used to enjoy them and the early Romans sold them as delicacies.

There are more than eighty species of poisonous mushrooms in this country, the most deadly type being the *Amanita phalloides*. It is responsible for more than 90 per cent of the deaths from mushroom poisoning.

MUSSEL POISONING—At certain times of the year the form of shellfish known as mussel is poisonous. Outbreaks of poisoning have been seen on the Pacific coast, Nova Scotia, Canada, and in Belgium. Now studies of such poisoning have been made by Drs. Hermann Sommer and K. F. Meyer of the University of California, who find that the original source of the poisoning is a microscopic organism that grows in the ocean. Like all plankton organisms, it is most abundant in the summer, and at times may multiply so largely that there will be 40,000,000 of these germs in a quart of water.

When the germs are present, the water develops a deep rust-red color, so that it is red in the daytime and beautifully luminescent at night. Ap-

parently the organism develops largely in the summer because of the strong radiation of the sun, which offers ideal conditions for the growth of these germs.

The poison developed by these germs has been analyzed and found to be one of the strongest poisons known. It is an alkaloid like strychnine, muscarine, and aconitine. So powerful is this poison that one millionth of a gram is sufficient to kill a mouse if it is injected into its body. A fatal dose by mouth for human beings is just a few milligrams, or a thousandth of a gram. It represents about one two hundred thousandth of a pound.

Plankton, which is found in the ocean, serves as a food for animals on the seashore. When the mussels take in the plankton, they store the poison in their digestive glands. This poison is not harmful to the mussels but is harmful to the person who eats them. The mussels gradually get rid of the poison in a few weeks, provided they do not absorb any additional organisms.

The muscular tissue, or white meat, of the shellfish does not contain much of this poisonous material because practically all of it is concentrated in the digestive gland—the dark central portion of the mussel.

The condition is not confined exclusively to the mussels, but may also be found in certain clams. The only shellfish which are entirely free from the poison are those which live far from the open ocean, such as the softshell clams, native oysters, and scallops. Abalones and crabs do not eat the plankton.

While death from this poisoning is not frequent, it occurs with sufficient regularity to warrant a warning. In July 1936 there were two deaths caused from this source. During 1939 there were several outbreaks on the Pacific coast.

Anyone who gets enough of the

poison feels first a prickly sensation in the lips, the tongue, and the finger tips, followed by numbness, then failure to co-ordinate properly in walking, and, finally, ascending paralysis, so that death may result from respiratory failure in from two to twelve hours after eating the poisonous shellfish.

Unfortunately we do not know of any antidote that will stop the action of the poison once it is absorbed. This means that prevention is most important. Drs. Sommer and Meyer suggest the following rules:

Do not eat the viscera (dark meat) or drink the juice from mussels, clams, or similar shellfish from the open Pacific coast between the first of May and the first of November. The white meat must be thoroughly washed before cooking. The addition of baking soda in cooking shellfish, which has been advocated, helps to reduce the toxicity but is no safeguard against poisoning if highly toxic whole shellfish are prepared.

NARCOTIC DRUG POISONING—Narcotic drugs are poisonous when taken in sufficiently large doses. When people are poisoned by these drugs, they incline to fall asleep and to sleep into death. It is customary to treat the patient by bringing about vomiting so as to get as much of the poison out of the body as possible. Strong black coffee is given to stimulate the higher centers of the brain. Frequently it may be necessary to pick the patient up, walk him about, and stimulate him in other ways in order to keep him awake. As long as he is awake, he will continue to breathe, but when he is asleep, breathing may stop.

THALLIUM POISONING—Thallium is related in its action to that of lead and arsenic. Among the first uses to which the product was put was to mix it with various grains and other substances in the form of a paste which permitted its sale as a rat poison. Its special value as a poison was due to the fact that it would not warn a rat away by any special odor or taste. It would severely depress the heart and injure the nervous system and thus produce death.

The very factors which made it especially useful as a rat poison made it dangerous to human beings and particularly to children.

Occasionally reports appear of thallium poisoning in children who have received overdoses.

There is unfortunately no certain antidote for thallium poisoning. The physician may administer sodium thiosulfate, which is found to be effective to some extent in poisoning by arsenic, and he may use all of the usual measures for supporting life while the body tries to overcome disease.

ZINC NOT POISONOUS—The feeding of animals with zinc has been the chief method used for determining the possible deleterious effects. No noticeable harmful changes were found, however, on the feeding of zinc. Through three generations of animals their chemical tests did not reveal any accumulation of this matter in the organs when the animals were examined after death.

Buttermilk normally contains a small amount of zinc, which increases after contact with zinc containers.

Zinc is regularly present in the internal organs of animals fed with ordinary foods. The amount present does not increase appreciably when the animals are fed with foods containing additional amounts of zinc. Apparently the zinc taken into the body is promptly excreted by the usual routes.

POISONING—albuminuria may result: See KIDNEY, article THE KIDNEY: ITS DISEASES AND DISTURBANCES.

POISONING—antidotes: See article FIRST AID.

Poisoning—arsenic: See article Occupation and Health.

Poisoning—blood: See Infectious Disease, article The Prevention and Treatment of Infectious Disease; article Digestion and Digestive Diseases; Kidney, article The Kidney: Its Diseases and Disturbances.

Poisoning—first aid: See article First Aid.

Poisoning—food: See article First Aid; Diet, article Advice on the Diet.

Poisoning—mercurial: See Kidney, article The Kidney: Its Diseases and Disturbances.

Poisoning—metallic: See article First Aid.

Poisoning—nicotine: See article Occupation and Health.

Poisoning—symptoms: See article First Aid.

Poisons—body's response: See Infectious Disease, article The Prevention and Treatment of Infectious Disease.

Poisons—dangerous, defined: See Medicine Chest, article The Family Medicine Chest.

Poisons—diarrhea caused by: See article Digestion and Digestive Diseases.

Poisons—germs develop: See Infectious Disease, article The Prevention and Treatment of Infectious Disease.

Poisons—industrial: See article Occupation and Health.

Poisons—mistaken for acute indigestion: See article Digestion and Digestive Diseases.

POLIOMYELITIS See *Infantile Paralysis.*

POLYCYTHEMIA When the red blood cells are increased far above the normal amount, the condition is called polycythemia. The average number of red blood cells is about 5,000,000 to 6,000,000 in each cubic millimeter of blood. In polycythemia the number may increase to reach as high as 15,000,000 in each cubic millimeter of blood. Too many red blood cells make it difficult for the blood to flow.

A slight increase in red blood cells is found in certain chronic diseases and is also associated with slight degrees of poisoning of various types. Usually such slight increases indicate that the body is trying to make up for lack of oxygen brought about by the interfering factor.

Sometimes the total number of red blood cells is not actually increased but they are concentrated in the blood to give a much higher red blood cell count. For example the blood may lose great amounts of water because of diarrhea as in cholera, or there may be failure to get sufficient water into the body.

It is said that hard exercise will increase the number of red blood cells in the circulation and also that massage may bring about this result.

In certain unusual tropical diseases the spleen becomes much enlarged and there is also a tremendous increase in the number of red blood cells. In such cases the person appears constantly flushed but with a blue rather than a red appearance, the small veins are prominent, and all of the blood vessels seem full because of the extra amount of red blood cells.

The symptoms associated with an excessive number of red blood cells are dizziness, fainting, a feeling of fullness in the head, nosebleed, and sometimes disturbances of vision and constant ringing in the ears. The condition usually affects older people rather than young ones, coming on rather gradually and increasing steadily. Headache is not an infrequent symptom because of the congested blood vessels. Frequently people with these conditions are told by their friends that they are getting dark-colored, and there may be some associated disturbances of the nervous system.

When these conditions occur, a careful examination of the blood will show the greatly increased number of red blood cells and lead to a prompt diagnosis. This is the type of condition in which a simple laboratory procedure gives a definite clue to the nature of the disorder.

Recently new methods of treatment have been developed. It has become possible to apply radium and the X ray to the spleen and to the long bones which are concerned with the manufacture of red blood cells, and certain drugs have been developed, like benzol, which seem definitely to reduce the large amount of red blood cells. In many instances the combination of the three methods of treatment seems to bring about cure.

It is, of course, important to know whether or not the condition is actual or is simply a temporary apparent increase in the red blood cells due to living at high altitudes, inhaling carbon monoxide over long periods of time, or some similar temporary factor.

POLYCYTHEMIA See BLOOD, article THE BLOOD AND ITS DISEASES.

PORES, DILATED (See also discussion under *Acne*) A dilated pore usually becomes filled with a plug of soggy material. If the material is squeezed out, the pore fills up again in about a month. Past treatment has usually included cauterization, freezing with carbon-dioxide snow, or surgical excision and closing. New research shows that a dilated pore results from growth of the lining of the hair follicle. The best way to eliminate the dilated pore permanently is by surgical excision and closing. Superficial measures attack only the surface of the dilated pore and will not eradicate it.

POSTURE The human body is in many ways a machine—probably the most efficient, complex, and intricate machine that was ever put together—but with all its efficiency it suffers with certain weaknesses and defects that result from the way in which the machine was evolved.

Fundamentalists are convinced that man sprang in his present form into life. Evolutionists are equally if not more convinced that the human being evolved from a species that once walked on all fours. After the human being began to straighten up so as to use two of the feet as hands, he put stresses and strains on parts of the body that were not constructed to bear that burden. The experts in orthopedic surgery say that the mechanics of the body resulting from this evolution make a good many people round-shouldered, stoop-shouldered, with sunken chests, twisted backs, protruding abdomens, and lame hips. Much of the difficulty arises because insufficient attention is given to strengthening the weak points during the years of growth.

When the little baby first reaches up a tiny hand to pull himself up to his feet, the stresses on certain portions of the body begin.

Good posture means that the body is held in the correct position when standing, sitting, or lying down, and also in motion. In standing, the human being must stand tall, the abdomen drawn in, the shoulders square and high, the chin straight back, the weight properly distributed on the feet, the curve of the back well within normal limitations.

In the correct sitting position the body is erect, the head poised to bring the center of gravity in the line joining the bones of the hips. It does good

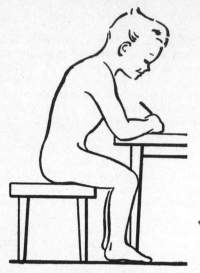

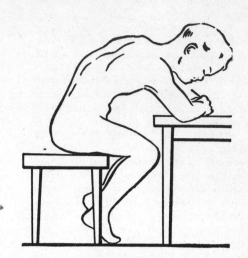

Correct posture

Incorrect posture

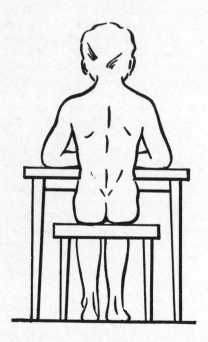

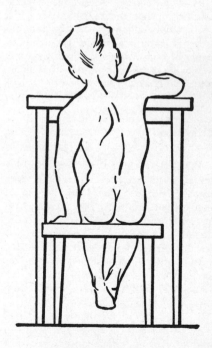

Correct Posture

Incorrect posture

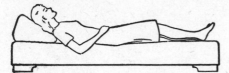

Lying down requires the least energy

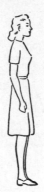

Standing requires 12 per cent more
energy than lying down

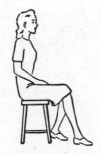

Sitting requires 4 per cent more
energy than lying down

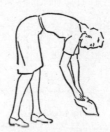

Bending requires 55 per cent more
energy than lying down

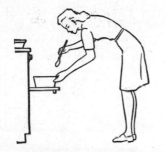

Incorrect posture for low oven

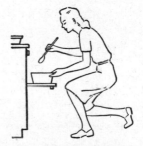

Correct posture for low oven

Handle too short

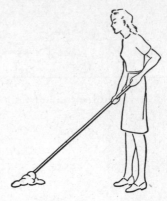

Longer handle eliminates stooping

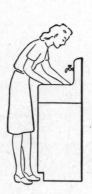

Sink too low

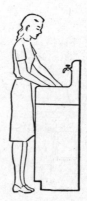

Correct height

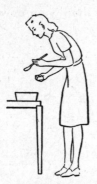

Table too low

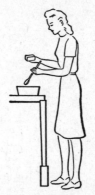

Table correct height

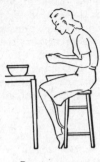

Poor posture

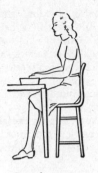

Good posture

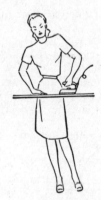

Standing is fatiguing

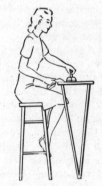

Sitting is more comfortable

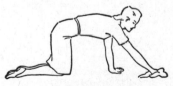

Kneeling is fatiguing

to practice this position while sitting. Constant assumption of a bent posture or a droopy position while at work or at rest results in stretching and relaxing of ligaments with a tendency toward permanent sagging. As a result, the back becomes rounded and the chin is shoved forward.

Here are some simple exercises which help to strengthen the muscles of the back and abdomen and thus improve posture:

1. Lie on the back, hands back of the neck. Take a deep breath and raise chest high; keep chest up and exhale by pulling abdomen in.

2. Same position; knees bent, feet pulled up. Pull abdomen in hard and then relax part way.

3. Sit in a chair, trunk bending forward. Incline trunk forward from the hips, keeping spine straight. This exercise may be done standing.

4. Standing; abdominal retraction. Stand with the heels four inches away from the wall but with the hips, shoulders, and head touching the wall; flatten the lower part of the back against the wall by pulling in the abdominal muscles. Holding this position, come away from. the wall with the weight well forward on the balls of the feet.

5. Standing; leg raising. Stand with hands on hips, back flat, and chin in; raise leg forward without bending the knee; lower it; repeat with other leg. This exercise teaches how to hold the back flat.

6. Carrying the head forward, clasp hands behind the head. Force the head back against their pressure, keeping chin in. This strengthens the muscles of the back of the neck.

7. Spinal curvatures. "Stand tall," holding the back straight. Rise on the toes with the arms extended forward and up, stretching the arms and the body.

8. Distended abdomen. This condition may be successfully prevented and largely overcome by doing exercises 2 and 4.

Posture

BY

MORRIS FISHBEIN, M.D.

Former Editor, *Journal American Medical Association,*
Chicago; Editor, *Excerpta Medica, Bulletin World Medical Assn.; Post-graduate Medicine.*

GOOD POSTURE will cure some conditions and certainly prevent many others. In infancy its preventive value has the greatest influence on the ensuing life of the baby, though much can be done, by means of persistent exercise, to overcome faults of posture in later life.

The home and school can coöperate effectively in training children to observe the rules of correct posture. In the school, however, most can be done in providing desks and seats of correct height and size, as well as the instruments for gymnastic exercises.

The need for proper seating cannot be too greatly emphasized, because of its direct effect on the spine. Desks should be designed to fit the abnormally large or small, as well as the normal-sized child. The seated pupil should not use a seat so low that his shoulders perforce become rounded, his head droops, and his chest is flattened. The elbows should be able to rest on the desk without stooping or unduly elevating the shoulders, and the edge of the desk should overlap the edge of the seat. Many schools have a certain number of specially adjustable desks and seats for the express use of children who are above or below the average size.

Perfectly fitting seats are not everything. A child cannot sit still long. It is not in his nature to do so. He will become weary unless sufficient opportunity is allowed for exercising and changing the posture during school hours. If he sits too long, the upper part of the body leans forward on or against the desk, constricting the chest, crowding the abdominal organs, and impeding the circulation in the veins. The weight is supported by the arms, and the head, neck, and spine hang by the muscles of the shoulder blades in abnormal curves. To relieve this overstrain of the back and shoulder muscles the pupil slumps back until his weight rests on the shoulder blades and lower end of the spine, leaving the center of the back unsupported. The back sags down in a single long curve, the chest contracts, the breathing is made shallow, and the circulation slows up. This position stretches the muscles and ligaments of the spine, rounds the back and shoulders, and shoves forward the chin.

CORRECT SITTING POSTURE.

The correct sitting posture is one in which the pupil sits erect, the pelvis resting equally on the seat, with the arms beside the hips and the head poised so as to bring the center of gravity within a line joining the seat bones. This posture makes a minimum demand on muscular energy, and is most conducive to correct carriage. But the demands of school life do not permit the pupil to keep it long. Reading, writing, and drawing are exercises that require deviations from the ideal. If we add to these requirements ill-fitting desks and long periods of sitting, in which bad posture becomes habitual, the mischievous result cannot long be in doubt. The work of the school day should be arranged with these things in mind. The first year of the child's school life should not have more than one third of the time in confinement at the desk.

KINDERGARTEN TRAINING

Short periods of sitting, followed by double that time spent in muscular activity out of the seat, should be the rule. This activity may in most cases consist of movements correlated with intellectual exercise. In the kindergarten exercise is admirably combined with mental culture by the teaching of imitative games in which the large muscle groups are exercised in hopping, jumping, and running, and in imitating with the arms the flight of birds and insects. The circulation is stimulated and postural faults are prevented, while at the same time the child is taught valuable lessons in natural history in which his interest never flags.

TRAINING IN HIGHER GRADES

The school day of children in the higher grades should have two five-minute periods of corrective exercise at least, in addition to the games of the recess, previously described. These exercises should be designed to promote quick, strong, muscular control; to expand and enlarge the chest by deep breathing; to bring the blood from the abdomen out into the extremities; to correct spinal fatigue, and to teach the proper carriage of the body.

It is not possible for a child to remain long at rest with the weight equally on both feet, because the tension on both legs being the same, the muscles rapidly tire. The pupil instinctively rests his weight on the right, placing his left leg with bent knee out to the side as a prop. This resting position lowers the right shoulder, curves the spine, and may start the first stage of a permanent scoliosis. The best resting pose to teach is that recommended by Dr. Eliza Mosher, in which the inactive foot is placed in front instead of at the side. In this the feet can be changed as the weight-bearing leg tires.

BAD POSTURE

What are the best rules and exercises for correct posture?

There is a test now widely used by which even the untrained teacher may form an accurate estimate of a child's posture. The first part of the test is designed to find the pupil's ability to take the erect attitude. The long axis of the trunk should continue the long axis of the head and neck. To assist the eye of the observer, a vertical line may be dropped from the front of the ear to the forward part of the foot. In poor posture the axes of the head, neck, and trunk will form a zigzag instead of a straight line.

Another simple way to estimate the extent of the deformity is to stand the child beside an upright pole or rod. The variations from correct posture are three: the so-called fatigue, or gorilla type, in which the head is thrust forward, the chest sunken, and the abdomen protruded; the round-back posture, in which the hollow at the small of the back is obliterated, a posture cultivated by faults of seating already described; and the bantam, or pouter-pigeon type, in which the chest is pushed forward and upward, and the lower spine over-extended, forming a marked exaggeration of the natural lumbar curve. This posture is always the result of faulty teaching and is an exaggeration of the correct standing posture caused by the mistaken efforts on the part of the teacher to overcorrect the first two faults.

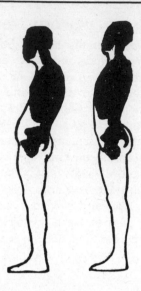

Left: The relation of the head, thorax and pelvis in the incorrect standing position. *Right:* The relation of the head, thorax and pelvis in the correct standing position.

ENDURANCE TEST

A child who can assume a good posture may not be able to sustain it. Some kind of endurance test is therefore an aid whereby faults of posture may be discovered and eliminated by having the children march. As the march proceeds, old muscle habits reassert themselves, and many pupils who could hold the correct posture for a few minutes fall back into habitual faults. Heads will drop forward, shoulders droop, and chests sink, as they march. As these faults appear, the child is taken out of the marching line. Those who pass the standing and marching tests are then put through the third test, designed to show the action and endurance of the muscles of the spine and shoulders that are usually the first to yield to fatigue. When the arms are raised upward these postural muscles, if weak, allow the chin to come forward and the chest to sink backward, so that a few minutes spent in raising the arms forward and upward fully extended, lowering them sidewise and downward to the position at the start, will bring this weakness to the surface.

PHYSICAL TRAINING

Physical training is not only a matter of health. It is necessary for the education of the fundamental nerve centers of the body and the building of character. During the whole of childhood these centers are developing, and their growth is not completed until adult life. For this reason not less than one hour in five should be devoted to training the motor area of the brain, in addition to the time allowed for free play. This should take the form of both gymnastics and athletics. Gymnastics, in addition to their corrective or medical character, have a value in discipline and also in the accurate application of exercise for a given purpose; they are less diffuse than athletics, more concentrated, and for this reason they cannot be applied closely or for long to the very young, except in the guise of play. For girls, the exercises most popular are the peasant dances of Ireland, Scotland, Spain, and Sweden, in which good posture is an integral part of the dance, and agility and grace are developed.

POSTURE OF STUDENTS OF COLLEGE AGE

The necessity for good posture at college age is a logical sequence to the valuable habits learned in childhood. The college student's remediable defects must be corrected, and his physical powers trained to the highest point of efficiency. He must be taught that graceful carriage characteristic of the well-bred man. His powers of self-preservation and efficiency must be increased. If he has not learned it already, he must be given the opportunity for physical recreation through a knowledge of sports and games, for athletic activity

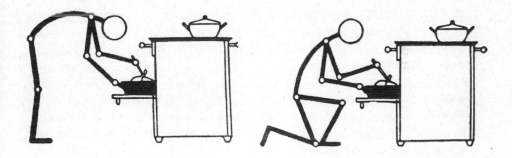

Left: Incorrect posture for low oven. *Right:* Correct posture for low oven.

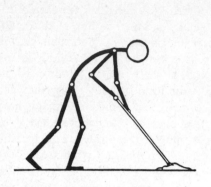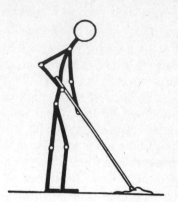

Left: Handle too short. *Right:* Longer handle eliminates stooping.

should be the safety valve of a sedentary life, and should also teach, in addition to those social and moral qualities which can be cultivated so well in no other way, the lesson of gracefully carrying the body. That is why a university course in physical education should begin with a careful examination to find the exact bodily condition of the student and so to give an intelligent foundation on which to base advice and instruction. Nor is the examination of the student complete without a test of his ability to accomplish certain muscular feats that cover the main activities of the body, in exercises of maximum effort and of endurance.

PHYSICAL EDUCATION FOR WOMEN

Physical education for women too often follows slavishly the scheme planned for men, not because it is best for women, but because it is the same. This is a deplorable mistake, because bodily training of the two sexes must differ radically in order to fit each for its own future life and environment. It cannot, with impunity, ignore the psychologic and physiologic differences between the boy and the girl and between man and woman.

In these days of professional freedom for women, with its consequent demand on their efficiency and endurance, there is much reason for women to practise good posture. Many women suffer from the effect of faulty attitude with its direct relation to pain, like backache and headache.

The first twelve years of a girl's life need differ little from that of a boy's in physical activity. She may lead the same outdoor life, climbing, swimming, running, playing ball, and nothing will prepare her so well for the great physical and mental change which takes place with the attainment of puberty. Outdoor games and exercises establish nervous stability and poise and give the best possible foundation on which to build her future womanhood.

GAMES FOR WOMEN

Women cannot stand prolonged physical or mental strain as well as men, but with frequent rests they can in the end accomplish almost as much. Certain games, such as football, boxing, pole vaulting, and heavy gymnastics, are obviously unsuited to them; but in dancing, swimming, calisthenics, archery, skating, and fencing they come much nearer to competing with men on equal terms. While they are less adapted to arduous muscular work, their vital endurance is better; so that the disadvantage they have in other activities is made up for by this greater tenacity to life. With a few exceptions, girls accustomed to athletics and gymnastics can continue exercise without detriment during menstruation, though they should refrain at that time from too exhausting contests or competitions.

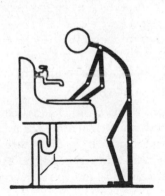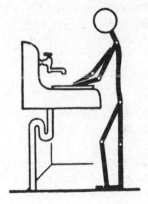

Left: Sink too low. *Right:* Correct height.

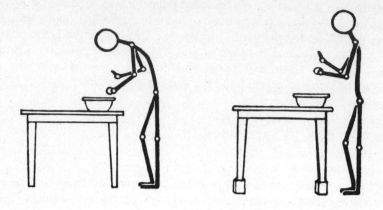

Left: Table too low. *Right:* Table correct height.

Swimming is one of the best exercises for women, calling into action most of the muscles of the body, but sparing those of the back so generally overworked in standing and sitting postures.

Finally, it is quite as important to take occasional hours of absolute rest, in the recumbent position, at it is to exercise, especially when the nervous and muscular system is overwrought.

Postural Effect of Clothing

The importance of proper clothing for men, women, and children has a high place in the promotion of good posture that cannot be overemphasized, although in these days of greater freedom and simplicity in dress there is not so much need to belabor the point as there was a few generations ago. Any tendency to return to the constricting, overweighted, and too numerous garments of a few decades past should be greatly deplored.

Proper shoes have a definite effect on posture, in both children and adults. It has been found that the ground plan of the human foot varies so that it may be straight, inflared, or outflared; therefore, no one type of shoe will be suited to all types of feet. Deformities of the feet, either from the construction of the footwear or from the breaking down of the longitudinal and lateral arches of the feet, have a vital influence on posture. The balance of the foot, either flat or on a high heel, also affects the posture, although this is not so serious as was formerly supposed, if the shoe is so made that the weight rests on the heel instead of slipping forward and crowding the toes into the forward part of the shoe.

The advantage of the upright position is somewhat offset by the frequency of deformities due to a yielding of the structures concerned with support. The body may yield at the spine, at the knee joints, or at the arch of the foot, which becomes broken down and flattened, causing the deformity known as flat-foot. A typical case of flat-foot shows a turning out of the line of the heel, a convexity of the inner contour of the foot, and a concavity of its outer margin. A tracing of the foot would show no instep. The great majority of such cases are what might be termed static and are found in nurses, clerks, waiters, barbers, motormen, and all others whose long hours of continued standing keep the muscles and ligaments of the foot constantly on the strain. The pernicious habit of standing with the toes turned out always makes it worse. Flat-foot is also found in the very fat, whose weight is too much for their ligaments. Bernard Roth, in his series of 1,000 cases of twisted spine, found flat-foot in 76 per cent of them. In an examination of 1,000 supposedly normal students I have found it in 217 cases. Lovett has found many

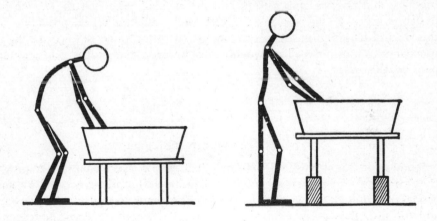

Left: Washtub too low. *Right:* Correct height obtained through blocks.

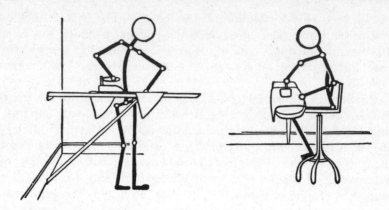

Left: Standing is fatiguing. *Right:* Sitting is more comfortable.

cases among hospital nurses, who are peculiarly susceptible to it. The symptoms are varied. A considerable degree of flat-foot may be present without causing much irritation, and again great pain may be caused by a comparatively slight degree of this deformity. In any case, the close association between footwear and posture must always be kept in mind. The Posture League has designed shoes of the straight, inflared, and outflared types, providing for this natural variation in the normal foot, and at the same time correcting or preventing a position which would tend to drop the arches and produce pain or deformity.

CLOTHING AND ROUND SHOULDERS

Another frequent postural deformity caused or aggravated by improper clothing is round or uneven shoulders. Clothing which is supported by suspenders bearing on the points of the shoulders tends to pull them downward and forward. It is a common deformity among school children, and occurs in almost 20 per cent of university students uncomplicated with other postural defects. It is frequently discovered in girls about the age of puberty, when especial attention is apt to be paid to their figure and carriage. Round shoulders are not likely to be outgrown, and patients usually become permanently and structurally set in the faulty posture, with flattened chest walls and distorted figure.

The clothing should be examined, and when found to be supported from the tip of the shoulders the garments should be altered to bring the pressure in toward the root of the neck, instead of out on the shoulders. It has been pointed out that the cut of most ready-made clothing causes pressure on the back of the neck and tip of the shoulders, constantly tending to produce this deformity. Such clothing, especially men's and boys' suit coats, and men's, women's, and children's top coats, should be bought with particular care that the shape of the shoulders and backs of these garments do not have a tendency to encourage poor posture.

Exercises for Faulty Posture

The following six exercises are recommended for the correction of the ordinary case of faulty posture:

1. With the patient standing in his habitual faulty position, place the hand about one inch in front of the sternum and tell him to raise the chest and shove it forward to touch the hand without swaying the body. He will at first try to

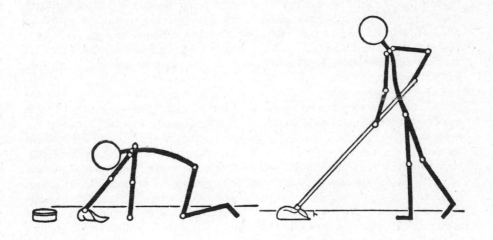

Left: Kneeling is fatiguing. *Right:* Suitable equipment saves strength.

draw the shoulders back, but this fault must be overcome at the very beginning, and the shoulder muscles must be kept relaxed. Gradually increase the distance to which he can bring the chest forward, repeating it again and again until he can take the position without difficulty and without contracting the muscles of the back. While in this position make him breathe deeply five times and then relax. This should be done before a mirror, so that he will recognize the feeling of the correct posture and associate it with the proper attitude as seen in the glass. He should then try to take it without looking at the mirror. This posture should be drilled into him until it becomes habitual and until he can maintain it without discomfort. R. J. Roberts, of Boston, used to tell his young men to press the backs of their necks against the collar button, considering this as the keynote of the position. In whatever way it is accomplished, the object is to get the proper relation between the thorax and the pelvis.

After repeating Exercise 1 twenty times, take:

2. Arms forward raise, upward stretch, rise on tiptoes, inhale. Sideward lower, slowly press the arms back, and exhale. This exercise, when done correctly, expands the chest, bringing in all the extensors of the back and levators of the shoulders.

3. The patient stands, arms downward and backward, fingers interlocked and palms outward. Extend the neck, roll the shoulders backward and forearms into supination, the palms being first in, then down, and then out. Reverse to starting position and relax. This exercise is valuable for projecting the chest forward, stretching the shortened ligaments, and drawing in the abdomen. Care should be taken to have the chin pressed backward when the arms are brought downward and turned outward. In resistant cases, where this exercise cannot be done with the fingers interlocked, a handkerchief tied in a loop may be substituted and held in the fingers.

4. Patient stands with the arms at the sides. Arms sideward raise, upward stretch, inhale, forward bend, and rise. Arms sideward, lower, exhale. In this exercise the lungs are filled when the chest is in the most favorable position for expansion. The breath is retained when the trunk is flexed, forcing the air into the cells of the lungs under pressure. The bending and rising bring into powerful action the extensors of the back and neck and the retractors of the shoulders.

5. Patient lies prone on a couch with the feet strapped, or upon the floor with the feet caught on the edge of a bureau or other article of furniture. Hands clasped behind the head. Raise the head and extend the spine, pressing the elbows backward. This exercise is a severe one on the back and shoulders. Follow with a deep breathing exercise.

6. Patient lies in similar position as in Exercise 5, arms at the sides. Raise head, bring arms forward and imitate the breast stroke.

In this exercise the spine is kept in static contraction, while the retractors of the shoulders are alternately contracted and relaxed.

ADDITIONAL EXERCISES

Here are some simple exercises which help to strengthen the muscles of the back and abdomen and thus improve posture:

1. Lie on the back, hands back of the neck. Take a deep breath and raise chest high; keep chest up and exhale by pulling abdomen in. *2.* Same position; knees bent, feet pulled up. Pull abdomen in hard and then relax part way. *3.* Sit in a chair, trunk bending forward. Incline trunk forward from the hips, keeping spine straight. This exercise may be done standing. *4.* Standing; abdominal retraction. Stand with the heels four inches away from the wall but with the hips, shoulders, and head touching the wall; flatten the lower part of the back against the wall by pulling in the abdominal muscles. Holding this position, come away from the wall with the weight well forward on the balls of the feet. *5.* Standing; leg raising. Stand with hands on hips, back flat, and chin in; raise leg forward without bending the knee; lower it; repeat with other leg. This exercise teaches how to hold the back flat. *6.* Carrying the head forward; clasp hands behind the head. Force the head back against their pressure, keeping chin in. This strengthens the muscles of the back of the neck. *7.* Spinal curvatures. "Stand tall," holding the back straight. Rise on the toes with the arms extended forward and up, stretching the arms and the body. *8.* Distended abdomen. This condition may be prevented and largely overcome by doing exercises 2 and 4.

PRECOCIOUS HAIR (See also *Hair*) Precocious hair around the sex organs is not an important symptom but may cause some anxiety. Twenty-nine children were studied at Johns Hopkins University to determine the significance of such growth. All but one of the children were girls. Most were taller than average and the growth of their bones was from one to four years ahead of that of ordinary children. Nothing was found in the blood or glandular activity in the bodies of the children of any significance. The investigators therefore reassured the parents that eventually the children would mature quite normally.

Investigators of glandular functions tested the rate of growth of hair under the arms. They found an increased growth during hot weather. In 18 patients with genital underdevelopments the men showed a low rate of hair growth. The women's rate was slow but increased when they took estrogenic hormones. When the function of the pituitary gland is low the underarm hair growth is low. After testing the rate of growth under a variety of conditions, the conclusion was reached that underarm growth in women depends largely on the adrenal glands which is activated by the pituitary gland. In men the rate of growth depends on both the adrenal and the sex glands.

PRECOCIOUS HAIR GROWTH (See also discussion under *Blood, Hair, Pituitary Gland*) Precocious growth of hair around the sex organs is usually just an unimportant variation in growth. Twenty-nine children were studied at Johns Hopkins University to determine the significance of such growth. All but one of the children were girls. Most were taller than average, and the growth of their bones was from one to four years ahead of that of ordinary children. However, nothing significant was found in the blood or glandular activities of the bodies of these children, so it seemed safe to reassure parents that eventually the children would mature quite normally.

PREGNANCY During 1943 there was an excess of several hundred thousand births in the United States over the number that would ordinarily have been expected. This situation was definitely related to the war and to the fact that some 10,000,000 men were removed from civilian life into a military career.

During the period of 280 days from the time when a child is conceived until his birth, many changes take place in the body of the prospective mother. While the greatest changes take place in the organs immediately concerned with childbirth, every organ of the body of the mother is influenced by the pregnancy. At the time the child is conceived, the egg cell which has come from the ovary of the mother is fertilized by the male cell. About the middle of the menstrual cycle an egg cell, or ovum, passes from the ovary of the woman down the fallopian tube to the uterus, or womb.

The time when the woman is most likely to become pregnant is the period between the tenth and seventeenth days after the first day of menstruation. This is now considered to be the period of greatest fertility.

When pregnancy occurs, the uterus becomes thickened and enlarges with the growth of the prospective child. The breasts of the mother begin to enlarge as early as the second month and in very young mothers who are having their first baby as early as the second or third week. These changes also increase during the course of pregnancy. The various glands of the body are affected by the pregnancy, since most of them have to increase their work by producing greater amounts of secretion. The whole rate of chemical changes going on in the body, measured by the basal metabolism, is also likely to be increased during pregnancy.

The mother needs extra calcium at this time because of the demands of the growing baby for this substance used in the building of bones and teeth.

In a healthy pregnant woman the number of red blood cells and the amount of red coloring matter also increase to the upper boundaries of normal. This is associated with increased nutrition and the demands of the growing baby.

DIAGNOSIS—There are certain definite signs by which the doctor can determine whether or not a woman is pregnant.

In the majority of cases the regular menstruation disappears after the woman has conceived and does not appear again during the course of pregnancy. Physicians, therefore, are likely to say that the first cause of the disappearance of menstruation is prospective childbirth. A discontinuance of menstruation in a woman who has always been regular before means in the vast majority of cases that she has become pregnant. In some instances, however, the woman may have a discharge of blood from the uterus once and occasionally twice after conception has occurred. The duration and the quantity are usually much less than normal.

A common sign of prospective motherhood is some nausea and vomiting in the morning. This usually develops during the second month and rarely lasts beyond the end of the fourth month. It may, however, appear during the first month and may extend beyond the fourth month in occasional cases. There are many variations in the appearance, intensity, and duration of this disorder. Some women are troubled several times a day. In rare instances the disturbance occurs only at night when the woman goes to bed.

Many women during this time become increasingly emotional. Peevishness, fretfulness, irritability, and unreasonableness are not uncommon. Some women are more or less depressed, but many are increasingly buoyant and joyful.

The craving for strange foods which appears is a manifestation of the mental changes that may occur. Indeed this

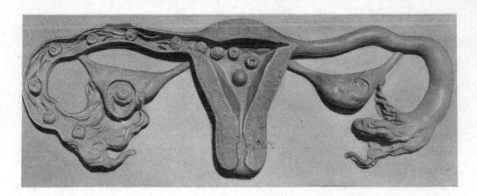

The single human ovum shown in thirteen stages on the way from ovary to implantation in the uterine cavity.   Cleveland Health Museum

mental state may be reflected not only in unusual appetites but by a complete change of habits, so that a woman who has been exceedingly cleanly and meticulous in her habits may suddenly become careless and slovenly.

Between the sixteenth and eighteenth week the prospective mother is likely to feel a feeble fluttering, which is called quickening. The symptom is not a certain one because there are many things that go on inside the abdomen related to digestion that might simulate movements of the prospective child. Women who are greatly worried as to whether or not they are actually pregnant frequently imagine they feel movements that are actually not there.

The usual changes in shape and size of the body are well known to most people as signs of pregnancy. There are, however, certain signs which are so positive that they do not permit any contradiction. One of these is an X-ray picture, which will show the presence of the child. Another is the hearing of the heartbeat of the child, which, incidentally, appears between the eighteenth and twentieth weeks and occasionally earlier. Finally, there are the laboratory tests like the Aschheim-Zondek test which have a very high degree of positiveness in making a diagnosis.

SUPERSTITIONS—There are many strange notions about pregnancy which persist and which are hard to destroy.

Of all the persistent notions not founded on fact, the one that prevails among people to the greatest extent is the idea that the mother can in some way mark the baby while carrying it. We know with certainty that there is no nervous connection between the mother and the unborn child. The mothers of Sparta in ancient Greece were commanded to look only on pictures and statues which showed the strong and beautiful so that their children would be strong and beautiful. We know today that it is not possible to affect the child, who is actually the sum of his parents, by any such activity.

The idea most widely prevalent is the belief that a shock to the mother will mark the child. Yet during all great wars, when mothers all over the

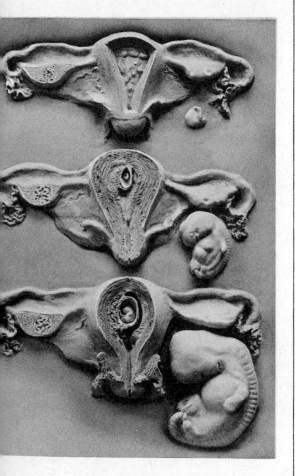

Uterus with the embryo four, six and seven weeks old. The embryo is enlarged eight times.   Cleveland Health Museum

world are exposed to unusual horrors, the number of babies born with markings is no greater than in normal times. Thousands of babies with birthmarks or defects have been born to mothers whose mentalities have not shown the slightest sign of any disturbance.

Many strange beliefs are associated with determining whether the baby will be a boy or a girl. Some people think that a girl's heart beats more rapidly than 140 times a minute and that a boy's heartbeat is likely to be slower. True, large babies usually have slower rates than small babies, and boys are generally slightly larger than girls; there is not enough difference, however, to make it possible for anyone to determine with certainty before birth which babies will be boys and which will be girls.

CONTINUED IN VOLUME 7

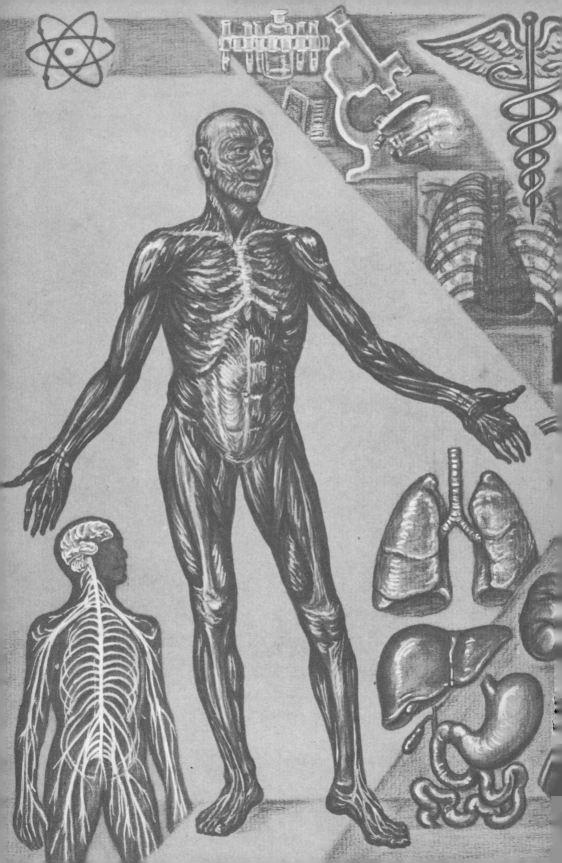